S0-EJV-394

ORGAN AND SPECIES SPECIFICITY IN CHEMICAL CARCINOGENESIS

BASIC LIFE SCIENCES

Alexander Hollaender, General Editor

Associated Universities, Inc., Washington, D.C.

Recent volumes in the series:

ORGAN AND SPECIES SPECIFICITY IN CHEMICAL CARCINOGENESIS

Edited by

ROBERT LANGENBACH
STEPHEN NESNOW
U.S. Environmental Protection Agency
Research Triangle Park, North Carolina

and

JERRY M. RICE
National Cancer Institute
Bethesda, Maryland

PLENUM PRESS • NEW YORK AND LONDON

Library of Congress Cataloging in Publication Data

Symposium on Organ and Species Specificity in Chemical Carcinogenesis (1981: Raleigh, N.C.)
Organ and species specificity in chemical carcinogenesis.

(Basic life sciences; v. 24)
"Proceedings of a Symposium on Organ and Species Specificity in Chemical Carcinogenesis, held during March 1981, in Raleigh, N.C."—Verso t.p.
Bibliography: p.
Includes index.
1. Carcinogenesis—Congresses. I. Langenbach, Robert, 1942– . II. Nesnow, Stephen, 1941– . III. Rice, Jerry M. IV. Title. V. Series.
RC268.5.S97 1981 616.99′4071 82-18919
ISBN 0-306-41184-9

This report has been reviewed by the Health Effects Research Laboratory, U.S. Environmental Protection Agency, and approved for publication. Approval does not signify that the contents necessarily reflect the views and policies of the U.S. Environmental Protection Agency, nor does mention of trade names or commercial products constitute endorsement or recommendation for use.

Proceedings of a Symposium on Organ and Species Specificity in Chemical Carcinogenesis, held during March 1981, in Raleigh, North Carolina

A Division of Plenum Publishing Corporation
233 Spring Street, New York, N.Y. 10013

Printed in the United States of America

PREFACE

The Symposium on Organ and Species Specificity in Chemical Carcinogenesis was held March 1981 in Raleigh, North Carolina. Dr. James Miller concluded this Symposium with these remarks:

"Without a doubt all of us would agree this has been a very successful symposium in illustrating a very wide range of chemical, stereochemical, biochemical, metabolic, molecular, and biological factors in chemical carcinogenesis. I think it is noteworthy that many of the discussions have dealt with pharmacodynamic, or toxicodynamic, factors that can influence the biological activities of the extremely wide range of structures that we choose to call chemical carcinogens.

I sincerely hope that after this symposium everyone here will realize the very great need we have for further information on these agents in the species we profess to be working for, the human species.

We badly need an adequate data base on human organs, human tissues, human cells, human subcellular preparations, and human body fluids.

I don't think we can rely on extrapolations of data on chemical carcinogenesis from experimental animals to humans, no matter how sophisticated or plausible these extrapolations may seem, until we know far more about chemical carcinogenesis in humans.

Now, I'd like to add a somewhat personal note. As many of you know, my wife and I have shared a joint career of some 40 years in this field, and I'd like to emphasize in these closing remarks the factor of youth.

Youth in science is well recognized as the source of new information, new daring, and new experimentation. My wife and I have often remarked to each other over these 40 years on the pleasure we've had in working with a succession of youthful people, both pre-doctorate and post-doctorate. If anything can keep you young, that is it.

I think we have a wonderful set of youthful people in the field of chemical carcinogenesis, and it gives me great confidence for the future in this field.

So I think the field's in good hands. I wish you all the best of luck."

James A. Miller
McArdle Laboratory for
Research on Cancer

ACKNOWLEDGMENTS

Our sincere thanks are extended to Leslie Silkworth, Olga Wierbicki, Barbara Elkins, Linda Cooper, Barbara Perillo, and Slate Raymond for assistance in preparing this book for publication.

Financial support for the Symposium on Organ and Species Specificity in Chemical Carcinogenesis by the U.S. Environmental Protection Agency and the National Cancer Institute is gratefully acknowledged.

CONTENTS

THE NATURE OF ORGAN SPECIFICITY IN CHEMICAL CARCINOGENESIS

Jerry M. Rice[1] and Charles H. Frith[2]

[1]Laboratory of Comparative Carcinogenesis, National Cancer Institute, Frederick, MD 21701, and [2]Department of Pathology, University of Arkansas for Medical Sciences, Little Rock, AR 72205 and Pathology Services Project, National Center for Toxicological Research, Jefferson, AR 72079

INTRODUCTION

One of the most central problems in human oncology, as well as in experimental carcinogenesis, is that of organ specificity. The most cursory inspection of human cancer morbidity tables (1) shows that not all tissues of man are equally at risk for neoplasia, and that for a given tissue, risk varies with age, sex, and genetic background (Table 1). Where a specific causative agent is known, characteristically it is linked with a relatively narrow spectrum of diseases, or even with a single clinical entity: 2-aminonaphthalene causes carcinoma of the urinary bladder (2); bis (2-chloromethyl) ether (BCME) causes oat-cell carcinoma of the lung (3); vinyl chloride induces hepatic angiosarcoma (4). Major determinants of organ specificity can be found in some cases in peculiarities of metabolism and excretion of the carcinogen, as in the case of the aromatic amines and the urinary bladder; or in a crude biological form of the chemical Law of Mass Action, that the site of highest local concentration is the most vulnerable, as with pulmonary carcinogenesis in those who inhale the volatile, highly reactive BCME. But neither consideration clearly explains why vinyl chloride, when inhaled, selectively induces tumors of the hepatic endothelium while sparing hepatocytes, in which it is presumably metabolized.

There are also interspecies differences in organ specificity and these complicate attempts to assess human risk from experiments on animals. Most organic chemicals that are carcinogenic to mice include tumors of liver cells (5) and/or pulmonary alveolar cells (6) among their effects. Both types of tumors are relatively frequent in mice, especially in certain inbred strains; both are distinctly rare in the human inhabitants of industrialized nations.

Table 1. Percent Distribution of Malignant Neoplasms Diagnosed in the United States in 1969-71 by Selected Primary Site, Race, and Sex[a]

	White			Black		
Primary Site	Total	Male	Female	Total	Male	Female
All sites	100	100	100	100	100	100
Respiratory	14.9	23.9	5.9	17.3	26.5	6.2
Digestive	25.0	26.2	23.8	25.9	27.5	24.0
Esophagus	0.9	1.4	0.5	3.1	4.5	1.5
Stomach	3.3	4.1	2.6	4.5	5.5	3.3
Small intestine	0.3	0.4	0.3	0.4	0.4	0.3
Colon	10.4	9.6	11.2	8.3	6.8	10.2
Rectum	4.6	5.2	4.1	3.5	3.7	3.2
Liver	0.7	0.9	0.5	1.1	1.5	0.6
Urinary	6.8	9.6	4.0	4.3	5.2	3.2
Bladder	4.5	6.8	2.3	2.3	3.0	1.5
Nervous system	1.7	1.9	1.5	1.4	1.2	1.6
Lymphoreticular[b]	7.8	8.6	6.8	7.3	7.5	6.8

[a]Modified from Reference 1.
[b]Including lymphomas, leukemias, and multiple myeloma, but not organ-specific lymphomas, which are distributed among the sites.

No one predicts that an agent that induces liver cell tumors or pulmonary adenomas in mice will do the same in man; but the capacity to do so is generally considered a valid, if nonspecific, indicator of human risk. 2-Aminonaphthalene, for example, causes only liver tumors in mice, and is inactive in rats (2). How then do we interpret the capacity of an agent such as the flame retardant tris (2,3-dibromopropyl)phosphate (TRIS) (7) to induce in mice tumors not only of liver and lung but also of the kidney, and to effect renal carcinogenesis in rats as well? Does the kidney tell us more than the lungs and the liver? Does this mean that the human kidney, or the urinary tract as a whole, is especially vulnerable to this agent, and that epidemiologists should look for increased incidence of renal carcinoma or Wilms' tumor in exposed human populations? This may or may not be valid and from bioassays alone we cannot make such interspecies extrapolations with assurance.

But species differences have their redeeming features. They provide for the experimentalist a highly useful approach to identifying metabolic pathways and other determinants of susceptibility to specific carcinogens, by comparing susceptible and resistant cells, tissues, and organ systems. In this opening session the existence and nature of species differences and organ specificity in tumor induction will be discussed for a number of major classes of chemical carcinogens. By way of introduction, we here discuss (a) the kinds of differences that are observed in tumor induction studies; (b) the limitations of induced tumors as experimental end points; and (c) the requirements for full pathologic identification and description of the effects of carcinogens in animals.

ORGAN AND SPECIES DIFFERENCES IN EXPERIMENTAL CARCINOGENESIS

In different species, a given substance may be carcinogenic to the same cells and tissues, or its effects may be partially or totally different. In the most extreme cases, a substance that is carcinogenic in one species may be completely inactive in another. More commonly, in different species a carcinogen may affect a different spectrum of organs, or a different cell type within an organ system.

All-or-None Effects

While relatively uncommon, all-or-none effects have provided conclusive evidence of the importance of specific metabolic paths for activation of procarcinogens to proximate and ultimate carcinogenic metabolites. In other cases, they constitute a source of considerable frustration for the experimentalist, who may be unable to study an agent for lack of a suitable experimental model. The best known example of the former is provided by aromatic amines; of the latter, by arsenic.

Aromatic amines. 2-Acetylaminofluorene (AAF) provides the classic illustration of how interspecies differences in carcinogenic effects can be utilized to identify metabolic pathways of activation (Figure 1). Study of this compound played a crucial role in development of the electrophilic theory of carcinogenesis (8-10), and revealed that species differences in both the N-hydroxylation (11-13) and conjugation (14) steps are important for tumor induction. Some species, such as the guinea pig, do not N-hydroxylate AAF, and consequently, are refractory to it by virtue of this single metabolic difference from other, susceptible, species.

Arsenic compounds. In contrast, the mechanism by which these inorganic salts cause skin cancer in man remains an enigma. No unequivocal carcinogenic effect has been experimentally

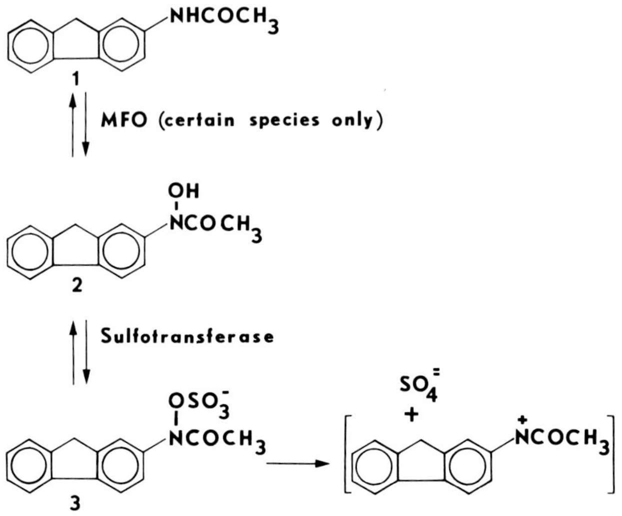

NHCOCH3
1
MFO (certain species only)
OH
NCOCH3
2
Sulfotransferase
OSO_3^-
NCOCH3
3
$SO_4^=$
+
$\overset{+}{N}COCH_3$

Figure 1. Hepatic activation of 2-acetylaminofluorene (AAF) to proximate and ultimate carcinogenic metabolites. For the procarcinogen AAF (1) to be carcinogenic for liver cells in the mouse, rat, hamster, and other species, it must be metabolized by a mixed-function oxidase (MFO) to its N-hydroxy derivative (2), a proximate carcinogen which is more carcinogenic than its precursor. In the guinea pig 1 is not efficiently metabolized to 2 and is not carcinogenic. Synthetic 2 induces non-hepatic tumors in this species, as do esters of 2. The sulfate, 3, which also is not efficiently generated by the guinea pig, in the liver of susceptible species is a reactive ultimate carcinogenic metabolite of 1. This simplified scheme disregards reversible deacetylation reactions and competing metabolic paths.

demonstrated in rodents or other laboratory species (15), although a complex mixture containing calcium arsenate has recently been shown to induce lung tumors in rats after intratracheal instillation (16). As a result, investigation of carcinogenesis by arsenic has been severely hampered.

Different Target Organs in Different Species

This is one of the most frequent patterns of species differences in chemical carcinogenesis by many classes of chemical carcinogens, including aflatoxins, nitrosamines, aromatic amines, and many others. Representative studies with aromatic amines (17) are illustrated in Table 2. Differences are seen both in major organ systems and in some target organs that are either unique to a single species, or so predominate among the sites of chemical carcinogenesis in a given species as to constitute a distinguishing feature.

Major organ systems. For aromatic amines, the major target organ is the urinary system, especially the urinary bladder. Table 2 shows clearly that different segments of the urinary system are affected in different species, and that different agents within the class vary in their patterns of carcinogenicity, both within and among species. 2-Aminonaphthalene is virtually restricted to the urinary bladder both in man and in the hamster, dog, and monkey; in the mouse, it does not affect the urinary bladder, but is carcinogenic for the liver. In contrast, AAF is carcinogenic for the urinary bladder in the rat, mouse, and rabbit, but not in the Syrian hamster, in which other (especially non-acetylated) aromatic amines are active. The ureter is a target of AAF chiefly in the rabbit, however, and the kidney only in the mouse. Further, there is extensive "spillover" to other major organ systems, especially in mice, in which AAF also induces tumors in the liver, intestine, and elsewhere. In the case of aromatic amines, these differences are generally ascribed to differences in metabolism, but detailed quantitative data to confirm this hypothesis are rarely both available and sufficient to provide mechanistic explanations for the spectrum of tumors observed.

Target organs unique to a single species. In the rat, the mouse, and other species used for carcinogenesis research, there are specific sites of tumor development, and specific, characteristic kinds of tumors that develop at those sites, which are involved frequently in response to many kinds of carcinogens. In the rat, Zymbal's gland -- a sebaceous gland of the external auditory canal -- is such an organ, in which squamous cell carcinomas commonly develop in response to many carcinogens, including AAF (Table 2). In the mouse, the retroorbital Harderian gland, in which adenomas and adenocarcinomas develop, is comparable

Table 2. Carcinogenic Activity of Selected Aromatic Amines in Different Species[a].

Species	Tumors Induced in						
	Bladder	Kidney	Liver	Intestine	Zymbal's Gland	Breast	Other
			2-Acetylaminofluorene				
Rat	+	−	+	−	+	+	
Mouse	+	+	+	+	−	+	
Hamster	−	−	+	−	−	−	
Rabbit	+	−	−	−	−	−	Ureter
Guinea pig	−	−	−	−	−	−	
			2-Aminonaphthalene				
Mouse	−	−	+	−	−	−	
Hamster	+	−	−	−	−	−	
Dog	+	−	−	−	−	−	
Monkey	+	−	−	−	−	−	
Man	+	−	−	−	−	−	
Rat	−	−	−	−	−	−	
Rabbit	−	−	−	−	−	−	
			4-(o-Tolylazo)-o-toluidine				
Hamster	+	−	+	−	−	+	
Mouse	+	−	+	−	−	−	Lung
Rat	−	−	+	−	−	−	
Dog	+	−	?	−	−	−	Gall bladder
Rabbit	?	−	−	−	−	−	

[a]Modified from Clayson and Garner (17).

in its frequent response to carcinogens. The mid-ventral sebaceous gland of the gerbil appears also to belong in this category (18). These unique target organs constitute one of the most extreme aspects of species differences in chemical carcinogenesis. The reason for the extraordinary susceptibility of such organs is not understood.

Different Target Cells within a Tissue or Organ

In general it is not enough to specify only the organ or tissue in which carcinogenesis occurs, since many different cell types combine to form these complex structures. In glands, for example, not only the parenchymal epithelium, but the supporting connective tissue stroma and its blood vessels may give rise to neoplasms. In complex glands, there may be several distinct kinds of epithelium: in the pancreas, for example, there are the acinar cells and the ducts of the exocrine pancreas, each of which can generate distinctive varieties of adenoma and carcinoma, as well as the several sub-types of endocrine cells of the islets of Langerhans. These also may give rise to tumors (and commonly do so in rats); such neoplasms must be distinguished from similar tumors of different histogenesis arising in the same organ. If detailed comparisons of the effects of an inducing agent in different species are to be valid, or if a given experimental system is to be utilized as a model of a human disease, convincing histopathologic evidence of the nature and origin of the tumors observed must be provided. It goes without saying that neoplasms must be distinguished from other lesions. Some of the organ systems in which these distinctions are commonly encountered in experimental animals are discussed below.

Liver. Liver is one of the most thoroughly studied of all tissues in both biochemistry and pathology and is the major target organ of a wide variety of chemical carcinogens. Tumors commonly arise in liver from the hepatic parenchymal cells (hepatocellular adenomas and carcinomas); the lining cells of the intrahepatic bile ducts (cholangiomas and cholangiocarcinomas); or the endothelial cells of the hepatic sinusoids (hemangiomas and hemangiosarcomas). The histologic features of each of these three major classes of tumor are compared with their respective cells of origin in Figure 2. The tumors illustrated in Figure 2 were all induced by the same metabolism-independent alkylating agent, nitrosoethylurea (ENU), but in three different species.

There are other carcinogens that are relatively specific for the liver in one or more species, but that selectively affect only one of these cell types. Vinyl chloride has already been mentioned as an example of an agent with specificity for hepatic sinusoidal endothelium in man; aflatoxin B_1, which will be discussed later in

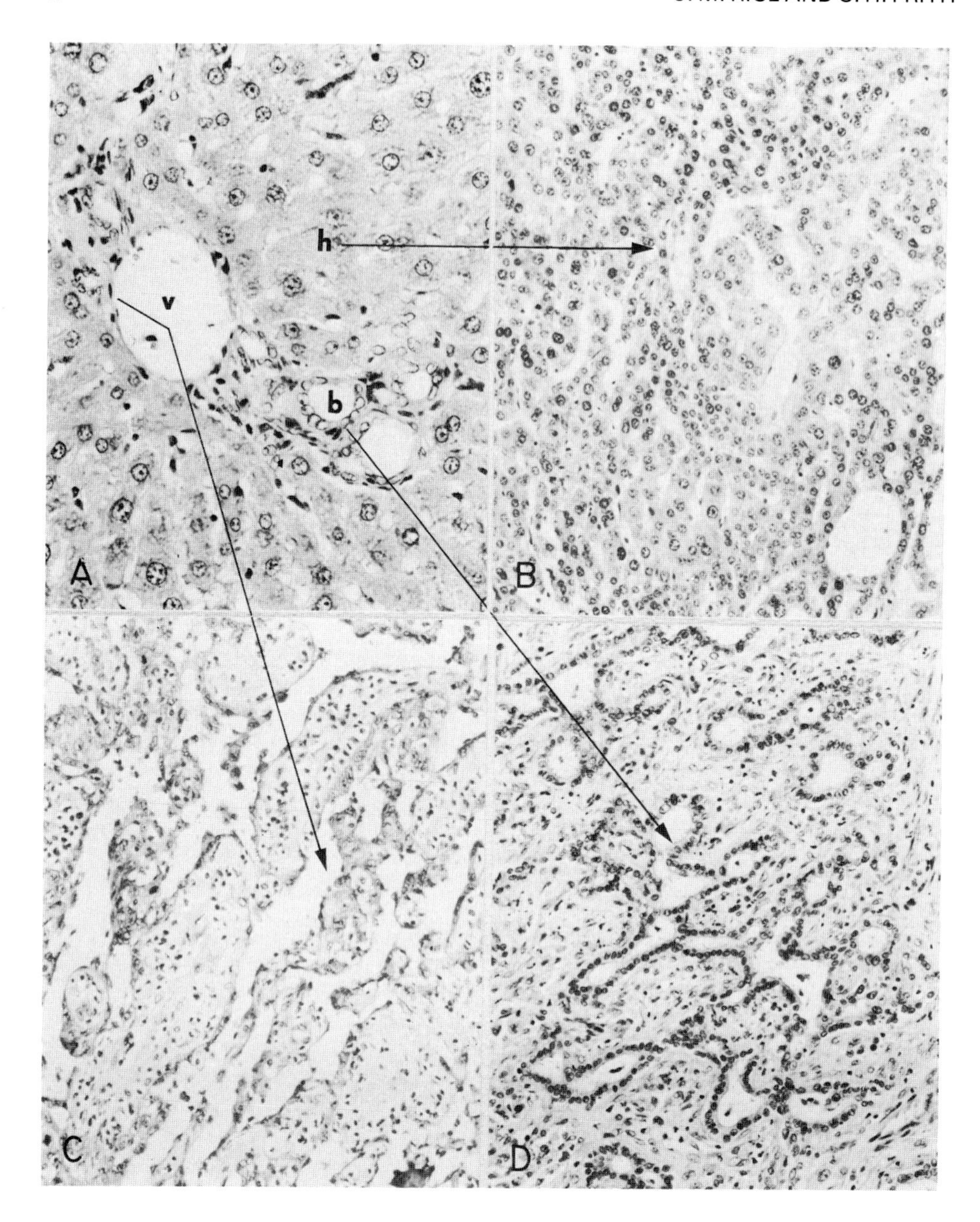

Figure 2. Tumors of the liver induced by nitrosoethylurea and the cells from which they originate. H & E. (A) Portal triad from normal liver, showing hepatocytes (h), bile ducts (b), and blood vessels (v), x 300; (B) hepatocellular carcinoma (mouse, x 220); (C) hemangiosarcoma (patas monkey, x 220); (D) cholangioma (rhesus monkey, x 220).

this session, is characteristically specific for hepatocytes in many diverse species, including rats and rainbow trout. Furthermore, these three general classes of neoplasm are not the only tumors that may arise in the liver; the supporting connective tissues, histiocytes, and occasionally other cell types may give rise to hepatic neoplasia.

In the liver, as elsewhere, different neoplasms are not always readily distinguishable, even by experienced observers. The inconsistencies in published descriptions of tumors induced in the rat liver by nitrosodimethylamine, and in the relative proportions of these that have been considered to originate from hepatocytes and from vascular endothelium, are instructive in this regard (19-21). Further, the biological properties and predictive value for carcinogenicity bioassays of hepatocellular neoplasms in mice remain an issue that many consider unresolved, even after decades of study (5,22).

Respiratory tract. In contrast to the liver, in which tumors of any kind may arise in any portion of the organ, the respiratory tract in rodents has anatomically distinct regions which vary from one species to another in susceptibility to a given carcinogen. In the mouse, tumors of the peripheral lung are readily induced by a wide variety of chemical carcinogens, to which exposure may occur either pre- or postnatally. Once thought to arise exclusively from one kind of alveolar lining cells, the type II (surfactant-secreting) pneumocytes (6), these neoplasms are now known to consist of two subclasses, the second arising from the non-ciliated clara cells of the terminal bronchiole (23). Tumors of the upper respiratory tract -- bronchi, trachea, larynx -- are virtually never seen in mice in response to systemically administered carcinogens, but in the Syrian hamster these are the very sites affected by certain agents, notably nitrosodiethylamine (DEN), even when exposure is both systemic and transplacental (24). The contrasting effects of DEN in the mouse (25) and hamster (24) are very striking and are not understood.

The nasal cavities of rodents may be affected by chemical carcinogens given either by inhalation or by other routes of administration, and several kinds of tumors can be induced. These neoplasms may kill the host by occlusion of the airways or by invasion of the brain without ever being grossly apparent, and may be overlooked without careful pathological examination.

Kidney. While tumors of the transitional epithelium of the renal pelvis are quite similar from one species to the next, neoplasms of the renal cortex vary markedly. The principal difference is in the nature of cellular differentiation in the tumors. In the mouse, chemically induced tumors of the renal cortex are almost always of adult epithelial morphology, arise from the proximal convoluted tubules, and are relatively benign; they are rarely the primary cause of death. This has been well shown for tumors induced by ENU (26) and is true whether the agent is administered either transplacentally or after birth. This is remarkable, since the kidney cortex evolves through differentiation of mesenchyme into epithelium; the ratio of undifferentiated mesenchyme to mature tubules is virtually infinite during early fetal life and becomes nearly zero by the time the postnatal mouse becomes adult. Yet in the mouse, mesenchymal or mixed mesenchymal/primitive epithelial tumors (nephroblastomas) are almost never seen, even in transplacental carcinogenesis experiments. In the rat, however, they are both common. Highly malignant, rapidly growing mesenchymal tumors characteristically develop as a consequence of exposing fetal or young rats to renal carcinogens, including ENU (27). These tumors do not arise from mature tubular epithelium, as in the mouse, but from undifferentiated interstitial mesenchyme. In the rabbit, the characteristic renal tumor is a nephroblastoma, a mixed tumor of mesenchyme and incompletely differentiated epithelium, which is characteristically induced in this species by ENU (28) and is the predominant naturally occurring renal tumor in old rabbits not given carcinogens. Renal cortical tumors, in parallel with liver tumors, may develop at any anatomical site within the cortical parenchyma, but vary markedly from species to species in morphology, behavior, and histogenesis.

LIMITATIONS OF TUMOR INDUCTION STUDIES

The preceding discussion illustrates the complexities involved in comparing the effects of carcinogens in different species on the basis of tumors that are actually observed in treated animals. Truly accurate quantitative and comprehensive qualitative comparisons are made very difficult by the fact that whatever tumors are actually observed in experimental animals must be considered only a fraction of those potentially present. This fraction can be increased by good detection techniques, but probably can never approach unity because of a number of factors that for convenience we group together under the term "variable latency."

Variable Latency

Not all neoplasms develop at the same rate. Even within one class of neoplasms, arising in a cohort of experimental animals that is completely uniform in genetics, age, sex, and extent of exposure, latency may vary by weeks or months, often a large fraction of the animals' life span. Furthermore, latency can be modified by factors extrinsic to the developing neoplasm, or the dormant potentially neoplastic cells from which they evolve.

Lethal versus non-lethal tumors. Dead animals grow no tumors. Frequently an experimental animal may be simultaneously at risk for one or more rapidly growing, highly malignant and lethal neoplasms, and also for less rapidly growing and generally benign tumors at other sites. Early death from mammary or intestinal carcinoma or malignant schwannoma in rats, or thymic lymphoma in mice, will preclude development of more slowly developing tumors such as renal or hepatocellular tumors in mice, or gliomas of the central nervous system or prostatic carcinoma in rats. The more slowly growing tumors will thus be underreported. This is an important consideration when a conclusion of the experiment is that a carcinogenic effect occurred only in certain tissues or organs. One should be wary of such statements; it is often safer to confine oneself to stating that an effect was observed only in certain organs.

Dormant tumor cells. It is well documented that potential tumor cells may persist in tissues long after exposure to a carcinogen has ceased. The presence of these cells may be revealed only by subsequent exposure to tumor-promoting agents, which are often not genotoxic and have great specificity for certain cell types. Tumor promotion has been reviewed recently (29) and will be discussed in relation to organ specificity in the next session of this Symposium. The very existence of the phenomenon of promoter-dependent tumor growth following exposure to chemical carcinogens is proof that only a fraction of potential tumor cells resulting from carcinogen exposure actually proceed to proliferate and form a tumor, at least in mouse skin and rat liver, where the persistence of such cells has been most clearly documented. There is no way at present to estimate this fraction, and it is reasonable to assume that dormancy is not exclusive to the organs and tissues in which it has so far been demonstrated. The actual tumor yield in a carcinogenesis experiment is, therefore, like the tip of an iceberg: only a small fraction of the effects of a carcinogen are actually measured by counting tumors.

Dormant tumor cells can also in some cases be unmasked by immune suppression of a carcinogen-treated host. One example of this is the appearance of transitional cell carcinomas of the urinary bladder in rats given anti-lymphocyte serum (ALS) after injection of nitrosomethylurea, a carcinogenic regimen that in rats not given ALS elicits tumor development chiefly in the nervous system (30). Immune suppression differs from tumor promotion in that it is a systemic effect on cells other than those from which tumors will arise, unlike tumor promotion, which appears to be a direct effect on dormant tumor cells.

Dose/Effect Relationships

Another aspect of latency is its inverse dependence on the dosage of carcinogen, which is one aspect of dose/effect relationships in chemical carcinogenesis. This concept was developed by Druckrey, who showed that in many systems, including single transplacental exposures to alkylating agents (31), data can be expressed in the form

$$\text{dose} \times (\text{latency})^{n} = \text{constant},$$

where the exponent n is characteristic of the tumor induction system, algebraically determined as the slope of a logarithmic plot of dose versus latency. At higher doses, tumors appear more rapidly; but each kind of tumor may have its own values of n and of the equation constant. One practical result of this is that at lower doses, one must observe experimental animals longer in order that the full range of observable effects can appear.

A less well documented, but potentially extremely important aspect of dose/effect relationships in carcinogenesis is that the degree of malignancy of the tumors observed, and even the classification of the tumors, may vary with dosage. This is illustrated in Figure 3 as an increasing ratio of hepatocellular carcinomas to adenomas as the duration of dietary exposure of mice to benzidine was increased (22), and in Figure 4 as a similarly increasing ratio with increasing dosage level (22). This phenomenon appears to be truly carcinogen-related, and not simply a natural evolution of adenomas into carcinomas with time; the degree of morphologic differentiation of the tumors also changes (22), and is inversely related to dosage (Figure 5). Similar trends have been documented (Figure 6) for increasing invasiveness of urinary bladder carcinomas with both dosage level and duration of exposure in mice fed AAF (32). One contributing mechanism for such effects, especially in chronic dietary exposure studies, may be direct mutagenic effects of the carcinogen on tumor cells that lead to clones of increasingly pleomorphic and malignant cells.

Adequacy of Experimental Observations

It is easy to overlook small tumors in hidden sites when necropsy protocols are focused exclusively on a few easily accessible organs or tissues; the history of chemical carcinogenesis is replete with instances of discovering induced tumors in sites such as the thyroid gland, brain, and urinary bladder only as a result of unusually painstaking technique. To be reasonably assured of completeness, one should examine virtually

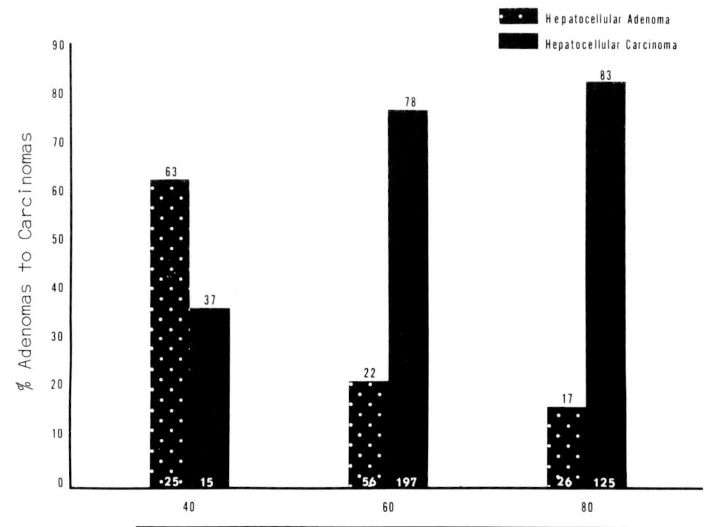

Length of Administration of Benzidine(Weeks)

Actual number of neoplasms is represented by number in bottom of each bar.

Figure 3. Ratio of hepatocellular adenomas to hepatocellular carcinomas with duration of administration of benzidine to female mice. From (22), by permission.

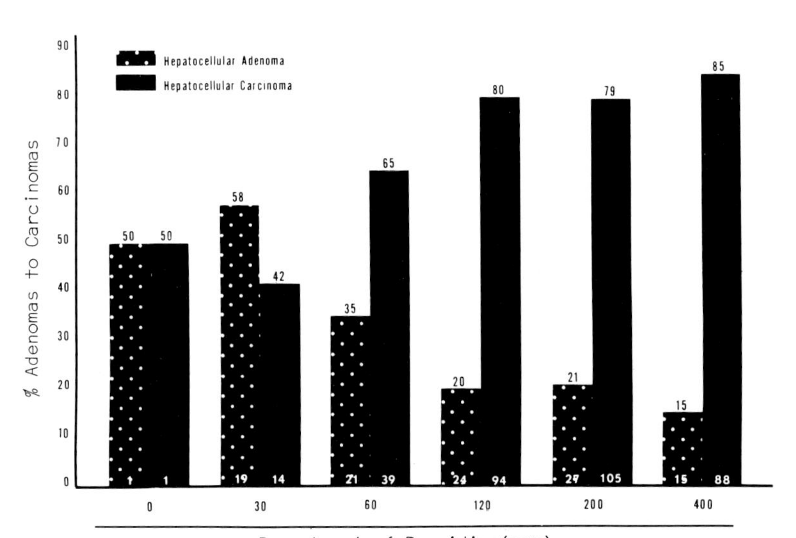

Actual number of neoplasms is represented by number in bottom of each bar.

Figure 4. Ratio of hepatocellular adenomas to hepatocellular carcinomas with dosage level of benzidine fed to female mice. From (22), by permission.

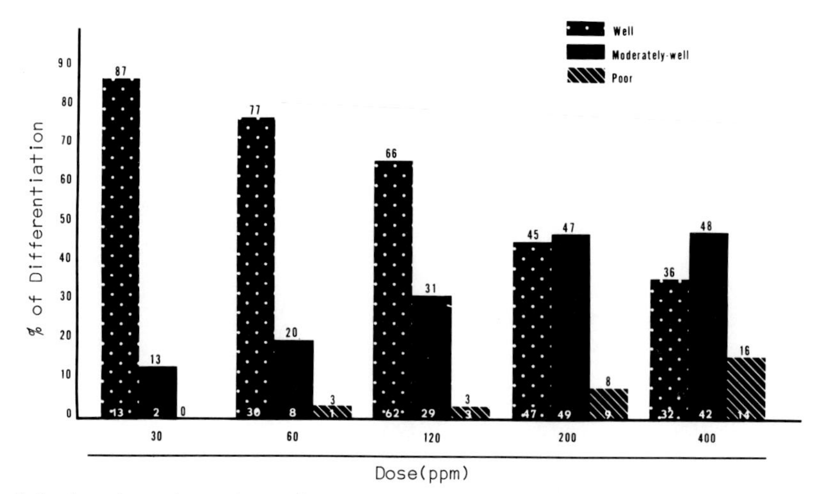

Actual number of neoplasms is represented by number in bottom of each bar.

Figure 5. Frequency of well, moderately, and poorly differentiated hepatocellular carcinomas in female mice fed benzidine at various dosage levels. From (22), by permission.

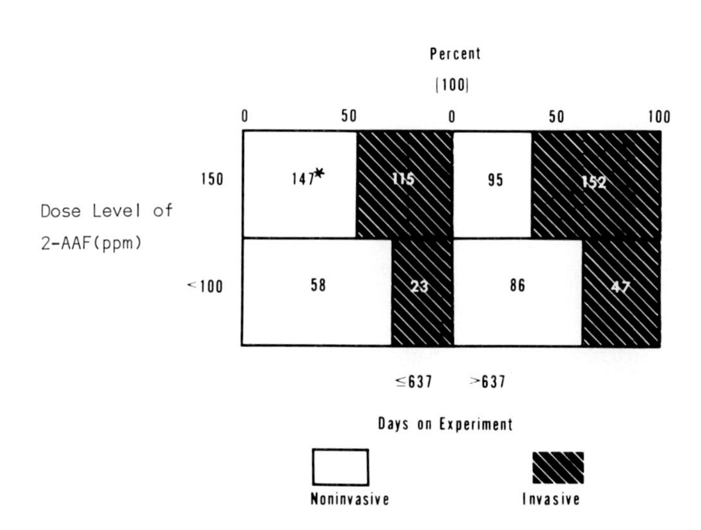

*Number represents the total number of mice with neoplasms.

Figure 6. Correlation of invasiveness of bladder carcinomas with dosage level and duration of administration of AAF in female BALB/c mice. From (32), by permission.

every tissue, a counsel of perfection that is time-consuming, expensive, and infrequently achieved in practice except at laboratories such as the National Center for Toxicological Research (NCTR). The extent of the necropsy examination of mice from carcinogenesis studies performed at NCTR is given in Figure 7 (33).

The importance of this approach was demonstrated by comparing gross and microscopic evaluations of these tissues (33). In some tissues and organs, notably liver and mammary gland, little improvement over gross observation of a mass was achieved by randomly slicing the organ and examining one section histologically. In other organs such as the Harderian gland, uterus, and adrenal cortex fully two thirds of the tumors detected microscopically were not observed grossly, and would have been overlooked had the protocol specified only histologic confirmation of grossly apparent lesions (Figure 8). An example of an adrenal cortical adenoma not seen on gross examination is illustrated in Figure 9. This is a small, benign tumor, and it might be argued that the detection of such lesions is of too little consequence to justify the effort; but it should be noted that even advanced carcinomas of the urinary bladder, especially those that produce no exophytic mass within the bladder lumen (Figure 10), were not detected grossly, even at NCTR, in a significant fraction (12%) of cases (33). In reading the presentations that follow, one should keep in mind the need for critical evaluation of the extent of the pathological examinations carried out in the various studies, as well as the kinds of differences between species - and between strains within a species -- that such examination might be expected to reveal.

A final word is in order about the nature of histopathologic data. Diagnostic histopathology, properly performed, is by no means as arbitrary and subjective as some who have had the experience of collaborating with several different pathologists may suspect. The discipline is, however, fundamentally descriptive rather than analytical, and, therefore, does retain an element of subjectivity. It also has its limitations, the most serious of which is the impossibility of separating the variables that may be present together in a given tissue. Inflammation and degenerative changes; necrosis and hemorrhage; infection; acute and chronic responses to toxic injury; regenerative hyperplasia and neoplasia may coexist, not only in the same organ, but together in the same lesion. When this occurs the kaleidoscopic superposition of images may render definitive diagnosis impossible, even if the tissue was fresh and no details have been lost through post-mortem autolysis. Tissues from small rodents dead more than a few hours before fixation may be uninterpretable in any case. The fewer the pathologic changes in a tissue, the better the chance that the precisely defined criteria that exist for identification and

Lung
Heart
Thymus
Skeletal Muscle
Kidney
Adrenal
Liver
Gall Bladder
Spleen
Pancreas
Cerebrum
Cerebellum
Spinal Cord
Stomach
Colon
Duodenum
Ileum

Lymph Nodes
Submaxillary Salivary Gland
Sublingual Salivary Gland
Parotid Salivary Gland
Lacrimal Gland
Harderian Gland
Eye
Thyroid
Trachea
Esophagus
Skin/Subcutis
Marrow
Bone
Testes
Epididymis
Seminal vesicle

Coagulating Gland
Preputial Gland
Penis
Ovary
Oviduct
Uterus
Mammary Tissue
Pituitary
Vagina
Prostate
Urethra
Bladder
Ureter
Aorta
Pulmonary Artery
Blood Smear

Figure 7. Organs collected from mice at necropsy for microscopic evaluation at the National Center for Toxicological Research (NCTR). From (33), by permission.

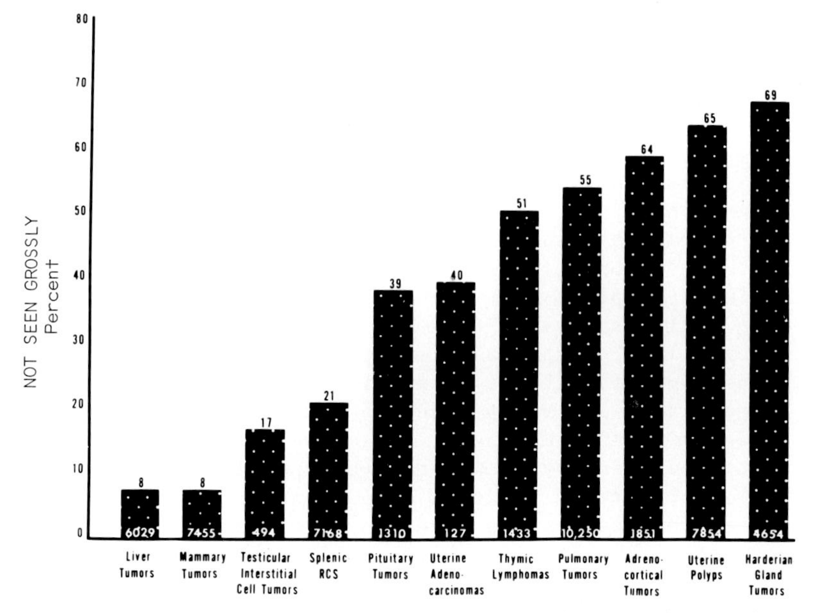

Figure 8. Comparison of gross and microscopic pathologic findings for selected tissues from mice fed AAF in the NCTR ED_{01} study. From (33), by permission.

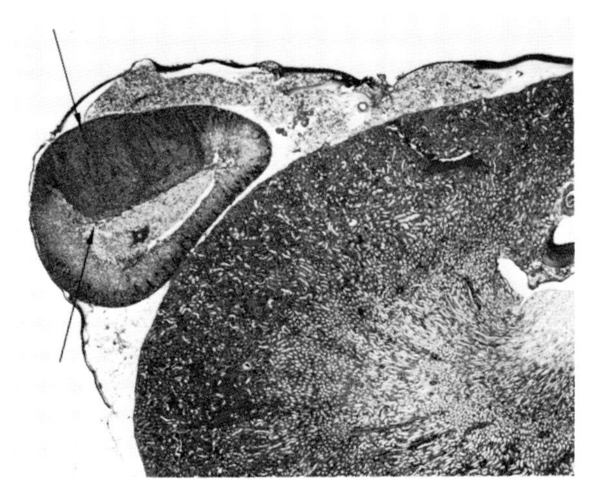

Figure 9. Arrows point to small adrenocortical adenoma not visible grossly. H & E, x 56. From (33), by permission.

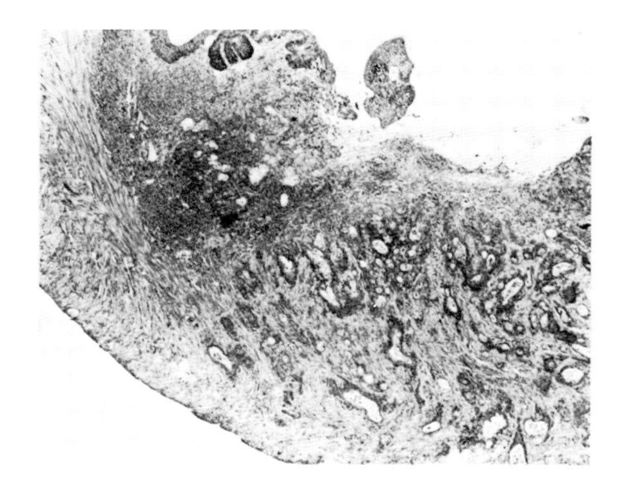

Figure 10. Deeply invasive transitional cell carcinoma which extends to the adventitia of the urinary bladder. Note that the wall is only slightly thickened and that the lumen of the bladder contains no neoplasm. Of such tumors, 12% were not seen grossly. H & E, x 56. From (33), by permission.

histogenetic classification of neoplasia can be properly applied by the pathologist.

The better the pathologic diagnoses, the more soundly established will be the foundation on which all efforts to understand organ and tissue specificity in chemical carcinogenesis must be based.

REFERENCES

1. Cutler, S.J., and J.L. Young, Jr. 1975. Third National Cancer Survey: Incidence Data. Department of Health, Education, and Welfare publication No. 75-787. National Cancer Institute Monograph 41. National Institutes of Health: Washington, DC. 454 pp.

2. IARC. 1974. Some Aromatic Amines, Hydrazine and Related Substances, N-Nitroso Compounds, and Miscellaneous Alkylating Agents. IARC Monographs on the Evaluation of Carcinogenic Risk of Chemicals to Man, Vol. 4. International Agency for Research on Cancer: Lyons, pp. 97-111.

3. IARC. 1974. Some Aromatic Amines, Hydrazine and Related Substances, N-Nitroso Compounds, and Miscellaneous Alkylating Agents. IARC Monographs on the Evaluation of Carcinogenic Risk of Chemicals to Man, Vol. 4. International Agency for Research on Cancer: Lyons, pp. 231-238.

4. IARC. 1974. Some Anti-thyroid and Related Substances, Nitrofurans and Industrial Chemicals. IARC Monographs, Vol. 7, pp. 291-305.

5. Tomatis, L., C. Partensky, and R. Montesano. 1973. The predictive value of mouse liver tumour induction in carcinogenicity testing -- a literature survey. Intl. J. Cancer 12:1-20.

6. Shimkin, M.B., and G.D. Stoner. 1975. Lung tumors in mice: application to carcinogenesis bioassay. Adv. Cancer Res. 21:1-58.

7. NCI. 1978. Bioassay of Tris (2,3-dibromopropyl)phosphate for Possible Carcinogenicity. Department of Health, Education, and Welfare publication No. 78-1326. National Cancer Institute Carcinogenesis Technical Report Series No. 76. National Institutes of Health: Washington, DC. 62 pp. and appendices.

8. Miller, J.A., and E.C. Miller. 1966. A survey of molecular aspects of chemical carcinogenesis. Laboratory Invest. 15:217-239.

9. Miller, E.C., and J.A. Miller. 1966. Mechanisms of chemical carcinogenesis: nature of proximate carcinogens and interactions with macromolecules. Pharmacol. Rev. 18:805-838.

10. Miller, E.C., and J.A. Miller. 1976. The metabolism of chemical carcinogens to reactive electrophiles and their possible mechanisms of action in carcinogenesis. In: C.E. Searle, ed. Chemical Carcinogens, ACS Monograph 173. American Chemical Society: Washington, DC. pp. 737-762.

11. Miller, J.A., J.W. Cramer, and E.C. Miller. 1960. The N- and ring-hydroxylation of 2-acetylaminofluorene during carcinogenesis in the rat. Cancer Res. 20:950-962.

12. Miller, E.C., J.A. Miller, and H.A. Hartmann. 1961. N-Hydroxy-2-acetylaminofluorene: a metabolite of 2-acetylaminofluorene with increased carcinogenic activity in the rat. Cancer Res. 21:815-824.

13. Miller, E.C., J.A. Miller, and M. Enomoto. 1964. The comparative carcinogenicities of 2-acetylaminofluorene and its N-hydroxy metabolite in mice, hamsters, and guinea pigs. Cancer Res. 24:2018-2031.

14. DeBaun, J.R., E.C. Miller, and J.A. Miller. 1970. N-Hydroxy-2-acetylaminofluorene sulfotransferase: its probable role in carcinogenesis and in protein-(methion-S-yl) binding in rat liver. Cancer Res. 30:577-595.

15. IARC. 1973. Some inorganic and organometallic compounds. IARC Monographs on the Evaluation of Carcinogenic Risk of Chemicals to Man, Vol. 2. International Agency for Research on Cancer: Lyons. pp. 48-73.

16. Ivankovic, S., G. Eisenbrand, and R. Preussmann. 1979. Lung carcinoma induction in BD rats after a single intratracheal instillation of an arsenic-containing pesticide mixture formerly used in vineyards. Int. J. Cancer 24:786-788.

17. Clayson, D.B., and R.C. Garner. 1976. Carcinogenic aromatic amines and related compounds. In: C.E. Searle, ed. Chemical Carcinogens, ACS Monograph 173. American Chemical Society: Washington, DC. pp. 366-461.

18. Haas, H., J. Hilfrich, N. Kmoch, and U. Mohr. 1975. Specific carcinogenic effect of N-methyl-N-nitrosourea on the midventral sebaceous gland of the gerbil (Meriones unguiculatus). J. Natl. Cancer Inst. 55:637-640.

19. IARC. 1978. Some N-Nitroso Compounds. IARC Monographs on the Evaluation of Carcinogenic Risk of Chemicals to Man, Vol. 17. International Agency for Research on Cancer: Lyons. pp. 125-175.

20. Taylor, H.W., W. Lijinsky, P. Nettesheim, and C.M. Snyder. 1974. Alteration of tumor response in rat liver by carbon tetrachloride. Cancer Res. 34:3391-3395.

21. Abanobi, S.E., E. Farber, and D.S.R. Sarma. 1979. Persistence of DNA damage during development of liver angiosarcomas in rats fed dimethylnitrosamine. Cancer Res. 39:1592-1596.

22. Frith, C.H., K.H. Baetcke, C.J. Nelson, and G. Schieferstein. 1979. Importance of the mouse liver tumor in carcinogenesis bioassay studies using benzidine dihydrochloride as a model. Toxicol. Lett. 4:507-518.

23. Kauffman, S.L. 1981. Histogenesis of the papillary clara cell adenoma. Amer. J. Pathol. 103:174-180.

24. Mohr, U., H. Reznik-Schuller, G. Reznik, and J. Hilfrich. 1975. Transplacental effects of diethylnitrosamine in Syrian hamsters as related to different days of administration during pregnancy. J. Natl. Cancer Inst. 55:681-683.

25. Diwan, B.A., and H. Meier. 1976. Transplacental carcinogenic effects of diethylnitrosamine in mice. Naturwissenschaften 63:487-488.

26. Lombard, L.S., J.M. Rice, and S.D. Vesselinovitch. 1974. Renal tumors in mice: light microscopic observations of epithelial tumors induced by ethylnitrosourea. J. Natl. Cancer Inst. 53:1677-1685.

27. Druckrey, H., B. Schagen, and S. Ivankovic. 1970. Erzeugung neurogener Malignome durch einmalige Gabe von "Äthylnitrosoharnstoff an neugeborene und junge BD-IX Ratten. Z. Krebsforsch. 74:141-161.

28. Fox, R.R., B.A. Diwan, and H. Meier. 1975. Transplacental induction of primary renal tumors in rabbits treated with 1-ethyl-1-nitrosourea. J. Natl. Cancer Inst. 54:1439-1448.

29. Slaga, T.J., A. Sivak, and R.K. Boutwell, eds. 1978. Mechanisms of Tumor Promotion and Carcinogenesis. Raven Press: New York. 588 pp.

30. Denlinger, R.H., J.A. Swenberg, A. Koestner, and W. Wechsler. 1973. Differential effect of immunosuppression on the induction of nervous system and bladder tumors by N-methyl-N-nitrosourea. J. Natl. Cancer Inst. 50:87-93.

31. Ivankovic, S., and H. Druckrey. 1968. Transplacentare Erzeugung maligner Tumoren des Nervensystems. I. Äthylnitrosoharnstoff an BD-IX Ratten. Z. Krebsforsch. 71:320-360.

32. Frith, C.H., J.H. Farmer, D.L. Greenman, and G.W. Shaw. 1980. Biologic and morphologic characteristics of urinary bladder neoplasms induced in BALB/c female mice with 2-acetylaminofluorene. J. Environ. Pathol. Toxicol. 3:103-119.

33. Frith, C.H., A.D. Boothe, D.L. Greenman, and J.H. Farmer. 1980. Correlations between gross and microscopic lesions in carcinogenic studies in mice. J. Environ. Pathol. Toxicol. 3:139-153.

DISCUSSION

Q.: If you supplement your histologic evaluation with biochemical markers, can you improve the accuracy and efficiency of your microscopic examination? Could you bridge the gaps that exist between gross identification and microscopic diagnosis by using biochemical markers?

A.: I think in some instances we could but I don't think that we would be completely successful. Jerry, do you want to comment on that?

A.: The issue is still one of finding the lesion. While a biochemical marker can be extremely useful, still if the lesion is not seen and the piece of tissue that contains it is not taken, the biochemistry will be no better than the histologic preparation. It's a matter of sampling.

Q.: Weren't bladder tumors also found in dogs given benzidine?

A.: There have been some studies, but the number of dogs was so small that I think it is equivocal whether benzidine really is a bladder carcinogen in the dog. It probably is.

Q.: Have you considered strain as well as species differences? Because if you look hard enough you can find rats that will get intestinal tumors or any other kind of tumor from acetylaminofluorene. I think strain differences are just as important in many cases as species differences.

A.: I agree very much.

SPECIES DIFFERENCES IN RESPONSE TO AROMATIC AMINES

Elizabeth K. Weisburger

Laboratory of Carcinogen Metabolism, National Cancer Institute, Bethesda, Maryland 20205

INTRODUCTION

Extensive studies on several species of laboratory animals have been done for only a few carcinogenic aromatic amines or amides; those so tested include benzidine, 4-aminobiphenyl, 2-acetylaminofluorene (AAF), and 2-aminonaphthalene (1). Even for these known carcinogens there are sizable variations in species response; the most striking occurs with AAF where at least 15 species have been tested (2). With this compound the guinea pig, cotton rat, monkey, steppe-lemming, and X/Gf mouse, among the mammals, have shown resistance to the carcinogenic effects. Metabolic studies, either *in vivo* or *in vitro*, have not always provided satisfactory explanations for these differences (3,4,5).

Likewise, 2',3-dimethyl-4-biphenylamine produces intestinal and ear duct tumors in rats but mainly leads to bladder tumors in hamsters (6). It is difficult to visualize such outstanding differences in metabolism that could alone account for this result. Instead, one presumes that a species or tissue specific system is more likely responsible.

In the course of the National Cancer Institute Bioassay Program, many environmental or industrial aromatic amines and derivatives as well as some of their nitro precursors were selected for carcinogenicity testing. The results from these studies afforded an extensive amount of material for structure-activity and species-susceptibility correlations.

MATERIALS AND METHODS

(C57BL/6 x C3H)F_1 mice (B6C3F_1) and F344 rats were the test animals, obtained from qualified laboratories. Animals were quarantined for two weeks prior to use in either the acute, prechronic, or chronic studies. The conditions of housing, maintenance, feeding, and all other details are given in the technical report on each compound. Most of the compounds tested were of high purity, as revealed by various spectral and chromatographic studies.

At the conclusion of the experimental or holding period, animals were killed for a thorough necropsy. Numerous tissues were removed for histopathological examination. Data were recorded in the Carcinogenesis Bioassay Data System (CBDS), which generated tables for verification of data and for statistical review. The NCI Technical Report on each compound provides a thorough discussion of the statistical methods employed and the reasons for concluding that an individual compound was or was not carcinogenic (Table 1).

RESULTS

The results are summarized in Tables 2 through 5. Table 2 shows the compounds that gave negative results in mice and rats; Table 3 shows the compounds that gave positive results in both mice and rats; Tables 4 and 5 give the data on those that showed carcinogenicity in mice only and in rats only, respectively.

Of the 53 aromatic amines or derivatives mentioned, approximately one-third, or 16, gave negative results in both mice and rats, while almost half, or 22, showed carcinogenicity in both mice and rats. Of those remaining, nine showed carcinogenicity in rats but had no such effect in mice. Six were active in mice but showed no effect in rats.

The majority of tumors induced by the compounds differed somewhat in mice and rats. In mice, liver tumors appeared most frequently, followed by those of the blood vessels (hemangioma or hemangiosarcoma), urinary bladder, hematopoietic system (lymphoma), and thyroid. More unusual tumors in mice were those of the Harderian or Zymbal's glands. In rats, liver tumors were also frequent, but the bladder, kidney, thyroid, skin and associated glands, Zymbal's gland, and other organs were frequently affected. Kidney tumors were induced in rats by o-anisidine, 1-amino-2-methylanthraquinone, and cinnamyl anthranilate. Phenazopyridine and 4,4'-thiodianiline led to colon tumors in rats, while cinnamyl anthranilate also caused pancreatic tumors, a relatively rare type of lesion, in male rats. In general, a greater variety of tumors was induced in rats by the compounds.

Table 1. Aromatic Amines Tested for Carcinogenicity in Rats and Mice in the NCI Bioassay Program

Compound [Common name]	Technical Report Number
2-Aminoanthraquinone	144
3-Amino-4-ethoxyacetanilide	112
3-Amino-9-ethylcarbazole·HCl	93
1-Amino-2-methylanthraquinone	111
4-Amino-2-nitrophenol	94
2-Amino-5-nitrothiazole	53
Aniline·HCl	130
o-Anisidine·HCl	89
p-Anisidine·HCl	116
o-Anthranilic acid	36
Azobenzene	154
4'-(Chloroacetyl)acetanilide	177
p-Chloroaniline	189
4-Chloro-m-phenylenediamine	85
4-Chloro-o-phenylenediamine	63
2-Chloro-p-phenylenediamine	113
4-Chloro-o-toluidine·HCl	165
5-Chloro-o-toluidine	187
3-Chloro-p-toluidine	145
Cinnamyl anthranilate	196
m-Cresidine	105
p-Cresidine	142
N-Nitrosophenylhydroxylamine [Cupferron]	100
4,4'-Sulfonyldianiline [Dapsone]	20
2,4-Diaminoanisole·H_2SO_4	84
2,4-Diaminotoluene	162
2,4-Dimethoxyaniline·HCl	171
3,3'-Dimethoxybenzidine-4,4'-diisocyanate	128
2,4-Dinitrotoluene	54
Hydrazobenzene	92
4,4'-Methylenebis(N,N-dimethyl)benzenamine [reduced Michler's Ketone]	186
2-Methyl-1-nitroanthraquinone	29
4,4'-bis (Dimethylamine)benzophenone [Michler's ketone]	181
5-Nitro-o-anisidine	127
4-Nitroanthranilic acid	109
6-Nitrobenzimidazole	117

(continued)

Table 1. (continued)

Compound [Common name]	Technical Report Number
1-Nitronaphthalene	64
4-Nitro-o-phenylenediamine	180
2-Nitro-p-phenylenediamine	169
Nitrosodiphenylamine	190
5-Nitro-o-toluidine	107
4,4'-Oxydianiline	205
Phenazopyridine·HCl	99
p-Phenylenediamine·2 HCl	174
1-Phenyl-3-methyl-5-pyrazolone	141
N-Phenyl-p-phenylenediamine	82
p-Quinone dioxime	179
2,3,5,6-Tetrachloro-4-nitroanisole	114
4,4'-Thiodianiline	47
2,5-Toluenediamine·H_2SO_4	126
2,6-Toluenediamine·2 HCl	200
o-Toluidine·HCl	153
2,4,5-Trimethylaniline	160

Table 2. Compounds Giving Negative Results in Mice and Rats at Two Dosage Levels

Compound	Structure	Levels (ppm) in Diet			
		Mice		Rats	
p-Anisidine·HCl	$NH_2 \cdot HCl$, OCH_3	5,000	10,000	3,000	6,000
Anthranilic acid	NH_2, COOH	25,000	50,000	15,000	30,000
4'-(Chloroacetyl) acetanilide	$NHCOCH_3$, $COCH_2Cl$	5,000	10,000	1,000	2,000
p-Chloroaniline	NH_2, Cl	2,500	5,000	250	500
2-Chloro-p-phenylene-diamine · H_2SO_4	NH_2, Cl, NH_2, $\cdot H_2SO_4$	3,000	6,000	1,500	3,000
3-Chloro-p-toluidine	NH_2, Cl, CH_3	600 300	1,200M[b] 600F[b]	1,635	3,269[a]

(continued)

Table 2. (continued)

Compound	Structure	Levels (ppm) in Diet			
		Mice		Rats	
2,4-Dimethoxyaniline· HCl	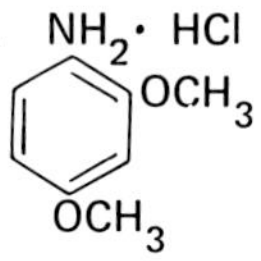 $NH_2 \cdot HCl$, OCH_3, OCH_3	2,500	5,000	1,500	3,000
4-Nitroanthranilic acid	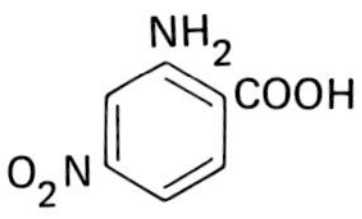 NH_2, COOH, O_2N	4,600	10,000	4,600	15,000[a]
1-Nitronaphthalene	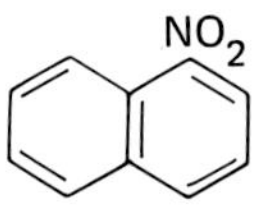 NO_2	600	1,200	600	1,800[a]
4-Nitro-o-phenylene-diamine	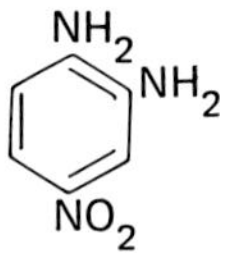 NH_2, NH_2, NO_2	3,750	7,500	375	750
p-Phenylenediamine· 2 HCl	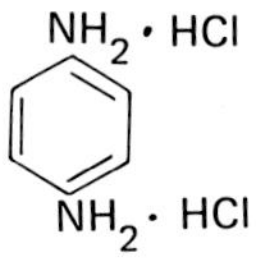 $NH_2 \cdot HCl$, $NH_2 \cdot HCl$	625	1,250	625	1,250
1-Phenyl-3-methyl-5-pyrazolone	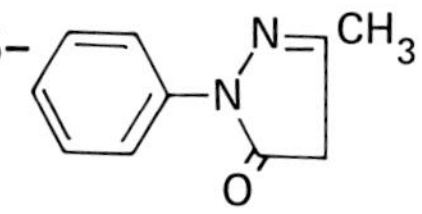 N, N, CH_3, O	7,500	15,000	2,500	5,000

(continued)

Table 2. (continued)

Compound	Structure	Levels (ppm) in Diet			
		Mice		Rats	
N-Phenyl-p-phenylenediamine·HCl	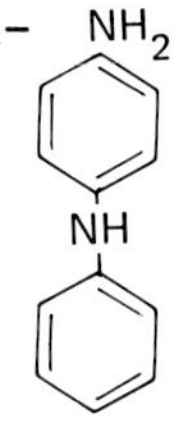 NH_2·HCl, NH (structure)	2,057 3,672	4,114[a]M[b] 8,170[a]F[b]	600	1,200
2,3,5,6-Tetrachloro-4-nitroanisole	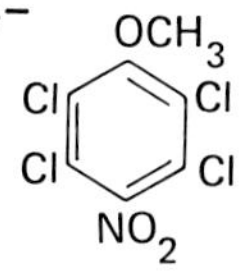 OCH_3, Cl, Cl, Cl, Cl, NO_2 (structure)	60	120	60	120
2,5-Toluenediamine·H_2SO_4	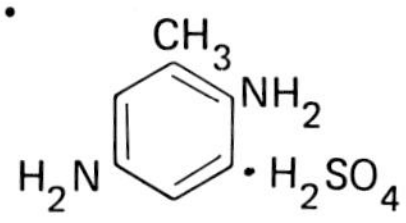 CH_3, NH_2, H_2N, ·H_2SO_4 (structure)	600	1,000	600	2,000[a]
2,6-Toluenediamine·2 HCl	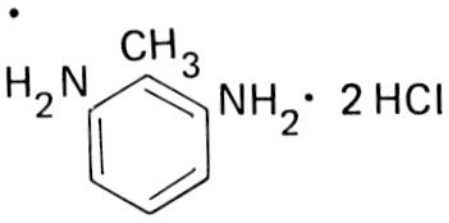 CH_3, H_2N, NH_2·2 HCl (structure)	50	100	250	500

[a]Time-weighted average concentration.
[b]M = Males; F = Females.

Table 3. Aromatic Amines Showing Carcinogenicity in Both Mice and Rats.

Compound	Structure	Levels (ppm) in Diet		Site Affected	
		Mice[a]	Rats[a]	Mice[a]	Rats[a]
2-Aminoanthraquinone		5,000 10,000	3,500 6,900[b]M 2,000F	Liver M&F Lymphoma F	Liver M
3-Amino-9-ethyl-carbazole·HCl		800 1,200	800 2,000	Liver M&F	Liver M&F Zymbal's gland M&F Uterus F Skin and subcutis M
1-Amino-2-methyl-anthraquinone		600[b]	1,000 2,000[b]	Liver F	Liver M&F Kidney M
o-Anisidine·HCl		2,500 5,000	5,000 10,000	Bladder M&F	Bladder M&F Kidney M Thyroid M

(continued)

Table 3. (continued)

Compound	Structure	Levels (ppm) in Diet				Site Affected	
		Mice		Rats		Mice	Rats
4-Chloro-o-phenylene-diamine	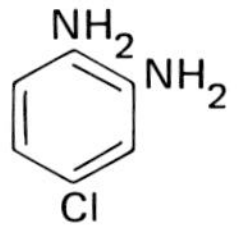 NH_2, NH_2, Cl	7,000	14,000[b]	5,000	10,000	Liver M&F	Bladder M&F Forestomach M&F
4-Chloro-m-phenylene-diamine	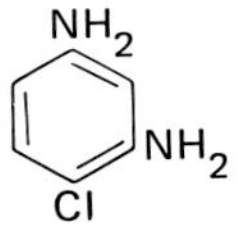 NH_2, NH_2, Cl	7,000	14,000[b]	2,000	4,000	Liver F	Adrenal M
Cinnamyl anthranilate	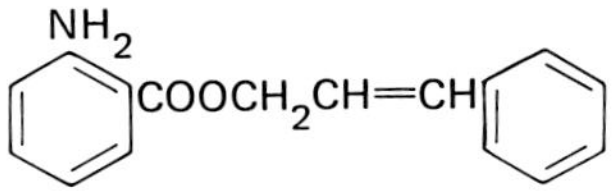 NH_2, $COOCH_2CH{=}CH$	15,000	30,000	15,000	30,000	Liver M&F	Pancreas M Kidney M
p-Cresidine	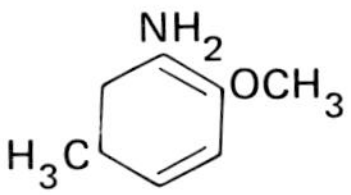 NH_2, OCH_3, H_3C	2,200 2,200	4,600[b]M 4,400[b]F	5,000	10,000	Bladder M&F Liver F	Bladder M&F Liver M Nasal cavity M&F

(continued)

Table 3. (continued)

Compound	Structure	Levels (ppm) in Diet				Site Affected	
		Mice		Rats		Mice	Rats
Cupferron	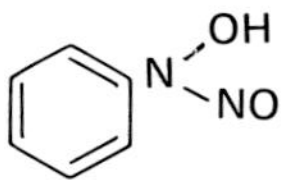 N, OH, NO	2,000	4,000[b]	1,500	3,000	Blood vessels M&F Liver F Zymbal's gland F	Blood vessels M&F Liver M&F Forestomach M&F Zymbal's gland F
2,4-Diaminoanisole· H_2SO_4	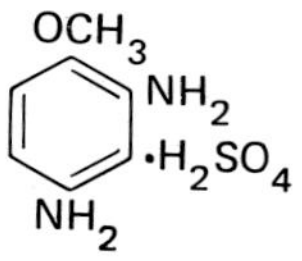 OCH_3, NH_2, $\cdot H_2SO_4$, NH_2	1,200	2,400	1,200	5,000[b]	Thyroid M&F	Skin and associated glands M&F Thyroid M&F
2,4-Diaminotoluene	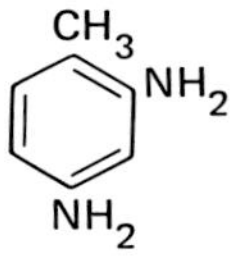 CH_3, NH_2, NH_2	100	200	79 79	176[b]M 171[b]F	Liver F Lymphoma F	Liver M&F Mammary gland F

(continued)

Table 3. (continued)

Compound	Structure	Levels (ppm) in Diet				Site Affected	
		Mice		Rats		Mice	Rats
Hydrazobenzene	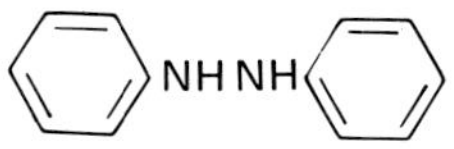 NH NH	80 40	400[b]M 400 F	80 40	300 M 100 F	Liver F	Liver M&F Mammary gland F Zymbal's gland M
4,4'-Methylenebis-(N,N-dimethyl)-benzenamine	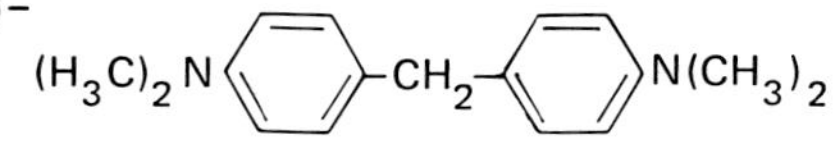 $(H_3C)_2N$ CH_2 $N(CH_3)_2$	1,250	2,500	375	750	Liver F	Thyroid M&F
2-Methyl-1-nitro-anthraquinone	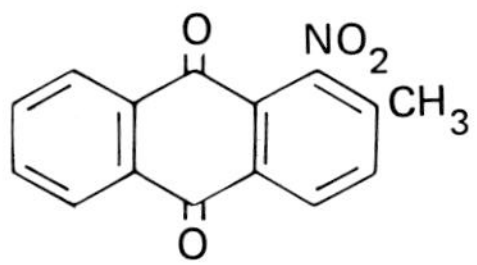 O NO_2 CH_3 O	300	600	600	1,200	Blood vessels M&F	Liver M Subcutaneous tissue M&F
Michler's ketone	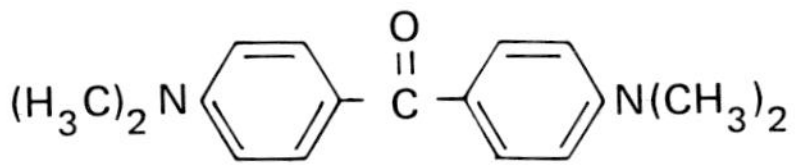 $(H_3C)_2N$ O C $N(CH_3)_2$	1,250	5,000	250 500	500 M 1,000 F	Blood vessels M Liver F	Liver M&F

(continued)

Table 3. (continued)

Compound	Structure	Levels (ppm) in Diet				Site Affected	
		Mice		Rats		Mice	Rats
5-Nitro-o-anisidine	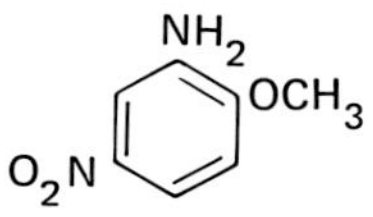 NH_2, OCH_3, O_2N	6,000	8,000[b]	4,000	8,000	Liver F	Skin, subcutis and associated glands M&F
p-Nitrosodiphenylamine	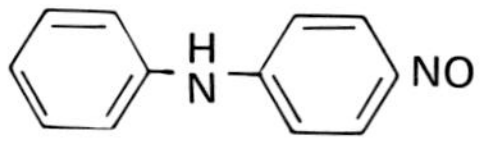 H N, NO	4,254[b]	9,000[b]	2,500	5,000	Liver M	Liver M
4,4'-Oxydianiline	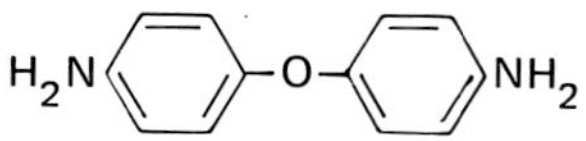 H_2N, O, NH_2	150 300 800		200 400 500		Liver M&F Thyroid F Harderian gland M&F	Liver M&F Thyroid M&F
Phenazopyridine·HCl	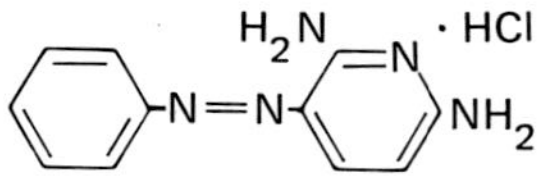 H_2N, N=N, N, ·HCl, NH_2	600	1,200	3,700	7,500	Liver F	Colon M&F

(continued)

Table 3. (continued)

Compound	Structure	Levels (ppm) in Diet				Site Affected	
		Mice		Rats		Mice	Rats
4,4'-Thiodianiline	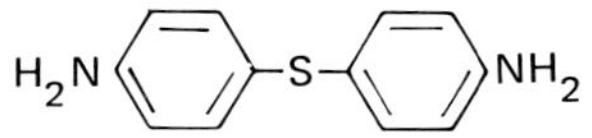 H_2N –S– NH_2	2,500	5,000	1,500	3,000	Liver M&F Thyroid M&F	Liver M Thyroid M&F Zymbal's gland M&F Colon M Uterus F
o-Toluidine·HCl	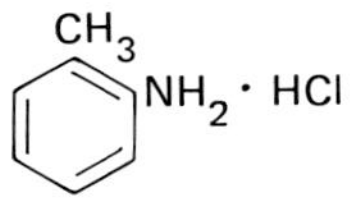 CH_3 $NH_2 \cdot HCl$	1,000	3,000	3,000	6,000	Liver F Blood vessels M	Spleen M&F Bladder F Subcutaneous tissue M Mammary gland F
2,4,5-Trimethylaniline	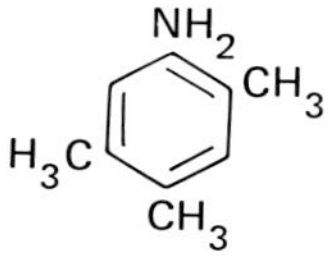 NH_2 CH_3 H_3C CH_3	50	100	200	800	Liver F	Liver M&F Bronchus F

[a]M = Male; F = Female.
[b]Time-weighted average concentration.

Table 4. Compounds Showing Carcinogenicity in Mice but Not in Rats.

Compound	Structure	Levels (ppm) in Diet[a]				Organ Affected[a] (Mice only)
		Mice		Rats		
3-Amino-4-ethoxy acetanilide	$NHCOCH_3$, NH_2, OC_2H_5	4,000	8,000	4,000	15,000	Thyroid M
4-Chloro-o-toluidine· HCl	$NH_2 \cdot HCl$, CH_3, Cl	3,750 1,250	15,000 M 5,000 F	1,250	5,000	Blood vessels M&F
5-Chloro-o-toluidine	NH_2, CH_3, Cl	2,000	4,000	1,250	5,000	Blood vessels M&F Liver M&F
6-Nitrobenzimidazole	O_2N, N, N	1,200	2,400	1,200	5,000	Liver M&F

(continued)

Table 4. (continued)

Compound	Structure	Levels (ppm) in Diet[a]				Organ Affected[a] (Mice Only)
		Mice		Rats		
2-Nitro-o-phenyl- enediamine	NH_2, NO_2, NH_2	2,200	4,400	550 1,100	1,100 M 2,200 F	Liver F
5-Nitro-o-toluidine	NH_2, CH_3, O_2N	1,200	2,300[b]	50	100[b]	Liver M&F Blood vessels M&F

[a]M = Males; F = Females.
[b]Time-weighted average concentration.

Table 5. Compounds Showing Carcinogenicity in Rats but Not in Mice.

Compound	Structure	Levels (ppm) in Diet				Organ Affected (Rats Only)
		Mice		Rats		
Aniline·HCl	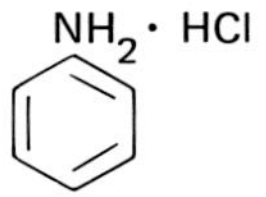 NH_2 · HCl	6,000	12,000	3,000	6,000	Blood vessels M&F Spleen M&F Multiple organs (sarcomas) M&F
4-Amino-2-nitrophenol	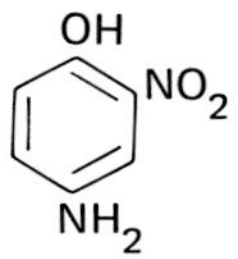 OH, NO_2, NH_2	1,250	2,500	1,250	2,500	Bladder M (F?)
2-Amino-5-nitrothiazole	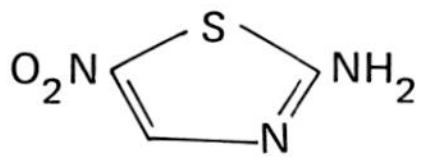 O_2N, S, N, NH_2	50	100	300	600	Lymphoma M Leukemia M
Azobenzene	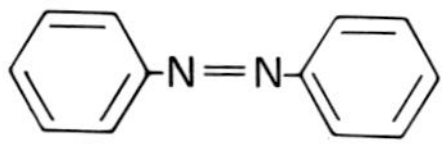 N=N	200; 208;	400 M 545[a]F	200;	400	Spleen M Abdominal cavity M&F

(continued)

Table 5. (continued)

Compound	Structure	Levels (ppm) in Diet				Organ Affected (Rats Only)
		Mice		Rats		
m-Cresidine	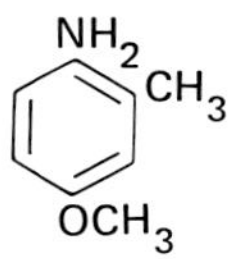 NH2, CH3, OCH3 (structure)	600	1,100[b]	800	1,600	Bladder M&F
Dapsone	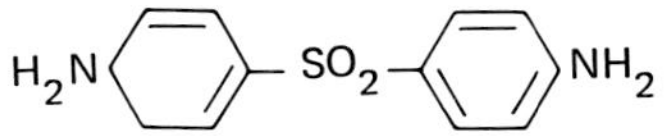 H2N–C6H4–SO2–C6H4–NH2 (structure)	500	1,000	600	1,200	Spleen and peritoneum M
3,3'-Dimethoxy-benzidine-4,4'-diisocyanate	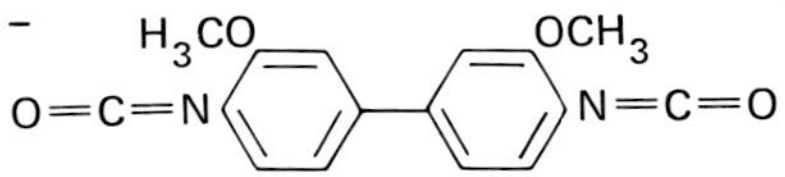 O=C=N, H3CO, OCH3, N=C=O (structure)	22,000 208	44,000 M 545[b]F	22,000	44,000	Skin M Zymbal's gland M&F Leukemia and lymphomas M&F Endometrium F

(continued)

Table 5. (continued)

Compound	Structure	Levels (ppm) in Diet				Organ Affected (Rats Only)
		Mice		Rats		
2,4-Dinitrotoluene	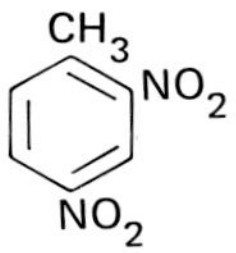 CH_3, NO_2, NO_2	80	400	80	200[b]	Skin and subcutaneous tissue M Mammary gland F
p-Quinone dioxime	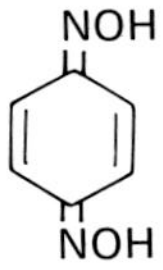 NOH, NOH	750	1,500	375	750	Bladder F

[a]M = Males; F = Females.
[b]Time-weighted average concentration.

In addition, 2,4-dinitrotoluene was somewhat unusual since only benign tumors as subcutaneous fibromas and mammary fibroadenomas were noted in rats after feeding this compound. Other relatively unusual lesions are the proliferative ones noted in the spleens of male rats given p-chloroaniline (7), even though the compound was finally classified as noncarcinogenic.

Thus, there was a diversity of responses, despite the fact that many of the compounds had originally been chosen for testing because of their structural similarity to known carcinogens, as well as their industrial use.

DISCUSSION

In this study, the diversity of structures examined often obscured the correlations that could be drawn. Although a previous publication listed the results of testing some of these aromatic amines (8), no attempt to derive structure-activity or species-specific correlations was made there. Overall, however, a few general statements can be made.

Thyroid tumors were usually caused by compounds that had an ether or thioether function. Among these were 3-amino-4-ethoxyacetanilide (male mice), o-anisidine (male rats), 2,4-diaminoanisole (male and female mice and rats), 4,4'-oxydianiline (male and female rats and female mice) (9), and 4,4'-thiodianiline (male and female mice and rats). An exception was reduced Michler's ketone which caused thyroid tumors in rats. However, the oxygen (-O-) and methylene ($-CH_2-$) groups are of approximately the same size. The ether function may simulate the corresponding part of the thyroxine molecule and thus deceive the organism into taking up these false or defective "thyroxines" into the thyroid. This effect is a matter for additional study. However, Evarts and Brown have shown that even after a few weeks of feeding 2,4-diaminoanisole to rats, there are goitrogenic effects in the thyroid and pigment that persists throughout the animals' lifespans (10,11).

Tumors of the ear duct (Zymbal's gland), induced by these compounds, were generally found in rats, but an exception was noted with cupferron which induced such tumors in both mice and rats. The model experimental compound to elicit Zymbal's gland tumors is 4-dimethylaminostilbene or its close derivatives (1). These types of tumors have also been induced in appreciable incidence by AAF, 2-aminoanthracene, and 3,3'-dimethylbenzidine (12), all aromatic amines with extended resonance systems of alternating double and single bonds. In the current series, 3-amino-9-ethylcarbazole and 3,3'-dimethoxybenzidine diisocyanate met such structural requirements. In addition, other compounds without the fully resonant structure, including thiodianiline, cupferron, hydrazobenzene, and 5-nitro-o-anisidine, also induced ear duct tumors. However, all may be considered to have a resonance structure somewhat extended over that of the benzene ring alone.

In man, the bladder is usually the primary organ affected by aromatic amines. However, 4-aminobiphenyl, 2-aminonaphthalene, and benzidine usually do not affect the bladder in rats or even in mice. The action of AAF on the bladder of rats or mice is often strain-dependent (13). In the current study, 4-amino-2-nitrophenol, o-anisidine, 4-chloro-o-phenylenediamine, m- and p-cresidine, p-quinone dioxime, and o-toluidine caused bladder tumors in rats; o-anisidine and p-cresidine affected the same organ in mice. Except for the quinone dioxime, these molecules are characterized by the presence of an amino or nitro group ortho to some other group (methoxy-, methyl-, hydroxyl-, or amino). Perhaps a dual approach to some bladder receptor is part of tumor initiation. More research is needed in this area.

Another type of tumor, although less frequent, was one affecting the blood vessels, generally of the spleen. These lesions, classified as hemangiomas or hemangiosarcomas, appeared in rats fed aniline hydrochloride, in mice or rats on cupferron, or in mice given Michler's ketone. Other cases of hemangiomas or hemangiosarcomas were noted in mice given o-toluidine or analogs thereof, including 4-chloro- and 5-chloro-o-toluidine, 5-nitro-o-toluidine and 2-methyl-1-nitroanthraquinone (14). However, other o-toluidine derivatives such as 2,5- and 2,6-toluenediamine and m-cresidine gave negative results in mice. Two compounds, 2,4-diaminotoluene and 2,4,5-trimethylaniline, led to liver tumors, rather than tumors of the blood vessels. In rats, illustrating the difference in susceptibility, only compounds with a single substituent on the aromatic ring caused this type of tumor.

The striking differences caused by changing the substituent groups are difficult to explain. In any event, little is known about the genesis of blood vessel tumors, and in mice their association with o-toluidine and derivatives may be purely fortuitous.

As for the liver, there was considerable variation between mice and rats in tumors in this organ. Of the 37 substances that caused tumors, only 13 led to liver tumors in rats; of the 9 compounds active in rats only, none led to liver tumors. On the other hand, 23 of the 37 carcinogens (62%) elicited liver tumors in mice. For those compounds active in mice only, 4 out of 6 (66%) led to liver tumors.

From the list of those active in both mice and rats, 19 out of 22 (86%) caused liver tumors in mice. Thus, for the majority of the active compounds, the induction of liver tumors in mice may serve as a fair indication of the degree of suspicion of the compounds (15).

In rats, the compounds more likely to affect the liver were bi- or tricyclic, or with methoxy or methyl groups that might simulate an additional ring, if monocyclic. In mice, the multiple ring compounds, plus many others, were active but it was difficult to determine any specific pattern.

Besides those attempts to correlate specific tumors in rats and mice with the structural features of the compounds tested, some consideration should be given to the features that led to compounds in the "negative" category. An amino group *para* to a methoxy, methyl, or amino group on an aromatic ring was more likely to afford a compound of little or no carcinogenic activity. However, similar combinations *ortho* or *meta* to each other generally showed varying degrees of carcinogenic activity. Of course, these premises are only guidelines to possible structure-activity correlations. The rate and type of metabolic interactions, solubility in biological media, and fit into a biological receptor may play a more prominent role than structure alone in determining the carcinogenicity of any one compound.

ACKNOWLEDGMENTS

The author wishes to thank members of SRI International for their assistance in collating some of the data and Mrs. Frances Williams for her secretarial assistance.

REFERENCES

1. Clayson, D.B., and R.C. Garner. 1976. Carcinogenic aromatic amines and related compounds. In: Chemical Carcinogens. C.E. Searle, ed. American Chemical Society: Washington, DC. pp. 366-461.

2. Weisburger, E.K. 1981. N-Substituted aryl compounds in carcinogenesis and mutagenesis. NCI Monograph 58:1-7.

3. Weisburger, E.K. 1981. Metabolic studies *in vivo* with arylamines. NCI Monograph 58:95-99.

4. Razzouk, C., M. Mercier, and M. Roberfroid. 1980. Biochemical basis for the resistance of guinea-pig and monkey to the carcinogenic effects of arylamines and arylamides. Xenobiotica 10:565-571.

5. Razzouk, C., M. Mercier, and M. Roberfroid. 1980. Induction, activation, and inhibition of hamster and rat liver microsomal arylamide and arylamine N-hydroxylase. Cancer Res. 40:3540-3546.

6. So, B.H., and E.L. Wynder. 1972. Induction of hamster tumors of the urinary bladder by 3,2'-dimethyl-4-aminobiphenyl. J. Nat. Cancer Inst. 48:1733-1738.

7. Ward, J.M., G. Reznik, and F.M. Garner. 1980. Proliferative lesions of the spleen in male F344 rats fed diets containing p-chloroaniline. Vet. Pathol. 17:200-205.

8. Van Duuren, B.L. 1980. Carcinogenicity of hair dye components. In: Cancer and the Environment. H.B. Demopoulos and M.A. Mehlman, eds. Pathotox Publishers, Inc.: IL. pp. 237-251.

9. Hayden, D.W., G.G. Wade, and A.H. Handler. 1978. Goitrogenic effect of 4,4'-oxydianiline in rats and mice. Vet. Pathol. 15:649-662.

10. Evarts, R.P., and C.A. Brown. 1980. 2,4-Diaminoanisole sulfate: Early effect on thyroid gland morphology and late effect on glandular tissues of Fischer 344 rats. J. Nat. Cancer Inst. 65:197-204.

11. Ward, J., S.F. Stinson, J.F. Hardisty, B.Y. Cockrell, and D.W. Hayden. 1979. Neoplasms and pigmentation of the thyroid gland in F344 rats exposed to 2,4-diaminoanisole sulfate, a hair dye component. J. Nat. Cancer Inst. 62:1067-1073.

12. Pliss, G.B., M.A. Zabezhinsky. 1970. Carcinogenic properties of orthotolidine (3,3'-dimethylbenzidine). J. Nat. Cancer Inst. 45:283-295.

13. Weisburger, E.K., and J.H. Weisburger. 1958. Chemistry, carcinogenicity, and metabolism of 2-fluorenamine and related compounds. Adv. Cancer Res. 5:331-431.

14. Krishna Murthy, A.S., J.R. Baker, E.R. Smith, and G.G. Wade. 1977. Development of hemangiosarcomas in $B6C3F_1$ mice fed 2-methyl-1-nitroanthraquinone. Intern. J. Cancer 19:117-121.

15. Ward, J.M., R.A. Griesemer, and E.K. Weisburger. 1979. The mouse liver tumor as an endpoint in carcinogenesis tests. Toxic. Appl. Pharmacol. 51:389-397.

DISCUSSION

Q.: First, in reference to the strains of mice and rats that were used for the testing, could you tell us why these particular strains have been selected?

A.: The Fischer rat was chosen because we had used it previously in a bioassay. We had also tried the Charles River and other Sprague-Dawley rats and came to the conclusion that the Fischer rat was preferable because it is smaller. The Sprague-Dawley rats became so large that after a while we needed one large rat cage for each rat. They became so large that it was difficult to do a necropsy on them. Fischer males do spontaneously develop testicular tumors, but these are a relatively benign type of tumor, seen in almost all the older rats. The (C57Bl/6 x C3H)F_1 or B6C3F_1 hybrid mouse was chosen for continuity with bioassays originally started by Dr. Hans Falk. He had used that hybrid mouse and found it was a relatively hardy but sensitive mouse, so we continued using it in the bioassay system.

Q.: The second question is in relation to control mice or control rats. I imagine that during this experiment, each laboratory has its own control group.

A.: Yes, they certainly do.

Q.: You will notice a great variation between the control groups in different laboratories. This, I think, is particularly relevant in relation to certain tests in which you find only a single type of tumor such as blood vessel tumors. Can you tell us how the kinds of tumors seen in control rats varies in different laboratories?

A.: I have not reviewed the variation between different laboratories in regard to control tumors, although it could be done, I'm sure. Perhaps some of the National Toxicology Program people who are looking at controls, like Dr. Jerrold Ward, might have data on that available.

Q.: In regard to the 16 negative compounds, were they also tested by _in vitro_ transformation assays or by bacterial mutagenicity tests, and if so, were they likewise negative there?

A.: I don't think a concerted effort is yet finished on testing all these compounds. The NTP has initiated mutagenicity, cell transformation, and other _in vitro_ tests on many of the bioassay compounds, but the results are not yet available. I think they're just finished with those.

Q.: I wonder if you'd get the same spectrum of effects if you could use a different treatment protocol; for example, if you gave your carcinogens transplacentally, or postnatally to animals of different ages.

A.: None of these alternatives has been explored with these compounds. After all, I have 53 compounds here and you can see the amount of work that would be required. But I'm sure that with many of the compounds, very interesting effects might be noted in different bioassay protocols. Except for two of the medicinals, all of the compounds were fed; the medicinals were injected. So there are great possibilities here.

Q.: Can this kind of experiment be correlated to wild animals?

A.: Do you mean the kinds of tumors seen?

Q.: Yes.

A.: I don't think any one has ever tried any of these specific compounds on wild rats or mice. But many of them were effective carcinogens in laboratory rodents and I have no doubt that, for example, some of those cresidines that caused a lot of tumors, could also cause various types of tumors in wild animals if they were properly tested.

AFLATOXIN B_1: CORRELATIONS OF PATTERNS OF METABOLISM AND DNA MODIFICATION WITH BIOLOGICAL EFFECTS

Robert G. Croy[1], John M. Essigmann[2], and Gerald N. Wogan[2]

[1]Sidney Farber Cancer Institute, Boston, Massachusetts 02114, and [2]Department of Nutrition and Food Science, Massachusetts Institute of Technology, Cambridge, Massachusetts 02139

INTRODUCTION

The molecular mechanisms by which aflatoxin B_1 (AFB_1) produces its biological effects are poorly understood. Many of the biochemical effects of the aflatoxins and other chemical carcinogens are mediated by activation through metabolism by one or more of the mixed-function oxidases and subsequent covalent modification of cellular macromolecules (1). Experimental evidence indicates that AFB_1-2,3-oxide is the ultimate reactive metabolite (2,3). It is reasonable that the sites and amount of macromolecular damage play essential roles determining molecular alterations and consequently observable biological effects. The consequences of covalent damage once formed will depend upon the ability of a cell or tissue to repair (correctly or incorrectly) or circumvent damage to essential cellular components before they are lethal or result in permanent change in the molecular program of the cell. For example, cells from patients with xeroderma pigmentosum that are defective in excision repair have increased sensitivity to ultraviolet (UV) light and some chemical agents. Conversely, cells competent for repair that are given adequate time to remove lesions from DNA before critical events exhibit increased survival (4). Thus, the kinetics of formation of this macromolecular damage and its repair are important. We have studied the covalent products formed in DNA of species sensitive and resistant to the biological effects of AFB_1 for correlations that may exist between the formation of these products, their removal, and biological responses to their presence.

ADDUCTS OF AFLATOXIN TO DNA

Metabolism of AFB_1 and Formation of DNA Adducts

Aflatoxin B_1 can undergo a variety of metabolic transformations (for review, see reference 5). Figure 1 presents a summary of the pathways that have been identified in a number of species. The presence of these pathways and their relative contributions to AFB_1 metabolism vary among species and may be influenced by inducers of the mixed-function oxidases such as phenobarbital, 3-methylcholanthrene, and AFB_1 itself (6,7). The formation of many of the more polar derivatives shown on the right of Figure 1 leads to their excretion in unconjugated forms as well as glucuronide and sulfate conjugates (5). Oxidation of the 2,3 bond of AFB_1 and at least two of its metabolites, aflatoxin M_1 (AFM_1) and aflatoxin P_1 (AFP_1) (8; Croy, unpublished data), produces electrophiles that can react with water to form dihydrodiols or with nucleophilic centers in cellular constituents, forming covalent adducts. The concentration of covalent adducts is highest in nucleic acids (3,9), and nucleic acid metabolism is most dramatically affected by AFB_1 in susceptible cells (10,11).

The covalent products formed in DNA have received particular attention as a result of biochemical studies that have demonstrated inactivation of DNA by AFB_1 (12,13) and AFB_1's potent mutagenic properties (14,15). The N^7 atom of guanine has been identified as the principal position modified in DNA both _in vitro_ and _in vivo_ (16-18). Acid hydrolysis of AFB_1-DNA produces a compound identified as 2,3-dihydro-3-hydroxy-(N^7-guanyl)AFB_1 (AFB_1-N^7-GUA). Like other N^7-guanine adducts, AFB_1-N^7-GUA is not stable in DNA as a result of the induced positive charge in the imidazole ring (11,19). This adduct can be removed from DNA by the spontaneous hydrolysis of either the glycosyl or N^7-C2 aflatoxin-guanine bonds, or undergo a chemical transformation through scission of the imidazole ring (17,20). The latter reaction forms a pyrimidine derivative containing the aflatoxin moiety still attached to the DNA backbone. Several investigators have reported that this ring-opened product is persistent in DNA _in vivo_, relative to the rapid rate of disappearance of the primary lesions through spontaneous or enzymatic processes (21,22). Recent evidence indicates that the covalent adducts formed at the N^7 atom of guanine by AFM_1 and AFP_1 undergo similar transformations producing analogous imidazole ring-opened adducts (Croy, unpublished results).

Rat, mouse, rainbow trout, and human tissues are capable of activating AFB_1 and producing AFB_1-N^7-GUA either _in vivo_ or _in vitro_ (16-18,23-25). However, no simple correlations seem to exist between the ability of a species to produce this product _in vivo_ or _in vitro_ and its sensitivity to AFB_1. For example, studies _in_

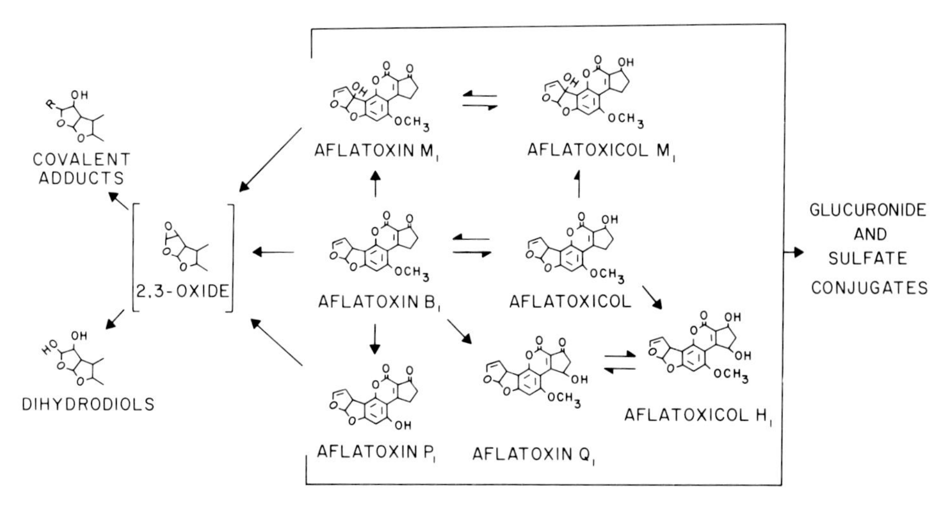

Figure 1. Metabolic transformations of AFB_1 that have been identified in various species.

vitro have found mouse and rat liver microsomes equally active in contrast to the differences in sensitivity of these species (26). Comparison of the covalent products that are formed *in vivo* in target and nontarget tissues of these two species has been more revealing as to the mechanisms underlying the differences in their sensitivities.

DNA Adducts in the Rat Liver In Vivo

The spectrum of DNA adducts produced by AFB_1 in the rat liver *in vivo* is more complex than that produced *in vitro* by hepatic microsomal activation of AFB_1 in the presence of calf thymus DNA. In the latter case, 95% of the covalent products are accounted for by AFB_1-N^7-GUA, and the remaining 5% are made up of its imidazole ring-opened derivatives (16).

Figure 2 shows the reversed-phase chromatographic pattern of [^{3}H]AFB_1 hydrolysis products isolated from rat liver DNA 2 h after a 1-mg/kg dose of [^{3}H]AFB_1. AFB_1-modified DNA was hydrolyzed by heating at 95°C in 0.1 N hydrochloric acid for 10 min, then neutralized and subsequently digested with nuclease P_1. Structures of products that have not been rigorously identified are enclosed in brackets. These compounds have been designated by letters A

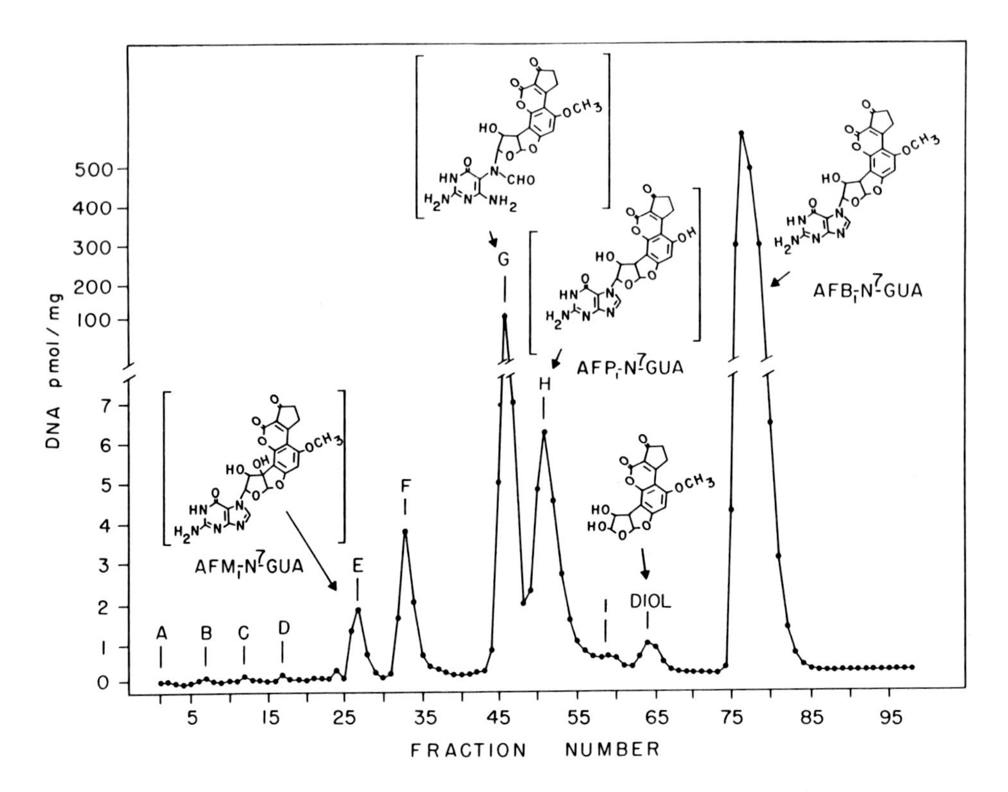

Figure 2. Reversed-phase chromatographic pattern of aflatoxin hydrolysis products from AFB_1-adducted DNA isolated from rat liver. Brackets indicate proposed structures of products not rigorously identified.

through I. The principal adduct, AFB_1-N7-GUA, eluted in fractions 75 through 86. Compounds eluted in peaks F and G are the products of chemical transformation of AFB_1-N7-GUA in DNA through imidazole ring scission. F was derived from G; however, their exact chemical relationship is unknown. Peaks H and E are N7-guanine adducts of AFM_1 and AFP_1, respectively. The imidazole ring-opened products of these adducts recently have been shown to elute in the region of peaks A through E.

AFLATOXIN-DNA ADDUCTS IN RELATION TO CARCINOGENESIS

Species Susceptibility and AFB_1-DNA Adduct Patterns

The Fischer rat and Swiss mouse represent extremes of sensitivity to both the toxic and carcinogenic effects of AFB_1. Hepatocellular carcinoma (HC) is induced in the rat by continuous feeding of levels as low as 1 ppb (27), while no response is seen in mice during exposure to dietary levels as high as 100 ppm (28). AFB_1 is acutely toxic to both species; however, they differ in sensitivity and organ specificity. The LD_{50} in the rat is approximately 1 mg/kg, and pathological effects are seen exclusively in the liver (29). The LD_{50} in the mouse is 14 mg/kg, and pathological effects are confined to the kidney (29,30).

The amount and identity of DNA adducts formed in both sensitive and resistant organs of the rat and mouse were compared. Two hours after administering an LD_{50} dose of [^3H]AFB_1 to either species, DNA was isolated from crude preparations of nuclei obtained from liver and kidney, and then hydrolyzed and analyzed by high pressure liquid chromatography (HPLC) as described above for the rat liver. Table 1 presents the quantitative relationships among the various AFB_1-DNA hydrolysis products obtained from the tissues. The greatest level of total modification (114 adducts/10^6 bases) was present in the target organ of the most sensitive species, the rat liver. DNA isolated from the kidney of this species was modified at one tenth of this level. Covalent damage to DNA in the mouse (7 AFB_1 adducts/10^6 bases) was also greatest in its target organ, the kidney. Mouse liver DNA was adducted at one third of this level.

The distribution of adducts among these tissues did not reveal possible relationships between pathological effects and the presence of specific lesions. AFB_1-N^7-GUA was the principal hydrolysis product obtained from adducted DNA in all tissues. Several minor products identified in the rat liver were absent or undetectable in the other tissues. As shown in Table 1, five of the nine major products detected in the rat liver were present in the kidney of this species. These minor products represented a higher proportion of total adducts in the kidney (30%) than in the liver (20%) with AFB_1-N^7-GUA (Peak H) increasing the largest amount. An opposite distribution of these minor products was seen in mouse tissues. The liver had a greater proportion of minor adducts with Peak H again accounting for most of the difference. Changes in the levels of AFB_1-N^7-GUA (Peak H) in these tissues were not large enough to account for the organotropism of AFB_1 in these species. However, its level may be indicative of the relative importance of metabolic pathways, such as O-demethylation, that do not primarily lead to AFB_1 activation. It is probable that these

Table 1. Quantitative Relationships of Acid Hydrolysis Products of DNA Modified by AFB_1 *In Vivo*

	Aflatoxin Residues/10^6 Bases			
	Liver		Kidney	
HPLC Peak	Rat	Mouse	Rat	Mouse
A	0.2	--	--	--
B	0.2	--	--	--
C	0.2	0.06	--	--
D	0.4	0.03	--	--
E	2.3	0.03	0.2	--
F	3.7	0.1	0.2	0.3
G	7.7	0.2	0.6	0.2
H,I	6.7	0.3	2.3	--
Diol	1.6	0.2	0.2	0.08
AFB_1-N^7-GUA	91	1.0	9.1	6.6
Total	114	2	13	7

other metabolic routes, such as those producing AFM_1 and AFP_1, would be more important in resistant tissues.

In summary, the total level of covalent modification of DNA by AFB_1 is correlated with the species sensitivity and organotropism of this mycotoxin in the Fischer rat and Swiss mouse. Qualitative differences in adduct patterns are not great enough to enable us to assign a particular role to any specific DNA adduct in production of toxic effects. However, the greater proportion of minor adducts in resistant tissues suggests that metabolic pathways other than direct 2,3-oxidation contribute a greater proportion to AFB_1 metabolism in these tissues, limiting AFB_1 activation. The absence of these minor products in DNA modified by AFB_1 activated by liver microsomal fractions *in vitro* indicates that the relationships between the various metabolic pathways are not accurately represented in these systems.

Kinetics of AFB_1 Metabolism and DNA Modification in Relation to Carcinogenesis

The effectiveness of aflatoxins as well as other chemical and physical agents as inducers of neoplasia in target tissues is dependent upon exposure level and frequency. Target tissues may change as a result of alterations in routes of administration or changes in the schedule of exposure to a particular agent. For example, single doses of AFB_1 are not effective in inducing HC in the rat in the absence of any further treatment, while administration of small multiple doses or continuous feeding at low levels, such as 1 ppm, in the diet is highly effective (28). In contrast, a high incidence (68%) of HC is induced in the rainbow trout after a single 1-h exposure to AFB_1 during embryogenesis (31). The physiology of these species is obviously quite different, and this difference is reflected in the kinetic patterns of AFB_1 adducts formed in DNA after a single dose of AFB_1.

In rat liver DNA was rapidly modified by AFB_1 (see Figure 3). The maximum level of AFB_1 products occurred at or slightly before 2 h after injection of a single subacute dose. The half-life of the principal adduct, AFB_1-N^7-GUA, was determined to be 7.5 h (21). This lesion initially represented 80% of covalent products formed in DNA. Its rapid disappearance was due to removal from DNA and conversion to imidazole ring-opened products. As a result of their persistence in DNA, these chemically altered derivatives of AFB_1-N^7-adducted guanines represented an increasing proportion of total AFB_1 adducts with time (e.g., 85% at 48 h). Approximately 20% of the initial amount of AFB_1-N^7-GUA was converted to these products. Minor adducts produced by AFM_1 and AFP_1 had the same kinetics of formation and removal at lower concentrations in DNA.

Figure 3 also shows the kinetics of modification of DNA by AFB_1 in the trout embryo. Rainbow trout embryos, 21 days old, were exposed to an aqueous solution containing 1 ppm [^{3}H]AFB_1 for 1 h. DNA was isolated from whole embryos after their separation from yolk and shell. Total levels of DNA modification and the concentrations of individual AFB_1 adducts in acid-hydrolyzed DNA were determined by HPLC, as previously described. The qualitative distribution of hydrolyzed AFB_1 products was essentially identical to that found in the rat liver. The major products were AFB_1-N^7-GUA and the two products formed by scission of its imidazole ring. Minor adducts formed between AFM_1 and AFP_1 with guanine also were present. In contrast to the rat, the levels of these products in embryo DNA increased continuously during the 24-h period after exposure and decreased slowly during the next 48 h. Whether this decrease is due to adduct removal or increased DNA content of the embryo has not been determined. The persistent, imidazole ring-opened products again accounted for a greater proportion of total adducts at longer times after exposure (50% at

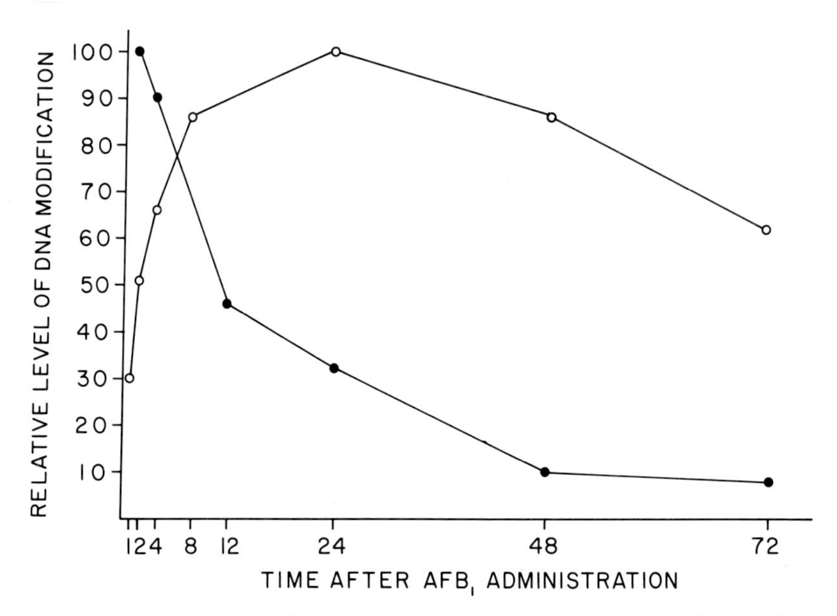

Figure 3. Kinetics of formation and disappearance of covalent AFB_1 modifications in DNA of rat liver (-●--●-) and the rainbow trout embryo (-0--0-) after exposure to a single dose of AFB_1.

72 h), indicating slow conversion of the initial N^7-guanine adduct to these derivatives.

The physical distribution of AFB_1 may be partly responsible for the extended period of DNA modification in the trout embryo. The hydrophobic AFB_1 molecule has been shown to be sequestered in the yolk of the embryo (31). This compartment may provide a reservoir of AFB_1 in the egg to which the embryo is exposed. A lower rate of metabolism or decreased rates of adduct removal from DNA may also contribute to the continued presence of these lesions.

Multiple exposures of the rat to AFB_1 produces a kinetic pattern of AFB_1-DNA adducts similar to the one described above for the trout embryo (21); this pattern correlates with the efficacy of AFB_1 in inducing HC in these species subjected to different treatment protocols. Rats subjected to administration of small multiple doses of AFB_1, shown to induce a 100% incidence of HC, accumulated persistent AFB_1 lesions in liver DNA that reached a steady-state level of 7 lesions/10^6 bases after one week (21). The concentration of these lesions in trout embryo DNA using the protocol described above is approximately one tenth this level (24). The high mitotic index in hepatic tissue of the trout embryo relative to the rat may partially explain its apparent increased sensitivity to AFB_1.

Since we do not know the exact biochemical effects of these adducts or the specific alterations needed to begin the neoplastic process, we can only speculate on the role that DNA modification or individual adducts have in the production of HC in these species. The presence of the primary AFB_1-N^7-GUA adduct in the trout embryo for an extended period of time may result in the greater probability of this lesion directly inducing changes in DNA or a larger proportion of it being converted to the persistent ring-opened form, which may subsequently induce these changes. Since these lesions can be present for a substantial portion of the time required for evolution of overt neoplasia, they may influence the progression of cells through separate stages of this process by different mechanisms.

In summary, predicting the species and organ specificity of carcinogenic agents such as AFB_1 on the basis of metabolic studies _in vitro_ or the similarities of covalent products produced in DNA is difficult. The susceptibility of the species in this investigation was dependent upon the amount and temporal distribution of total covalent damage to cellular macromolecules. Presently, determining the significance of either labile or persistent AFB_1 adducts in neoplastic transformation is impossible. Persistent lesions may be important if events responsible for initiating neoplasia are temporally separate from exposure. However, since the molecular events responsible for neoplastic transformation of a cell are unknown and the specific consequences of these lesions in DNA are not fully understood, progress at this time has been limited to establishing correlations between those two phenomena. Further investigations undoubtedly will provide clues as to the identity of these events and elucidate the complex interactions that determine the susceptibility of various species to aflatoxins and other agents.

REFERENCES

1. Miller, E.C. 1978. Some current perspectives on chemical carcinogenesis in humans and experimental animals: Presidential address. Cancer Res. 38:1479-1496.

2. Swenson, D.H., E.C. Miller, and J.A. Miller. 1974. Aflatoxin B_1-2,3-oxide: Evidence for its formation in rat liver in vivo and by human microsomes in vitro. Biochem. Biophys. Res. Comm. 60:1036-1043.

3. Swenson, D.H., J. Lin, E.C. Miller, and J.A. Miller. 1977. Aflatoxin B_1-2,3-oxide as a probable intermediate in the covalent binding of aflatoxins B_1 and B_2 to rat liver DNA and ribosomal RNA in vivo. Cancer Res. 37:172-181.

4. Heflich, R.H., R.M. Hazard, L. Lommel, J.D. Scribner, V.M. Maher, and J.J. McCormick. 1980. A comparison of the DNA binding, cytotoxicity, and repair synthesis induced in human fibroblasts by reactive derivatives of aromatic amide carcinogens. Chem. Biol. Interact. 29:43-56.

5. Wogan, G.N., and W.F. Busby. 1980. Naturally occurring carcinogens. In: Toxic Constituents of Plant Foodstuffs, second edition. I.E. Leiner, ed. Academic Press: New York. pp. 329-369.

6. Gurtoo, H.L., and R.P. Dahms. 1979. Effects of inducers and inhibitors on the metabolism of aflatoxin B_1 by rat and mouse. Biochem. Pharmacol. 28:3441-3449.

7. Schabort, J.C., and M. Steyn. 1969. Substrate and phenobarbital inducible aflatoxin 4-hydroxylation and aflatoxin metabolism by rat liver microsomes. Biochem. Pharmacol. 18:2241-2252.

8. Croy, R.G., and G.N. Wogan. 1979. Identification of an aflatoxin P_1-DNA adduct formed in vivo in rat liver. Proc. Am. Assoc. Cancer Res. 20:182.

9. Garner, R.C., and C.M. Wright. 1975. Binding of [^{14}C]Aflatoxin B_1 to cellular macromolecules in the rat and hamster. Chem. Biol. Interact. 11:123-131.

10. Gelboin, H.V., J.S. Wortham, R.G. Wilson, M. Friedman, and G.N. Wogan. 1966. Rapid and marked inhibition of rat liver RNA polymerase by aflatoxin B_1. Science 154:1205-1206.

11. Clifford, J.I., and K.R. Rees. 1966. Aflatoxin: a site of action in the rat liver cell. Nature 209:312-313.

12. Edwards, G.S., and G.N. Wogan. 1970. Aflatoxin inhibition of template activity of rat liver chromatin. Biochim. Biophys. Acta 224:597-607.

13. Yu, F. 1977. Mechanism of aflatoxin B_1 inhibition of rat hepatic nuclear RNA synthesis. J. Biol. Chem. 252:3245-3151.

14. Wong, J.J., and D.P. Hsieh. 1976. Mutagenicity of aflatoxins related to their metabolism and carcinogenic potential. Proc. Natl. Acad. Sci. USA 73:2241-2244.

15. Krahn, D.F., and C. Heidelberger. 1977. Liver homogenate-mediated mutagenesis in Chinese hamster V79 cells by polycyclic aromatic hydrocarbons and aflatoxins. Mutat. Res. 46:27-44.

16. Essigmann, J.M., R.G. Croy, A.M. Nadzan, W.F. Busby, V.N. Reinhold, G. Buchi, and G.N. Wogan. 1977. Structural identification of the major DNA adduct formed by aflatoxin B_1 in vitro. Proc. Natl. Acad. Sci. USA 74:1870-1874.

17. Lin, J., J.A. Miller, and E.C. Miller. 1977. 2,3-dihydro-2-(guan-7-yl)-3-hydroxy-aflatoxin B_1, a major acid hydrolysis product of aflatoxin B_1-DNA or -ribosomal RNA adducts formed in hepatic microsome-mediated reactions and rat liver in vivo. Cancer Res. 37:4430-4438.

18. Croy, R.G., J.M. Essigmann, V.N. Reinhold, and G.N. Wogan. 1978. Identification of the principal aflatoxin B_1-DNA adduct formed in vivo in rat liver. Proc. Natl. Acad. Sci. USA 75:1745-1749.

19. Singer, B. 1975. The chemical effects of nucleic acid alkylation and their relation to mutagenesis and carcinogenesis. In: Progress in Nucleic Acid Research and Molecular Biology, Volume XV. W.E. Cohn, ed. Academic Press: New York. pp. 219-284.

20. Wang, T.V., and P. Cerutti. 1980. Spontaneous reactions of aflatoxin B_1 modified deoxyribonucleic acid in vivo. Biochemistry 19:1692-1698.

21. Croy, R.G., and G.N. Wogan. 1981. Temporal patterns of covalent DNA adducts in rat liver after single and multiple doses of aflatoxin B_1. Cancer Res. 41:197-203.

22. Wang, T.V., and P. Cerutti. 1979. Formation and removal of aflatoxin B_1-induced DNA lesions in epitheloid human lung cells. Cancer Res. 39:5165-5170.

23. Croy, R.G., and G.N. Wogan. 1981. Quantitative comparison of covalent aflatoxin-DNA adducts formed in rat and mouse livers and kidneys. J. Natl. Cancer Inst. 66:761-768.

24. Croy, R.G., J.E. Nixon, R.O. Sinnhuber, and G.N. Wogan. 1980. Investigation of covalent aflatoxin B_1-DNA adducts formed in vivo in rainbow trout (Salmo gairdneri) embryos and liver. Carcinogenesis 1:903-909.

25. Autrup, H., J.M. Essigmann, R.G. Croy, B.F. Trump, G.N. Wogan, and C.C. Harris. 1979. Metabolism of aflatoxin B_1 and identification of the major aflatoxin B_1 adducts formed in cultured human bronchus and colon. Cancer Res. 39:694-698.

26. Godoy, H.M., and G.E. Neal. 1976. Some studies on the effects of aflatoxin B_1 in vitro on nucleic acid synthesis in the rat and mouse. Chem. Biol. Interact. 13:257-277.

27. Wogan, G.N., S. Pagialunga, and P.M. Newberne. 1974. Carcinogenic effects of low dietary levels of aflatoxin B_1 in rats. Food Cosmet. Toxicol. 12:681-685.

28. Wogan, G.N. 1973. Aflatoxin carcinogenesis. In: Methods in Cancer Research, Volume VII. H. Busch, ed. Academic Press: New York. pp. 309-344.

29. McGuire, R.A. 1969. Factors affecting the acute toxicity of aflatoxin B_1 in the rat and mouse. M.S. thesis. Massachusetts Institute of Technology, Cambridge, MA.

30. Akoa, M., K. Kuroda, and G.N. Wogan. 1971. Aflatoxin B_1: The kidney as a site of action in the mouse. Life Sci. 10:495-501.

31. Wales, J.H. R.O. Sinnhuber, J.D. Hendricks, J.E. Nixon, and T.A. Eisele. 1978. Aflatoxin B_1-induction of hepatocellular carcinoma in the embryos of rainbow trout (Salmo gairdneri). J. Natl. Cancer Inst. 60:1133-1139.

DISCUSSION

Q.: In trying to explain the difference in susceptibility between rats and mice in terms of differences in activation, I have concluded that it is really inactivation that is different. Dr. Degen in our group showed that one of the major metabolic pathways is conjugation with glutathione. If you study aflatoxin metabolism in mouse liver, you find that mouse liver is even more capable of oxidative metabolism of aflatoxin than rat liver; but it is also even better capable of inactivating the epoxide with glutathione. So I would say the species difference could be largely due to differences in inactivation.

In studies of this kind one often ignores formation of the water-soluble conjugation products. In many of these cases it is really the competition between activation and inactivation that makes a difference in species and in tissue specificity.

Q.: I wanted to mention the effects of aflatoxin on the cellular level as a specific point that has a bearing on our general discussion. We have been doing some work with Dr. Cortesi on transformation of the 3T3 clone 831-1-1 cells, in which we get a very good dose-response for transformation with aflatoxin. However, other investigators have looked at transformation in other systems _in vitro_ and have not found very good transformation by aflatoxin. In particular, Dr. Schechtman, at Microbiological Associates, working with another of the subclones of the 831 clone, found no transformation with aflatoxin unless he added separate metabolic activation.

The point is that there will be differences of response down to the cellular level, not only between different species or different strains of the same species. Even subclones of the same clone seem to react differently in some ways.

It may be that some cell systems would be good indicators of the response of their respective strain of origin. In our case, for example, we have been working on BALB-3T3-derived fibroblasts. I wanted to ask you, if you remember, what were the mouse strains that have been tested so far that gave negative evidence of carcinogenicity _in vivo_, and whether the BALB strain was in fact tested? It may turn out to be more susceptible than, say, the C3H strain, from which 10T1/2 cells are derived.

A.: I am only aware of studies in the Swiss mouse.

Q.: You showed us a pattern of quite a large number of DNA adducts formed _in vivo_ with aflatoxin. Have you or has anybody else been able to compare this pattern with what you get when aflatoxin is activated _in vitro_ by microsomal systems?

A.: Yes. In microsomal systems you get almost exclusively N^7 guanine adduct from direct alkylation by aflatoxin B_1; you don't find any of the P-1 or M-1 derivatives activated. So the *in vitro* pattern consists almost exclusively of the B_1, N^7 guanine adduct. It is much simpler than the *in vivo* pattern.

Q.: You show that in a two-hour period you get a very high level of binding to the N^7 and then after a week, you're down a hundred-thousand-fold. Have you looked at the composition of the DNA at these two stages to see if the repair process is in any way involved? Is there a change in the composition of the DNA? With that large an amount of change from, say, 1 out of every 10 residues being modified to 1 out of every 10 , one might expect a considerable number of mistakes.

A.: In terms of nearest neighbors, things like that, no, we haven't looked at those.

SPECIES SPECIFICITY IN NITROSAMINE CARCINOGENESIS

William Lijinsky

Chemical Carcinogenesis Program, Frederick Cancer Research Center, Frederick, Maryland 21701

INTRODUCTION

Many types of carcinogens show pronounced differences in effect in different species, often inducing tumors of a certain site in one and being inactive in another. N-Nitroso compounds, on the other hand, are commonly carcinogenic in all species examined, but induce tumors of different cell types and in different organs from one species to the next. This variability is particularly true of nitrosamines, whose organ and species specificity are probably due to differences in routes of metabolism and activation. These differences are open to study using biochemical and chemical methods and should afford a means of approaching an understanding of the mechanisms of nitrosamine carcinogenesis.

Early studies with nitrosodimethylamine (DMN) and nitrosodiethylamine (DEN) in rats and mice showed that both compounds mainly induce liver tumors after chronic administration, although tumors of other organs, such as the esophagus, are often seen after DEN treatment. A considerable incidence of tumors of the upper respiratory tract, particularly the trachea, occurs in Syrian hamsters following treatment with DEN, but no good correlation between this biological effect and DNA alkylation or tissue activation to bacterial mutagens is available comparing the hamster with the rat (1). This lack of a correlation suggests that simple measurement of bacterial mutagenesis is not a good indicator of carcinogenic effectiveness in whole animals. Neither is merely the measurement of the extent of DNA alkylation a means of assessing carcinogenic effectiveness, because of what is now so widely known as the requirement of alkylation at specific sites and the stability of the alkylated portions of DNA to excision repair.

A number of steps occur between administration of the carcinogen and the appearance of a neoplasm. Even if the initiation of the chain of events leading to tumor development is alkylation of DNA in target cells, or some other type of macromolecular interaction, many modifiers of the administered compound control the outcome, whether measured as incidence of tumors or tumors in a specific organ. If one excepts locally acting carcinogens, such as nitrosoalkylamides, a major factor in determining the action of carcinogens is the pharmacodynamics of their metabolism _in vivo_ and especially their metabolism in various organs and tissues, including activation to their "proximate carcinogenic forms."

Even in the case of locally acting N-nitroso compounds that alkylate DNA without a need for metabolic activation, some findings cast doubt on the directness of the relation between DNA alkylation and carcinogenesis. For example, nitrosomethylurea methylates DNA in rat liver, but does not ordinarily induce liver tumors in that species (2). Nitrosoethylurethane induces tumors of the forestomach when given by gavage to rats (3), but gives rise to liver tumors when given by gavage to guinea pigs and induces no tumors at all when applied to mouse skin in acetone solution, in contrast to the skin tumors produced in mice painted with nitrosoethylurea (4) or nitrosoethylnitroguanidine (5). Thus, the differences in response of several species to even direct-acting N-nitroso compounds can be quite marked and leaves open to question any simple mechanisms proposed.

SYMMETRIC NITROSODIALKYLAMINES

The observation was made that the liver is the main target of DMN and DEN in most species examined. In the case of DEN, as many as 25 species are responsive, including rat, mouse, gerbil, Syrian hamster, Chinese hamster, European hamster, guinea pig, hedgehog, rabbit, cat, dog, pig, chicken, frog, parakeet, fish, newt, and monkey. However, accepting this observation is difficult, because the response depends on the dose and dose rate of DEN administered. A recent dose-response study of this compound revealed that the liver is the main target only at relatively high dose rates (which produce considerable liver toxicity), while at low dose rates the main targets are the organs of the upper gastrointestinal tract, principally the esophagus, tongue, and forestomach.

In Fischer rats, the main target organ of nitrosodi-n-propylamine is the esophagus, with liver tumors also induced under certain conditions of dosage. Nitrosodi-n-butylamine induces both liver and bladder tumors in rats and only bladder tumors in both mice and Syrian hamsters. The mechanism of induction of bladder tumors in rats has been thoroughly investigated by Okada and his co-workers (6), who have produced convincing evidence that one of the butyl groups is oxidized in the 4-position successively to alcohol and carboxylic acid. The alcohol and carboxylic acid are excreted in the urine and assumed to be the proximate carcinogen for the bladder. However, the next steps, assumed to involve at some point oxidation at a carbon atom alpha to the nitroso function (as seems to be the case for most nitrosamines), are unknown. Neither is it known whether the induction of bladder tumors by nitrosodi-n-butylamine in other species involves the same sequence of metabolism.

Although a great deal of attention has been devoted to those nitrosamines that induce liver tumors, the liver is not a common target of most carcinogenic N-nitroso compounds. The most common target, at least in rats, is the upper gastrointestinal tract, particularly the esophagus. Unfortunately the esophagus is not an easy organ in which to study metabolic activation because of the paucity of active cells in that small organ. This lack of active cells explains our lack of progress in understanding why the esophagus is so favored.

CYCLIC NITROSAMINES

The seemingly easy explanation of carcinogenesis by aliphatic nitrosamines as generation of a simple alkylating agent that alkylates DNA fails to satisfy the carcinogenesis studies using cyclic nitrosamines in which little binding to DNA of target cells is measured, and with the exception of nitrosomorpholine, alkylation of specific bases in DNA has not been reported. Figure 1 shows the interspecies differences in response to a number of cyclic nitrosamines. Accompanying the considerable differences in the target organ are very large differences in carcinogenic potency among the compounds. In particular, nitrosopyrrolidine is a much weaker carcinogen than nitrosopiperidine or nitrosohexamethyleneimine (7). Nitrosopyrrolidine has induced liver tumors in rats, but lung tumors in mice and Syrian hamsters; nitrosopiperidine induced mainly esophageal tumors in rats, the same in mice, and lung tumors in hamsters; nitrosohexamethyleneimine induced tumors of the esophagus and liver in rats, lung tumors in mice, and tracheal tumors in hamsters. Nitrosoheptamethyleneimine, on the other hand, induced squamous lung tumors in rats, together with esophageal tumors, while in the hamster it induced mainly tumors of the forestomach and esophagus.

Although considerable study of the metabolism of these cyclic compounds has been done, especially in rats, very little indication of the mechanism by which they induce tumors exists. Notably, their binding to DNA *in vivo* is orders of magnitude smaller than that of the simple aliphatic nitrosamines, even in the case of

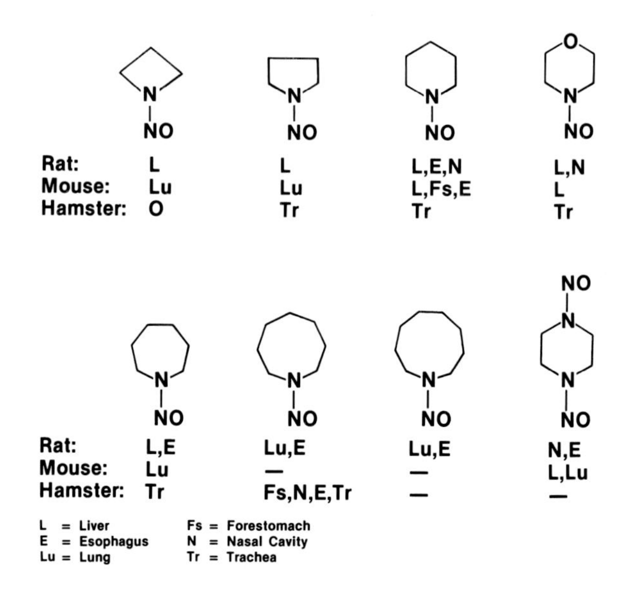

Figure 1. Interspecies differences in response to some cyclic nitrosamines.

those cyclic nitrosamines that induce liver tumors. They are metabolized at different rates in the rat, but this seems insufficient to explain their markedly different carcinogenic potencies. It is probable, however, that alpha oxidation is one step in the process of carcinogenesis by these compounds because, in the case of both nitrosomorpholine (8) and nitrosoheptamethyleneimine, labeling of the alpha carbon atoms with deuterium markedly decreases the carcinogenic potency, indicating that carbon-hydrogen cleavage is a rate-limiting step in carcinogenesis.

In the attempt to find explanations of the carcinogenicity of nitrosamines, activation by tissue microsomes to bacterial mutagens, particularly in the Ames test, has been investigated. Rao et al. have observed that many potent carcinogens for the rat are not mutagenic in the Ames test when activated by rat liver microsomes, even some compounds that are liver carcinogens (9). On the other hand, several of these compounds are mutagenic when hamster liver microsomes are used, even though the hamster is often less susceptible to the compound than is the rat, and the target organ in the hamster is usually not the liver. These discrepancies seem to show that the mutagenic moiety produced by microsomal activation is not necessarily on the pathway leading to carcinogenesis.

ASYMMETRICAL NITROSODIALKYLAMINES

Extending our investigations to a number of nitrosamines unlikely to yield simple alkylating moieties, we examined the carcinogenic activity of a series of nitrosomethyl-n-alkylamines (Figure 2), following the finding that nitrosomethyl-n-dodecylamine induced bladder tumors in the rat. This finding is an exception to the general rule proposed by Druckrey et al. (10) that asymmetric nitrosamines have the esophagus as their target in the rat. Based on his studies with nitrosodibutylamine, Okada (11) suggested that omega oxidation of the dodecyl chain is followed by successive beta oxidation, in the manner of fatty acid catabolism, to nitroso-methyl-3-carboxypropylamine, which might be the proximate carcinogen. Indeed, Okada found that this nitrosamino acid is a metabolite in the urine of rats given a single dose of nitrosomethyldodecylamine. The corresponding product of metabolism of a nitrosomethylalkylamine with an odd-numbered carbon chain would be nitrosomethyl-2-carboxyethylamine; in fact, nitroso-methyl-n-undecylamine gave rise to tumors of the liver and lung but no bladder tumors in rats. The single weakness in Okada's argument is that nitrosomethyl-3-carboxypropylamine has not been shown to be carcinogenic in rats.

The response of rats to the series of nitrosomethylalkylamines shown in Figure 2 has a considerable regularity. The tetradecyl, decyl, and octadecyl compounds, like the dodecyl, give rise to bladder tumors, although the octyl compound is much more potent than the larger molecules and also induces liver tumors (12). The hexyl and butyl analogs induced esophageal tumors in rats, while those with odd-numbered carbon chains, nitrosomethylheptylamine and nitrosomethylnonylamine, induced liver tumors.

In an effort to see whether this regularity holds in other species, we have begun to examine the carcinogenicity of nitrosomethylalkylamines in other species, beginning with

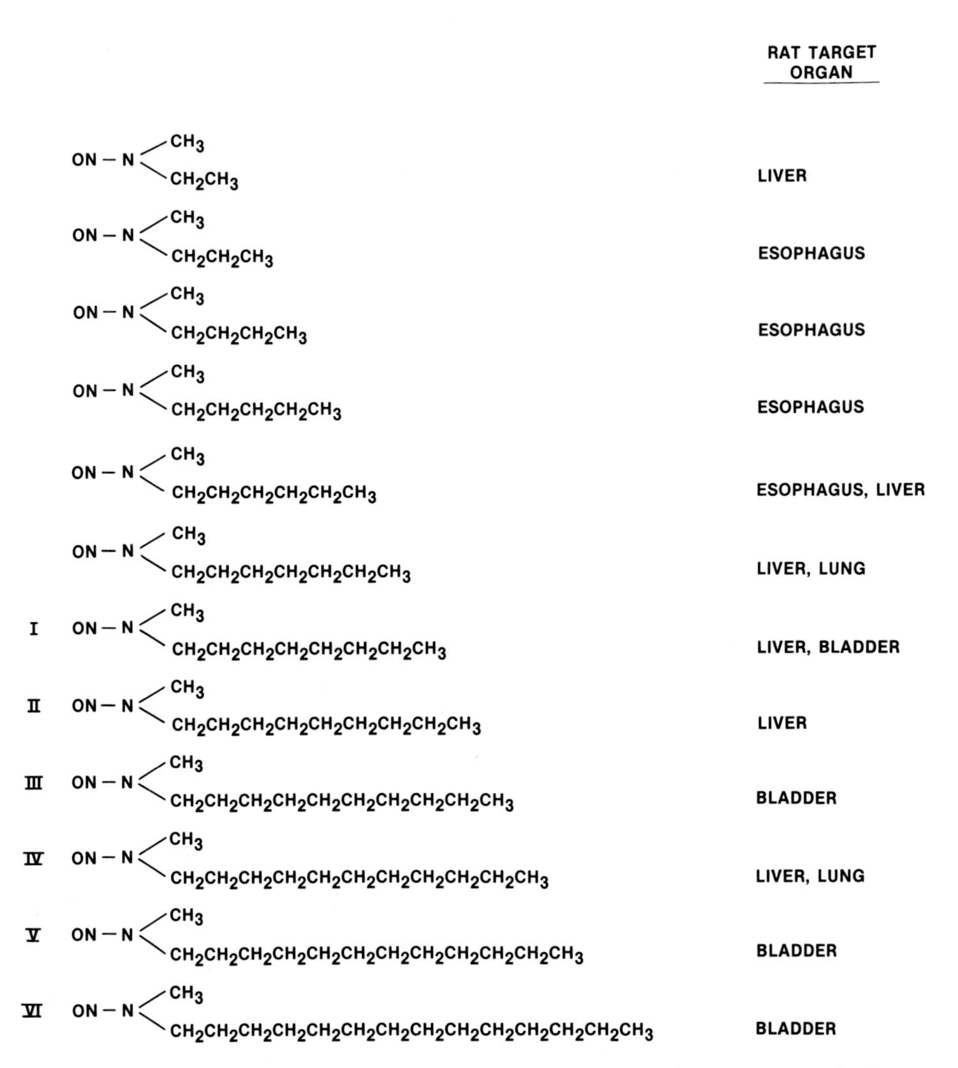

Figure 2. Carcinogenic activity of a series of nitrosomethyl-n-alkylamines.

nitrosomethyldodecylamine. In both Syrian and European hamsters this compound induces tumors of the bladder (13,14), but in guinea pigs it gives rise only to liver tumors (15). Nitrosomethyl-n-butylamine, an extremely potent esophageal carcinogen in rats. induced no esophageal tumors in mice or Syrian hamsters. A common finding is that the rat esophagus is very sensitive to many nitrosamines that do not induce esophageal tumors in other species. This suggests that the rat esophagus itself is sensitive to the nitrosamines and that there is not necessarily any gross difference between species in metabolism (for example, in the liver).

The response of the guinea pig liver to nitrosomethyldodecylamine suggests some unique route of metabolism of the compound in the guinea pig might exist that differentiates it from the other species. Alternatively, the liver of the guinea pig might be responsive to whatever carcinogenic metabolite is produced, while the bladder is not sensitive. The uniqueness of the guinea pig is also indicated in Table 1, in which a variety of nitrosamines appear to induce only liver tumors in the guinea pig, whatever the target organ is in other species. Thus, dinitroso-2,6-dimethylpiperazine and nitroso-2,6-dimethylmorpholine, that have a wide spectrum of targets in other species, only affect the liver in guinea pigs (15), as does nitrosomethylurethane already mentioned. On the other hand, the potent carcinogens nitrosoheptamethyleneimine and nitrosomethyldiethylurea, that induce tumors of the central nervous system in rats (16), appeared to be inactive in the guinea pigs. These findings would provide a basis for some interesting studies of metabolism of these compounds in guinea pigs, compared with rats and hamsters, although it is unlikely that the nitrosamines inactive in the guinea pig are not metabolized at all. In a broader sense, these findings might be important if man resembles the guinea pig rather than the rat or hamster.

NITROSODIETHANOLAMINE

One environmentally significant nitrosamine that has been studied in rats and hamsters is nitrosodiethanolamine, which is found at considerable concentrations in synthetic cutting oils and cosmetics as well as tobacco smoke. This nitrosamine, once considered a relatively weak carcinogen (10), on reexamination appears to be moderately potent in inducing liver tumors in rats (17). In the Syrian hamster, it induces mainly tumors of the nasal cavity (18). The risk it might pose to humans is unknown and little study of its mechanism of action has been done, apart from the observation that much of the administered dose is excreted unchanged in the urine of rats (19). Another significant finding is that nitrosodiethanolamine does not appear to be mutagenic to bacteria, even when activated by rat liver microsomes (9).

METABOLIC STUDIES

The observation that substitution of methyl groups for hydrogen at the positions beta to the nitroso group in nitrosomorpholine greatly increases the potency to rats and changes the target organ from liver (in the unsubstituted compound) to the esophagus (20) has led to a large number of studies relevant to interspecies variation in carcinogenic activity. The reason is that nitroso-2,6-dimethylmorpholine demonstrates this variation to a very high degree. As shown in Table 1, this nitrosamine induced esophageal tumors in rats, pancreas and liver tumors in Syrian hamsters, pancreas tumors in European hamsters, forestomach tumors in mice, and liver tumors (angiosarcomas) in guinea pigs. No large difference in potency of the compound between the species exists, as measured by the total dose required to produce almost 100% tumor response within six months to one year. Therefore, the differences in response can be expected to relate either to differences in metabolism and activation between the species or to biological differences in susceptibility of the several organs in the different species. Since almost nothing is known about the latter, we have focused on studying possible differences in metabolism that might relate to the observed biological effects.

Some preliminary biological experiments have provided some excellent leads, notably those comparing the carcinogenic effectiveness of the cis and trans isomers of nitroso-2,6-dimethylmorpholine (Me_2-NO-MORPH) and those examining the effect of deuterium labeling at the alpha or beta positions on carcinogenic potency. In the rat the trans isomer is considerably more effective inducing esophageal tumors than the cis isomer (21). On the other hand, in the Syrian hamster in which nitrosodimethylmorpholine induces tumors of the pancreas and liver, the cis isomer is more potent than the trans (22). In the guinea pig, the cis isomer is also more potent than the trans, to the extent that only the cis induced a significant incidence of liver tumors (23).

Similar differences in effect between rats and hamsters are seen with deuterium-labeled nitrosodimethylmorpholine. The derivative labeled in the alpha position to the nitroso group (Me_2-NO-MORPH-d_4) is less carcinogenic than the unlabeled compound in the rat, while the derivative labeled in the beta position (Me_2-NO-MORPH-d_2) is more carcinogenic than the unlabeled compound (24). This finding is consistent with the concept that oxidation takes place at both alpha and beta carbons, but that only alpha oxidation is a rate-limiting step in induction of esophageal tumors in the rat. In contrast, Me_2-NO-MORPH-d_4 is more carcinogenic than the unlabeled compound in the Syrian hamster (22), suggesting that in inducing pancreas and liver tumors in this species, beta oxidation is the rate-limiting step, rather than alpha oxidation.

These results imply that the pathways of metabolism of Me_2-NO-MORPH leading to carcinogenesis in the rat and hamster are entirely different, although it has been suggested elsewhere that

Table 1. Carcinogenic Action of Nitrosamines in Organs of Different Species.

	Rat	Syrian Hamster	Guinea Pig	Mouse	European Hamster
Nitroso- dimethylamine	Liver, Kidney	Liver, Nose	Liver	Liver	Liver
diethylamine	Liver, Esophagus	Trachea, Liver	Liver	Liver, Esophagus	Liver, Lung
di-n-butylamine	Bladder, Liver	Lung, Bladder		Bladder, Liver	
methyldodecylamine	Bladder	Bladder	Liver		Bladder
morpholine	Liver, Stomach	Trachea, Lung		Liver	
dimethylmorpholine	Esophagus	Pancreas, Liver	Liver	Stomach	Pancreas
bis-oxopropylamine	Liver	Pancreas	Liver		
bis-hydroxypropylamine	Esophagus	Pancreas, Liver	Liver		
heptamethyleneimine	Lung, Esophagus	Stomach, Esophagus	-		Lung
Dinitrosodimethylpiperazine	Esophagus	Lung	Liver		

they are similar, involving formation of nitrosohydroxypropyloxo-propylamine (25). Examination of the urinary metabolites of Me_2-NO-MORPH in rats, hamsters, and guinea pigs does not show major qualitative differences that might relate to the greatly different biological effects in the three species with the exception of one metabolite in hamster urine that is virtually absent from rat and guinea pig urine. This metabolite appears to be an acid, but is not yet identified. Its formation suggests that a pathway of metabolism of Me_2-NO-MORPH exists in the hamster that is absent in the rat and guinea pig.

Comparison of urinary metabolites arising from the cis and trans isomers of Me_2-NO-MORPH show that in all three species most of the metabolites excreted are quantitatively similar, but a few are formed in greater quantity from one isomer than from the other. Complete characterization of these metabolites might indicate which routes of metabolism are related to the differences in carcinogenic effect observed. This, in turn, might shed light on the large differences in carcinogenic effectiveness of other nitrosamines between species. Similar studies with other nitrosamines showing such differences are planned, together with examination of the metabolism of some of these compounds in organ or tissue culture *in vitro*.

REFERENCES

1. Bartsch, H., C. Malaveille, and R. Montesano. 1975. *In vitro* metabolism and microsome-mediated mutagenicity of dialkyl nitrosamines in rat, hamster, and mouse tissues. Cancer Res. 35:644-651.

2. Lijinsky, W., H. Garcia, L. Keefer, and J. Loo. 1972. Carcinogenesis and alkylation of rat liver nucleic acids by nitrosomethylurea and nitrosoethylurea administered by intraportal injection. Cancer Res. 32:893-897.

3. Lijinsky, W., and H.W. Taylor. 1976. Carcinogenesis in Sprague-Dawley rats of N-nitroso-N-alkylcarbamate esters. Cancer Lett. 1:275-279.

4. Lijinsky, W., and C. Winter. (in press). Skin tumors induced by painting nitrosoalkylureas on mouse skin. Cancer Res. Clin. Oncol.

5. Takayama, S., N. Kuwabara, Y. Azama, and T. Sugimura. 1971. Skin tumors in mice painted with N-methyl-N'-nitro-N-nitrosoguanidine and N-ethyl-N'-nitro-N-nitrosoguanidine. J. Natl. Cancer Inst. 46:973-980.

6. Okada, M., and M. Ishidate. 1977. Metabolic fate of N-n-butyl-N-(4-hydroxybutyl) nitrosamine and its analogues. Xenobiotica 7:11-24.

7. Lijinsky, W., and M.D. Reuber. 1981. Carcinogenic effect of nitrosopyrrolidine, nitrosopiperidine and nitrosohexamethyleneimine in Fischer rats. Cancer Lett. 12:99-103.

8. Lijinsky, W., H.W. Taylor, and L.K. Keefer. 1976. Reduction of rat liver carcinogenicity of nitrosomorpholine by alpha deuterium substitution. J. Natl. Cancer Inst. 57:1311-1313.

9. Rao, T.K., J.A. Young, W. Lijinsky, and J.L. Epler. 1979. Mutagenicity of aliphatic nitrosamines in *Salmonella typhimurium*. Mutat. Res. 66:1-9.

10. Druckrey, H., R. Preussmann, S. Ivankovic, and D. Schmähl. 1967. Organotrope Wirkungen bei 65 verschiedenen N-Nitroso-Verbindungen an BD-Ratten. Z. Krebsforsch. 69:103-201.

11. Okada, M., E. Suzuki, and M. Mochizuki. 1976. Possible important role of urinary N-methyl-N-(3-carboxypropyl)-nitrosamine in the induction of bladder tumors in rats by N-methyl-n-dodecylnitrosamine. Gann 67:771-772.

12. Lijinsky, W., J.E. Saavedra, and M.D. Reuber. (in press). Carcinogenesis in Fischer rats by methylalkylnitrosamines. Cancer Res.

13. Althoff, J., and W. Lijinsky. 1977. Urinary bladder neoplasms in Syrian hamsters after administration of N-nitroso-N-methyl-N-dodecylamine. Z. Krebsforsch. 90:227-231.

14. Ketkar, M.B., J. Althoff, and W. Lijinsky. 1981. The carcinogenic effect of nitrosomethyldodecylamine in European hamsters. Cancer Lett. 13:165-168.

15. Cardy, R.H., and W. Lijinsky. 1980. Comparison of the carcinogenic effects of five nitrosamines in guinea pigs. Cancer Res. 40:1879-1884.

16. Lijinsky, W., M.D. Reuber, and B.N. Blackwell. 1980. Carcinogenicity of nitrosotrialkylureas in Fischer rats. J. Natl. Cancer Inst. 65:451-453.

17. Lijinsky, W., M.D. Reuber, and W.B. Manning. 1980. Potent carcinogenicity of nitrosodiethanolamine in rats. Nature 288:589-590.

18. Hilfrich, J., I. Schmeltz, and D. Hoffman. 1978. Effects of N-nitrosodiethanolamine and 1,1-diethanolhydrazine in Syrian golden hamsters. Cancer Lett. 4:55-60.

19. Preussmann, R., G. Wurtele, G. Eisenbrand, and B. Spiegelhalder. 1978. Urinary excretion of N-nitrosodiethanolamine administered orally to rats. Cancer Lett. 4:207-209.

20. Lijinsky, W., and H.W. Taylor. 1975. Increased carcinogenicity of 2,6-dimethylnitrosomorpholine compared with nitrosomorpholine in rats. Cancer Res. 35:2123-2125.

21. Lijinsky, W., and M.D. Reuber. 1980. Comparison of carcinogenesis by two isomers of nitroso-2,6-dimethylmorpholine. Carcinogenesis 1:501-503.

22. Rao, M.S., D.G. Scarpelli, and W. Lijinsky. (in press). Carcinogenesis in Syrian hamsters by N-nitroso-2,6-dimethylmorpholine, its cis and trans isomers, and the effect of deuterium labeling. Carcinogenesis.

23. Lijinsky, W., and M.D. Reuber. 1981. Comparative carcinogenicity of two isomers of nitroso-2,6-dimethymorpholine in guinea pigs. Cancer Lett. 14:7-11.

24. Lijinsky, W., J.E. Saavedra, M.D. Reuber, and B.N. Blackwell. 1980. The effect of deuterium labeling on the carcinogenicity of nitroso-2,6-dimethylmorpholine in rats. Cancer Lett. 10:325-331.

25. Gingell, R., L. Wallcave, D. Nagel, R. Kupper, and P. Pour. 1976. Common metabolites of N-nitroso-2,6-dimethylmorpholine and N-nitrosobis(2-oxopropyl)amine in the Syrian hamster. Cancer Lett. 2:47-52.

DISCUSSION

Q.: Your work with the alpha deutero-substituted nitrosomorpholine indicated a fivefold decrease in tumor formation. It's interesting that isotope effects occurring in substitutions are typically about one-half that. This may suggest that what you've got here is a bifunctional agent, and therefore you would have to have two alpha substitutions, hydroxylations, in order to get an active species. Is there any indication that bifunctionality is a feature of cyclic nitrosamines?

A.: Perhaps I overstated the precision of our measure of potency. It could easily be from 2 to 7, because unless you do a very extensive dose-response study with large numbers of animals, you really can't say. My measure of 5 was based on the fact that the one dose of the unlabeled compound was as effective as five times the dose of the deuterium-labeled compound. But that doesn't mean that there wasn't considerable variation. So I wouldn't dwell on that too much. And in fact, deuterium isotope effects, chemical kinetic effects, have been stated to be from 2 to 13; I've seen figures.

Unfortunately, the biological studies are not very precise tools. But they're what we have and they're very much closer to man than the reaction in the test tube is. That's the reason we rely on it. I think the animal experiments are the bottom line.

ORGAN SPECIFICITY AND INTERSPECIES DIFFERENCES IN CARCINOGENESIS BY METABOLISM-INDEPENDENT ALKYLATING AGENTS

Jerry M. Rice and Alan Perantoni

Laboratory of Comparative Carcinogenesis, National Cancer Institute, Fort Detrick, Frederick, Maryland 21701

INTRODUCTION

The metabolism-independent or "direct-acting" alkylating agents comprise a structurally diverse group of chemically reactive organic compounds that include some of the most potent known mutagens and carcinogens. Their conversion to reactive intermediates requires no enzyme-mediated catalysis, and in this respect these compounds differ from the great majority of organic chemical carcinogens. Many of the direct-acting alkylating agents have been used in chemical syntheses for decades, and their chemistry is accordingly well known. The carcinogenicity of a number of these compounds has been studied extensively in both rodent and non-rodent species, and the results of such studies provide a remarkable illustration of qualitative interspecies differences in susceptibility to carcinogenesis that cannot be ascribed to differences in metabolism of xenobiotic compounds.

Much of the literature on carcinogenesis by alkylating agents is of relatively recent origin. In 1962, in his book on chemical carcinogenesis, D.B. Clayson concluded that at that time, with few exceptions, it was difficult to accept that the carcinogenic activity of these substances had been firmly established (1). By the end of that decade there remained little doubt, due in large part to studies on the biological effects of substances newly recognized as carcinogens, especially from laboratories working primarily on nitroso compounds (2). Extensive reviews of carcinogenesis by alkylating agents are now available, notably the chapter by Lawley (3) and the continuing series of International Agency for Research on Cancer (IARC) Monographs on the Evaluation of Carcinogenic Risks of Chemicals to Man. This survey will cover only those aspects that are directly pertinent to the problems of species differences and organ specificity.

Chemistry of Metabolism-Independent Alkylating Agents

Reaction mechanisms. All such agents participate in nucleophilic substitution reactions as donors of simple or substituted alkyl groups to a receptor, usually a heteroatom with an unshared electron pair. These alkylations result in formation of a covalent bond and are usually irreversible. Compounds are generally classified as S_N1- or S_N2-type agents, according to whether the initial step in model reactions involving them appears to proceed by a unimolecular or a bimolecular mechanism (3). The alkylating agent (R-X) and receptor Y react to form the alkylated product ($R\text{-}Y^+$) by a unimolecular mechanism as follows:

$$S_N1: \quad R\text{-}X \overset{k_1}{\rightarrow} R^+ + X^-; \; R^+ + Y \overset{k_2}{\rightarrow} R\text{-}Y^+$$

The initial step in the reaction sequence involves only a change in the alkylating agent R-X. When the rate-determining step of a reaction involves collision of two reacting molecular species, the reaction is bimolecular:

$$S_N2: \quad R\text{-}X + Y \overset{k_1}{\rightarrow} (X\text{-}R\text{-}Y) \overset{K_2}{\rightarrow} R\text{-}Y^+ + X^-$$

The initial step in this reaction sequence involves a collision between one molecule of (R-X) and one molecule of Y.

A large number of compounds act as model S_N2 reagents as above, including epoxides, lactones, sulfonate and sulfate esters, aziridines, phosphotriesters, and alkyl halides (especially iodides and bromides), as in the case of methyl methanesulfonate (MMS) (Figure 1). Another group of compounds, including many nitrosamides, under *in vivo* conditions undergo an S_N2 reaction with thiols such as cysteine or glutathione which causes their decomposition, in the process of which a highly reactive alkylating intermediate is liberated. Thiols thus accelerate alkylation of, e.g., DNA by compounds such as 1-nitroso-1-methyl-3-nitroguanidine (MNNG) (4) and nitrosomethylurethane (5) (Figure 2) by non-enzymatic means. Comparisons of the effects of such agents in different tissues must take this mechanism of activation into account.

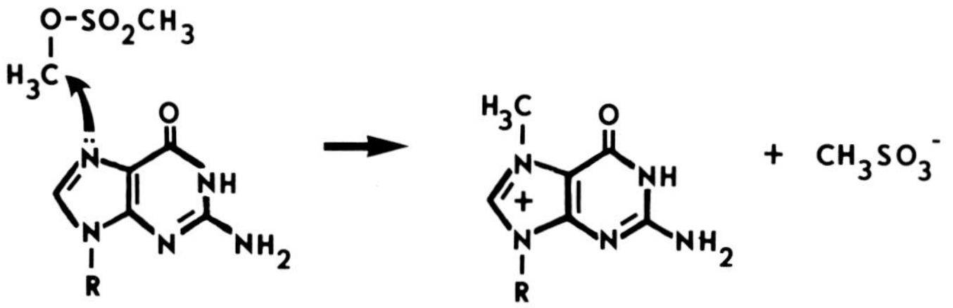

Figure 1. Methylation of the N-7 position of guanosine by methyl methanesulfonate: an S_N2 reaction.

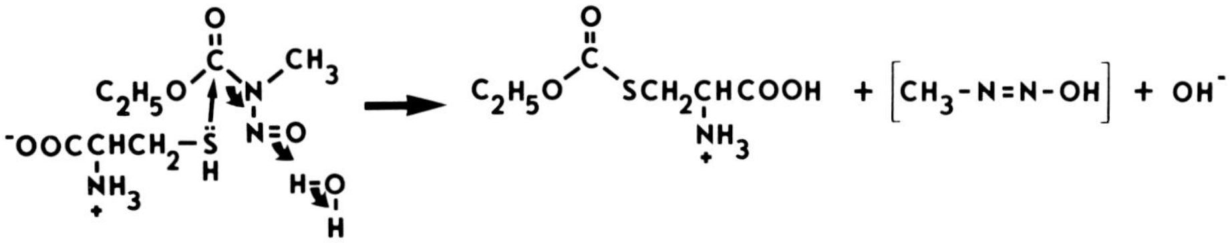

Figure 2. S_N2 reaction of cysteine with nitrosomethylurethane in aqueous solution, liberating a highly reactive methyldiazonium hydroxide moiety as a decomposition product.

True S_N1 reagents are less common and are best represented by the nitrosoalkylureas (Figure 3). The compounds in this series, especially the lower homologs nitrosomethylurea (MNU), nitrosoethylurea (ENU), and nitrosopropylurea, are appreciably acidic, and their decomposition (and reactivity) are base-catalyzed (6); the conjugate base is the molecular species that undergoes unimolecular decomposition to a reactive intermediate. Nitrosotrialkylureas, in which all replaceable hydrogen atoms have been substituted by alkyl groups, cannot be activated by this mechanism and are not direct-acting; they require enzyme-mediated metabolic activation (7). Alkylation by nitroso compounds is thought to proceed via the alkyldiazonium hydroxide intermediate since the alkyl group is transferred intact, whether via enzyme-catalyzed metabolism of nitrosamines (8) or by S_N1 decomposition of nitrosoalkylureas (9). There is no hydrogen exchange with the aqueous medium as would be necessitated by an alternative mechanism that postulates formation of a diazoalkane intermediate (5). Both toxicity (10) and carcinogenesis (11) at the site of application of the ethyl homolog, ENU, are also increased by concomitant administration of salts of heavy metals, particularly copper and cobalt, which catalyze decomposition of nitrosoalkylureas.

$$\text{MNU} \xrightarrow{-H^+} [\ldots]^- \xrightarrow{-NCO^-} [CH_3\text{-}N{=}N\text{-}OH] \xrightarrow[-N_2,\ -OH^-]{X:} \overset{+}{X}\text{-}CH_3$$

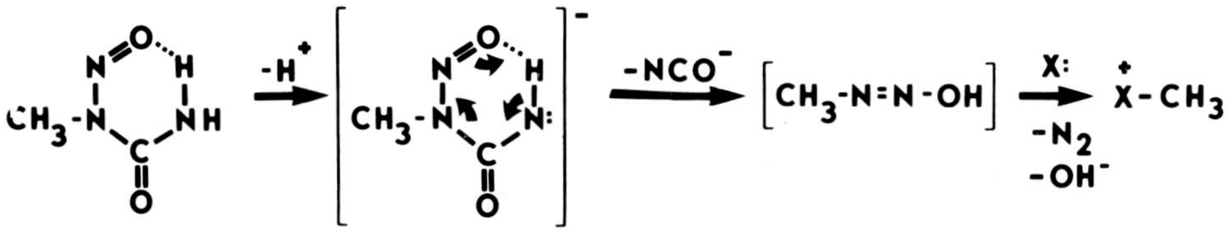

Figure 3. Base-catalyzed S_N1 decomposition of MNU to a reactive methyldiazonium hydroxide product, and subsequent reaction as a methylating agent.

Reaction products. The products of reaction of mutagenic and carcinogenic alkylating agents with cellular components, especially nucleic acids, are numerous and have been extensively studied and comprehensively reviewed (12). Table 1 shows some data of particular importance for comparing effects of alkylating agents in different tissues. These support several general conclusions.

First, agents differ quantitatively in the relative proportions of specific reaction products formed. Major differences are seen even when one compares different sources of the same alkyl group (e.g., the methyl donors MMS and MNU) or successive members of a homologous series the members of which vary in the size of the alkyl group (MNU, ENU, etc.) (13-16).

Table 1. Major Products of Reaction of Selected Alkylating Agents with DNA *In Vivo* and *In Vitro*.

Agent	DNA Source	3-Alkyladenine	O^6-Alkylguanine	7-Alkylguanine	Alkylphosphate	Ref.
MMS	Salmon sperm[a]	9.8	0.3	82	1.0[e]	13,14
EMS	Salmon sperm[a]	5.6	2.0	70	15[e]	13,14
	HeLa cell[a]	4.4	0.2	75	13	15
	HeLa cell[b]	2.2	0.3	81	8.0	15
MNU	HeLa cell[a]	8.0	4.0	60	25	15
ENU	HeLa cell[a]	4.2	12	11	70	15
	HeLa cell[b]	4.6	7.5	17	66	15
	Fetal rat brain cell[b]	4.7	7.6	12	49	16
	Human fibroblast[c]	4.1	5.7	6.5	60	16
	Human fibroblast[d]	5.4	6.3	9.0	58	16

[a]Alkylated *in vitro*.
[b]Alkylated *in vivo*.
[c]Alkylated *in vitro* with 6 ethyl groups/10^5 DNA-phosphate.
[d]Alkylated *in vitro* with 700 ethyl groups/10^5 DNA-phosphate.
[e]See Reference 14.

Secondly, similar ratios of reaction products are found in DNAs exposed to a given agent, largely irrespective of source and dose (and hence of the overall extent of alkylation). DNAs isolated from different cell types from different species exposed to the same alkylating agent *in vivo* have comparable proportions of reaction products; these proportions in turn are comparable to the proportions of reaction products in isolated DNA from any source exposed to the same agent under physiological conditions *in vitro*.

The nature of the interactions between a given agent and the DNA, and presumably other components, of any target cell thus appear to be determined by the chemical properties of the agent. Accordingly it appears reasonable to compare the effects of a given compound in different tissues or different species under similar conditions of exposure, with the working hypothesis that any differences in biological effects such as carcinogenesis are due to differences in the properties of the various target cells.

Carcinogenesis by Alkylating Agents

As a result of the intrinsic chemical reactivity of direct-acting alkylating agents, these substances are locally carcinogenic, inducing tumors at the site of application. The most reactive agents decompose too rapidly to be transported to distant sites in significant quantity; thus, their carcinogenicity and "organ specificity" is highly dependent on the route of administration. Bis(chloromethyl)ether (BCME), for example, induces tumors of the skin when applied cutaneously (17), tumors of lung and nasal cavity when inhaled (18,19), and of the skin and soft connective tissues when injected subcutaneously (20,21) (Table 2). BCME also induces tumors at a remote site (the lung), but only when given by the last mentioned route, and then only in mice, the more highly susceptible species (20). A large proportion of all carcinogenic direct-acting alkylating agents have been tested only by one or two routes in one or at most two species and yield similar results. In addition, tumors of the oral cavity, esophagus, and/or forestomach have frequently been induced in mice or rats exposed by feeding or gastric intubation (3). The potential of most of these substances for systemic tumor induction is limited also by their slight to negligible solubility in aqueous media.

A number of direct-acting alkylating agents, however, have chemical properties compatible with uniform, systemic distribution throughout the body when administered by an appropriate route. Such compounds not only induce tumors directly at the site of application, but regularly do so at remote sites when given in a manner that allows efficient distribution. For example (Table 3), MNU induces exclusively local tumors when given by repeated

Table 2. Dependence on Route of Administration of Local and Systemic Carcinogenesis by a Highly Reactive Alkylating Agent, Bis(chloromethyl)ether ($ClCH_2OCH_2Cl$)

		Site of Tumor Development		
Route	Species	Local	Systemic	Ref.
Percutaneous	Mouse	Skin	--	17
Inhalation	Mouse	Lung	--	18
	Rat	Lung, nasal cavity	--	19
Subcutaneous	Mouse	Skin, soft tissues	Lung	20
	Rat	Soft tissues	--	21

percutaneous (22), intrarectal (23,24), transurethral (25), and in some species by oral (26,27) and intraperitoneal (28) administration, but tends progressively toward induction of neoplasms at multiple remote sites when given by subcutaneous (29,30), oral (31), intraperitoneal (32), and especially intravenous (33-36) routes. This tendency is even more pronounced when this compound is given as a single exposure (9,37-40).

Nitrosomethylurea. MNU is a crystalline solid, soluble freely in polar organic solvents and in water to the extent of approximately 14 g/l. Its chemical stability is markedly pH-dependent (Figure 3); the half-life of MNU is 72 min at pH 7.0 and 6 min at pH 8 (41). At blood pH (7.4), this half-life is sufficiently long for distribution throughout an experimental animal, once MNU has been absorbed into the bloodstream. In rats, the compound is widely and quite uniformly distributed shortly after intravenous injection (42), and can no longer be detected in the blood 15 min later (43). ENU has similar properties (41,44). A single administration of either MNU or ENU over a wide range of dosages is sufficient for carcinogenesis in small rodents. Therefore, the latency period for tumor development in such experiments can be defined with great precision because of the extraordinarily brief period of exposure.

Representative effects in adult rodents of a single intraperitoneal or intravenous exposure are presented in Table 4; additional studies are briefly summarized in IARC Monographs on the

Table 3. Dependence on Route of Administration of Local and Systemic Carcinogenesis by Nitrosomethylurea ($CH_3N(NO)CONH_2$).

Route	Species	Site of Tumor Development		Ref.
		Local	Systemic	
Multiple exposures				
Percutaneous	Rat, mouse	Skin	--	22
Intrarectal	Rat, mouse	Colon	--	23
	Guinea pig	Colon	--	24
Transurethral	Rat	Urinary bladder	--	25
Subcutaneous	Chinese hamster	Soft tissue	Stomach	29
	European hamster	Soft tissue, skin	Stomach	30
Oral	Rhesus monkey	Oropharynx, esophagus	--	26
	Minipig	Stomach	--	27
	Rat	Stomach	Brain, nerves	31
Intraperitoneal	Mouse	--	Lymphoid	32
	Rat	Mesothelium, nerves, mesentery	--	28
Intravenous	Rat	--	Brain, nerves	33,34
		--	Mammary glands	35,36
Single exposures				
Oral	Rat	Stomach	Kidney, intestine, skin, odontogenic	37
Intraperitoneal	Rat	--	Kidney, intestine, mammary, lymphoid, vessels	38
Intravenous	Rat	Blood vessels	Kidney, intestine, mammary, lymphoid, odontogenic, stomach, lung, brain	39,40

Table 4. Carcinogenesis in Adult Animals Following a Single Injection of an Alkylating Agent.

				Organs in Which Tumors Develop[a]									
Species	Strain	Dose (mg/kg)	Path.[b]	CNS[c]	PNS[c]	Marrow or Lymphoid	Kidney	Intestine	Blood Vessels	Lung	Liver	Mammary	Other	Ref.
MNU, i.p.														
Rat	Wistar	50	2	-	-	3/20	8/20	2/20	1/20	-	-	2/20	5/20	38
Mouse	B6C3F1	50	2	-	-	32/80	2/80	-	-	2/80	-	-	20/80 stomach; 11/80 other	38
Rat		45-90[d]	2	-	+[f]	13/80	7/80	7/80	-	-	20/80	9/80	24/80 sarcoma; 1/80 other	45
MNU, i.v.														
Rat	Wistar	70	3	-	-	8/51	16/51	4/51	1/51	8/51	-	18/51	1/51 odonto-genic; 11/51 other	39
Rat	BD	70-100	2	1/16	-	1/16	7/16	5/16	-	-	-	1/16	15/16 stomach; 2/16 jaw; 1/26 other	40
ENU, i.p.														
Mouse	B6C3F1	60[e]	3	-	2/120	26/120	7/120	+[f]	-	97/120	18/120	+[f]	28/120 Harderian gland; 17/120 stomach	46
Gerbil		50	3	-	-	-	-	-	-	-	-	-	9/23 cutaneous melanoma	48
ENU, i.v.														
Rat	BD	20	2	10/29	7/29	-	-	-	-	-	-	-	6/29	47
		40	2	10/18	8/18	-	3/18	-	-	-	-	-	1/18	47
		80	2	9/17	7/17	-	7/17	-	-	-	-	-	5/17	47

[a]Animals with tumors per animals at risk.
[b]Extent of histologic examination: 1 = gross tumors only; 2 = gross tumors and selected tissues only; 3 = complete.
[c]CNS = central nervous system; PNS = peripheral nervous system.
[d]Treatment following partial hepatectomy.
[e]Trioctanoin used as vehicle.
[f]Tumors seen at this site; numbers not specified.

Evaluation of Carcinogenic Risk of Chemicals to Humans, Vol. 17 (44). When MNU is given intraperitoneally, local tumors (in this case, intraabdominal sarcomas) are seen in rats given relatively high doses (45), but the majority of neoplasms occur in remote sites, frequently the gastric and intestinal mucosa and lymphoreticular tissues in which a large population of proliferating cells normally exists. Liver cell tumors develop in rats only when MNU is given while the liver is in a state of regenerative hyperplasia immediately following partial hepatectomy (45). Tumors also develop in both rats and mice in organs and tissues in which cell proliferation is less active, notably the kidney, mammary glands, lung, and peripheral nervous system (38,45). An even wider spectrum of tumors was seen when comparable doses are given intravenously (39,40). Tumors of blood vessels, to be expected as "local" tumors resulting from intravenous exposure, are conspicuously rare in rats given MNU.

Nitrosoethylurea. More marked interspecies differences are apparent in mice, rats, and other species subjected to a single intraperitoneal or intravenous injection of ENU (Table 4). In mice, ENU induces tumors of the Harderian gland and high multiplicities of primary epithelial tumors of the liver and the peripheral lung (46). None of these tumors occur in rats, in which species tumorigenesis is most rapid and pronounced in the central and peripheral nervous systems (47). In the gerbil, a completely different result is obtained: no tumors occur in any of the sites commonly affected in either rats or mice, and only cutaneous melanomas are seen, after a latency of nearly two years (48).

Effect of dose on tumor latency. A reasonable hypothesis is that some or all of these differences in organ specificity could be due to differences in the magnitude of the dose actually reaching the target tissues in the different species. Single exposures are limited by acute toxicity, and the effects of multiple repeated exposures to these agents have also been extensively studied in mice, rats, and several other species. In evaluating the results of such studies in the context of species differences and organ specificity, however, increases in tumor incidence and multiplicity with increasing doses are not the only dose/effect relationships that must be considered, as these can be overshadowed by the inverse relationship between tumor latency and dose.

Table 5 illustrates this effect for both single exposures to ENU in rats (47) and multiple exposures to MNU in mice (32). Both the neurogenic and renal tumors induced in rats and the lymphomas induced in mice in these studies are rapidly growing, lethal neoplasms. The mean latency for lymphomas in mice decreases from 218 days, when 5 weekly injections of 10 mg/kg were given, to 87 days when 40 mg/kg were given at each injection. The 87-day period appears to be an irreducible minimum that was not further

Table 5. Inverse Relationship Between Tumor Latency and Magnitude of Exposure to Carcinogenic Nitrosoalkylureas

Single Dose (mg/kg)	Total Injections x Inj./Week	Number of Animals	% With Tumor	Tumors/ Animal[a]	Mean Latency (days)
MNU: Lymphomas in Adult Female Mice (32)					
0		30	0	--	--
10	5 x 1	29	7	--	218
20	5 x 1	30	93	--	147
30	5 x 1	28	89	--	97
40	5 x 1	29	93	--	87
50[b]	5 x 1	18	83	--	90
ENU: Neurogenic Plus Renal Tumors in Newborn Rats (47)					
5	1	28	32	0.3	500
10	1	16	69	1.3	310
20	1	16	100	2.2	240
40	1	15	100	2.3	205
80	1	16	100	2.9	183

[a]Total tumors per total animals at risk.
[b]Toxic; some early deaths occurred before the first tumor was seen.

shortened when the dose was increased to a higher (and acutely toxic) level (32). Similarly, in rats, the latency for neurogenic and renal tumors in rats given a single injection of ENU at 80 mg/kg was less than half as long as in rats given only 5 mg/kg.

Latency varies markedly among and within species for different kinds of tumors. It is quite certain that tumors with long latencies will not be seen in animals subjected to a carcinogenic regimen that causes their early death from lethal kinds of tumors that develop much more rapidly. Consequently, at higher doses, a narrower range of organ sites may be observed than at lower doses. Examples of rapidly lethal experimental tumors include schwannomas, renal mesenchymal tumors, intestinal carcinomas and certain mammary tumors in rats, thymic lymphomas in mice, and tracheal adenomas and carcinomas in Syrian hamsters.

Multiple injections. The effects of multiple intraperitoneal or intravenous injections of MNU or ENU in adult animals of various species are summarized in Table 6. Depending on the dose level and schedule, carcinogenesis in the rat may be largely restricted under these conditions to a single organ system, notably the lymphoreticular system (41,49,50), mammary gland (35,36), or nervous system (34). This restriction is probably due in large part to the rapid development of these lethal neoplasms. Other results are also consistent with this view. For example, adenocarcinomas of the intestinal mucosa develop frequently in rats given a single intravenous injection of MNU (39,40) but are rare or absent in rats given multiple injections (34-36). In other species, the spectrum of organs affected was often quite different under similar conditions of exposure. Epithelial tumors of the lung are common only in the mouse after either MNU (51,52) or ENU; these are never seen in the rat (34-36,41,49,50,53,54), Syrian hamster (55), guinea pig (56), or patas monkey (57) under these conditions of exposure, and only rarely in the European hamster (58) or gerbil (59). Tumors of the blood vessels appear more frequently in larger species; in experiments with intravenous MNU, these were seen with great frequency in the rabbit (60,61) and one breed of dog (62,63), but rarely or not at all in the rat (34-36), mouse (51), European hamster (58), or gerbil (59). Hepatocellular tumors were recorded only in the mouse (51) and European hamster (58). Renal tumors differed markedly from one species to another, consisting exclusively of epithelial tumors of the renal cortex in mice (46), but predominately of mesenchymal tumors in rats (47). Occasionally, tumor sites unique to a species were observed, such as the predilection of MNU for the heart in European hamsters (58) and for the mid-ventral sebaceous gland in gerbils (59).

Age dependence. Many organ systems vary in susceptibility to the carcinogenic effects of alklating agents during pre-and postnatal development. A qualitative summary of these effects for ENU in the prenatal, neonatal, suckling, and adult rat (47,64) and mouse (46,65) is presented in Table 7. Some organ systems, such as the central nervous system (CNS) and peripheral nervous system (PNS), are more susceptible during very early life in both species, while others, such as the stomach and kidney, are more susceptible during later life. The overall trend within a species, however, is toward quantitative changes in susceptibility during development. The spectrum of tissues affected differs between species at all times. Liver and lung parenchyma in rats, for example, remain refractory to ENU even during the perinatal period, while in the mouse both are more susceptible during the perinatal period than during adulthood.

Table 6. Carcinogenesis Following Repeated Intravenous or Intraperitoneal Injection of Nitrosoalkylureas.

Species	Strain	Treatment[b]	Path.[c]	Organs in Which Tumors Develop[a]										Ref.
				CNS[d]	PNS[d]	Marrow or Lymphoid	Kidney	Intestine	Blood Vessels	Lung	Liver	Mammary	Other	
ENU, i.p.														
Rat	Wistar	10/M/3 or 5M	2	-	-	17/30	-	-	-	-	-	-	3/30	49
ENU, i.v.														
Rat	BD	10/W/25W	2	5/16	-	9/16	-	-	-	-	-	-	-	41
Rat[e]	Wistar	15/W/15W	1	9/200	8/200	95/200	-	-	-	-	-	-	18/200	50
Patas monkey		12/2W/104W	3	-	-	3/13	-	4/13	5/13	-	-	-	8/13	57
MNU, i.p.														
Rat	F344; SD	5/W/36W	3	12/26	5(18?)/26	1/26	-	-	5/26	-	-	-	-	54
Rat	BD	5/W/36W	2	15/21	1/21	1/21	1/21	-	-	-	-	-	3/21	53
		5,10/W/26W	2	9/15	3/15	-	1/15	-	-	-	-	-	2/15	53
Mouse	A;C3H	5,15/W/44W	2	-	-	-	-	-	-	21/80	-	-	-	52
Syrian hamster		2.5/M/4M 1/W/22W	1	-	-	-	-	10/10	-	-	-	-	odonto-genic	55
Guinea pig	NIH 13	10/W/18W	2	-	-	-	-	1/22	2/22	-	1 (angio-sarcoma)	-	7/22	56

[a]Expressed as animals with tumors per animals at risk.
[b]Expressed as dose in mg/kg body weight/given per week (W) or month (M)/for a number of weeks or months or for the life (L) of the animal.
[c]Extent of histopathologic examination: 1 = gross tumors only; 2 = gross tumors and selected tissues only; 3 = complete.
[d]CNS = central nervous system; PNS = peripheral nervous system.
[e]All male animals.
[f]All female animals.

(continued)

Table 6. (continued)

Species	Strain	Treatment[b]	Path.[c]	Organs in Which Tumors Develop[a]										Ref.
				CNS[d]	PNS[d]	Marrow or Lymphoid	Kidney	Intestine	Blood Vessels	Lung	Liver	Mammary	Other	
MNU, i.v.														
Rat	F344; SD	5/W/36W	3	17/35	13/35	4/35	-	-	-	-	-	-	8/35	34
Rat[f]	Buffalo	50/M/3M	1	-	-	-	-	-	-	-	-	34/38	-	35
Rat	Lewis	25/M/6M	1	6/20[e]	-	-	-	-	-	-	-	23/35[f]	-	36
Mouse[e]	C3HeB/ FeJ	25/W/7W	3	2/19	-	3/19	-	-	-	9/19	2/19	-	7/19 stomach	51
European hamster		2.5,5,10/ W/18W	3	-	28/90 heart	-	-	-	-	2/90	3/90	-	29/90 stomach; 16/90 oral; 5/90 nasal	58
Gerbil		2.5,5/ W/15W	3	-	-	1/48	-	-	-	1/48	-	-	14/48 oral; 19/48 mid-ventral sebaceous gland; 1/48 Zymbals gland	59
Rabbit		10-20/ 2-4W/L	3	31/127	-	-	-	61/127	34/27	-	-	-	17/127 local (ear)	60,61
Dog	Mongrel	20/M/L	2	2/10	4/10	-	-	-	1/10	-	-	-	-	62
Dog	Boxer	5/W/36W	3	-	14/20	5/20	-	1/20	7/20	1/20	-	-	7/20	63

[a]Expressed as animals with tumors per animals at risk.
[b]Expressed as dose in mg/kg body weight/given per week (W) or month (M)/for a number of weeks or months or for the life (L) of the animal.
[c]Extent of histopathologic examination: 1 = gross tumors only; 2 = gross tumors and selected tissues only; 3 = complete.
[d]CNS = central nervous system; PNS = peripheral nervous system.
[e]All male animals.
[f]All female animals.

Table 7. Age Dependence of Organ-Specific Carcinogenesis Following a Single Exposure to ENU.

Dose (mg/kg)	Age Exposed	Route[b]	No. of Animals	Major Sites of Tumor Development[a]							
				CNS[c]	PNS[c]	Kidney	Female Genital	Lung	Liver	Stomach	Lymph
BD-IX Rats (47,64)											
60	Prenatal, day 12	T	25	+	-	-	-	-	-	-	-
60	Prenatal, day 16	T	26	+++	+++	-	-	-	-	-	-
80	Day 1	SC	16	++	++	+	-	-	-	-	-
80	Day 10	PO	16	+	+	++	-	-	-	-	-
80	Day 30	IV	17	+	+	++	-	-	-	-	-
$B6C3F_1$ Mice (46,65)											
60	Prenatal, day 12	T	161	++	++	+	+++	+	+	+	-
60	Prenatal, day 16	T	108	++	++	+	++	+++	+++	+	-
60	Day 1	IP	120	+	+	++	++	++	++	+	+
60	Day 15	IP	120	-	-	++	++	++	++	++	++
60	Day 42	IP	120	+	+	+	++	++	+	++	++

[a]The number of (+) signs is used only to indicate trends within a site for a given species.
[b]T = transplacental; SC = subcutaneous; PO = oral intubation; IV = intravenous.
[c]CNS = central nervous system; PNS = peripheral nervous system.

Strain dependence. Within a species, quantitative differences in susceptibility of a given organ system to carcinogenesis by direct-acting alkylating agents also varies from strain to strain. Again, taking ENU as a model compound and comparing its transplacental effects on fetal mice (66) and rats (67) of different inbred strains (see Table 8), it is evident that major quantitative differences in susceptibility of the major target organs, often exceeding a decimal order of magnitude, exist among strains of mice with respect to tumors of the lung, liver, and lymphoid tissues, and among strains of rats with respect to tumors of the nerves and central nervous system. The pattern of tumor development, however, is in each case determined by the species; in all strains of mice, the major sites of tumor development are the pulmonary and hepatic epithelia and the lymphoid tissues, while tumors of the brain, spinal cord, and nerves predominate in rats, regardless of strain.

Sex differences. Organs other than the gonads, breast, and reproductive tract are in some cases significantly more susceptible to direct-acting alkylating agents in one sex. This trait is especially evident in the mouse liver (68), which is more susceptible in males. Hepatocellular tumors, readily induced in high multiplicity in some strains of mice by a single transplacental exposure to ENU, have a latency of nearly a year, and during at least the initial 10 weeks of postnatal life there are no histologically evident neoplastic or preneoplastic changes in the liver. When litter mates from C3HfB/HeN litters prenatally exposed to ENU are randomly paired, and some gonadectomized six to eight weeks after birth, the resulting radical alteration in hormonal environment in gonadectomized mice significantly modifies the yield of liver cell tumors in both sexes at 40 weeks, decreasing the multiplicity in males and increasing it in females. This trend could be intensified by administering exogenous estradiol to gonadectomized males and testosterone to gonadectomized females (68). The inhibitory effect of exogenous estrogen on development of liver cell tumors in genetic males is nearly absolute, while exogenous androgen significantly promotes development of liver cell tumors in genetic females (see Table 9).

DISCUSSION

Adequate data are available to confirm that major qualitative and quantitative interspecies differences exist in organ specificity for carcinogenesis by direct-acting alkylating agents, at least the S_N1-type agents typified by MNU and ENU. In addition, less extreme differences, generally quantitative in nature, exist among sexes, strains, and individuals of different ages within a species.

Table 8. Strain Dependence of Transplacental Carcinogenesis by Single Exposure to ENU

	Offspring		Major Sites of Tumor Development							
Strain	At Risk	% With Tumor	CNS[a]	PNS[a]	Kidney	Lymphoma	Lung	Liver	Ovary	Mean Latency (days)
Rats with tumors/rats at risk: BD rats, 50 mg/kg i.v., day 15 of gestation (67)										
I	14	100	0.86	0.79	-	-	-	-	-	285
II	14	100	1.00	0.21	-	-	-	-	-	250
III	25	96	1.00	0.04	-	-	-	-	-	325
IV	18	56	0.72	0.06	-	-	-	-	-	550
V	14	100	1.14	0.07	-	-	-	-	-	320
VI	14	100	0.71	1.00	0.14	-	-	-	-	205
VII	19	89	0.63	0.74	-	0.05	-	-	0.05	365
VIII	20	80	0.70	0.35	-	0.05	-	-	0.05	400
IX	16	94	0.75	1.06	+[b]	-	-	-	0.05	180
X	25	96	0.76	0.44	-	-	-	-	-	260
Mice with tumors/mice at risk: Jackson Laboratory mice, 60 mg/kg i.p., day 18 of gestation (66)										
AKR/J	20	95	-	-	-	0.85	0.40	-	-	
SWR/J	24	83	-	-[c]	-	0.67	0.58	-	0.04	
DBA/2J	27	67	-	-	-	0.44	0.07	0.22	-	
C57BL/6J	29	62	-	-	-	0.55	0.24	0.06	-	
C57L/J	24	63	-	-	-	0.42	0.17	0.08	0.13	

[a]CNS = central nervous system; PNS = peripheral nervous system.
[b]Tumor seen at this site in previous experiments.
[c]Tumor seen at this site when exposure occurred earlier in gestation.

Table 9. Effect of Sex on Development of Hepatocellular and Pulmonary Epithelial C3HfB/HeN Mice and Its Modification by Gonadectomy and Exogenous Hormone Administration[a]

Offspring			Tumors/Mouse[b]	
Genetic Sex	Postnatal Treatment	Number	Lung	Liver
Male	Gonadectomy, estrogen	8	13.5	0.1
	Gonadectomy	8	17.9	9.6
	Sham surgery	9	13.3	22.8
Female	Gonadectomy, androgen	6	15.8	4.8
	Gonadectomy	4	9.5	3.5
	Sham surgery	5	11.0	1.0

[a]After a single transplacental exposure to ENU (60 mg/kg) on day 16 or 17 of gestation (68).
[b]Forty weeks after birth.

Major Interspecies Differences in Organotropism

Nervous system. All species studied appear more susceptible during the perinatal period. The rat is the most highly susceptible species; both the glia of the brain and spinal cord and the Schwann cells of the nerves are highly vulnerable. The mouse displays largely the same distribution of tumors as the rat, but is two to three decimal orders of magnitude less susceptible, while the gerbil, which has not been studied during the perinatal age period, appears totally refractory. Other species exhibit extremely variable proportions of tumors in the central and peripheral nervous systems: tumors of the nerves, but not the CNS, were seen in boxer dogs; tumors of the CNS, but not the nerves, have been described in other species including the opossum.

Liver cells. The rat is totally resistant except when the adult liver is regenerating after partial hepatectomy. Hepatocellular tumors are not induced transplacentally by alkylating agents in the rat, but they are in the mouse, which is highly susceptible. Fetal and neonatal mice are more susceptible than older animals, and males are more susceptible than females. Most other species are highly but not totally resistant, including the Syrian hamster, guinea pig, gerbil, rabbit, and dog.

Vascular endothelium. Larger animals appear to develop a higher relative incidence of vascular tumors. Such neoplasms are frequent in the patas monkey, dog, and rabbit, but are much less common in smaller species, especially the mouse and rat.

Respiratory tract. The peripheral lung of the mouse is extremely susceptible to direct-acting alkylating agents, especially in certain strains and during prenatal development. Tumors at this site are rarely encountered in other species. In rats and hamsters, the upper respiratory tract, especially the trachea, is susceptible to carcinogenesis following direct application of these agents, but is much less susceptible when administration is by intravenous injection or other systemic application. Larger species, including the rabbit, dog, and patas monkey, are highly resistant.

Urinary system. The renal cortex is often affected in many species, while the renal pelvis, ureter, and bladder are generally spared. The cortical cell of origin and the histologic pattern of the resulting tumors vary markedly from species to species. Renal tumors induced by direct-acting alkylating agents in the mouse invariably arise from the proximal convoluted tubular epithelium, and are adenomas and adenocarcinomas. This also occurs in the rat, especially in older animals, but in addition in this species, mesenchymal and undifferentiated cells may give rise respectively to sarcomas and nephroblastomas especially during the perinatal period. Characteristically, only nephroblastic tumors develop in the rabbit.

Possible Mechanisms of Interspecies Differences

Effective dose. While extensive bioassays for carcinogenic activity have provided clear evidence of differing degrees of susceptibility to direct-acting alkylating agents, both from one cell type to another within a species and for a given cell type among different species, comparatively little detailed pharmacodynamic data exist in most cases to support the hypothesis that the same effective dose of carcinogen is delivered to a given population of target cells in any two different species receiving the same weight-adjusted exposure to a given agent, or to target and non-target cells within an organ in which some, but not all, types of cells give rise to tumors. Most of the current data has been obtained as an average for the total population of all cells of different kinds within an organ. Relatively few demonstrations exist like that of Kleihues et al. (69) who showed that alkylation by MNU of glial cells (which readily give rise to tumors) and neurons (which rarely do so) in the highly susceptible rat brain proceeds to the same extent *in vivo*, so that explanations of the differing susceptibilities of the two cell types must be found elsewhere. Until such data become available, the assertion that the potential precursors of tumors and adjacent refractory cells within an organ in fact have received an equivalent exposure must remain indirect and inferential.

The possible role of differing capacitites for repair of carcinogen-inflicted intracellular damage, especially to DNA, as a determinant of susceptibility and of species and organ differences in susceptibility likewise appears to require refinement beyond the whole-organ level of analysis (70-72).

Inhibition and promotion of expression of the neoplastic phenotype. A second approach to the question of organ specificity concerns the phenomenon of tumor promotion and the potential of at least some kinds of potential tumor cells to persist, quiescent, for prolonged periods without proliferating. The capacity for promoting agents to stimulate such cells, and the apparent restriction on promoting activity of a given agent to specific kinds of cells (73), suggests that this phenomenon may be of general significance, and that some of the current dilemmas in organotropism of chemical carcinogens may ultimately be resolved by new discoveries in the field of tumor promotion.

It remains a reasonable hypothesis that direct-acting agents that are widely and apparently uniformly distributed when given systemically induce the initial stage of neoplastic transformation in cells of virtually all tissues throughout the organism. This may be necessary for tumor development, but not sufficient, except in highly permissive tissues in which barriers to subsequent progression towards autonymous neoplastic proliferation are very low. The rat nervous system and the mouse liver may be examples of such highly permissive tissues; to be precise, one should specify the glia of the rat central nervous system, the Schmann cells of the rat peripheral nervous system, and the mouse hepatocyte. The squamous epithelium of the mouse epidermis may represent the other extreme, a refractory cell whose neoplastic phenotype is rarely expressed unless the barriers to expression are lowered by exposure to a promoting agent. All cell types in all species may fall somewhere in a continous spectrum between the rat glial cell and mouse cutaneous squamous epithelium in the extent of their dependence on tumor promoting agents --of the nature of which in most cases, we are quite ignorant --to allow proliferation of potentially neoplastic clones. If so, this could explain the enormous differences among species in response to the same metabolism-independent carcinogens, and could be a very good thing: a phenomenon exploitable for the prevention of some cancer in man.

REFERENCES

1. Clayson, D.B. 1962. Chemical Carcinogenesis. Little, Brown, and Co.: Boston. p. 181.

2. Van Duuren, B.L., ed. 1969. Biological Effects of Alkylating Agents. Ann. N.Y. Acad. Sci., 163, Article 2. pp. 589-1029.

3. Lawley, P.D. 1976. Carcinogenesis by alkylating agents. In: Chemical Carcinogens, ACS Monograph 173. C.E. Searle, ed. American Chemical Society: Washington, DC. pp. 83-244.

4. Wheeler, G.P., and B.J. Bowdon. 1972. Comparison of the effects of cysteine upon the decomposition of nitrosoureas and of 1-methyl-3-nitro-1-nitrosoguanidine. Biochem. Pharmacol. 21:265-267.

5. Schoental, R. 1961. Interaction of the carcinogenic N-methylnitrosourethane with sulfhydryl groups. Nature 192:670.

6. Garrett, E.R., G. Shigeru, and J.F. Stubbins. 1965. Kinetics of solvolyses of various N-alkyl-N-nitrosoureas in neutral and alkaline solutions. J. Pharm. Sci. 54:119-123.

7. Lijinsky, W., M.D. Reuber, and B.N. Blackwell. 1980. Carcinogenicity of nitrosotrialkylureas in Fischer 344 rats. J. Natl. Cancer Inst. 65:451-453.

8. Lijinsky, W., J. Loo, and A.E. Ross. 1968. Mechanism of alkylation of nucleic acids by nitrosodimethylamine. Nature 218:1174-1175.

9. Lijinsky, W., H. Garcia, L. Keefer, J. Loo, and A.E. Ross. 1972. Carcinogenesis and alkylation of rat liver nucleic acids by nitrosomethylurea and nitrosoethylurea administered by intraportal injection. Cancer Res. 32:893-897.

10. Zeller, W.J., and S. Ivankovic. 1972. Steigerung der toxischen Wirkung von Alkylnitrosoharnstoffen durch Schwermetalle. Naturwissenschaften 59:82.

11. Ivankovic, S., W.J. Zeller, and D. Schmähl. 1972. Steigerung der carcinogenen Wirkung von Äthylnitrosoharnstoff durch Schwermetalle. Naturwissenschaften 59:369.

12. Singer, B. 1975. The chemical effects of nucleic acid alkylation and their relation to mutagenesis and carcinogenesis. In: Progress in Nucleic Acid Research and Molecular Biology, Volume 15. W.E. Cohn, ed. Academic Press: New York. pp. 219-284, 330-332.

13. Lawley, P.D., D.J. Orr, and M. Jarman. 1975. Isolation and identification of products from alkylation of nucleic acids: ethyl- and isopropylpurines. Biochem. J. 145:73-84.

14. Bannon, P., and W. Verly. 1972. Alkylation of phosphates and stability of phosphate triesters in DNA. Eur. J. Biochem. 31:103-111.

15. Sun, L., and B. Singer. 1975. The specificity of different classes of ethylating agents toward various sites of HeLa cell DNA in vitro and in vivo. Biochemistry 14:1795-1802.

16. Singer, B., W.J. Bodell, J.E. Cleaver, G.H. Thomas, M.F. Rajewsky, and W. Thon. 1978. Oxygens in DNA are main targets for ethylnitrosourea in normal and xeroderma pigmentosum fibroblasts and fetal rat brain cells. Nature 276:85-88.

17. Van Duuren, B.L., C. Katz, M. Goldschmidt, K. Frenkel, and A. Sivak. 1972. Carcinogenicity of halo-ethers, II. Structure-activity relationships of analogs of bis(chloromethyl)ether. J. Natl. Cancer Inst. 48:1431-1439.

18. Leong, B.K.J., H.N. MacFarland, and W.H. Reese, Jr. 1971. Induction of lung adenomas by chronic inhalation of bis(chloromethyl)ether. Arch. Environ. Hlth. 22:663-666.

19. Laskin, S., M. Kuschner, R.T. Drew, V.P. Cappiello, and N. Nelson. 1971. Tumors of the respiratory tract induced by inhalation of bis(chloromethyl)ether. Arch. Environ. Hlth. 23:135-136.

20. Gargus, J.L., W.H. Reese, Jr., and H.A. Rutter. 1969. Induction of lung adenomas in newborn mice by bis(chloromethyl)ether. Toxicol. Appl. Pharmacol. 15:92-96.

21. Van Duuren, B.L., A. Sivak, B.M. Goldschmidt, C. Katz, and S. Melchionne. 1969. Carcinogenicity of halo-ethers. J. Natl. Cancer Inst. 43:481-486.

22. Graffi, A., F. Hoffmann, and M. Schütt. 1967. N-Methyl-N-nitrosourea as a strong topical carcinogen when painted on skin of rodents. Nature (London) 214:611.

23. Narisawa, T., C.-Q. Wong, R.R. Maronpot, and J.H. Weisburger. 1976. Large bowel carcinogenesis in mice and rats by several intrarectal doses of methylnitrosourea and negative effect of nitrite plus methylurea. Cancer Res. 36:505-510.

24. Narisawa, T., C.-Q. Wong, and J.H. Weisburger. 1975. Induction of carcinoma of the large intestine in guinea pigs by intrarectal instillation of N-methyl-N-nitrosourea. J. Natl. Cancer Inst. 54:785-787.

25. Hicks, R.M., and J.St.J. Wakefield. 1972. Rapid induction of bladder cancer in rats with N-methyl-N-nitrosourea, I. Histology. Chem.-Biol. Interact. 5:139-152.

26. Adamson, R.H., F.J. Krolikowski, P. Correa, S.M. Sieber, and D.W. Dalgard. 1977. Carcinogenicity of 1-methyl-1-nitrosourea in non-human primates. J. Natl. Cancer Inst. 59:415-422.

27. Stavrou, D., E. Dahme, and J. Kalich. 1976. Gastroonkogene Wirkung von Methylnitrosoharnstoff beim Miniaturschwein. Res. Exp. Med. 169:33-343.

28. Thomas, C., J.L. Sierra, and G. Kersting. 1968. Neurogene Tumoren bei Ratten nach intraperitonealer Applikation von N-Nitroso-N-methylharnstoff. Naturwissenschaften 55:183.

29. Reznik, G., U. Mohr, and N. Kmock. 1976. Carcinogenic effect of different nitroso-compounds in Chinese hamsters: N-dibutylnitrosamine and N-nitrosomethylurea. Cancer Lett. 1:183-188.

30. Mohr, U., H. Haas, and J. Hilfrich. 1974. The carcinogenic effects of dimethylnitrosamine and nitrosomethylurea in European hamsters (Cricetus cricetus L.). Brit. J. Cancer 29:359-364.

31. Schreiber, D., and W. Jänisch. 1967. Geschwulste bei Ratten nach wiederholter Applikation von N-Methyl-N-nitrosoharnstoff durch die Magensonde. Exp. Path. 1:331-338.

32. Joshi, V.V., and J.V. Frei. 1970. Effects of dose and schedule of methylnitrosourea on incidence of malignant lymphoma in adult female mice. J. Natl. Cancer Inst. 45:335-339.

33. Denlinger, R.H., A. Koestner, and J.A. Swenberg. 1973. An experimental model for selective production of neoplasms of the peripheral nervous system. Acta Neuropath. (Berlin) 23:219-228.

34. Swenberg, J.A., A. Koestner, and W. Wechsler. 1972. The induction of tumors of the nervous system with intravenous methylnitrosourea. Lab. Invest. 26:74-85.

35. Gullino, P.M., H.M. Pettigrew, and F.H. Grantham. 1975. N-Nitrosomethylurea as mammary gland carcinogen in rats. J. Natl. Cancer Inst. 54:401-444.

36. Bots, G.T.A.M., and R.G.T. Willighagen. 1975. Tumors in the mammary gland induced in Lewis rats by intravenous methylnitrosourea. Brit. J. Cancer 31:372-374.

37. Leaver, D.D., P.F. Swann, and P.N. Magee. 1969. The induction of tumours in the rat by a single oral dose of N-nitrosomethylurea. Brit. J. Cancer 23:177-187.

38. Terracini, B., and M.C. Testa. 1970. Carcinogenicity of a single administration of N-nitrosomethylurea: a comparison between newborn and 5-week-old mice and rats. Brit. J. Cancer 24:588-598.

39. Murthy, A.S.K., G.F. Vawter, and A. Bhaktaviziam. 1973. Newplasms in Wistar rats after an N-methyl-N-nitrosourea injection. Arch. Pathol. 96:53-57.

40. Druckrey, H., D. Steinhoff, R. Preussmann, and S. Ivankovic. 1964. Erzeugung von Krebs durch eine einmalige Dosis von Methylnitrosoharnstoff und verschiedenen Dialkylnitrosaminen an Ratten. Z. Krebsforch. 66:1-10.

41. Druckrey, H., R. Preussmann, S. Ivankovic, and D. Schmahl. 1967. Organtrope carcinogene Wirkungen bei 65 verschiedenen N-Nitroso-Verbindungen an BD-Ratten. Z. Krebsforsch. 69:103-201.

42. Kleihues, P., and K. Patzschke. 1971. Verteilung von N-[^{14}C]-Methyl-N-nitrosoharnstoff in der Ratte nach systemischer Applikation. Z. Krebsforsch. 75:193-200.

43. Swann, P.F. 1968. The rate of breakdown of methyl methane sulphonate, dimethyl sulphate and N-methyl-N-nitrosourea in the rat. Biochem. J. 110:49-52.

44. International Agency for Research on Cancer. 1978. Some Nitroso Compounds. IARC Monographs on the Evaluation of the Carcinogenic Risk of Chemicals to Humans, Volume 17. Lyons, France. pp. 191-215, 227-255.

45. Craddock, V.M., and J.V. Frei. 1974. Induction of liver cell adenomata in the rat by a single treatment with N-methyl-N-nitrosourea given at various times after partial hepatectomy. Brit. J. Cancer 30:503-511.

46. Vesselinovitch, S.D., K.V.N. Rao, N. Mihailovich, J.M. Rice, and L.S. Lombard. 1974. Development of broad spectrum of tumors by ethylnitrosourea in mice and the modifying role of age, sex, and strain. Cancer Res. 34:2530-2538.

47. Druckrey, H., B. Schagen, and S. Ivankovic. 1970. Erzeugung neurogener Malignome durch einmalige Gabe von Äthyl-nitrosoharnstoff (ÄNH) an neugeborene und junge BD IX-Ratten. Z. Krebsforsch. 74:141-161.

48. Kleihues, P., J. Bucheler, and U.N. Riede. 1978. Selective induction of melanomas in gerbils (Meriones unguiculatus) following postnatal administration of N-ethyl-N-nitrosourea. J. Natl. Cancer Inst. 61:859-863.

49. Hadjiolov, D. 1972. Thymic lymphoma and myeloid leukemia in the rat induced with ethylnitrosourea. Z. Krebsforsch. 77:98-100.

50. Zeller, W.J., and D. Schmähl. 1979. Leukemias induced by ethylnitrosourea in Wistar rats: Incidence and chemotherapy. Leuk. Res. 3:239-248.

51. Denlinger, R.H., A. Koestner, and W. Wechsler. 1974. Induction of neurogenic tumors in C3HeB/F3J mice by nitrosourea derivatives: Observations by light microscopy, tissue culture, and electron microscopy. Int. J. Cancer 13:559-571.

52. Eckert, V.H., and E. Seidler. 1971. Zur tumorerzeugendem Wirkung von Methylnitrosoharnstoff an der Maus. Arch. Geschwulstforsch. 38:7-9.

53. Druckrey, H., S. Ivankovic, and R. Preussmann. 1965. Selektive Erzeugung maligner Tumoren in Gehirn und Rückenmark von Ratten durch N-Methyl-N-Nitrosoharnstoff. Z. Krebsforsch. 66:389-408.

54. Swenberg, J.A., A. Koestner, W. Wechsler, M.N. Branden, and H. Abe. 1975. Differential oncogenic effects of methylnitrosourea. J. Natl. Cancer Inst. 54:89-96.

55. Herrold, K.M. 1969. Adenocarcinomas of the intestine induced in Syrian hamsters by N-methyl-N-nitrosourea. Path. Vet. 6:403-412.

56. Rao, M.S., and J.K. Reddy. 1977. Pathology of tumors developed in guinea pigs given intraperitoneal injections of N-methyl-N-nitrosourea. Neoplasma 24:57-61.

57. Rice, J.M., W.T. London, A.E. Palmer, D.L. Sly, and G.M. Williams. 1977. Direct and transplacental carcinogenesis by ethylnitrosourea in the patas monkey (Erythrocebus patas). Proc. Am. Assoc. Cancer Res. 18:53.

58. Ketkar, M., G. Reznik, H. Haas, J. Hilfrich, and U. Mohr. 1977. Tumors of the heart and stomach induced in European hamsters by intravenous administration of N-methyl-N-nitrosourea. J. Natl. Cancer Inst. 58:1695-1699.

59. Haas, H., J. Hilfrich, N. Kmoch, and U. Mohr. 1975. Specific carcinogenic effect of N-methyl-N-nitrosourea on the midventral sebaceous gland of the gerbil (Meriones unguiculatus). J. Natl. Cancer Inst. 55:637-640.

60. Schreiber, V.D., and W. Janisch. 1973. Tumoren des Gefass systems bei Kaninchen nach Applikation von Methylnitrosoharnstoff (MNH). Zbl. allg. Path. 117:99-105.

61. Schreiber, D., A. Lageman, and M. Geyer. 1972. Erzeugung von Dünndarmkarzinomen bei Kaninchen mit Methylnitrosoharnstoff. Zbl. allg. Path. 115:40-47.

62. Stavrou, D., K.G. Haglid, and W. Weidenbach. 1975. Experimentelle Induktion neurogener Tumoren beim Hund durch chronische parenterale Applikation von Methylnitrosoharnstoff. In: Proc. VII International Congress of Neuropathology, Budapest, 1974. Excerpta Medica: Amsterdam. pp. 425-431.

63. Denlinger, R.J., A. Koestner, and J.A. Swenberg. 1978. Neoplasms in purebred boxer dogs following long-term administration of N-methyl-N-nitrosourea. Cancer Res. 38:1711-1717.

64. Ivankovic, S., and H. Druckrey. 1968. Transplacentare Erzeugung maligner Tumoren des Nervensystems. I. Äthylnitrosoharnstoff (ÄNH) an BD IX-Ratten. Z. Krebsforsch. 71:320-360.

65. Vesselinovitch, S.D., M. Koka, K.V.N. Rao, N. Mihailovich, and J.M. Rice. 1977. Prenatal multicarcinogenesis by ethylnitrosourea in mice. Cancer Res. 37:1822-1828.

66. Diwan, B.A., and H. Meier. 1974. Strain- and age-dependent transplacental carcinogenesis by 1-ethyl-1-nitrosourea in inbred strains of mice. Cancer Res. 34:764-770.

67. Druckrey, H., C. Landschütz, and S. Ivankovic. 1970. Transplacentare Erzeugung maligner Tumoren des Nervensystems. II. Äthylnitrosoharnstoff an 10 genetisch definierten Rattenstämmen. Z. Krebsforsch. 73:371-386.

68. Rice, J.M. 1973. Biological behaviour of transplacentally induced tumours in mice. In: Transplacental Carcinogenesis. L. Tomatis and U. Mohr, eds. IARC Scientific Publications No. 4. International Agency for Research on Cancer: Lyons, France. pp. 71-83.

69. Kleihues, P., P.N. Magee, J. Austoker, D. Cox, and A.P. Mathias. 1973. Reaction of N-methyl-N-nitrosourea with DNA of neuronal and glial cells _in vivo_. FEBS Lett. 32:105-108.

70. Kleihues, P., and G.P. Margison. 1974. Carcinogenicity of N-methyl-N-nitrosourea: Possible role of excision repair of O^6-methylguanine from DNA. J. Natl. Cancer Inst. 53:1839-1841.

71. Pegg, A.E., and J.W. Nicoll. 1976. Nitrosamine carcinogenesis: The importance of the persistence in DNA of alkylated bases in the organotropism of tumour induction. In: Screening Tests in Chemical Carcinogenesis. R. Montesano, H. Bartsch, and L. Tomatis, eds. IARC Scientific Publications No. 12. International Agency for Research on Cancer: Lyons, France. pp. 571-592.

72. Bücheler, J., and P. Kleihues. 1977. Excision of O^6-methylguanine from DNA of various mouse tissues following a single injection of N-methyl-N-nitrosourea. Chem.-Biol. Interact. 16:325-333.

73. Slaga, T.J., A. Sivak, and R.K. Boutwell, eds. 1978. Mechanisms of Tumor Promotion and Cocarcinogenesis. In: Carcinogenesis, a Comprehensive Survey, Volume 2. Raven Press: New York. 588 pp.

DISCUSSION

Q.: I think one should be cautious in accepting some of these long-term carcinogenicity data as clear evidence for species specificity. There are limitations we must recognize. For example, you mentioned that the gerbil appears very resistant to the induction of brain tumors, but I notice that in some studies, there was a high incidence of local tumors in animals given methylnitrosourea. The absence of brain tumors might be due to reduced survival of the animals.

My other concern is uncertainty whether the animal is resistant to carcinogenicity in general or to an agent specifically; in the case of methylnitrosamine, you can get liver tumors after a single dose.

I think it's really dangerous to oversimplify this.

A.: Dr. Kleihues, who did the experiments, can tell you many of the gerbils lived well into their second year, and I don't think that their failure to yield tumors of the nervous system is due to premature death.

In the case of the hamster, as you pointed out, it is susceptible to hepatic carcinogenesis by other classes of compounds. The nitrosamines, of course, are metabolism-dependent, and that may bring other factors into play.

A.: I would like first to comment on this criticism by Dr. Montesano. I think with respect to the long-term and repeated treatment with methylnitrosourea, his criticism is correct; the experimenters found "local" tumors in the mid-ventral sebaceous gland and on the whole, these animals did not survive very long. They were killed at a fairly early time. I think we cannot prove whether the gerbil nervous system was indeed resistant under these circumstances. On the other hand, in our studies, gerbils were treated with single doses of alkylnitrosoureas; the animals survived for almost three years, and there has not been a single tumor of the nervous system, so far.

ORGAN AND SPECIES SPECIFICITY IN NICKEL SUBSULFIDE CARCINOGENESIS

F. William Sunderman, Jr.

Departments of Laboratory Medicine and Pharmacology, University of Connecticut School of Medicine, Farmington, Connecticut 06032

INTRODUCTION

The carcinogenic effects of metal compounds in man and experimental animals have been comprehensively reviewed in several recent articles and monographs (1-7). Four metals (arsenic, cadmium, chromium, and nickel) have been established as human carcinogens on the basis of epidemiological investigations, and compounds of 13 metals (aluminum, beryllium, cadmium, cobalt, chromium, copper, iron, manganese, nickel, lead, platinum, titanium, and zinc) have been shown to induce cancers in experimental animals (5-7). Nickel subsulfide (Ni_3S_2) is the most potent metallic carcinogen that has been identified to date; Ni_3S_2 has been evaluated for carcinogenicity much more thoroughly and extensively than any other metal compound (3,8-10). Consequently, Ni_3S_2 has been selected as the focal point for this exposition of organ and species specificity in metal carcinogenesis.

During the past decade, several carcinogenicity studies of Ni_3S_2 have been performed in the author's laboratory. These tests, involving more than a thousand animals, have included several species and strains of rodents, diverse routes of administration, and various dosages. The experiments have been conducted with similar protocols, and the test animals have been maintained under uniform conditions. Many of these experiments have been published (11-20), but several investigations (chiefly those with negative outcomes) have not been reported until now. In the present article, every carcinogenesis test of Ni_3S_2 performed in the author's laboratory has been reexamined and tabulated in a consistent fashion to facilitate deductions about organ and species specificity.

MATERIALS AND METHODS

Nickel subsulfide dust (αNi_3S_2, median particle diameter <2 µm, Ni = 73.4%, S = 25.6%) was donated by Louis Renzoni, Sc.D., and J. Stuart Warner, Ph.D., of INCO Ltd., Toronto, Canada. Chemical and physical properties of the Ni_3S_2 dust and criteria of its purity have been previously described (13,15). The experimental animals were rats of the Fischer 344, Wistar-Lewis, and Long-Evans Hooded strains (Charles River Breeding Laboratories, Inc., North Wilmington, MA) and NIH Black strain (National Cancer Institute, Bethesda, MD); Syrian golden hamsters of the LVG/LAK strain (Charles River Breeding Laboratories, Inc.); mice of the DBA/2 and C57BL/6 strains (Charles River Breeding Laboratories, Inc.); and rabbits of the albino New Zealand strain (Charles River Breeding Laboratories, Inc.). The rats and rabbits were housed in stainless-steel mesh cages, and the hamsters and mice were housed in polypropylene cages. The animals were given tap water and laboratory chows (Ralston-Purina Co., St. Louis, MO) *ad libitum*. The rabbit diet was supplemented with fresh vegetables.

Except for the transplacental and intraocular carcinogenesis tests, the animals were two to three months old when the experiments were initiated. In the transplacental carcinogenesis test, Ni_3S_2 was administered to pregnant Fischer rats by intramuscular injection (20 mg/rat) on the sixth day of gestation. In the intraocular carcinogenesis test, Ni_3S_2 was injected into the vitreous cavity of the right eye of Fischer rats (0.5 mg/rat) when approximately one month old.

The vehicle for injections varied. For intramuscular injections in rats, mice, and rabbits, the vehicle was 0.1 to 0.5 ml penicillin G procaine suspension (Wycillin, 300,000 units/ml) (Wyeth Laboratories, Inc., Philadelphia, PA). The vehicle for intrarenal, intrahepatic, intratesticular, and intraocular injections in rats and for intramuscular and intratesticular injections in hamsters was 0.02 to 0.5 ml sterile saline (sodium chloride solution, 0.15 mol/l). The vehicle for injections into the submaxillary gland of rats and for applications of Ni_3S_2 onto the cheek pouches of hamsters was glycerol (certified reagent) (Fisher Scientific Co., Pittsburgh, PA).

Techniques for intramuscular, intrarenal, intrahepatic, and intraocular injections of single doses of Ni_3S_2 have been described elsewhere (13,15-17,20). Injection of Ni_3S_2 (2.5 mg in 0.2 ml glycerol) into the right submaxillary gland of Fischer rats was performed after surgical exposure of the gland under ether anesthesia. Applications of Ni_3S_2 (2 mg in 0.2 ml glycerol or 2.5 mg in 0.1 ml glycerol) onto the mucosa of hamster cheek pouches was performed with a camel's hair brush, without anesthesia (21). Intratracheal insufflation of Ni_3S_2 (1, 2, 5, or 10 mg in 0.1 or 0.2 ml sterile saline) was performed in hamsters by means of a curved, smooth-tipped canula (#18 gauge) during ether anesthesia.

Groups of control animals were included in each experiment, except for the study of submaxillary gland injections in rats, the comparison of intrarenal injections of Ni_3S_2 in four rat strains, and the study of intramuscular injections in rabbits. Control animals received injections or treatments with the vehicle, according to identical schedules.

Mice, rats, hamsters, and rabbits were housed in separate animal rooms and isolated from other experimental animals during the carcinogenesis tests. Animals that died within two months were excluded from computations of tumor incidences and mortality ratios. Animals were weighed and examined at weekly or biweekly intervals. The animals either died spontaneously or were killed when they had become so cachectic that they could not move around in their cages, and hence could not obtain food or water. Most experiments were terminated two years after the initial administration of the test compound. In the intratesticular carcinogenesis experiment in rats, controls were killed at 20 months, coincident with the death of the last Ni_3S_2-treated rat. In the intraocular carcinogenesis experiment, control rats and the sole surviving Ni_3S_2-treated rat were killed 10 months after the intraocular injection. In the transplacental carcinogenesis study in rats, surviving progeny of Ni_3S_2-treated and control dams were killed at 26 months of age. The intramuscular carcinogenesis study in rabbits was terminated at 72 months.

Except for rare instances when rats were cannibalized, all animals were autopsied. Tissue specimens were fixed in 10% neutral buffered formalin, and paraffin-embedded sections were stained with hematoxylin and eosin for examination by light microscopy. In most experiments, selected tumors were diced in 4% cacodylate-buffered glutaraldehyde and post-fixed in cacodylate-buffered 2% osmium tetroxide. The tissues were embedded in epoxy resin for ultrathin sectioning, and the sections were stained with lead citrate and uranyl acetate. Electron microscopy was performed with a Phillips 300 microscope at 6 kV.

Statistical tests of null hypotheses for tumor incidences were performed by the χ^2 test with Yates' correction, if the total sample size was >30, or by Fischer's exact test, if the total sample size was <30 (22). Median survival periods in control and Ni_3S_2-treated groups were compared by the Brown-Mood median test (22). Two-tailed estimates of probability were computed.

RESULTS

Carcinogenesis Tests in Rats

Tests of the carcinogenicity of Ni_3S_2 in male Fischer rats are summarized in Tables 1 and 2. Tumor incidences at the site of intramuscular injection of Ni_3S_2 ranged from 24% at a dose of 0.6 mg/rat to 100% at a dose of 20 mg/rat. The incidences of local sarcomas 14 months after intramuscular injections were linearly related to the reciprocals of Ni_3S_2 dosages (Figure 1). As indicated in Table 2, tumors at the injection site were mostly rhabdomyosarcomas, fibrosarcomas, or undifferentiated sarcomas. Distant mestastases were found in 43% of these tumor-bearing rats. In order of decreasing frequency, the sites of the metastases were: retroperitoneal and mediastinal lymph nodes, lung, kidney, heart, liver, spleen, bone, salivary gland, adrenal gland, and testis.

After intrarenal injection of Ni_3S_2, renal tumors developed only at doses of 5 and 10 mg/rat (28 and 75% incidences, respectively). The renal neoplasms included spindle cell tumors (probably fibrosarcomas) and mixed cell and undifferentiated cell tumors (probably carcinomas). Since the histological findings were ambiguous, these renal tumors could not be classified definitely as sarcomas or carcinomas (15).

No local tumors developed after a 5-mg/rat intrahepatic injection of Ni_3S_2; one hepatic tumor developed at a dose of 10 mg/rat. This hepatic tumor was an adenocarcinoma that arose at the injection site and metastasized to lung, pancreas, spleen, and retroperitoneal lymph nodes.

After intratesticular injection of Ni_3S_2 at a dose of 10 mg/rat, malignant tumors (fibrosarcomas, rhabdomyosarcomas, and malignant fibrous histiocytomas) developed in the injected testes of 84% of the rats. Metastases to lung, kidney, or abdominal lymph nodes were found in 25% of tumor-bearing rats.

Malignant tumors of the eye developed in 93% of the rats within eight months after a 0.5-mg/rat intraocular injection of Ni_3S_2. One third of the injected eyes of Ni_3S_2-treated rats contained multiple primary tumors. The ocular neoplasms included malignant melanomas, retinoblastomas, gliomas, a phakocarcinoma, and unclassified malignant tumors. Extraocular invasion was seen in three rats with melanomas; metastases to lung and brain were found in one rat with a melanoma. After injection of Ni_3S_2 into the submaxillary gland at a dose of 2.5 mg/rat, no tumors developed at the injection site.

Based upon the data in Table 1, the relative susceptibilities of Fischer rat organs to induction of neoplasms following a single

Table 1. Carcinogenicity of Ni_3S_2 in Male Fischer Rats.

Route of Single Injection	Dose (mg/rat)	Rats With Local Tumors	Median Tumor Latent Period (mo)	Tumors With Distant Metastases	Survivors at End of Study	Median Survival Period (mo)
Intramuscular	0	0/142[a]			69/142	23
	0.6	7/29[a]	11	4/7	7/29	14
	1.2	23/30[a]	10	5/23	5/30[b]	15
	2.5	105/112[a]	10	37/105	2/112[a]	12[c]
	5.0	35/38[a]	7	17/35	1/38[a]	9[a]
	10.0	22/23[a]	6	27/22	0/23[a]	7[a]
	20.0	9/9[a]	7	6/9	0/9[a]	8[a]
Intrarenal	0	0/35			26/35	>24
	0.6	0/11			10/11	>24
	1.2	0/12			7/11	>24
	2.5	0/12			8/12	>24
	5.0	5/18[c]	11	1/5	9/18[b]	23
	10.0	18/24[a]	9	13/18	2/24[a]	14[a]
Intrahepatic	0	0/6			1/6	17
	5.0	0/13			3/13	18
	10.0	1/6	13	1/1	0/6	13
Intratesticular	0	0/18			10/18	18
	10.0	16/19[a]	10	4/16	0/19[c]	11[c]
Intraocular	0	0/11			d	
	0.5	14/15[a]	8	1/14	d	
Submaxillary gland	2.5	0/11			3/11	17

[a] $p < 0.001$ versus corresponding controls.
[b] $p < 0.05$ versus corresponding controls.
[c] $p < 0.01$ versus corresponding controls.
[d] The intraocular carcinogenesis study was terminated at 10 months.

Table 2. Classification of Tumors Induced by Ni_3S_2 in the Male Fischer Rats.

Route of Single Injectionn	Histologic Type	Number of Tumors	Percent of Total
Intramuscular	Rhabdomyosarcoma	104	52
	Fibrosarcoma	45	22
	Undifferentiated sarcoma	45	22
	Liposarcoma	5	2
	Neurofibrosarcoma	1	<1
	Hemangiosarcoma	1	<1
Intrarenal	Spindle cell tumor	9	39
	Mixed cell tumor	8	35
	Undifferentiated cell tumor	4	17
	Rhabdomyosarcoma	2	9
Intrahepatic	Hepatocarcinoma	1	100
Intratesticular	Fibrosarcoma	10	63
	Rhabdomyosarcoma	3	19
	Malignant fibrous histiocytoma	3	19
Intraocular[a]	Melanoma	11	50
	Retinoblastoma	4	18
	Glioma	3	14
	Unclassified malignant tumor	3	14
	Phakocarcinoma	1	4

[a]Twenty-two ocular tumors were found in 14 rats.

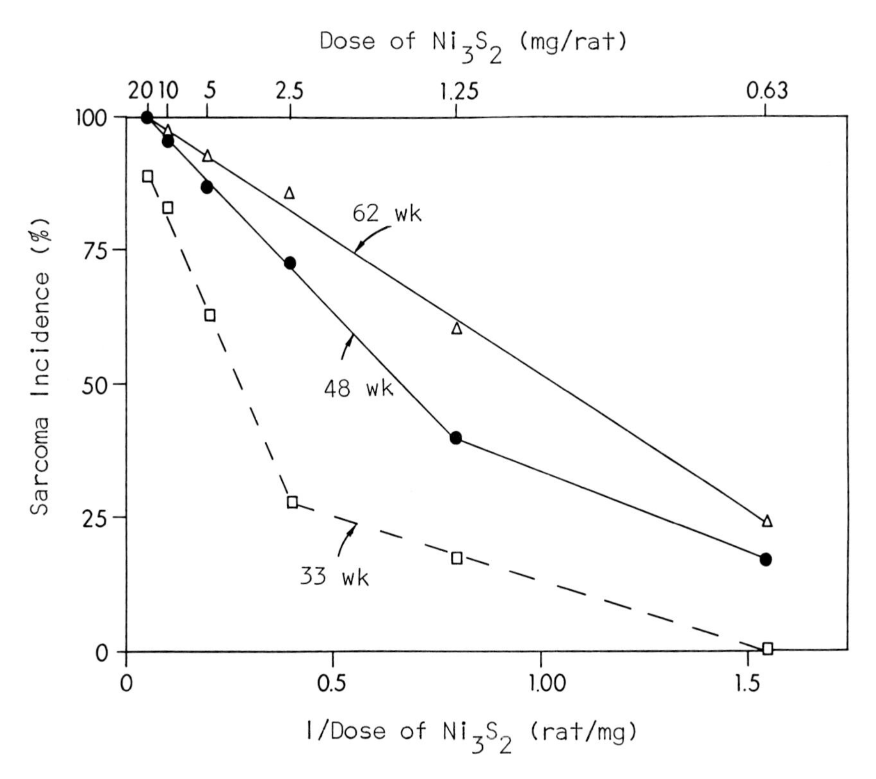

Figure 1. Reciprocal plot of sarcoma incidences at specific intervals following intramuscular injection of Ni_3S_2 in Fischer rats. The numbers of rats tested at each dosage are given in Table 1.

injection of Ni_3S_2 are ranked as follows: eye > muscle > testis ≃ kidney > liver. The submaxillary gland is omitted from this ranking.

Transplacental carcinogenicity of Ni_3S_2 was tested by intramuscular administration of Ni_3S_2 (20 mg/rat) to pregnant dams on the sixth day of gestation; control dams received a similar injection of the vehicle. By age 26 months, two malignant and two benign tumors developed in progeny of Ni_3S_2-treated dams, compared to three malignant and two benign tumors in progeny of control dams (Table 3). Hence, administration of Ni_3S_2 to pregnant rats had no significant effect upon tumor incidence in the progency (19).

Table 3. Negative Test for Transplacental Carcinogenicity of Ni_3S_2 in Fischer Rats.

Category	Sex[a]	Dose[b] (mg/dam)	Tumor Bearing Progeny	Median Tumor Latent Period (mo)	Tumors With Distant Metastases	Survivors at End of Study	Median Survival Period (mo)
Progeny of control dams	M	0	1/29[c]	26	0/1	2/29	19
	F	0	4/24[d]	25	0/4	6/24	23
	M+F	0	5/53	25	0/5	8/53	20
Progeny of Ni_3S_2-treated	M	20	0/17			2/17	21
	F	20	4/33[e]	25	1/4	5/33	24
	M+F	20	4/50	25	1/4	7/50	23

[a]M = male; F = female.
[b]Single intramuscular injections of 0 or 20 mg Ni_3S_2 in groups of eight pregnant dams on the sixth day of gestation.
[c]Subcutaneous neurofibroma.
[d]Myelogenous leukemia; uterine endometrial carcinoma; basal cell carcinoma of skin; uterine endometrial polyp.
[e]Pancreatic adenocarcinoma; myelogenous leukemia; pulmonary bronchial adenoma; uterine endometrial polyp.

Table 4 shows the incidences of renal cancer in four rat strains following a 5-mg/rat intrarenal injection of Ni_3S_2. No renal tumors developed in Long-Evans Hooded rats; the tumor incidences in Fischer, NIH Black, and Wistar-Lewis rats were 29, 50, and 64%, respectively. Based upon the data in Table 4, the relative susceptibilities of rat strains to induction of renal neoplasms following intrarenal injection of Ni_3S_2 are ranked as follows: Wistar-Lewis > NIH Black > Fischer > Long-Evans Hooded. No significant differences occurred in tumor incidences of male versus female rats of any strain.

Carcinogenesis Tests in Hamsters

Carcinogenesis tests of Ni_3S_2 in male Syrian hamsters are summarized in Table 5. Dose-response relationships were observed for induction of local sarcomas following administration of Ni_3S_2 to hamsters by intramuscular and intratesticular injections. The tumor incidences in hamsters were lower than the corresponding tumor incidences in Fischer rats following intramuscular or intratesticular injections of Ni_3S_2. Intratracheal administration of Ni_3S_2 at a dose of 2.5 mg/hamster for four successive months (total dose = 10 mg/hamster) did not induce any tumors of the respiratory tract. Intratracheal administration of Ni_3S_2 at a dose of 2 mg/hamster for 18 successive weeks (total dose = 36 mg/hamster) caused excessive mortality. The hamsters in the Ni_3S_2-treated group all died within 7 months; the hamsters in the control group all died within 21 months. No neoplasms of the respiratory tract or other organs were found in the Ni_3S_2-treated or control hamsters.

To ascertain whether topical or oral administration of Ni_3S_2 might induce cancers, Ni_3S_2 in glycerol was painted onto the buccal pouch mucosa of Syrian hamsters three times a week for 18 or 36 weeks, according to the dosage schedules given in Table 5. No tumors were found in the buccal pouch, oral cavity, or gastrointestinal tract of Ni_3S_2-treated or control hamsters. A pleural mesothelioma developed in one of the Ni_3S_2-treated hamsters (total dose = 540 mg/hamster), and a fibrosarcoma of the leg developed in one of the control hamsters (18-week treatment group). Squamous cell carcinomas of the buccal pouch developed in all 4 hamsters in a positive control group (not shown in Table 5) that received buccal pouch applications of 1 mg 7,12-dimethylbenz[*a*]anthracene in glycerol three times a week for 18 weeks (total dose = 54 mg/hamster).

Table 4. Carcinogenicity of Ni_3S_2 After a Single Intrarenal Injection in Four Rat Strains.

Rat Strain	Sex[a]	Dose (mg/rat)	Rats With Renal Tumors	Median Tumor Latent Period (mo)	Tumors With Distant Metastases	Survivors at End of Study	Median Survival Period (mo)
Long-Evans	M	5	0/6			4/6	>24
	F	5	0/6			4/6	>24
	M+F	5	0/12			8/12	>24
Fischer	M	5	5/18	11	1/5	9/18	23
	F	5	4/13	17	1/4	3/13	22
	M+F	5	9/31[b]	13	2/9	12/32	23
NIH Black	M	5	3/6	12	2/3	1/6	11
	F	5	3/6	10	3/3	3/6	12
	M+F	5	6/12[c]	11	5/6	4/12	11[b]
Wistar-Lewis	M	5	2/5	10	2/2	0/5	12
	F	5	5/6[c]	17	3/5	1/6	13
	M+F	5	7/11[c]	14	5/7	1/11[c]	13[b]

[a] M= male; F = female.
[b] $p < 0.05$ versus corresponding value for Long-Evans Hooded rats.
[c] $p < 0.01$ versus corresponding value for Long-Evans Hooded rats.

Table 5. Carcinogenicity of Ni_3S_2 in Male Syrian Hamsters.

Route of Administration	Total Dose (mg/hamsters)	Hamsters With Local Tumors	Median Tumor Latent Period (mo)	Tumors With Distant Metastases	Survivors at End of Study	Median Survival Period (mo)
Intramuscular[a]	0	0/14			1/14	16
	5	4/15	10	2/4	4/15	15
	10	12/17[b]	11	8/12	0/17	12
Intratesticular[a]	0	0/10			1/10	19
	2.5	1/10	17	0/1	2/10	20
	10	4/13	12	0/4	0/13	12
Intratracheal	0[c]	0/15			3/15	14
	10[c]	0/12			4/12	14
	0[d]	0/21			0/21	9
	36d	0/15			0/15	4[b]
Buccal pouch	0[e]	0/6			0/6	15
	54[e]	0/6			0/6	15
	108[e]	0/7			2/7	19
	0[f]	0/15			4/15	19
	540[f]	0/15			4/15	19
	1080[f]	0/13			1/13	17

[a]Single injection.
[b]$p < 0.05$ versus corresponding controls.
[c]Monthly intratracheal insufflations of 0 or 2.5 mg Ni_3S_2 in 0.2 ml NaCl vehicle for 4 months.
[d]Weekly intratracheal insufflations of 0 or 2 mg Ni_3S_2 in 0.1 ml NaCl vehicle for 18 weeks.
[e]Thrice-weekly buccal pouch applications of 0, 1, or 2 mg Ni_3S_2 in 0.1 ml glycerol for 18 weeks.
[f]Thrice-weekly buccal pouch applications of 0, 5, or 10 mg Ni_3S_2 in 0.1 ml glycerol for 36 weeks.

Carcinogenesis Tests in Mice

Results of intramuscular carcinogenesis tests of Ni_3S_2 in DBA/2 and C57BL/6 strains of mice are listed in Table 6. Administration of a 2.5-mg/mouse dose of Ni_3S_2 induced local sarcomas in 60% of DBA/2 mice and 50% of C57BL/6 mice.

Carcinogenesis Tests in Rabbits

Ni_3S_2 was administered to the hind legs of four male New Zealand albino rabbits (two months old) by bilateral intramuscular injections (25 mg/site, total dose = 50 mg/rabbit). The rabbits died after 16, 49, 69, and 72 months. No tumors were found at the injection sites or elsewhere.

DISCUSSION

Dose-Response Relationships

Establishment of dose-response relationships is a prerequisite for inferences about organ and species susceptibilities to Ni_3S_2 carcinogenesis. Gilman (23) observed direct correlation between the incidence of sarcomas in Fischer rats and the intramuscular dose of Ni_3S_2 (ranging from 0.25 to 10 mg/site). In Gilman's study, the dose-response curve levels off at approximately 80% tumor incidence when Ni_3S_2 doses exceed 10 mg/site (23). The present report documents dose-response relationships for tumor induction by Ni_3S_2 following intramuscular and intrarenal injections in Fischer rats and intramuscular and intratesticular injections in Syrian hamsters.

Relative Susceptibilities of Animal Species

Gilman (24) reported that Wistar rats are more susceptible than C3H or Swiss mice to induction of local sarcomas following intramuscular injection of Ni_3S_2. Hildebrand and coworkers (25-27) observed rhabdomyosarcomas and leiomyosarcomas in Wistar rats and albino rabbits after intramuscular injection of Ni_3S_2 (20 mg/rat and 80 mg/rabbit), but they did not furnish information about the numbers of experimental animals or the tumor incidences. Jasmin and coworkers (28,29) induced renal cancers in Sprague-Dawley and Fischer rats by intrarenal injection of Ni_3S_2; they were unsuccessful in similar attempts to induce renal tumors in mice, hamsters, or rabbits. Based upon the present report and these observations from other laboratories, no absolute species specificity for Ni_3S_2 carcinogenesis appears to exist, albeit rats are more susceptible than mice, hamsters, or rabbits.

Table 6. Carcinogenicity of Ni_3S_2 After a Single Intramuscular Injection in Two Mouse Strains.

Mouse Strain	Sex[a]	Dose (mg/mouse)	Mice With Local Tumors	Median Tumors Latent Period (mo)	Tumors With Distant Metastases	Survivors at End of Study	Median Survival Period (mo)
DBA/2	M	0	0/5			0/5	19
	F	0	0/4			0/4	20
	M+F	0	0/9			0/9	19
	M	2.5	1/4	14	0/1	0/4	12
	F	2.5	5/6	13	0/5	0/6	14
	M+F	2.5	6/10[b]	13	0/6	0/10	13
C57BL/6	M	0	0/5			0/5	21
	F	0	0/4			0/4	17
	M+F	0	0/9			0/9	19
	M	2.5	2/5	13	0/2	0/5	20
	F	2.5	3/5	14	0/3	0/5	14
	M+F	2.5	5/10[c]	14	0/5	0/10	17

[a] M = male; F = female.
[b] $p < 0.01$ versus corresponding controls.
[c] $p < 0.05$ versus corresponding controls.

Relative Susceptibilities of Rat Strains

Daniel (30) compared the incidences of sarcomas in Long-Evans Hooded and NIH Black rats after bilateral intramuscular injections of Ni_3S_2 at a dose of 20 mg/site. Within 14 months, tumors occurred at one or both injection sites in 14/23 (61%) of NIH Black rats, compared to 28/28 (100%) of Long-Evans Hooded rats. Yamashiro et al. (31) compared the incidences of sarcomas in Long-Evans Hooded and Fischer rats following a single 10-mg/rat intramuscular injection of Ni_3S_2. Within 10 months, the proportion of tumor-bearing rats was 11/18 (61%) in the Long-Evans Hooded strain compared to 59/63 (94%) in the Fischer strain. The present report indicates the following ranking of four rat strains in susceptibility to induction of renal neoplasms after intrarenal injection of Ni_3S_2: Wistar-Lewis > NIH Black > Fischer > Long-Evans Hooded. The results reported by Daniel (30), Yamashiro et al. (31), and the present author should not be compared directly, because different rat substrains were tested and different experimental conditions prevailed. Nonetheless, these studies indicate that significant differences are encountered in the susceptibilities of rat strains to Ni_3S_2 carcinogenesis.

Influence of Routes of Administration

The present report suggests the following ranking for susceptibilities of organs of Fischer rats to tumor induction following direct injection of Ni_3S_2: eye > muscle > testis ≈ kidney > liver. These findings are consistent with observations of Jasmin and coworkers (28,29) that Fischer and Sprague-Dawley rats are more susceptible to Ni_3S_2 induction of tumors in muscle than in the kidney. Jasmin and Solymoss (29) did not observe any hepatic tumors in eight rats after intrahepatic injection of Ni_3S_2 (10 mg/rat). In a group of 20 rats that received intravenous injections of Ni_3S_2 (10 mg/rat), Jasmin and Solymoss (29) found one rat with myeloid leukemia and eight rats with mammary carcinomas or adenomas; no tumors were observed in an unspecified number of controls.

Ottolenghi et al. (32) exposed 226 Fischer rats to inhalation of Ni_3S_2 (6 h/day, 5 days/week for 72 weeks) at an average atmospheric concentration of 1 mg/m^3. A control group of 241 rats was exposed to filtered room air under the same conditions. Within two years after initiation of the experiment, 14 malignant lung tumors (10 adenocarcinomas, 3 squamous cell carcinomas, and 1 fibrosarcoma) were found in the Ni_3S_2-exposed rats, compared to 1 malignant lung tumor (an adenocarcinoma) in the controls. Yarita and Nettesheim (33) confirmed the carcinogenicity of Ni_3S_2 for respiratory tract mucosa by injecting Ni_3S_2 into heterotopic tracheal transplants in Fischer rats. At a dose of 1 mg

Ni_3S_2/trachea, the carcinoma incidence was 10%, and the sarcoma incidence was 10%. When the dose of Ni_3S_2 was increased to 3 mg/trachea, the carcinoma incidence fell to 1.5%, and the sarcoma incidence increased to 67%. The much higher proportion of sarcomas at the dose of 3 mg/trachea may be attributed to Ni_3S_2 toxicity for tracheal epithelial cells, manifested by widespread epithelial atrophy and necrosis (33).

The observations cited demonstrate that most organs of rats are susceptible to Ni_3S_2 carcinogenesis following direct exposure by injection or inhalation, and that the intraocular and intramuscular routes of administration yield the highest tumor incidences. Administration of Ni_3S_2 to Syrian hamsters by buccal pouch painting did not induce any tumors of the buccal pouch, oral cavity, or gastrointestinal tract. This finding suggests that Ni_3S_2 may not be carcinogenic by the oral route of administration. Chronic feeding tests of Ni_3S_2 in mice, rats, and hamsters are needed to confirm or refute this speculation.

Morphologic Transformation in Tissue Culture

DiPaolo and Casto (34) incubated Syrian hamster fetal cells in tissue culture media that contained Ni_3S_2 in concentrations of 0 (control), 1, 2.5, or 5 mg/l. After eight days, the percentages of colonies that showed morphological transformation were 0.0, 1.5, 5.2, and 11.5, respectively. Costa et al. (35) incubated Syrian hamster fetal cells *in vitro* for two days in tissue culture media that contained Ni_3S_2 in concentrations of 0 (control), 0.1, 1, or 5 mg/l. After the cells were replanted in fresh media and incubated for two weeks, the percentages of colonies that showed morphological transformation were 0.1, 4.2, 6.8, and 8.9, respectively. Five clones of the Ni_3S_2-transformed cells were administered to nude mice by subcutaneous injection; undifferentiated sarcomas developed in 26/27 (96%) of the nude mice at the injection site (35). Costa and Mollenhauer (36) reported a correlation between the uptake of Ni_3S_2 particles by Syrian hamster fetal cells *in vitro* and the proportion of colonies that developed morphological transformation. The findings of DiPaolo and Casto (34) and Costa et al. (35) are indicative of *in vitro* carcinogenicity of Ni_3S_2 for Syrian hamster fetal cells. Such studies have not been performed with Ni_3S_2 in fetal cells from other species.

SUMMARY AND CONCLUSIONS

In summary, dose-response relationships have been demonstrated for Ni_3S_2 carcinogenesis in rats and hamsters and for transformation of Syrian hamster fetal cells by Ni_3S_2 *in vitro*.

Absolute species specificity has not been observed in Ni_3S_2 carcinogenesis, although rats are apparently more susceptible than mice, hamsters, or rabbits. Also, significant variations have been reported in susceptibilities of rat strains to Ni_3S_2 carcinogenesis. Most organs of rats have been found to be susceptible to Ni_3S_2 carcinogenesis following direct exposure by injection or inhalation; intraocular and intramuscular routes of administration have yielded the highest tumor incidences. Finally, an experiment in hamsters has indicated that Ni_3S_2 may be noncarcinogenic by the oral route; further studies are needed to confirm or refute this speculation. For discussions of molecular mechanisms that may be involved in carcinogenesis by Ni_3S_2 and other nickel compounds, readers are referred to recent review articles (8-10).

ACKNOWLEDGMENTS

The author is grateful to the pathologists Daniel M. Albert, M.D., Ivan Damjanov, M.D., Peter J. Goldblatt, M.D., Bernard Gondos, M.D., Thomas J. Lau, M.D., Ronald M. Maenza, M.D., Kilmer S. McCully, M.D., Arun M. Pradhan, M.D., and Sheldon Taubman, M.D. and to the research assistants Patricia R. Allpass, Leopold Delaney, John M. Mitchell, Marilyn C. Reid, and Lois A. Rinehimer who participated in the carcinogenesis studies that are included in this report.

This research was supported by grant no. EY-03140 from the U.S. Department of Energy and grant no. ES-01337 from the National Institute of Environmental Health Sciences.

REFERENCES

1. Flessel, C.P., A. Furst, and S.B. Radding. 1980. A comparison of carcinogenic metals. In: Metal Ions in Biological Systems, Volume 10. H. Sigel, Ed. Marcel Dekker, Inc.: New York. pp. 23-54.

2. Kazantis, G., and L.J. Lilly. 1979. Mutagenic and carcinogenic effects of metals. In: Handbook on the Toxicology of Metals. L. Friberg, G.F. Nordberg, and V.B. Vouk, eds. Elsevier/North Holland Biomedical Press: New York and Amsterdam. pp. 237-272.

3. Sunderman, F.W., Jr. 1977. Metal carcinogenesis. In: Advances in Modern Toxicology, Volume 2. R.A. Goyer and M.A. Mehlman, eds. Hemisphere Publishing Corp.: Washington, DC. pp. 257-295.

4. Sunderman, F.W., Jr. 1978. Carcinogenic effects of metals. Fed. Proc. 37:40-46.

5. Sunderman, F.W., Jr. 1979. Carcinogenicity and anti-carcinogenicity of metal compounds. In: Environmental Carcinogenesis. P. Emmelot and E. Kriek, eds. Elsevier/North Holland Press: New York and Amsterdam. pp. 165-192.

6. IARC Monographs on the Evaluation of the Carcinogenic Risk of Chemicals to Humans: Some Metals and Metal Compounds (Arsenic, Beryllium, Chromium, and Lead), Volume 23. 1980. International Agency for Research on Cancer: Lyons, France. pp. 39-415.

7. IARC Monographs on the Evaluation of the Carcinogenic Risk of Chemicals to Man: Cadmium and Nickel. Volume 11. 1976. International Agency for Research on Cancer: Lyons, France. pp. 39-112.

8. Sunderman, F.W., Jr. 1979. Mechanisms of metal carcinogenesis. Biol. Trace Element Res. 1:63-86.

9. Sunderman, F.W., Jr. 1981. Recent research on nickel carcinogenesis. Environ. Hlth. Perspect. 40:131-144.

10. Furst, A., and S.B. Radding. 1980. An update on nickel carcinogenesis. In: Nickel in the Environment. J.O. Nriagu, ed. Wiley-Interscience Publishing Co.: New York. pp. 585-600.

11. Maenza, R.M., A.M. Pradhan, and F.S. Sunderman, Jr. 1971. Rapid induction of sarcomas in rats by combination of nickel sulfide and 3,4-benzopyrene. Cancer Res. 31:2067-2071.

12. Sunderman. F.W., Jr., T.J. Lau, and L.J. Cralley. 1974. Inhibitory effect of manganese upon muscle tumorigenesis by nickel sulfide. Cancer Res. 34:92-95.

13. Sunderman, F.W., Jr., K.S. Kasprzak, T.J. Lau, P.P. Minghetti, R.M. Maenza, N. Becker, C. Onkelinx, and P.J. Goldblatt. 1976. Effects of manganese on carcinogenicity and metabolism of nickel subsulfide. Cancer Res. 36:1790-1800.

14. Sunderman, F.W., Jr., and R.M. Maenza. 1976. Comparisons of carcinogenicities of nickel compounds in rats. Res. Comm. Chem. Pathol. Pharmacol. 14:319-330.

15. Damjanov, I., F.W. Sunderman, Jr., J.M. Mitchell, and P.R. Allpass. 1978. Induction of testicular sarcomas in Fischer rats by intratesticular injection of nickel subsulfide. Cancer Res. 38:268-276.

16. Sunderman, F.W., Jr., R.M. Maenza, P.R. Allpass, J.M. Mitchell, I. Damjanov, and P.J. Goldblatt. 1978. Carcinogenicity of nickel subsulfide in Fischer rats and Syrian hamsters after administration by various routes. In: Inorganic and Nutritional Aspects of Cancer. G.N. Schrauzer, ed. Plenum Publishing Corp.: New York. pp. 57-67.

17. Sunderman, F.W., Jr., R.M. Maenza, S.M. Hopfer, J.M. Mitchell, P.R. Allpass, and I. Damjanov. 1979. Induction of renal cancers in rats by intrarenal injection of nickel subsulfide. J. Environ. Pathol. Toxicol. 2:1511-1527.

18. Sunderman, F.W., Jr., E.A. Trudeau, Jr., E. Horak, J.M. Mitchell, and P.R. Allpass. 1979. Serum ceruloplasmin concentrations in rats with primary and transplanted sarcomas induced by nickel subsulfide. Ann. Clin. Lab. Sci. 9:60-67.

19. Sunderman, F.W., Jr., K.S. McCully, and L.A. Rinehimer. 1981. Negative test for transplacental carcinogenicity of nickel subsulfide in Fischer rats. Res. Comm. Chem. Pathol. Pharmacol. 31:555-564.

20. Albert, D.M., J.R. Gonder, J. Papale, J.L. Craft, H.G. Dohlman, M.D. Reid, and F.W. Sunderman, Jr. 1980. Induction of ocular neoplasms in Fischer rats by intraocular injection of nickel subsulfide. In: Nickel Toxicology. S.S. Brown and F.W. Sunderman, Jr., eds. Academic Press: New York. pp. 55-58.

21. Morris, A.L. 1961. Factors influencing experimental carcinogenesis in the hamster cheek pouch. J. Dental Res. 40:3-15.

22. Siegel, S. 1956. Nonparametric Statistics for the Behavioral Sciences. McGraw-Hill Book Company: New York. pp. 95-116.

23. Gilman, J.P.W. 1965. Muscle tumourigenesis. Proceedings of the Sixth Canadian Cancer Research Conference. Pergamon Press: Oxford, England. pp. 209-223.

24. Gilman, J.P.W. 1962. Metal carcinogenesis II. A study on the carcinogenic activity of cobalt, copper, iron, and nickel compounds. Cancer Res. 22:158-165.

25. Hildebrand, H.F., and G. Biserte. 1979. Nickel subsulfide-induced leiomyosarcoma in rabbit white skeletal muscle. Cancer 43:1358-1374.

26. Hildebrand, H.F., and G. Biserte. 1979. Cylindrical laminated bodies in nickel subsulfide-induced rhabdomyosarcoma in rabbits. Eur. J. Cell Biol. 19:276-280.

27. Hildebrand, H.F., J-P. Kerckaert, and G. Biserte. 1980. Tumoral myosins of Ni_3S_2-induced rhabdomyosarcomas in rat and rabbit: Comparative studies with adult and fetal myosins of skeletal muscle. Eur. J. Cell. Biol. 20:240-248.

28. Jasmin, G., and J.L. Riopelle. 1976. Renal carcinomas and erythrocytosis in rats following intrarenal injection of nickel subsulfide. Lab. Invest. 35:71-78.

29. Jasmin, G., and B. Solymoss. 1978. The topical effects of nickel subsulfide on renal parenchyma. In: Inorganic and Nutritional Aspects of Cancer. G.N. Schrauzer, ed. Plenum Press: New York. pp. 69-83.

30. Daniel, M.R. 1966. Strain differences in the response of rats to the injection of nickel sulphide. Brit. J. Cancer. 20:886-895.

31. Yamashiro, S., J.P.W. Gilman, T.J. Holland, and H.M. Abandowitz. 1980. Nickel sulphide-induced rhabdomyosarcomata in rats. Acta Pathol. Jap. 30:9-22.

32. Ottolenghi, A.D., J.K. Haseman, W.W. Payne, H.L. Falk, and H.N. MacFarland. 1975. Inhalation studies of nickel sulfide in pulmonary carcinogenesis of rats. J. Natl. Cancer Inst. 54:1165-1172.

33. Yarita, T., and P. Nettesheim. 1978. Carcinogenicity of nickel subsulfide for respiratory tract mucosa. Cancer Res. 38:3140-3145.

34. DiPaolo, J.A., and B.C. Casto. 1979. Quantitative studies of _in vitro_ morphological transformation of Syrian hamster cells by inorganic metal salts. Cancer Res. 39:1008-1013.

35. Costa, M., J.S. Nye, F.W. Sunderman, Jr., P.R. Allpass, and B. Gondos. 1979. Induction of sarcomas in nude mice by implantation of Syrian hamster fetal cells exposed _in vitro_ to nickel subsulfide. Cancer Res. 39:3591-3597.

36. Costa, M., and H.H. Mollenhauer. 1980. Phagocytosis of nickel subsulfide particles during the early stages of neoplastic transformation in tissue culture. Cancer Res. 40:2688-2694.

DISCUSSION

Q.: Your focus has been on the nickel in Ni_3S_2; yet you showed experiments where this substance was present and yet was not able to produce tumors. Has there been a corresponding study of other nickel salts to see whether or not tumor formation is subsulfide-dependent rather than nickel-dependent?

A.: Yes, the best control is NiS, nickel sulfide, which has the same constituents as the Ni_3S_2. Amorphous nickel sulfide, itself, has not produced any. Nickel metal, by itself, produces a small incidence of tumors.

Q.: What about other subsulfides which might have a different solubility?

A.: There are eight different nickel sulfides. Is that what you were referring to?

Q.: No; I meant subsulfides of other metals.

A.: We are studying subsulfides of several other metals. Primarily, we're looking at the effects on erythrocytosis. That work hasn't been extended yet to carcinogenesis. We haven't found any effects on the erythrocytosis. We're also looking at mixed sulfides; nickel-iron sulfide is being studied.

Q.: In a recent report on combined effects of nickel and benzo[a]pyrene *in vitro*, synergism was present in the amount of cell transformation. Are you perhaps looking at a co-carcinogenesis or promotion-type event with the combination of the nickel and sulfur?

A.: We're also concerned with that. I think it's too complex a problem to discuss here.

Q.: I'm wondering about the correlation between the hematocrit and a species' susceptibility to tumorigenesis. Do you think that oxygen is involved in the mechanism of nickel carcinogenesis?

A.: There is correlation between species susceptibility to Ni_3S_2 tumorigenesis and erythrocytosis. Yes, I think oxygen may be involved. Heme oxygenase is a microsomal enzyme that degrades heme to liberate carbon monoxide, iron, and biliverdin. Heme oxygenase activity is induced by nickel chloride. We are presently studying the effects of carcinogenic nickel compounds on heme oxygenase activity in rat tissues.

CHEMICAL CARCINOGENESIS STUDIES IN NONHUMAN PRIMATES

R. H. Adamson and S. M. Sieber

Laboratory of Chemical Pharmacology, National Cancer Institute, National Institutes of Health, Bethesda, Maryland 20205

INTRODUCTION

A wide variety of chemicals has been shown to be capable of inducing malignant tumors in rodents. However, rodent data are difficult to extrapolate to man, and the problem of risk assessment for humans remains largely unsolved. Extrapolation of rodent carcinogenesis data to man is particularly difficult because of known species differences in metabolic pathways (both activation and detoxification), involving potentially carcinogenic chemicals. Nonhuman primates are phylogenetically closer to man than rodents, and many metabolic pathways in monkeys parallel those in humans (1,2). For this reason, nonhuman primates may provide a more suitable model for the study of potential carcinogens, particularly those requiring metabolic activation and those detoxified by various enzyme systems.

Chemical carcinogenesis studies in nonhuman primates have been conducted for the past 20 years in this laboratory. During this time a considerable amount of information on the spontaneous tumor incidence in a closed colony of nonhuman primates, primarily Old World monkeys, has been amassed. In addition, the carcinogenicity of chemicals and other substances has been assessed. The results of these ongoing studies are described below.

METHODS

Animals

The present colony, consisting of 545 animals, is comprised of four species: *Macaca mulatta* (rhesus), *Macaca fascicularis* (cynomolgus), *Cercopithecus aethiops* (African green), and *Galago crassicaudatus* (bush babies). Fifty-four of these monkeys are adult breeders that supply the newborns for experimental studies. The original goal of this program was to establish whether selected carcinogens would have any effect in primates of any species, and as wide a range of species as was practical was deliberately chosen. African green (Gr), cynomolgus (Cy), rhesus (Rh), and occasionally (Cy x Rh)F_1 hybrids were generally included in each protocol, and were assigned randomly as they became available. Accordingly, different numbers of each species were used from one study to the next. The majority of the animals are housed in an isolated facility that contains only animals committed to this study, and with the exception of the breeding colony, most animals are housed in individual cages. Details of maintenance and management procedures and the method used to rear neonates have been described elsewhere (3). Newborns produced by the breeding colony are taken within 12 hours of birth to a nursery staffed on a 24-hour basis. The administration of test compounds is usually initiated within 24 hours of birth and continues until a tumor is diagnosed or until a predetermined exposure period has been completed.

A variety of clinical, biochemical, and hematological parameters is monitored weekly or monthly, not only to evaluate the general health status of each animal, but also for the early detection of tumors. Surgical procedures are performed under phencyclidine hydrochloride, Ketamine, or sodium pentobarbital anesthesia. All animals that die or are sacrificed are carefully necropsied and the tissues subjected to histopathologic examination.

Compounds Under Evaluation

A wide variety of substances has been or is being evaluated (Table 1). The compounds are administered subcutaneously (sc), intravenously (iv), intraperitoneally (ip), or orally (po). For po administration to newborn monkeys, the compound is added to Similac formula at feeding time; when the monkeys are six months old, carcinogens given po are generally incorporated into a vitamin mixture given to the monkeys as a vitamin sandwich on a half slice of bread. The dose level chosen is dependent on the chemical under evaluation. The therapeutic agents under test are administered at doses likely to be encountered in a clinical situation. Other

Table 1. Substances Tested for Carcinogenic Activity in Nonhuman Primates.

Common Name	Alternate or Chemical Name(s)
Therapeutic Agents	
Procarbazine	N-Isopropyl-α-(2-methylhydrazino)-p-toluamide
Adriamycin	Daunorubicin
Melphalan	L-p-Bis(2-chloroethyl)aminophenyl-alanine; phenylalanine mustard
Azathioprine	6-[(1-Methyl-4-nitroimidazol-5-yl-thio]purine; Imuran
Cyclophosphamide	2-[Bis(2-chloroethyl)amino]tetrahydro-2H-1,3,2-oxazaphosphorine-2-oxide; Cytoxan
Food Additives and Environmental Contaminants	
Aflatoxin B_1	--
MAM acetate[a]	Methylazoxymethanol acetate
Sterigmatocystin	
Cyclamate	Cyclohexane sulfamic acid, sodium salt
Saccharin	2,3-Dihydro-3-oxobenzisosulfonazole; 2-sulfobenzoic acid imide
DDT	1,1,1-Trichloro-2,2-bis(p-chlorophenyl)ethane
Arsenic	Sodium arsenate
Cigarette smoke condensate	--
Model Rodent Carcinogens	
Urethane	Ethyl carbamate
3-Methylcholanthrene	--
Dibenzo[a,i]pyrene	
Dibenz[a,h]anthracene	
2-Acetylaminofluorene	
2,7-Bis(acetylamino)fluorene	
4-Dimethylaminoazobenzene	Butter yellow
3'-Methyl-4-dimethylaminoazobenzene	--
N-Nitroso Compounds	
Nitrosomethylurea	1-Methylnitrosourea
1-Nitroso-1-methyl-3-nitroguanidine	N-Methyl-N'-nitro-N-nitrosoguanidine
Nitrosopiperidine	1-Nitrosopiperidine
Nitrosodimethylamine	Dimethylnitrosamine
Nitrosodiethylamine	Diethylnitrosamine
Nitrosodi-n-propylamine	Dipropylnitrosamine

[a]Some animals also received cycasin, methyl azoxymethanol-β-D-glucopyranoside, or crude cycad meal containing cycasin.

substances, such as environmental contaminants and food additives, are usually given at levels 10 to 40 times higher than the estimated human exposure level. The remainder of the chemicals tested are administered at maximally tolerated doses that, on the basis of weight gain, blood chemistry, hematology findings, and clinical observations, appear to be devoid of acute toxicity.

RESULTS

Therapeutic Agents

Of the cancer chemotherapeutic agents under test, only procarbazine (4) and adriamycin (5) have thus far provided evidence of being carcinogens in nonhuman primates. Table 2 compares the tumor incidence in a group of 50 monkeys receiving long-term procarbazine treatment with that in a control population of 219. The group of 50 monkeys received procarbazine by ip, sc, and/or po routes, and 41 have been necropsied. Thirteen of the necropsied monkeys were diagnosed with tumor, yielding an overall tumor incidence of 26%. In contrast, 7 out of 219 (3.2%) control monkeys have developed spontaneous tumors over the past 20 years. Controls consisted of 45 Gr, 91 Rh, and 83 Cy monkeys; among these, tumors have developed in 3 Gr, 3 Rh, and 1 Cy. Approximately half of the procarbazine-induced neoplasms were acute leukemia, chiefly myelogenous (see Table 3), that arose in monkeys after latent periods ranging between 16 and 143 months (average 77 months). The monkeys developing leukemia had ingested an average cumulative procarbazine dose of 45.53 g (range 2.69 to 103.68 g). Table 4 lists the six solid tumors induced by procarbazine; half of these tumors were osteosarcomas, two were hemangiosarcomas, and one was a lymphocytic lymphoma. The solid tumors arose in monkeys ingesting an average cumulative procarbazine dose of 56.88 g (range 23.85 to 154.37 g) and were diagnosed after an average latent period of 98 months (range 68 to 148 months).

An evaluation of the carcinogenic potential of adriamycin was initiated approximately 6 years ago in a group of 10 monkeys. The original plan was to administer 30 doses of adriamycin at 1 mg/kg (30 mg/kg); when this total dose was attained, the monkeys were to be observed for the remainder of their lives. However, a monkey died with acute clinical signs of congestive heart failure (ascites, periorbital edema, and rapid and labored respiration) after receiving 26 doses of adriamycin (26 mg/kg). Dosing of all monkeys in this group was terminated approximately one month later, but in the following two months, five more monkeys developed congestive heart failure and died, and two additional monkeys died three and four months later, respectively. Necropsy and histopathologic examination of tissue from all eight animals revealed lesions typical of adriamycin cardiomyopathy. These

Table 2. Summary of Control and Procarbazine-Treated Monkeys[a]

Group	No. Alive	No. Dead			No. of Monkeys
		Without Tumor	With Tumor	(%)	
Procarbazine	9	28	13	(26)	50[b]
Control[c]	129	83	7	(3.2)	219

[a]From 1961 to 1981.
[b]23 Rh, 16 Cy, and 11 Gr.
[c]Includes non-treated animals, breeders, and vehicle-treated controls.

monkeys had received an average cumulative adriamycin dose of 74.4 mg divided among 23 to 27 monthly doses (see Table 5). Another monkey was sacrificed because of marked weight loss and anorexia of approximately five weeks duration. Although no specific abnormalities were noted at necropsy of this monkey except for enlarged mesenteric lymph nodes, histological examination of sections of bone marrow yielded a diagnosis of acute myeloblastic leukemia. This animal had received a cumulative adriamycin dose of 77.8 mg, and the leukemia was diagnosed two months after the last dose of adriamycin. The tenth monkey in this series is alive and without evidence of illness; it received 25 injections of adriamycin (72 mg), the last administered 42 months ago.

We are currently repeating this study, using 2 groups of 10 monkeys each; the monkeys are receiving monthly intravenous injections of adriamycin at 0.2 and 0.4 mg/kg, and dosing will be terminated when the monkeys have received a cumulative adriamycin dose of 60 mg. To date, the monkeys receiving adriamycin at 0.2 and 0.4 mg/kg have been given cumulative drug doses of 15.6 and 21.8 mg, respectively. None of the monkeys has developed signs of congestive heart failure or other indications of ill health.

The remainder of the chemotherapeutic agents under test (melphalan, azathioprine, and cyclophosphamide) have not as yet provided any indication of carcinogenicity. Twenty monkeys are receiving melphalan po at a dose of 0.1 mg/kg, 5 days/week. The first group of 10 monkeys was put on test 64 months ago, and since that time has ingested an average cumulative melphalan dose of 128 mg/kg. The second group of 10 monkeys was put on test 10 months later, and the average cumulative melphalan dose ingested

Table 3. Acute Leukemias Induced in Monkeys by Procarbazine.

Monkey No.	Species[a]	Sex	Dose (mg/kg)	Route[b]	Months Dosed	Total Dose (gm)	Latent Period (mo)[c]	Type of Leukemia
267D	Rh	F	50 10	sc po	15 1	2.69	16	Myelogenous
733I	Cy	M	20	ip	57	7.29	57	Undifferentiated
726I	Cy	M	20	ip	68	16.24	68	Myelogenous
313E	Rh	F	5-50 10	sc po	35 33	37.25	68	Myelogenous
567G	Rh	F	10-25 10	sc po	6 71	49.99	77	Myelogenous
13T	Rh	M	25-50 10	sc po	36 73	101.64	109	Myelogenous
336E	Rh	F	10-50 10	sc po	33 110	103.68	143	Myelogenous
Average						45.53	77	

[a]Rh = rhesus; Cy = cynomolgus.
[b]Doses for sc and ip given 1 day/week; po doses given 5 days/week.
[c]Latent period is the number of months from first dose to diagnosis of leukemia.

Table 4. Solid Tumors Induced in Monkeys by Procarbazine.

Monkey No.	Species[a]	Sex	Dose (mg/kg)	Route[b]	Months Dosed	Total Dose (gm)	Latent Period (mo)[c]	Tumor(s) Diagnosed
734I	Rh	M	10-20 10	ip po	62 5	23.85	71	Hemangioendothelial sarcoma; kidney
731I	Rh	F	10-20 10	ip po	63 5	24.22	68	Osteosarcoma; humerus
314E	Cy	F	5-50 10	sc po	35 62	32.88	97	Hemangiosarcoma; spleen
315E	Cy	M	5-50 10	sc po	35 63	50.18	98	Lymphocytic lymphoma
333E	Cy	F	10-50 10	sc po	33 70	57.05	103	Osteosarcoma; jaw
557G	Cy	F	10-50 10	sc po	7 140	154.37	148	Osteosarcoma; humerus
Average						56.88	98	

[a]Rh = rhesus; Cy = cynomolgus.
[b]Doses for sc and ip given 1 day/week; po doses given 5 days/week.
[c]Latent period is the number of months from first dose to diagnosis of leukemia.

Table 5. Effects of Adriamycin in Monkeys[a]

No. of Monkeys	No. of Doses[b]	Avg. Total Dose (mg)	Cause of Death
8[c]	23-27	74.4[d]	Congestive heart failure
1 (Rh)	27	77.8	Acute myeloblastic leukemia (Rh)
1 (Rh)	25	72.0	None

[a]Summary of first study.
[b]Monkeys were given monthly iv doses of adriamycin (1 mg/kg) beginning at two months of age.
[c]4 Cy, 4 Rh.
[d]Range is 66.2 to 80.6.

by this group of monkeys is 108 mg/kg. None of the monkeys has died, and none has demonstrated any clinical signs of ill health.

Two groups of monkeys are being given azathioprine po, 5 days/week. A group of 14 monkeys has been receiving the compound at 2.0 mg/kg for an average of 38 months (range 9 to 43 months). During this period the monkeys have received a cumulative azathioprine dose averaging 1.52 g/kg (range 0.36-1.72 g/kg). A second group of 10 monkeys began receiving azathioprine (5.0 mg/kg) an average of 28 months ago (range 25 to 29 months); these monkeys have ingested an average of 2.8 g/kg azathioprine (range 2.5-2.9 g/kg). All monkeys receiving azathioprine appear healthy and are without clinical signs of ill health.

A study of the potential carcinogenicity of cyclophosphamide was recently initiated. A group of 20 monkeys is receiving cyclophosphamide po 5 days/week. Dosing (3 mg/kg) begins when the monkeys are six months old, and the dose is increased to 6 mg/kg when the monkeys are one year old. The study has been under way for an average of only six months; during this period an average cumulative cyclophosphamide dose of 0.78 g (range 0.04 to 2.25 g) has been administered. Thus far, none of the monkeys has died, and there is no evidence of toxicity on this dosage schedule.

Food Additives and Environmental Contaminants

Despite prolonged treatment with most of the food additives and environmental contaminants listed in Table 1, only aflatoxin B_1 (AFB_1) and methylazoxymethanol-acetate (MAM-acetate) have induced tumors in monkeys. AFB_1 has been under evaluation for the past 15 years (6). A total of 45 monkeys, chiefly rhesus and cynomolgus, has received AFB_1 ip (0.125 to 0.25 mg/kg) and/or po (0.1 to 0.8 mg/kg) for two months or longer, and six are currently alive and without evidence of tumor. Eighteen of the 39 monkeys necropsied to date developed one or more malignant neoplasms, yielding an overall tumor incidence of 40% (see Table 6). A summary of the tumors diagnosed in these monkeys is shown in Table 7. Seven of the 18 tumor-bearing monkeys developed hemangioendothelial sarcomas of the liver, five had bile duct or gallbladder adenocarcinomas, and two developed hepatocellular carcinomas. One monkey had an osteosarcoma and three were found at necropsy to have multiple primary tumors. Adenocarcinoma of the pancreas occurred in all monkeys with multiple primary tumors, coincident with urinary bladder carcinoma, adenocarcinoma of the bile ducts, or osteosarcoma. The tumors diagnosed in the 18 monkeys developed after an average latent period of approximately 10 years (range 5 to 12 years) and after an average cumulative AFB_1 dose of 820 mg (range 292 to 1103 mg).

Table 6. Summary of Control and AFB_1-Treated Monkeys[a]

		No. Dead			
Group	No. Alive	Without Tumor	With Tumor	(%)	No. of Monkeys
AFB_1[b]	6	21	18	(40.0)	45[c]
Control	129	83	7	(3.2)	219

[a]From 1961 to 1981.
[b]Monkeys received AFB_1 by po (0.1 to 0.8 mg/kg) and/or ip (0.125 to 0.25 mg/kg) routes; dosing began within one month of birth.
[c]25 Rh, 18 Cy, 2 Gr.

The carcinogenic potential of cycads (crude cycad meal, purified cycasin, and synthetic MAM-acetate) administered by po or ip routes has been under investigation for the past 12 years (7). Eighteen monkeys survived longer than two months after the first dose of cycasin (50 to 75 mg/kg) or MAM-acetate (1.5 to 3.0 mg/kg) given po, 5 days/week. Eleven of these animals have been necropsied and three had tumors (see Table 8). A group of 10 monkeys received MAM-acetate by weekly ip injections (3 to

Table 7. Tumors Induced by AFB_1

Tumor Type[a]	No. of Monkeys	Avg. Total Dose (mg)	Avg. Latent Period (mo)
Hemangiosarcoma: liver	7 (5 Rh, 2 Cy)	978	140
ACA: bile duct or gallbladder	5 (2 Rh, 3 Cy)	959	137
CA: hepatocellular	2 Rh	478	60
Osteosarcoma	1 Cy	412	115
CA: pancreas and urinary bladder	1 Gr	292	107
ACA: pancreas and bile duct; osteosarcoma	1 Rh	353	117
ACA: pancreas and bile duct	1 Rh	1103	142
Average		820	126

[a]ACA = adenocarcinoma; CA = carcinoma.

Table 8. Summary of Control and Cycad-Treated Monkeys[a]

Group	No. Alive	No. Dead: Without Tumor	No. Dead: With Tumor	(%)	No. of Monkeys[b]
Cycad[c]					
po	7	8	3 (2 Rh, 1 Cy)	(16.7)	18
ip	2	3	5 (1 Gr, 3 Rh, 1 Cy)	(50.0)	10
Control	129	83	7	(3.2)	219

[a]From 1961 to 1981.
[b]17 Rh, 9 Cy, 2 Gr.
[c]Monkeys received cycads (crude cycad meal, purified cycasin or synthetic methylazoxymethanol acetate) within three days of birth.

10 mg/kg). Eight of these animals have been necropsied, and five had tumors. In addition, one of the two surviving monkeys in the ip treatment group developed a hepatocellular carcinoma that was surgically resected approximately eight years ago. Table 9 lists the tumors diagnosed in monkeys receiving cycad products by ip or po routes. All five of the necropsied monkeys treated with MAM-acetate by the ip route developed hepatocellular carcinoma, and two of the five had multiple primary tumors. In one monkey, a liver hemangiosarcoma, renal carcinoma, and esophageal squamous cell carcinoma were diagnosed in addition to hepatocellular carcinoma; the other monkey developed a renal carcinoma, adenocarcinoma of the small intestine, and esophageal squamous cell carcinoma. The tumors developing in the monkeys treated by the ip route were diagnosed after an average latent period of 80 months (range 63 to 88 months) and after an average cumulative MAM-acetate dose of 6.65 g (range 3.88 to 9.66 g).

Three monkeys on po cycads have thus far developed tumors (see Table 9). One monkey developed multiple primary tumors (hepatocellular carcinoma, bile duct adenocarcinoma, and renal carcinoma), and the other two had hepatocellular carcinoma and pancreatic adenocarcinoma, respectively. These tumors developed after latent periods of 107, 69, and 179 months and after the ingestion of considerably more cycad material than the tumor-bearing monkeys in the ip treatment group had been given.

Sterigmatocystin has been under test for the past five years. It is being administered po, 1 day/week at 1 mg/kg (15 monkeys) and 2 mg/kg (15 monkeys)). Thus far, only one monkey in the 2-mg/kg group has been necropsied, and histopathologic examination of tissue from this animal revealed no evidence of tumor development, although severe toxic hepatitis with hyperplastic nodules was noted. The remaining 29 animals are in good health.

Our studies have failed to implicate either cyclamate or saccharin as carcinogens in nonhuman primates (8). Cyclamate has been administered po 5 days/week at 100 mg/kg (12 monkeys) and 500 mg/kg (11 monkeys) for the past 10 and one-half years. The 100-mg/kg dose corresponds, on an equivalent surface area basis, to a daily intake of 2.3 g/day/70 kg man. With an average of 384 mg cyclamate in a 10-oz diet drink, this dose is equivalent to drinking about 6 diet drinks/day; correspondingly, the 500-mg/kg dose is equivalent to ingesting approximately 30 diet drinks/day. Two monkeys at each of the dose levels have died, but no evidence of tumor was found at necropsy or after histological examination of their tissue.

Saccharin has been administered to 2 groups of 10 monkeys each at 25 mg/kg, 5 days/week. One group of monkeys has been receiving saccharin for an average of 122 months (range 120 to 124 months),

Table 9. Tumors Induced by Cycads

Species[a]	Sex	Total Dose (gm)	Latent Period (mo)	Tumor(s) Diagnosed[b]
IP Dosing[c]				
Gr	M	3.88	63	HCA
Cy	F	5.06	80	HCA Hemangiosarcoma: liver CA: kidney SCA: esophagus
Rh	F	6.27	87	HCA
Rh	F	8.38	88	HCA CA: kidney ACA: small intestine SCA: esophagus
Rh	M	9.66	86	HCA
PO Dosing				
Rh	M	13.71[d] 28.62[c]	107	HCA ACA: bile duct CA: kidney
Cy	M	43.0[e] 30.41[d] 18.10[c]	69	HCA
Rh	M	53.5[e] 74.99[d]	179	ACA: pancreas

[a]Gr = African green; Cy = cynomolgus; Rh = rhesus.
[b]HCA = hepatocellular carcinoma; CA = carcinoma; ACA = adenocarcinoma; SCA = squamous cell carcinoma.
[c]MAM-acetate.
[d]Cycasin.
[e]Cycad meal.

and the second group was entered on study approximately three years ago. The 25-mg/kg dose corresponds, on an equivalent surface area basis, to a daily intake of 5 cans of diet soda (120 mg saccharin/can) or 15 packages of Sweet'N Low® (40 mg saccharin/package)/day. Since the inception of the saccharin study, none of the animals has died, and there is no evidence of toxicity in any of the animals thus far.

Similarly, long-term DDT administration has not yielded tumors in our nonhuman primates. A total of 24 animals has received DDT by the po route (20 mg/kg), 5 days/week, in a study that has been under way for the past 134 months. Administration of DDT is discontinued after a dosing interval of 130 months is completed. Although five of the monkeys have died thus far, none was found to have developed tumor. The apparent cause of death in these animals was DDT-induced central nervous system toxicity, as all experienced severe tremors and convulsions immediately prior to death. The 19 surviving monkeys appear to be in good health.

The carcinogenic potential of arsenic has been under evaluation for approximately six years. A total of 20 monkeys has received sodium arsenate po (0.1 mg/kg) 5 days/week, and three monkeys in the group have died. The cause of death in the monkeys was unrelated to arsenic treatment, and the surviving monkeys are well and without signs of toxicity. Nine monkeys have received lung implants containing tobacco smoke condensate in a beeswax matrix; all are well and without evidence of toxicity approximately eight years after implantation of the material.

Model Rodent Carcinogens

With the exception of urethane (ethyl carbamate), no compound listed in Table 1 as a "model rodent carcinogen" has induced tumors in Old World monkeys. Starting within one month of birth, urethane (250 mg/kg) was given po, 5 days/week, to rhesus and cynomolgus monkeys. Urethane treatment was continued for a maxmimum of five years, during which time some animals also received whole body irradiation in 3 to 10 weekly courses (50 rads/course). Urethane treatment was discontinued 11 to 14 years ago, and since that time all monkeys have been observed. Of 40 monkeys receiving urethane, 30 survived 6 months or longer after the first dose, and 22 of them have been necropsied (see Table 10). Thus far, eight malignant tumors have been found in five (16.7%) of the 30 treated monkeys; two of the five monkeys with tumors had received irradiation in addition to urethane. One or more primary liver tumors (three cases of hemangiosarcomas and one case each of adenocarcinoma of intrahepatic bile ducts and hepatocellular carcinoma) were diagnosed in four monkeys in which additional tumors present included an ependymoblastoma and a pulmonary adenocarcinoma (see

Table 11). An adenocarcinoma of the jejunum was diagnosed in the fifth monkey. The animals with tumors had received an average cumulative urethane dose of 260 g (range 230 to 339 g); the latent period for tumor induction averaged 171 months (range 142 to 229 months).

Table 10. Summary of Control and Urethane-Treated Monkeys[a]

Group	No. Alive	No. Dead Without Tumor	No. Dead With Tumor	(%)	No. of Monkeys
Urethane[b]					
Irr[c]	3	10	2	(13.3)	15[d]
Not Irr	5	7	3	(20.0)	15[d]
Controls	129	83	7	(3.2)	219

[a]From 1961 to 1981.
[b]Monkeys received urethane (250 mg/kg) 5 days/week for a maximum of five years, and treatment was discontinued 11 to 14 years ago. Some monkeys also received 3 to 10 weekly courses of whole body irradiation (50 rads/course).
[c]Irr = irradiated.
[d]8 Rh, 7 Cy.

Earlier studies from this laboratory (9) demonstrated that single sc doses (10 mg) of 3-methylcholanthrene (3-MC) produced fibrosarcomas in the primitive prosimian, Tupaia glis (tree shrew). Of six treated animals, three died within four months, and the three survivors developed fibrosarcomas within 14 to 16 months. A similar study in Old World monkeys was initiated 20 years ago in which 3-MC was administered po (14 animals) and by sc injection (7 animals). Animals treated po received the compound at a dose of 20 to 120 mg/kg 5 to 7 days/week; sc injections were given at 10 to 40 mg/kg for a total of 1 to 12 doses. Dosing was discontinued after 5 years, and the animals have been observed for up to 15 years. Although 8 of the 14 animals in the po treatment group, and 5 of the 7 in the sc group have died, no tumors have been detected at necropsy or upon histopathologic examination of their tissue.

Table 11. Tumors in Monkeys Given Urethane

Species[a]	Sex	Irradiation (No. of Courses)	Total Dose (gm)	Latent Period (mo)	Tumor(s) Diagnosed[b]
Rh	M	10	230.1	155	ACA: bile duct ACA: lung
Rh	M	9	243.0	181	Hemangiosarcoma: liver Ependymoblastoma
Cy	M	None	244.1	142	Hemangiosarcoma: liver
Rh	F	None	245.8	149	HCA Hemangiosarcoma: liver
Rh	F	None	339.2	229	ACA: jejunum
Average			260.4	171	

[a]Rh = rhesus; Cy = cynomolgus.
[b]ACA = adenocarcinoma; HCA = hepatocellular carcinoma.

Similarly, our previous studies with benzo[a]pyrene (BP) showed that fibrosarcomas developed in the prosimian *Galago crassicaudatus* (bush baby) at the site of a single sc injection (9). However, no tumors have developed in a group of Old World monkeys that received multiple sc injections of BP (30 to 90 mg/kg); 9 out of a total of 17 animals have survived treatment with this compound and have been under observation for up to 18 years. Other model rodent carcinogens, that after prolonged administration to Old World monkeys have failed thus far to induce tumors, include dibenz[a,h]anthracene; 2-acetylaminofluorene; 2,7-bis(acetylamino)fluorene; 4-dimethylaminoazobenzene; and 3'-methyl-4-dimethylaminoazobenzene.

N-Nitroso Compounds

The nitroso compounds as a class appear to be potent carcinogens in nonhuman primates; all but one of these compounds (N-nitrosodimethylamine [DMNA]) have induced tumors in monkeys. A summary of results obtained with nitrosomethylurea (MNU) is shown in Table 12. A group of 43 monkeys received MNU (10 to 20 mg/kg) by the po route in 5 doses/week. Eighteen monkeys have been necropsied, and nine were diagnosed with malignant tumors, yielding an overall tumor incidence of 21% (10). All tumors induced by MNU were squamous cell carcinomas of the esophagus and oropharynx (see Table 13), and developed after latent periods ranging between 57 and 133 months (average 93 months).

Table 12. Summary of Control and MNU-Treated Monkeys[a]

		No. Dead			
Group	No. Alive	Without Tumor	With Tumor	(%)	No. of Monkeys
MNU	25	9	9	(20.9)	43[c]
Controls[b]	129	83	7	(3.2)	219

[a]From 1961 to 1981.
[b]Includes non-treated animals, breeders, and vehicle-treated controls.
[c]18 Rh, 19 Cy, 2 (Rh x Cy)F_1, and 4 Gr.

A rough parallel has been observed between the cumulative MNU dose ingested and the degree of esophageal damage found at necropsy of the treated monkeys (see Table 14). No esophageal lesions were found in two monkeys that had ingested an average of 15.34 g MNU for a period averaging 26 months, whereas esophagitis accompanied by candidiasis and chronic inflammatory infiltrates were noted in the esophageal mucosa of two monkeys receiving an average of 19.90 g MNU for an average of 58 months. In five monkeys necropsied after having ingested an average of 47.40 g MNU for an average of 54 months, esophageal lesions were more severe and included esophageal epithelial atrophy, hyper- or dyskeratosis, and dysplasia. The nine monkeys with squamous cell carcinomas of the esophagus had received MNU for an average of 93 months (range 57 to 133 months); during this period they had ingested an average cumulative MNU dose of 120.0 g (range 53.2 to 180.6 g). Only one monkey receiving in excess of 53.2 g MNU was found at necropsy to be without a carcinoma; this monkey had ingested 201.41 g MNU over the course of 124 months, and histopathologic examination of sections of esophagus revealed chronic esophagitis and extensive esophageal dysplasia.

Table 13. Tumors in Monkeys Receiving MNU Orally

Monkey No.	Species[a]	Sex	Total Dose (gm)[b]	Latent Period (mo)[c]	Histological Diagnosis
617H	Cy	M	53.21	63	SCA[d]: pharynx and esophagus with invasion of mediastinal lymph nodes; squamous metaplasia: trachea
622H	Rh	F	65.74	57	SCA: soft palate, tongue, and esophagus with invasion into stomach
539G	Rh	F	108.14	72	SCA: mouth; SCA *in situ*: pharynx; squamous papillomas: tongue, pharynx, and esophagus; dyskeratosis: esophageal mucosa
540G	Rh	M	129.29	83	SCA: mouth and esophagus; squamous papilloma and hyperkeratosis: buccal mucosa; SCA: esophagus
627H	Rh	M	129.91	133	SCA: esophagus
538H	Rh	M	133.80	72	SCA: mouth, pharynx, and esophagus; multiple squamous papillomas: pharynx and esophagus
569G	Gr	M	137.21	124	SCA: mouth, pharynx, and esophagus
624H	Rh	F	142.32	129	SCA: gingiva and esophagus
579G	Rh	M	180.65	107	SCA: mouth and esophagus

[a]Cy = cynomolgus; Rh = rhesus; Gr = African green.
[b]MNU (10 to 20 mg/kg) was incorporated into a vitamin sandwich and given 5 times/week; dosing was initiated within one week of birth.
[c]Latent period is the time in months from the first dose of MNU until the clinical diagnosis of tumor.
[d]SCA = squamous cell carcinoma.

Table 14. Esophageal Lesions Found at Necropsy in Nonhuman Primates Given MNU

No. of Monkeys	Avg. Total Dose (gm)[a]	Months Dosed	Esophageal Pathology
2	15.34	26	None
2	19.90	58	Esophagitis, candidiasis
5	47.40	54	Hyper- or dyskeratosis
9	120.00	93	Squamous cell carcinoma

[a]MNU (10 to 20 mg/kg) was given po 5 days/week.

1-Nitroso-1-methyl-3-nitroguanidine (MNNG) is also being administered by the po route (0.4 mg/kg, 5 days/week). A group of 21 monkeys has received this compound for periods of up to eight years; thus far, two animals have died of causes unrelated to treatment with MNNG. The remaining 19 animals appear to be in good health and without signs of toxicity. However, three additional monkeys were given MNNG as a colon implant; two monkeys have been necropsied, and one monkey was diagnosed with a well-differentiated adenocarcinoma of the rectosigmoid junction. The latter monkey had received a total MNNG dose of 8.65 g, administered in gelatin cubes containing 5.3 to 42.7 mg MNNG, which were inserted into the colon 2 days/week.

Another nitroso compound, 1-nitrosopiperidine (PIP), is carcinogenic in nonhuman primates (see Table 15), regardless of whether it is administered by po or ip routes. Thus 11 out of 12 monkeys (92%) receiving PIP po (400 mg/kg), 5 days/week, developed tumors, as did 5 of the 11 (46%) animals given PIP by weekly ip (40 mg/kg) injection. All tumors induced by PIP were hepatocellular carcinomas. Although the latent period for tumor development was similar in the po and ip treatment groups (87 and 76 months, respectively), the average total PIP dose ingested by monkeys receiving po treatment (1742.5 g) was approximately 45-fold greater than that of monkeys in the ip treatment group (39.4 g).

Table 16 summarizes resulted obtained in two small groups of six monkeys each, treated with N-nitrosodipropylamine (DPNA) and DMNA. All monkeys given weekly ip injections of DPNA (40 mg/kg) have been necropsied and found to have hepatocellular carcinomas. In contrast, four of the six monkeys treated with bimonthly ip injections of DMNA (10 mg/kg) have been necropsied, and none have developed tumors. Although histopathologic examination of tissue

Table 15. Summary of Control and PIP-Treated Monkeys[a]

Group	No. Alive	No. Dead: Without Tumor	No. Dead: With Tumor	(%)	No. of Monkeys[b]
PIP					
PO[b]	0	1 (Rh)	11	(91.7)[d]	12
IP[c]	2 (1 Rh, 1 Cy)	4 (2 Gr, 2 Rh)	5	(4.5)[e]	11
Controls	129	83	7	(3.2)	219

[a]From 1961 to 1981. 23 Monkeys given PIP comprised 13 Rh, 7 Cy, and 3 Gr.
[b]PO doses of PIP (400 mg/kg) were given 5 days/week.
[c]IP doses (40 mg/kg) were given 1 day/week.
[d]6 Rh, 5 Cy.
[e]3 Rh, 1 Cy, 1 Gr.

Table 16. Summary of Control and DPNA- and DMNA-Treated Monkeys[a]

Group	No. Alive	No. Dead: Without Tumor	No. Dead: With Tumor	(%)	No. of Monkeys
DPNA[b]	0	0	6	(100.0)[c]	6
DMNA[d]	2	4	0	(0.0)	6
Controls	129	83	7	(3.2)	219

[a]From 1961 to 1981. 4 Rh and 2 Cy received DPNA; 2 Cy and 4 Rh received DMNA.
[b]DPNA (40 mg/kg) was given 1 day/week by ip injection.
[c]All six tumors were HCA and developed after an average total dose of 7.0 g and after an average latent period of 28 months.
[d]DMNA (10 mg/kg) was given 1 day/2 weeks by ip injection

from these animals revealed severe hepatotoxicity (e.g., toxic hepatitis, cirrhosis, and hyperplastic nodules), no tumors were detected.

Nitrosodiethylamine (DENA) is a potent and predictable hepatocarcinogen in Old World monkeys, inducing tumors when given either by the ip or po route of administration (see Table 17). Twenty-nine out of 41 monkeys receiving po doses of DENA (40 mg/kg) 5 days/week developed hepatocellular carcinomas. Bimonthly ip injections of DENA (40 mg/kg) induced hepatocellular carcinomas in 106 out of 131 monkeys. When administered po, DENA induced tumors earlier and at a lower cumulative dose in cynomolgus monkeys, as compared to African greens, with the group of rhesus monkeys intermediate between the two species. This apparent species difference was not observed, however, when DENA was given by the ip route.

Table 17. Hepatocellular Carcinoma Induced by DENA

Species[a]	No. of Animals	Avg. Total Dose (gm)[b]	Avg. Latent Period (mo)
PO			
Cy	14	18.0	26
Rh	12	25.4	49
Gr	3	55.1	105
IP			
Cy	38	1.56	17
Rh	51	1.95	17
Gr	12	1.32	16
Cy x rh	5	1.84	15

[a]Cy = cynomolgus; Rh = rhesus; Gr = African green.
[b]DENA (40 mg/kg) was given po 5 days/week and ip bimonthly.

Table 18 shows DENA as carcinogenic in the prosimian *Galago crassicaudatus* (bush baby). The tumors induced in this species are primarily muco-epidermoid carcinoma of the nasal cavity rather than the hepatocellular carcinomas found in Old World monkeys. All 10 bush babies given bimonthly ip doses of DENA (10 to 30 mg/kg) developed tumors of the nasal cavity. In two of these animals, carcinoma of the liver was also present, and in both cases metastases to the lungs or to intestinal lymph nodes were noted.

The average total dose of DENA inducing tumors in the bush babies (0.75 g) is considerably lower than that required to induce tumors in Old World monkeys and reflects the lower body weight of

Table 18. Muco-Epidermoid Carcinoma (M-E CA) of the Nasal Mucosa Induced in Bush Babies by DENA

Group	No. With M-E CA/Total	No. With Liver CA/Total	Avg. Total Dose (gm)[a]	Avg. Latent Period (mo)
DENA	10/10	2/10	0.75	23
Controls	0/13	0/13	-	-

[a]DENA was administered by bimonthly ip injections at 10 to 30 mg/kg.

the bush babies. The average latent period for tumor induction in this species (23 months) is comparable to that in Old World monkeys. No obvious reason exists for the marked difference in the site of DENA-induced tumors noted between Old World monkeys and the bush babies. Possibly, it is related to differences in the metabolism or distribution of DENA, and this possibility is currently being investigated in our laboratory.

At this time, we are employing DENA as a model hepatocarcinogen in Old World monkeys to examine the relationship between chronic (milligrams per kilograms) dose, cumulative dose, and latent period for tumor induction. To this end, groups of monkeys are being given bimonthly ip injections of DENA at doses of 0.1, 1, 5, 10, 20, and 40 mg/kg and are observed for the appearance of tumor. In the four groups of monkeys in which tumors have developed, we have found that the latent period increases as the milligram-per-kilogram dose decreases (see Table 19). The study is incomplete; consequently, a precise value for the minimum carcinogenic dose for DENA cannot be given. However, it appears that this value will be approximately 1.4 g. Table 19 also shows the total dose and observation period for DENA-treated monkeys that are currently alive and without evidence of tumor. The 10 monkeys in the 0.1-mg/kg group have been studied only eight months and have received a total DENA dose of approximately 1 mg. In the 1-mg/kg group, the 80-month observation period exceeds the latent period required by the 5-mg/kg dose, but the total DENA dose administered (0.768 g) is below the apparent carcinogenic dose (1.4 g). The four tumor-free monkeys in the 5-mg/kg group, however, have received an average total DENA dose that exceeds the apparent carcinogenic dose, and they have been observed for seven months longer than the average latent period for tumor induction at this dose level. The single tumor-free monkey at the 10-mg/kg dose level has received a total DENA dose (4.101 g) that is well in excess of the apparent carcinogenic dose. This monkey has been observed for a period that is approximately twice the latent period for tumor induction by DENA at that dose.

DISCUSSION

The rodent has traditionally been the system in which bioassays for chemical carcinogenesis are carried out, and the results of such bioassays have provided much of the basis for estimating the risk that chemicals may pose to man. However, a number of problems exist when extrapolating rodent carcinogenesis data to man. These problems include the necessity of administering exceedingly high doses of the test chemical to compensate for the relatively short life span of mice and rats (11), the high incidence of spontaneous tumors in some rodent colonies in which bioassays are carried out (12), and the observation that rodents metabolize many chemicals via pathways that differ from those found in the human.

On the other hand, nonhuman primates are employed infrequently in long-term carcinogenesis studies, chiefly because of the expense of such an undertaking, the time period required to complete a lifetime study, the unavailability of sufficient numbers of animals, and the relatively large quantity of test chemical required. Nevertheless, a number of advantages exist when performing chemical carcinogenesis studies in nonhuman primates rather than in rodents. These advantages include the comparatively low incidence of spontaneous tumors arising in monkeys, the similarity of many of their metabolic pathways to those of the human (1,2), and the fact that their relatively long life span and large size enable the experimenter to administer chemicals by routes and by dosage schedules that closely parallel human exposure patterns. Thus, although nonhuman primates will never supplant rodents as the primary screening system for potentially carcinogenic chemicals, they can provide important information on the carcinogenic potential of chemicals in wide use, chemicals to which large numbers of humans are exposed, or chemicals for which data from rodents are ambiguous or conflicting.

The carcinogenic potential in nonhuman primates of a variety of chemicals, differing widely in chemical structures and properties, has been under investigation in this laboratory for the past 20 years. Prior to the inception of this study, nonhuman primates, unlike the rodent, were believed to be relatively resistant to tumor induction by chemicals. Therefore, an early objective of the present study was to evaluate the response of monkeys to chemicals known to be carcinogenic in rodents. A series of model rodent carcinogens, including 3-MC, BP, dibenz[a,h]anthracene, 2-acetylaminofluorene, and urethane, was accordingly tested. With the exception of urethane, none of these

Table 19. Induction of Hepatocellular Carcinoma (HCA) in Monkeys by Bimonthly IP Injections of DENA.

DENA Dose (mg/kg)	No. HCA/No. Treated	Monkeys with HCA		Monkeys Without HCA	
		Avg. Total Dose (gm)	Avg. Latent Period (mo)	Avg. Total Dose (gm)	Months Observed
0.1	0/10 (4 RH, 6 Cy)	-	-	0.001	8
1	0/10 (7 Rh, 1 Cy, 2 Gr)	-	-	0.768	80
5	6 (4 RH, 2 Cy)/10 (6 Rh, 3 Cy, 1 Gr)	3.128	65	2.872	72
10	9 (5 Rh, 4 Cy)/10 (5 Rh, 5 Cy)	1.780	34	4.101	63
20	11/11 (6 Rh, 5 Cy)	2.177	26	-	-
40	10/10 (5 Rh, 3 Cy, 1 F_1, 1 Gr)	1.430	17	-	-

model rodent carcinogens has proved to be carcinogenic in the Old and New World species of monkey employed in our studies, although both 3-MC and BP produced tumors in more primitive primates (bush babies and tree shrews), as they do in rodents (9). These results suggest that prosimian primates resemble the rodent more closely than they do macaques in their response to a carcinogenic stimulus.

Many of the chemicals classified in the present study as "food additives and environmental contaminants" are reported to be rodent carcinogens. Thus the artificial sweeteners cyclamate and saccharin as well as DDT have been (or may be) withdrawn from public use on the basis of their carcinogenicity in rodents. Nevertheless, neither the artificial sweeteners nor DDT have induced tumors in nonhuman primates despite extensive testing over prolonged time periods. The mold product sterigmatocystin is another example of a rodent carcinogen (13) that thus far is apparently devoid of carcinogenicity in nonhuman primates. However, both AFB_1 and cycad (particularly MAM-acetate) are potent carcinogens in rodents (14,15) and are carcinogenic in nonhuman primates as well. Although arsenic is suspected of being a human carcinogen (16), it has not induced tumors in rodents and has not as yet proved to be carcinogenic in nonhuman primates.

Many of the clinically useful antineoplastic and immunosuppressive agents are potent rodent carcinogens (17); however, they were tested in our monkey colony because of the increasing suspicion that they are etiologic agents in second malignant tumors arising in successfully treated cancer patients and in tumors arising in patients receiving chronic immunosuppressive therapy for collagen vascular disease or for renal homografts (18). Five chemotherapeutic agents have been evaluated for carcinogenic activity in our colony of nonhuman primates, but only one of these (procarbazine) has as yet demonstrated unequivocable carcinogenic properties. Adriamycin may be a leukemogen, but further studies are needed and are in progress. The other three drugs, azathioprine, melphalan, and cyclophosphamide, have probably not been tested long enough for their carcinogenic potential to become manifested.

With the exception of DMNA, all of the nitroso compounds induced tumors in nonhuman primates. MNU is a direct-acting carcinogen; the fact that po doses of this compound induced tumors of the oropharynx and esophagus is no surprise. However, another direct-acting carcinogen, MNNG, has not as yet induced tumors when administered po, although a colon implant containing this chemical produced an adenocarcinoma at the site of implantation. The remainder of the carcinogenic nitroso compounds are hepatocarcinogens in Old World monkeys, inducing a high yield of hepatocellular carcinoma in the treated animals. The chemical that we have acquired the most information about, DENA, is a predictable and reproducible carcinogen, inducing tumors following either ip or po treatment. Extensive studies with this chemical have provided information pertaining to the relationship between chronic dose, cumulative dose, and latent period for tumor induction.

Our results indicate that the latent period for tumor induction increases as the chronic milligram-per-kilogram dose decreases and that the cumulative carcinogenic dose for DENA is approximately 1.4 g. Assuming an average body weight of 8 kg, the monkeys in the 1-mg/kg treatment group would receive approximately 208 mg of DENA/year. Taking the value 1.4 g as the carcinogenic dose for DENA, the latent period for tumor induction in these animals would be about six to seven years, a time interval well within the average life span (25 to 30 years) of Old World monkeys in captivity. However, in the 0.1-mg/kg group, the maximum total DENA dose that could be given over a 25- to 30-year period is approximately 0.52 to 0.62 g, a cumulative dose that is considerably lower than the apparent carcinogenic dose for DENA.

Some insight into low-dose extrapolation of carcinogenic risk may be gained by considering a semilog plot of the milligram-per-kilogram dose of DENA against the latent period for tumor induction (Figure 1; Table 19). The 40, 20, and 10 mg/kg points fall on a straight line that intersects the ordinate at 88 months. This point on the ordinate corresponds to a DENA dose of 0.1 mg/kg. Thus, animals in the 0.1-mg/kg group should develop tumors after a latent period of 88 months if the relationship between milligram-per-kilogram dose and latent period is strictly linear; however, the animals receiving this dose have only been under observation for eight months (Table 19). The line passes through the ordinate at 60 months for the 1-mg/kg group, although this group remains tumor free after 80 months of observation. The tumors developing in the six animals receiving the 5-mg/kg dose required a latent period of 65 months, a figure that shows a marked deviation from the value (42 months) expected if the relationship between dose and latent period is indeed linear.

ACKNOWLEDGMENTS

This work is being supported in part by National Cancer Institute contract NO1-CM-33708 with Hazleton Laboratories America, Inc., Vienna, Virginia.

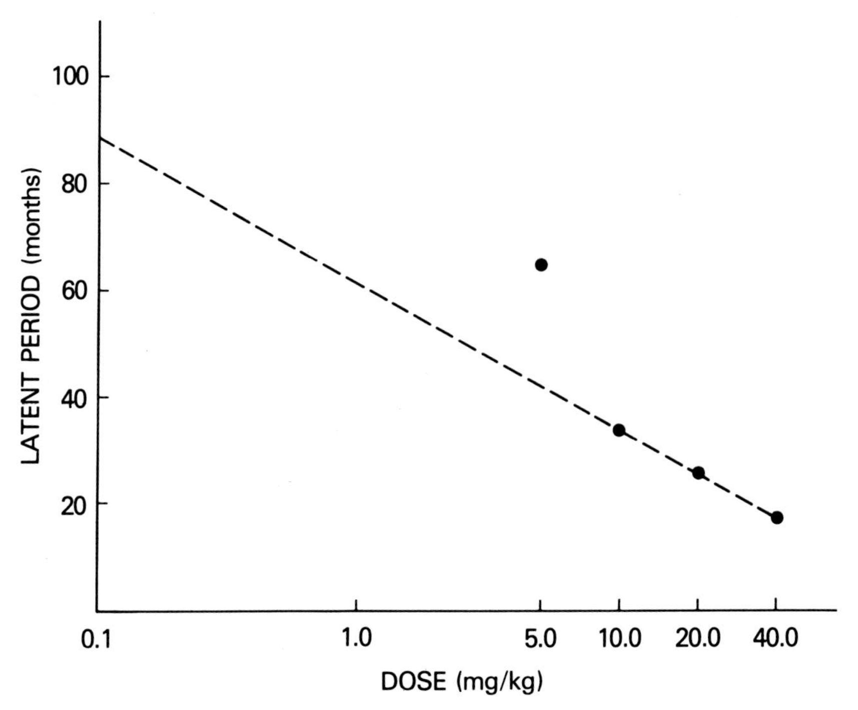

Figure 1. Relationship between chronic (milligram-per-kilogram) DENA dose and latent period for tumor induction in Old World monkeys receiving bimonthly ip injections of DENA at 0.1, 1, 5, 10, 20, and 40 mg/kg.

REFERENCES

1. Smith, R.L., and R.T. Williams. 1974. Comparative metabolism of drugs in man and monkeys. J. Med. Primatol. 3:138-152.

2. Smith, R.L., and J. Caldwell. 1977. Drug metabolism in non-human primates. In: Drug metabolism - from microbe to man. D.V. Parke, and R.L. Smith, eds. Taylor and Francis Ltd.: London. pp. 331-356.

3. Adamson, R.H. 1972. Long-term administration of carcinogenic agents to primates. In: Medical Primatology 1972, Part III. E.I. Goldsmith, and J. Moor-Jankowski, eds. S. Karger: Basel, Switzerland. pp. 216-225.

4. Sieber, S.M., P. Correa, D.W. Dalgard, and R.H. Adamson. 1978. Carcinogenic and other adverse effects of procarbazine in nonhuman primates. Cancer Res. 38:2125-2134.

5. Sieber, S.M., P. Correa, D.M. Young, D.W. Dalgard, and R.H. Adamson. 1980. Cardiotoxic and possible leukemogenic effects of adriamycin in nonhuman primates. Pharmacol. 20:9-14.

6. Sieber, S.M., P. Correa, D.W. Dalgard, and R.H. Adamson. 1979. Induction of osteogenic sarcomas and tumors of the hepatobiliary system in nonhuman primates with aflatoxin B_1. Cancer Res. 39:4545-4554.

7. Sieber, S.M., P. Correa, D.W. Dalgard, K.R. McIntire, and R.H. Adamson. 1980. Carcinogenicity and hepatoxicity of cycasin and its aglycone, methylazoxymethanol-acetate in nonhuman primates. J. Natl. Cancer Inst. 65:177-189.

8. Sieber, S.M., and R.H. Adamson. 1978. Long-term studies on the potential carcinogenicity of artificial sweeteners in nonhuman primates. In: Health and Sugar Substitutes. B. Guggenheim, ed. S. Karger: Basel, Switzerland. pp. 266-271.

9. Adamson, R.H., R.W. Cooper, and R.W. O'Gara. 1970. Carcinogen-induced tumors in primitive primates. J. Natl. Cancer Inst. 45:555-559.

10. Adamson, R.H., F.J. Krowlikowski, P. Correa, S.M. Sieber, and D.W. Dalgard. 1977. Carcinogenicity of 1-methyl-1-nitrosourea (MNU) in nonhuman primates. J. Natl. Cancer Inst. 59:415-422.

11. Sontag, J.M. 1977. Aspects in carcinogen bioassay. In: Origins of Human Cancer, Book C. H.H. Hiatt, J.D. Watson, and J.A. Winsten, eds. Cold Spring Harbor Laboratory: New York. pp. 1327-1338.

12. Weisburger, J.H., D.P. Griswold, J.D. Prejean, A.E. Casey, H.B. Wood, and E.K. Weisburger. 1975. The carcinogenic properties of some of the principle drugs used in clinical cancer chemotherapy. Recent Results Cancer Res. 52:1-17.

13. Purchase, I.F.H., and J.J. Van der Watt. 1970. Carcinogenicity of sterigmatocystin. Food Cosmet. Toxicol. 8:289-293.

14. Butler, W.H. 1965. Liver injury and aflatoxin. In: Mycotoxins in Foodstuffs. G.N. Wogan, ed. Massachusetts Institute of Technology Press: Cambridge, MA. pp. 175-186.

15. Laqueur, G.L. 1964. Carcinogenic effects of cycad meal and cycasin (methylazoxymethanol glycoside) in rats and effects of cycasin in germfree rats. Fed. Proc. 23:1386-1388.

16. Hernberg, S. 1977. Incidence of cancer in population with exceptional exposure to metals. In: Origins of Human Cancer, Book A. H.H. Hiatt, J.D. Watson, and J.A. Winsten, eds. Cold Spring Harbor Laboratory: New York. pp. 147-157.

17. Sieber, S.M., and R.H. Adamson. 1975. The clastogenic, mutagenic, teratogenic, and carcinogenic effects of various antineoplastic agents. In: Pharmacological Basis of Cancer Chemotherapy. Williams and Wilkins Co.: Baltimore, MD. pp. 401-468.

18. Sieber, S.M., and R.H. Adamson. 1975. Toxicity of antineoplastic agents in man: Chromosomal aberrations, antifertility effects, congenital malformations, and carcinogenic potential. Adv. Cancer Res. 22:57-155.

ORGAN SPECIFICITY AND TUMOR PROMOTION

Stuart H. Yuspa, Henry Hennings,
Ulrike Lichti, Molly Kulesz-Martin,

In Vitro Pathogenesis Section, Laboratory of Cellular Carcinogenesis and Tumor Promotion, Division of Cancer Cause and Prevention, National Cancer Institute, Bethesda, Maryland 20205

INTRODUCTION AND BACKGROUND

The modification of experimental carcinogenesis by agents that are not carcinogenic alone has been studied for over 40 years. Much attention has centered on compounds termed tumor promoters. Tumor promoters cause or allow the expression of the latent tumor phenotype induced in some cells by limited doses of carcinogens. Both chemical and physical stimuli can act as tumor promoters. Interest in tumor promotion is appropriate since this phase of carcinogenesis accounts for most of the latent period. For many years research in tumor promotion was confined to studies in mouse skin and limited to the use of impure reagents such as croton oil. During the last decade, broad interest in this aspect of carcinogenesis has developed largely due to the discovery of specific agents that act as tumor promoters and to the development of experimental models other than mouse skin in which promotion-like events contribute to tumor formation. Perhaps of equal importance, epidemiological studies in human cancer have suggested that a promotion phase is important in lung cancer, colon cancer, and cancer in hormonally-regulated target tissues.

When one examines a list of model systems where tumor promotion has been demonstrated (see Table 1), it is clear that the phenomenon occurs in the epithelium of complex tissues. Most commonly, target epithelial cells are organized in a stratifying or maturing arrangement, usually in a terminally differentiating lining epithelium. Such epithelia are often composed of more than one cell type or of cells in differing biological states. It is unclear whether tissue complexity is a fundamental requirement for a multistage mechanism or if other, less complex, organ sites have simply not been adequately explored.

Table 1. *In Vivo* Model Systems Demonstrating a Promotion Stage in Carcinogenesis

Mouse skin	Rat breast
Rat liver	Mouse and rat stomach
Rat esophagus	Rat trachea
Rat colon	Mouse lung
Rat bladder	

The list of known promoting agents or stimuli has rapidly expanded, as model systems to assay for promotion have been developed. Table 2 provides a relatively current listing of promoting agents. Promoting activity has been identified in both natural and synthetic chemical agents. The general properties associated with promoting agents are as follows:

1) Most appear to be tissue specific.

2) Not carcinogenic alone; must be given after initiating agent to exert effect.

3) Action of individual exposures reversible and not cumulative; repeated exposures required.

4) In general, biological activity strictly determined by molecular structure for chemical promoters.

5) Appear to act directly without requiring metabolism or covalent binding to macromolecules.

6) Most not mutagenic.

7) Usually induce proliferation in target tissue (although proliferation alone is not sufficient promoting stimulus).

8) Induced changes progressive and intermediate preneoplastic stages may be observed prior to overt malignancy.

In most cases promoting agents are tissue specific although phorbol esters have effects on many cell types (1) and wounding or injury may promote in several tissues. Promoting events must occur after initiation, and promoting stimuli must be repeatedly administered at frequent intervals, suggesting that reversible mechanisms are involved in promotion. Structural specificity exists among biologically active promoters so that minor changes in structure markedly affect promoting activity for phorbol esters (2) and barbiturates (3). Many nonmutagens are promoters but mutagenic agents may also act as promoters, as in the examples of ultraviolet (UV) light (4) and bromomethylbenz[a]anthracene (5) in skin. Induced proliferation in target cells appears to be a common effect of most promoters, yet a number of agents that induce proliferation in specific target tissues are not active as promoters (6). Characteristically, tumor induction involving a promotion phase results in progressive preneoplastic changes prior to the formation of cancer. Many of these preneoplastic lesions are reversible.

Table 2. Examples of Experimental Promoting Agents

Media	Promoting Agent
Mouse skin	Phorbol esters (croton oil) Anthralin Cigarette smoke condensate Dihydroteleocidin (fungal product) 7-Bromomethylbenz[a]anthracene UV light Wounding
Rat liver	Phenobarbital DDT Polychlorinated biphenyl
Rat bladder	Saccharin Cyclamate Tryptophan
Rat colon	Bile acids Cholestyramine High fat diets Wounding
Hamster lung	Chronic irritation (saline lavage)
Hormone-dependent tissues	Hormones

In the two most extensively studied multistage models, mouse skin and rat liver, basic biological observations have yielded clues to the mechanism of tumor promotion. Studies in skin comparing tumor induction by initiator-promoter or by repeated initiator application have suggested that the mechanism of cancer induction by each protocol may be different (see Table 3). One-stage protocols generally yield de novo carcinomas or persistent papillomas while two-stage protocols yield mostly papillomas that regress (7,8). Carcinomas arise from papillomas late in the two-stage process often independently of continuous promoter treatment (9). This difference in the pattern of induction of preneoplastic and malignant lesions is shown graphically in Figure 1 where data from three separate reports of skin tumorigenesis (7,9,10) are compared. When promoters are employed to induce skin cancer there is a preponderance of benign lesions. Figure 1 also indicates that preneoplastic lesions predominate when promoters are employed to induce liver tumors. In this case, limited exposure of rats to acetylaminofluorene (AAF) resulted in about 30% with liver cancers and only 8% with adenomas at 292 days. When AAF was followed by phenobarbital or DDT, virtually all animals had preneoplastic lesions and the percentage with carcinomas was actually diminished at this time. Considerably later, the carcinoma incidence increased in the promoted group, suggesting that adenomas converted to malignant liver lesions in these animals as was the case for papillomas converting to carcinomas in mouse skin. In skin, carcinogenesis involving promoters also differs from repeated initiator application in strain susceptibility and in the types of chemicals that modify each process (see Table 3). Mechanistic studies in tumor promotion, therefore, must be directed at defining pathogenesis based upon the biology of cancer induction by the two-stage protocol, particularly with regard to the formation of benign lesions.

Phorbol esters and particularly the potent analogue 12-O-tetradecanoylphorbol-13-acetate (TPA) have been useful for defining the biology and biochemistry of promotion in mouse skin. The biological characteristics of promotion as produced by applications of phorbol esters are summarized below.

1) Produces tumors only in initiated skin.

2) Produces primarily benign tumors (papillomas) which commonly regress.

3) Malignant tumors are rare, arise in papillomas, occur late, and may occur independently of promoter exposure.

4) Tumors are monoclonal.

5) Biochemical changes appear to occur in many cells, not just initiated cells.

Table 3. Comparison of Mouse Skin Carcinogenesis by Repeated Application of Initiator (One-Stage) or Initiation and Promotion (Two-stage)

Characteristic	One-Stage	Two-Stage
Primary tumor type	Papillomas and squamous cell carcinomas (1:1)	Papillomas (carcinomas occur late and infrequently)
Latent period	Papillomas and carcinomas: 20-50 wks	Papillomas: 10-20 wks Carcinomas: 50 wks
Strain susceptibility	BALB/c > Swiss > A > C57BL > AKR	BALB/c > C57Bl > A > Swiss > AKR
Tumor regression	Uncommon	Common
Inhibited by:		
Retinoids	No	Yes
Steroids	Partial	Yes
7,8-Benzoflavone	Yes	No
Enhanced by prostaglandin F_2	No	Yes

6) Cell selection or tissue sensitization leads to enhanced responses with multiple applications.

The tumor spectrum has been discussed earlier. Several other aspects of phorbol ester action are of particular interest. While a requirement for prior initiation for tumor production exists, promoters seem to induce biochemical changes in many or all epidermal cells, not just initiated cells. Repeated promoter exposures sensitize the tissue for certain responses to a subsequent exposure such as stimulation of DNA synthesis (11), stimulation of ornithine decarboxylase (ODC) induction (12,13), and elevation of cyclic guanosine monophosphate levels (14). This result suggests a selection of sensitive cells during promotion, a change more likely to occur in complex tissues where a variety of

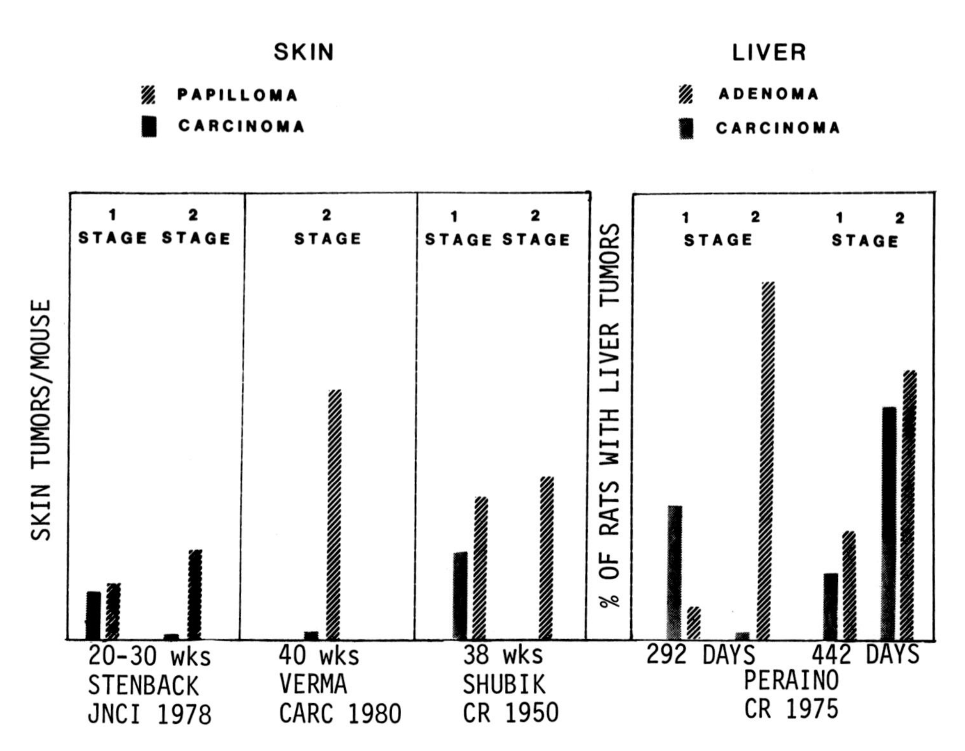

Figure 1. Compilation of data on relative incidence of benign or malignant tumors produced by particular carcinogenesis protocols in mouse skin or rat liver models. One-stage protocols utilize repeated exposures to a polycyclic aromatic hydrocarbon in mouse skin or a limited repeated exposure to AAF for rat liver. Two-stage protocols involve a single exposure to a polycyclic aromatic hydrocarbon followed by croton oil or TPA for mouse skin. The rat liver studies employed phenobarbital following AAF administration. For details of these studies see References 3,7,9,10.

target cells exists. The skin tumors produced by two-stage protocols are monoclonal (15), indicating an origin from a single (presumably) initiated cell, without recruitment of normal cells into the tumor mass. The monoclonal origin of tumors, the suggestion of tissue remodeling with repetitive promoter exposure, and the requirement for repeated promoting stimuli prior to the development of tumors strongly suggest that cell selection is involved in promotion.

Analysis of the biochemical changes produced by phorbol esters in mouse skin has also been useful in formulating working hypotheses on the mechanism of promotion (see Table 4). A large number of changes occur in response to TPA. Several occur within a few minutes (cyclic nucleotides, prostaglandins); others take hours (changes in RNA and protein synthesis, polyamine synthesis, transglutaminase and histidase activity, histone phosphorylation, and phospholipid synthesis) or up to 24 h (DNA synthesis and synthesis of a histidine-rich protein [HRP]). The hyperplasia induced by phorbol esters in mouse skin may persist for weeks. Mediation of some responses via action at the cell membrane is likely, and a receptor for TPA has been identified in mouse skin (16). Table 4 divides the pleiotrophic responses of skin into major functional groups relating to epidermal differentiation or proliferation. Many of these changes occur with the same temporal sequence. Since differentiation and proliferation are thought to be mutually exclusive in epidermis, and basal cells appear to the principal target for TPA action (17), considerable heterogeneity must exist among basal cells in their program of induced responses. It is these biochemical and biological observations that have guided our studies to elucidate the mechanism of tumor promotion and to develop an understanding of two-stage skin carcinogenesis.

Experimental Studies

While conceptual advances in the biology of carcinogenesis have come from whole animal studies, mechanistic studies are better performed under less complex circumstances. For this reason we felt it essential to develop an epithelial cell culture model for carcinogenesis research. Since mouse epidermis was so widely studied *in vivo*, was readily available, and had clearly separable stages in the transformation process, it seemed an appropriate system to study *in vitro*. Over the last decade, results from this and other laboratories have shown that mouse epidermal cell culture is both a valid and useful model system to study normal epidermal function as well as alterations associated with tumor initiation and promotion (18,19). To facilitate experimental work, a major advance in epidermal cell culture came with the discovery that extracellular ionic calcium is a key regulator of epidermal growth and differentiation (20). In medium with reduced calcium concentrations (0.02 to 0.09 mM), epidermal basal cells are selectively cultivated. These cells have morphological, cell kinetic, and marker protein characteristics of basal cells and grow as a monolayer with a high proliferation rate. When the calcium concentration of culture medium is elevated to levels found in most commercial preparations (1.2 to 1.4 mM), proliferation ceases and terminal differentiation rapidly ensues with squamous differentiation and sloughing of cells occurring by 72 to 96 h. This simple physiological manipulation has been useful in approaching questions regarding initiation and promotion.

Table 4. Effects of Phorbol Esters on Mouse Epidermis *In Vivo* and *In Vitro*.

Differentiative Functions	Unknown Function	Proliferative Functions
↓DNA synthesis	Cyclic nucleotide changes	↑DNA synthesis
↑RNA and protein synthesis	Protease induction	↑RNA and protein synthesis
↑Synthesis of HRP (27 K)	13.5 K, 25 K, 35 K, 50 K proteins	↑Polyamine biosynthesis
↑Epidermal transglutaminase	↑Phospholipid synthesis	↑Prostaglandin synthesis
↑55 K and 70 K protein	Histone phosphorylation	↓Histidase activity
↑Ca^{++}-induced differentiation	Dark cells	↓Chalone responsiveness
		↓Ca^{++}-induced differentiation

The biological nature of initiation. In order to extrapolate experimental results in phorbol ester research to a mechanism of tumor promotion, we must understand the nature of the initiated cell. It seems logical that in a terminally differentiating tissue such as skin, an alteration in terminal differentiation must accompany tumorigenesis. This theory seems likely because proliferating cells in epidermal tumors are observed away from the basement membrane area whereas cells in normal epidermis cease proliferation upon leaving the basement membrane. The ability to proliferate under conditions where normal cells are obligated to differentiate would likely be an early event in transformation, perhaps a key change in initiation. The responses of cultured basal cells to increases in extracellular calcium resemble the changes observed in basal cells *in vivo* as they migrate away from the basement membrane and commit to differentiate. In cell culture, therefore, it might be expected in analogy to *in vivo* data that carcinogens could alter the basal cell response to calcium-induced terminal differentiation. Our laboratory has been studying this model and the results are summarized in Table 5.

Table 5. Summary of Initiation Studies

Cultures derived from skin initiated *in vivo* and basal cells exposed to initiators *in vitro* yield foci that grow under conditions where normal cells differentiate.

Cells from these foci initially are nontumorigenic but on prolonged subculture produce squamous cell carcinomas when injected into syngeneic or nude mice.

The commitment to terminally differentiate is also altered in cultured malignant epidermal cells.

Malignant cells can be selected from a large excess of normal cells in culture by growth in medium favoring terminal differentiation.

Basal cells exposed to carcinogens *in vitro* and subsequently induced to differentiate by calcium formed foci which resisted terminal differentiation (21). Colony number was proportional to carcinogen dose. Cells obtained from these colonies were typical keratinocytes; they expressed differentiative functions but failed to cease proliferation when signaled to differentiate. Such cells were not tumorigenic but on prolonged subculture yielded tumorigenic cell lines. Similar foci were derived from cell cultures of mouse skin initiated *in vivo* by exposure to 7,12-dimethylbenz[*a*]anthracene and cultured in 0.02 mM calcium medium for several weeks followed by selection in 1.2 mM calcium. In these experiments control skin did not yield colonies (22). Malignant epidermal cells cultured in the presence of a large excess of normal basal cells in 0.02 mM calcium medium also continued to proliferate and form colonies when switched to 1.2 mM calcium, while all normal cells died by terminal differentiation (21). These results suggest that initiation of carcinogenesis results in the ability of initiated cells to resist the signal to cease proliferation in association with terminal differentiation. In normal skin such a trait alone could not result in a tumor, due to the strong regulatory influences of surrounding normal cells (23-25).

The biological nature of promotion. *In vivo* data on mouse skin have indicated that cell selection is involved in tumor promotion. Our studies have been designed to elucidate the cellular basis for selection with the hope that the results could explain a selective clonal expansion of differentiation-altered initiated cells. These studies are summarized in Table 6. Since basal cells were the presumed target for initiators, it was important to determine whether basal cells were particularly responsive to TPA when compared to more differentiated cells in the epidermis. The induction of ODC was used as a marker for responsiveness. Ornithine decarboxylase activity in basal cells cultured in 0.07 mM calcium medium and exposed to TPA was as much as 20-fold greater than activity in TPA-exposed cells cultured in 1.2 mM calcium for just one day (17). In fact, basal cells lost responsiveness to TPA within several hours of culture in 1.2 mM calcium medium, indicating that phorbol esters can no longer influence ODC activity in epidermal cells very shortly after they commit to differentiation (17). These changes in responsiveness were not due to a direct effect of extracellular calcium on ODC induction since UV light induced ODC equally at all calcium concentrations.

When the responsiveness of basal cells to TPA was studied by other parameters, it became clear that a portion of the population was induced to differentiate by the promoter. This result could be detected by morphological changes, measurement of the formation of cornified squames, and increase in the activity of the differentiation-specific enzyme epidermal transglutaminase (26). As terminally differentiated cells sloughed from the culture dish, transglutaminase activity decreased. Remarkably, the basal cells remaining after a brief TPA exposure were shown to be transiently resistant to terminal differentiation when cultured in 1.2 mM calcium or when exposed to TPA a second time (27). However, these cells were stimulated to proliferate by the second TPA exposure and appeared to be more sensitive to the induction of ODC activity.

Table 6. Summary of Promotion Studies

Basal cells are the target cell for phorbol esters.
Epidermal cells become unresponsive to phorbol esters shortly after they commit to differentiate.
Heterogeneity for responsiveness to phorbol esters exists among subpopulations of basal cells.
Certain basal cells are induced to differentiate by phorbol esters while others are stimulated to proliferate and transiently resist differentiation signals.
Heterogeneity with regard to differentiation and proliferation would result in selective regenerative hyperplasia.

Thus, two types of response occur in epidermal basal cells exposed to phorbol esters. In one population the induction of terminal differentiation occurs. In a second population, TPA stimulates proliferation and produces a transient block in response to a differentiation stimulus. The latter cell type cannot be induced to differentiate by a second TPA exposure if the interval between exposures is short. This response is similar to that of mouse skin *in vivo* after several TPA exposures where proliferative stimulation is the principal response. If the culture interval between TPA exposures is prolonged (10 days), then heterogeneity in responsiveness is restored (Yuspa, unpublished data). This finding is similar to those *in vivo* where treatment intervals are prolonged.

The results obtained from studies in epidermal basal cell cultures suggest that phorbol esters produce a balanced and programmed heterogeneous response with regard to differentiation and proliferation. The net effect of this type of heterogeneity is to select for and to expand the proliferating population with each promoter exposure, thus remodeling the target tissue. Clonal selection of carcinogen-altered (differentiation-altered) cells would result if normal basal cells were induced to differentiate while altered (initiated) cells were among those that are stimulated to proliferate. Clonal expansion of initiated cells (with an altered program of differentiation) resulting from phorbol ester-regulated cell selection would yield benign tumors that are the major product of two-stage skin carcinogenesis. This model requires that a subsequent change in a papilloma cell is necessary for carcinoma development.

ACKNOWLEDGMENT

The technical assistance of Theresa Ben and secretarial assistance of Maxine Bellman are appreciated.

REFERENCES

1. Diamond, L., T.G. O'Brien, W.M. Baird. 1980. Tumor promoters and the mechanism of tumor promotion. Adv. Cancer Res. 32:1-74.

2. Yuspa, S.H., U. Lichti, T. Ben, E. Patterson, H. Hennings, T.J. Slaga, N. Colburn, and W. Kelsey. 1976. Phorbol-esters stimulate DNA synthesis and ornithine decarboxylase activity in mouse epidermal cell cultures. Nature 262:402-404.

3. Peraino, C., R.J.M. Fry, E. Staffeldt, and J.P. Christopher. 1975. Comparative enhancing effects of phenobarbital, amobarbital, diphenylhydantoin and dichlorodiphenyltrichloroethane on 2-acetylaminofluorene-induced hepatic tumorigenesis in the rat. Cancer Res. 35:2884-2890.

4. Epstein, J.H. 1978. Photocarcinogenesis: A review. Natl. Cancer Inst. Monograph 50:13-25.

5. Scribner, N.K., and J.D. Scribner. 1980. Separation of initiating and promoting effects of the skin carcinogen 7-bromomethylbenz[a]anthracene. Carcinogenesis 1:97-100.

6. Marks, F., S. Bertsch, and J. Schweizer. 1978. Homeostatic regulation of epidermal cell proliferation. Bull. Cancer 65:207-222.

7. Shubik, P. 1950. The growth potentialities of induced skin tumors in mice. The effects of different methods of chemical carcinogenesis. Cancer Res. 10:713-717.

8. Saffiotti, U., and P. Shubik. 1956. The effects of low concentrations of carcinogen in epidermal carcinogenesis. A comparison with promoting agents. J. Natl. Cancer Inst. 16:961-969.

9. Verma, A.K., and R.K. Boutwell. 1980. Effects of dose and duration of treatment with the tumor promoting agent, 12-O-tetradecanoylphorbol-13-acetate on mouse skin carcinogenesis. Carcinogenesis 1:271-276.

10. Stenback, F. 1978. Life history and histopathology of ultraviolet light-induced skin tumors. Natl. Cancer Inst. Monograph 50:57-70.

11. Raick, A.N., K. Thumm, and B.R. Chivers. 1972. Early effects of 12-O-tetradecanoylphorbol-13-acetate on the incorporation of tritiated precursor into DNA and the thickness of the interfollicular epidermis, and their relation to tumor promotion in mouse skin. Cancer Res. 32:1562-1568.

12. O'Brien, T.G. 1976. The induction of ornithine decarboxylase as an early, possibly obligatory, event in mouse skin carcinogenesis. Cancer Res. 36:2644-2653.

13. Lichti, U., S.H. Yuspa, and H. Hennings. 1978. Ornithine and S-adenosylmethionine decarboxylases in mouse epidermal cell cultures treated with tumor promoters. In: Mechanisms of Tumor Promotion and Cocarcinogenesis. T.J. Slaga, A. Sivak, and R.K. Boutwell, eds. Raven Press: New York. pp. 221-232.

14. Garte, S.J., and S. Belman. 1978. Effects of multiple phorbol myristate acetate treatments on cyclic nucleotide levels in mouse epidermis. Biochem. Biophys. Res. Comm. 84:489-494.

15. Iannaccone, P.M., R.L. Gardner, and H. Harris. 1978. The cellular origin of chemically induced tumors. J. Cell Sci. 29:249-269.

16. Delclos, K.B., D.S. Nagle, and P.M. Blumberg. 1980. Specific binding of phorbol ester tumor promoters to mouse skin. Cell 19:1025-1033.

17. Lichti, U., E. Patterson, H. Hennings, and S.H. Yuspa. 1981. The tumor promoter 12-O-tetradecanoylphorbol-13-acetate induces ornithine decarboxylase in proliferating basal cells but not in differentiating cells from mouse epidermis. J. Cell Physiol. 107:261-270.

18. Yuspa, S.H., U. Lichti, D. Morgan, and H. Hennings. 1980. Chemical carcinogenesis studies in mouse epidermal cell cultures. In: Biochemistry of Normal and Abnormal Epidermal Differentiation. I.A. Bernstein and M. Seiji, eds. University of Tokyo Press: Tokyo. pp. 171-188.

19. Yuspa, S.H., P. Hawley-Nelson, J.R. Stanley, and H. Hennings. 1980. Epidermal cell culture. Transplant. Proc. 12, Suppl. 1:114-122.

20. Hennings, H., D. Michael, C. Cheng, P. Steinert, K. Holbrook, and S.H. Yuspa. 1980. Calcium regulation of growth and differentiation of mouse epidermal cells in culture. Cell 19:245-254.

21. Kulesz-Martin, M., B. Koehler, H. Hennings, and S.H. Yuspa. 1980. Quantitative assay for carcinogen altered differentiation in mouse epidermal cells. Carcinogenesis 1:995-1006.

22. Yuspa, S.H., and D.L. Morgan. 1981. Initiation of carcinogenesis in mouse skin is associated with alterations in commitment for terminal differentiation. Nature 293:72-74.

23. Yuspa, S.H., H. Hennings, M. Kulesz-Martin, and U. Lichti. (in press). The study of tumor promotion in a cell culture model for mouse skin, a tissue which exhibits multistage carcinogenesis _in vivo_. In: Cocarcinogenesis and Biological Effects of Tumor Promoters. E. Hecker, ed. Raven Press: New York.

24. Yuspa, S.H., H. Hennings, and U. Lichti. (in press). Initiator and promoter induced specific changes in epidermal function and biological potential. J. Supramol. Struct.

25. Potten, C.S., and T.D. Allen. 1975. Control of epidermal proliferative units. Differentiation 3:161-165.

26. Yuspa, S.H, T.B. Ben, H. Hennings, and U. Lichti. 1980. Phorbol ester tumor promoters induce epidermal transglutaminase activity. Biochem. Biophys. Res. Comm. 97:700-708.

27. Yuspa, S.H., T. Ben, H. Hennings, and U. Lichti. 1981. Heterogeneous response in epidermal basal cells exposed to the tumor promoter 12-O-tetradecanoylphorbol-13-acetate. Submitted for publication.

DISCUSSION

Q.: It was first reported that neoplastic cells from the human cervix had increased growth capacity *in vitro*; recently Marchak and Nettesheim have reported similar observations for carcinogen-altered cells in the rat trachea, and others have also shown the same thing for liver cells. I think this general phenomenon is a quite universal one, and provides a very nice trick for studying cellular changes in carcinogenesis. The combined *in vivo/in vitro* approach offers certain advantages.

I would like to ask, can you immediately select these initiated cells in a high calcium-containing medium, or must you grow the cells for some time before attempting selection?

A.: In our *in vitro* experiments, there is about a three-week period after treating cells *in vitro* with carcinogens before we can see any colonies in the treated dishes, and under those conditions we get almost no colonies in the controls.

The experiment that you're really asking about is the *in vivo* experiment; that is, when we initiate *in vivo*, should we then immediately be able to detect initiated cells by cultivation *in vitro*. That experiment is in progress right now but I don't know the results.

Q.: It is not clear to me whether you're saying that the initiated cell has a greater potential for spontaneous genetic change than the precursor population from which it was derived.

A.: I think probably on an individual cell basis, no; but since in papillomas there is a large population of cells that are continuously proliferating, I think the chance is certainly much greater that a cell that would undergo a spontaneous change would be located in the papilloma.

Q.: So it is really a change in the numbers --

A.: In the number of cells at risk, yes. Let's say probably by a factor of 10.

SKIN TUMOR PROMOTION: A COMPARATIVE STUDY OF SEVERAL STOCKS AND STRAINS OF MICE

John Reiners, Jr., Kowetha Davidson, Kay Nelson, Mark Mamrack, and Thomas Slaga

Biology Division, Oak Ridge National Laboratory, Oak Ridge, Tennessee 37830

INTRODUCTION

Topical application of some chemical carcinogens will induce skin tumors on mice. In general, most chemical carcinogens have to be given repeatedly to induce a large number of tumors (complete carcinogenesis). Skin tumors also can be induced by the sequential application of a single subthreshold dose of a carcinogen (initiation phase) followed by repeated treatment with a noncarcinogenic promoter (promotion phase). This second procedure employing initiation and promotion is referred to as two-stage carcinogenesis.

The objectives of this review are threefold. We hope to provide evidence for the multistage nature of promotion, correlate promotion-associated morphological and biochemical responses with specific stages of promotion, and present concepts relevant to promotion that can be inferred from investigations with mouse stocks and strains which vary in their response to complete and two-stage carcinogenesis.

RESULTS

Mouse Skin Two-Stage Carcinogenesis

Evidence for chemical promotion was first provided by Berenblum (1), who reported that a regimen of croton oil applied alternately with small doses of benzo[a]pyrene (BP) to mouse skin induced a large number of tumors. Subsequently, Mottram (2) found that a single subcarcinogenic dose of BP followed by multiple applications of croton oil could induce skin tumors. Our present understanding of the promotional phase of two-stage carcinogenesis encompasses almost four decades of research. During this period, a large number of promoting reagents were identified, and their efficacy was determined through a quantitative analysis. In addition, chemicals that inhibit promotion were identified, as well as early morphological and biochemical responses resulting from treatment of skin with promoting chemicals.

Promoting reagents. The promotion phase of two-stage skin carcinogenesis in mice can be accomplished by repeated treatment with a variety of chemicals. Compounds such as anthralin (3), iodoacetic acid (4), citrus oil (5), some surface-active chemicals such as Tween 60 (6) and sodium dodecyl sulfate (6), extracts of unburned tobacco and tobacco smoke condensate (7,8), benzoyl peroxide (9), and some phenolic compounds (10) have weak to moderate promoting ability. The most potent tumor promotion compounds are certain phorbol esters found in croton oil and some synthetic phorbol ester derivatives (11,12,13). The most potent of the naturally occurring tumor promoters is the phorbol ester 12-O-tetradecanoylphorbol-13-acetate (TPA). The importance of structure to efficacy as a promoting chemical is demonstrated by the findings that the parent alcohol, phorbol, and 4-O-methyl TPA are relatively inactive as skin tumor promoters (14).

Markers for promotion. Much of our present knowledge of the cellular and biochemical responses induced in mouse skin by tumor promoters has been derived from investigations using phorbol esters as the promoting agent. Although the phorbol esters induce a variety of responses in mouse skin (15,16), the induction of epidermal hyperplasia, ornithine decarboxylase activity (ODC), and dark basal keratinocytes (dark cells) appear to correlate best with promotion (16).

Dark cells were first described by Raick (17,18) and are a subpopulation of skin epidermal basal cells. The term "dark cell" was derived from their electron density and the preferential dark staining of these cells by toluidine blue in semi-thin sections. Approximately 2% of adult SENCAR mouse epidermal basal cells are dark cells. The percentage of dark cells in SENCAR skin increases to 20 to 25% within 24 h after a single topical application of TPA (16). Because dark cells represent a high percentage of the basal cells in embryonic mouse skin, papillomas, and squamous cell carcinomas (17,18, Slaga, unpublished data), it is thought that they represent a less differentiated embryonic or stem cell population.

Inhibitors of promotion. A variety of chemicals that can modify the promotion process recently have been reviewed in depth (16,19). The most potent of the promotion phase inhibitors are the anti-inflammatory steroids, some retinoids, and protease inhibitors. Table 1 summarizes the relative inhibitory effects of representative compounds of these three classes on tumor response in two-stage carcinogenesis. The anti-inflammatory steroid fluocinolone acetonide (FA) is an extremely potent inhibitor of phorbol ester tumor promotion in mouse skin. The inhibitory effect is dose-responsive, and as little as 0.01 μg of FA can almost completely counteract skin tumorigenesis. FA effectively inhibits the induction of hyperplasia and dark cells (see Table 1). Retinoic acid (RA) and the protease inhibitor tosyl phenylalanine chloromethyl ketone (TPCK) also inhibit phorbol ester promotion but not all of the biochemical and morphological responses inhibited by FA. Specifically, RA inhibits the induction of ODC but has no effect on the induction of dark cells and hyperplasia. Conversely, TPCK inhibits the induction of dark cells but not hyperplasia or ODC. The differences in their effects on cellular responses and their efficacy as promotion inhibitors suggests that hyperplasia, ODC, and dark cells might be markers for different stages of the promotion process.

Table 1. Effects of FA, RA and TPCK on Tumor Response in Two-Stage Carcinogenesis[a]

	Relative Ability to Counteract (%)			
Inhibitor	TPA Promotion	TPA-Induced Hyperplasia	TPA-Induced Dark Cells	TPA-Induced ODC and Polyamine Levels
FA	100	100	100	20
RA	80	0	0	85
TPCK	70	0	70	10

[a]The abilities of FA, RA and TPCK to counteract the various TPA responses are expressed from 100% (complete suppression) to 0% (no effect). The effects of the inhibitors were determined from dose-response studies (16,14,20).

Two-Stage Promotion

Strong evidence for the existence of multi stages in promotion was first provided by Boutwell (21). He reported that skin tumors could be induced by limited topical application of croton oil to initiated skin followed by numerous treatments with turpentine (a non-promoting agent). These results led him to postulate that the promotional phase of two-stage carcinogenesis could be subdivided into two phases, conversion and propagation. However, similar experiments by Raick (18) and Slaga et al. (14), using hyperplastic agents such as turpentine, ethylphenylpropiolate, and acetic acid, did not show a two-stage promotion. In subsequent experiments, Slaga and coworkers (14,16, 19,20) corroborated and refined the original promotion model using mezerein, a very weak promoter that induces many biochemical and morphological activities similar to those seen after TPA treatment.

TPA, applied topically to initiated mice (DMBA, 10 nmol) twice a week for 16 continuous weeks at a dose of 2 μg, gives a significant tumor response in which 100% of the mice develop 8 or more papillomas/mouse (see Table 2). However, if TPA is given for only two weeks and subsequently followed by treatment with acetone, a non-promoter, no tumor response is detected. Mezerein, a diterpene structually similar to TPA, is not an efficient complete promoter (see Table 2). However, if mezerein is administered after two weeks of TPA treatment, it complements the TPA treatments and results in a tumor response equivalent to that in which TPA is given as a complete promoter. In such an experimental procedure, TPA effectuates stage 1 of promotion and mezerein facilitates stage 2 of promotion.

The ability of mezerein to act as a second-stage promoter, but not a complete promoter, has facilitated other experiments whose results corroborate the existence of multi-stages in promotion. The calcium ionophore A23187 or 4-O-methyl TPA are poor complete promoters but very effective first-stage promoters (see Table 2). When applied topically to mouse skin prior to the administration of TPA (stage 1) or mezerein (stage 2), the anti-inflammatory steroid FA can effectively inhibit the tumor response (see Table 3). RA does not inhibit the first stage of promotion but is an effective inhibitor of the second stage. Conversely, the protease inhibitor TPCK effectively inhibits the first stage of promotion but is not an inhibitor of the second stage.

The data obtained from inhibitor studies have facilitated the construction of a model for multi-stage promotion in SENCAR mouse skin (see Figure 1). Stage 1 of promotion can be accomplished by topical application of a complete promoter such as TPA, or specific first-stage promoters such as 4-O methyl TPA or the calcium ionophore A23187. Stage 1 can be inhibited by FA and the protease inhibitor TPCK. To date, the only morphological marker assignable to the first stage of promotion is the induction of dark cells.

Table 2. Relative Tumor Response with Two-Stage Promotion[a]

Initiator[b]	Promoter		Normalized Tumor Response
DMBA	TPA[c]		100
DMBA	Mezerein[c]		2
	Stage 1[d]	Stage 2[e]	
DMBA	TPA	Acetone	0
DMBA	TPA	Mezerein (1 μg)	35
DMBA	TPA	Mezerein (2 μg)	50
DMBA	TPA	Mezerein (4 μg)	85
DMBA	TPA	Mezerein (6 μg)	120
DMBA	4-O-methyl TPA (80 μg)	Mezerein (2 μg)	40
DMBA	TPA	4-O-methyl TPA (80 μg)	0
DMBA	A23187 (80 μg)	Mezerein (2 μg)	60
DMBA	TPA	A23187 (80 μg)	0

[a]The mice were initiated with 10 nmol of DMBA and promoted with 2 μg of TPA or as shown above.
[b]Initiation period was 1 week.
[c]Administered twice a week for 16 weeks.
[d]Administered twice a week for 2 weeks.
[e]Administered twice a week for 14 weeks.

Two types of data provide evidence for assigning dark cells to the first stage of promotion. First, mezerein, a second-stage promoter, causes all of the known TPA-induced morphological and biological responses except dark cells (14,16). Second, RA inhibits second-stage promotion (see Table 3) and does not inhibit the induction of dark cells (see Table 1). Correspondingly, TPCK inhibits the first stage of promotion and the induction of dark cells (see Tables 1 and 3).

The second stage of promotion can be accomplished with complete promoters and some chemicals such as mezerein that are specific for the second stage. Stage 2 can be inhibited specifically by RA and is characterized by hyperplasia and the induction of ODC, followed by increased levels of polyamines. It is important to emphasize that not all hyperplastic reagents are second-stage promoters in mouse skin (16).

Table 3. The Effects of Tumor Promotion Inhibitors on Two-Stage Promotion[a]

	Promoter		
Initiator[b]	Stage 1[c]	Stage 2[d]	Normalized Tumor Response
DMBA	TPA	Mezerein	100
DMBA	TPA + FA	Mezerein	0
DMBA	TPA	Mezerein + FA	20
DMBA	TPA + RA	Mezerein	95
DMBA	TPA	Mezerein + RA	20
DMBA	TPA + TPCK	Mezerein	25
DMBA	TPA	Mezerein + TPCK	94

[a]The mice were initiated with 10 nmol of DMBA and promoted with 2 g of TPA and 2 g of mezerein. FA (1 g), RA (10 g), and TPCK (10 g) were applied simultaneously with TPA or mezerein.
[b]Initiation period was 1 week.
[c]Administered twice a week for 2 weeks.
[d]Administered twice a week for 14 weeks.

Complete and Two-Stage Carcinogenesis in Different Mouse Stocks and Strains

The model for two-stage promotion depicted in Figure 1 was primarily derived from experiments performed with the SENCAR mouse. The SENCAR stock was selectively bred for sensitivity to skin tumor induction by polycyclic aromatic hydrocarbon (PAH) initiation followed by promotion (20,21). Consequently, the SENCAR mouse is extremely sensitive to two-stage carcinogenesis and coincidentally, sensitive to complete carcinogenesis. However, several other mouse stocks and strains exist that are refractory to promotion or that differ in their susceptibility to complete and two-stage carcinogenesis. The following ranking indicates the susceptibility of several mouse strains and stocks to complete and two-stage carcinogenesis:

with complete carcinogenesis

SENCAR > CD-1 $\geqslant$ C57BL/6 $\geqslant$ BALB/c $\geqslant$ ICR/Ha Swiss > C3H

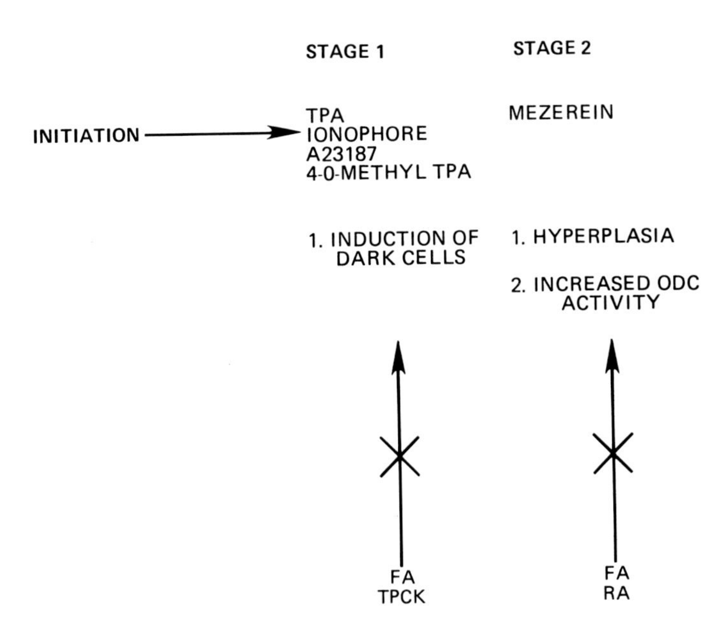

Figure 1. Two-stage promotion in mouse skin.

with two-stage carcinogenesis (initiation-promotion)

SENCAR >> CD-1 > ICR/Ha Swiss > BALB/c > C57BL/6 > C3H > DBA/2

It is important to emphasize the limitations of these rankings. First, only the responses to BP and DMBA were included in the analyses. Second, dose-response data for both the carcinogen and the promoter were not available for many of the mouse strains and stocks. Although these rankings represent subjective analyses, the differences between mice at the extremes of the rankings are significant (20-28).

Complete carcinogenesis. For any individual mouse stock or strain, an excellent correlation has been observed between the amount of PAH bound to DNA and the skin tumor response (22,23). However, this correlation between DNA binding and tumor response breaks down when a comparison is made between mouse strains or stocks that differ in their tumor response to complete carcinogenesis (24). Sims and coworkers (24) have demonstrated that the kinetics of binding of DMBA to the DNAs of C57BL/6, DBA/2, and Swiss mice are virtually identical. Although the possibility exists that a specific metabolite of the DMBA was responsible for the tumor response and was undetected in this study, recent investigations suggest that the major metabolites of DMBA and BP are qualitatively similar in mouse strains that vary in their response to complete carcinogenesis with PAHs (20,25,26). Although these data are far from conclusive, they suggest that some aspects of initiation are probably similar in strains of mice that differ in their response to complete carcinogenesis. Presumably, complete carcinogenesis has the equivalent of a promotion phase built into it. Differences in the promotional phase of complete carcinogenesis might be responsible for the variations in sensitivity found in different mouse stocks and strains.

Two-stage carcinogenesis. As discussed previously, present evidence suggests that some aspects of initiation with PAHs are qualitatively and quantitatively similar in mouse stocks and strains that differ in their response to complete carcinogenesis. Furthermore, initiation is probably similar or identical in complete and two-stage carcinogenesis. C57BL/6 mice were refractory to two-stage carcinogenesis but responsive to complete carcinogenesis. ICR/Ha Swiss mice responded poorly to complete carcinogenesis but did respond to initiation-promotion. This unequal susceptibility to complete and two-stage carcinogenesis within a stock or strain of mice strongly suggests that the promotional phases of complete and two-stage carcinogenesis are dissimilar. In addition, differences in sensitivity to initiation and promotion between mice may be due to alterations in the promotional phase of two-stage carcinogenesis.

The results of promotion in SENCAR and C57BL/6 mice are summarized as follows:

1. Repeated applications of various dose levels of TPA for 52 weeks without initiation in SENCAR mice gave a low level of papillomas (5 to 20%) and carcinomas (<15%) but did not show a dose-response relationship.

2. Repeated applications of various dose levels of TPA with initiation in SENCAR mice gave a dose-response in terms of papillomas (early) and carcinomas (late).

3. Repeated applications of various dose levels of TPA for 52 weeks without initiation in C57BL/6 mice did not give any tumors.

4. Repeated applications of various dose levels of TPA with initiation in C57BL/6 mice gave a very low level of papillomas (<5%) and carcinomas (<15%). (In this experiment BP doses of 50 to 1600 nmol were used to initiate the mice.)

(These experiments were done in collaboration with Dr. Stephen Nesnow, U.S. Environmental Protection Agency, Research Triangle Park, North Carolina.) Approximately 100% of the SENCAR mice developed a large number of papillomas over the course of the experiment in contrast to the C57BL/6 mice which did not give a tumorigenic response with BP as an initiator and TPA as a promoter. Since the C57BL/6 mice responded to complete carcinogenesis with BP, the data suggest that TPA is not effective as a tumor promoter in this strain of mice and that the promotional phase of two-stage carcinogenesis is defective or altered in C57BL/6 mice relative to the SENCAR mice.

To further investigate promotion in C57BL/6 mice, we examined the biochemical and morphological responses assumed to be markers for multi-stage promotion (see Table 4). Blumberg and coworkers (29) have reported that C57BL/6 mice contain specific receptors for TPA. As in the case of SENCAR mice, TPA induces hyperplasia, ODC, dark cells, and changes in the SDS-DTT extractable proteins of C57BL/6 mice (see Table 4). In addition, we examined two parameters that could modulate promotion. TPA induced a two- to threefold increase in a cytoplasmic cAMP independent protein kinase that phosphorylated the stratum corneum basic protein, a structural protein important in the terminal differentiation of skin (Mamrack, Oak Ridge National Laboratories [ORNL], Oak Ridge, Tennessee, unpublished data). However, this enzyme was induced to the same level in both SENCAR and C57BL/6 mice. In addition, we examined the effects of TPA on the levels and affinity of the glucocorticoid receptors (Davidson, ORNL, Oak Ridge, Tennessee, unpublished data). Within 6 h, TPA treatment inhibited dexamethasone binding to glucocorticoid receptors by 60% in both SENCAR and C57BL/6 mice. The dissociation constant for dexamethasone binding was not altered by TPA treatment in either stock of mice.

Compared with SENCAR mice, C57BL/6 mice have large adrenal glands. Trainin's (30) observation that adrenalectomy enhances tumor promotion by croton oil suggests that endogenous glucocorticoids can modulate promotion. We do not currently know if the differences in sensitivity to two-stage promotion are related to the size of the adrenal glands.

Based upon the analyses reported in Table 4, we postulate the following explanation for the failure of the C57BL/6 mice to respond to promotion. First, the data in Table 4 show that some of the responses assayed are qualitatively but not quantitatively similar in the SENCAR and C57BL/6 mice. Possibly a threshold level exists that needs to be exceeded to obtain promotion. Second, the data in Table 4 represent the results obtained after only one topical application of TPA. Susskin and Barret (31) have shown that the hamster, a species that is refractory to two-stage

Table 4. Morphological and Biological Responses Induced by TPA in Sensitive (SENCAR) and Resistant (C57BL/6) Mice[a]

Skin Response	SENCAR	C57BL/6
Hyperplasia	++++	++
Stimulation of ODC activity	++++	++
Changes in keratin proteins resembling embryonic pattern	+++	++
Induction of dark cells	++++	++
Stimulation of protein kinases	++	++
Decrease in glucocorticoid receptors	++	++
Presence of TPA receptor[b]	+	+

[a]Slaga, unpublished results.
[b]Data from reference 29.

carcinogenesis, responds to a single treatment of TPA but loses its responsiveness in repeated treatments. In this respect, we presently do not know if C57BL/6 mice retain their responsiveness to TPA after multiple treatments. Third, although the parameters listed in Table 4 are the best known markers for promotion, other critical, but presently cryptic, processes important to promotion may exist.

DISCUSSION

Investigations using inhibitors of promotion and complementary combinations of stage 1 and 2 promoters have provided evidence for multi-stages in skin tumor promotion. Stage 1 of promotion is characterized by an increase in the number of dark cells, a subpopulation of epidermal basal cells, and can be specifically blocked by the protease inhibitor TPCK. Stage 2 of skin promotion is characterized by hyperplasia and the induction of ODC activity. Stage 2 of promotion can be specifically inhibited by retinoic acid.

Several conjectures concerning promotion can be postulated from comparisons of stocks and strains of mice that vary in their susceptibility to complete and two-stage carcinogenesis. First, complete carcinogenesis may have an intrinsic promotion phase. Second, differences in susceptibility to complete and/or two-stage carcinogenesis may be due to differences in the promotional stage. Third, the mechanisms of promotion are not identical in complete and two-stage carcinogenesis.

Preliminary experiments comparing mice that are susceptible and refractory to promotion suggest that (1) the quantitative degree of response or (2) the retention of responsiveness to multiple treatments with promoter are important in the promotion process; alternately, (3) there exist events critical to promotion that have not been recognized.

The availability of mice that differ in their susceptibilities to complete and/or two-stage carcinogenesis will allow further dissection of the mechanisms involved in tumor promotion.

ACKNOWLEDGMENTS

Research was supported by NIH Grant CA-20076 and by the Department of Energy, under Contract W-7405-eng-26 with the Union Carbide Corporation.

REFERENCES

1. Berenblum, I. 1941. The cocarcinogenic action of croton resin. Cancer Res. 1:44-48.

2. Mottram, J.C. 1944. A developing factor in experimental blastogenesis. J. Pathol. Bacteriol. 56:181-187.

3. VanDuuren, B.L., and B.M. Goldschmidt. 1978. Structure-activity relationships of tumor promoters and cocarcinogens and interaction of phorbol myristate acetate and related esters with plasma membranes. In: Carcinogenesis: A comprehensive survey, Volume 2. Mechanisms of Tumor Promotion and Cocarcinogenesis. T.J. Slaga, A. Sivak, and R.K. Boutwell, eds. Raven Press: New York. pp. 491-508.

4. Gwynn, R.H., and N.H. Salamon. 1953. Studies on cocarcinogenesis. SH-reactons and other substances tested for cocarcinogenic action in mouse skin. Brit. J. Cancer 7:482-489.

5. Roe, F.J.C., and W.E.H. Pierce. 1960. Tumor promotion by citrus oils: Tumors of the skin and urethral orifice in mice. J. Natl. Cancer Inst. 24:1389-1403.

6. Boutwell, R.K., and D.K. Bosch. 1957. Studies on the role of surface active agents in the formation of skin tumors in mice. Proc. Am. Assoc. Cancer Res. 2:190-191.

7. Bock, F.G., G.E. Moors, and S.K. Crouch. 1964. Tumor-promoting activity of extracts of unburned tobacco. Science 145:831-833.

8. VanDuuren, B.L., A. Sivak, L. Langseth, B.M. Goldschmidt, and A. Segal. 1964. Initiators and promoters in tobacco carcinogenesis. Natl. Cancer Inst. Monogr. 28:173-204.

9. Slaga, T.J., A.J.P. Klein-Szanto, L.L. Triplett, L.P. Yotti, and J.E. Trosko. 1981. Skin tumor promoting activity of benzoyl peroxide, a widely used free radical-generating compound. Science 213:1023-1025.

10. Boutwell, R.K., and D.K. Bosch. 1959. Tumor promoting action of phenol and related compounds for mouse skin. Cancer Res. 19:413-424.

11. VanDuuren, B.L. 1969. Tumor promoting agents in two-stage carcinogenesis. Progr. Exptl. Tumor Res. 11:31-68.

12. Hecker, E. 1978. Structure-activity relationships in diterpene esters irritant and cocarcinogenic to mouse skin. In: Carcinogenesis: A Comprehensive Survey, Volume 2. Mechanisms of Tumor Promotion and Carcinogenesis. T.J. Slaga, A. Sivak, and R.K. Boutwell, eds. Raven Press: New York. pp. 11-48.

13. Slaga, T.J., J.D. Scribner, S. Thompson, and A. Viaje. 1974. Epidermal cell proliferation and promoting ability of phorbol esters. J. Natl. Cancer Inst. 57:1145-1149.

14. Slaga, T.J., S.M. Fischer, K. Nelson, and G.L. Gleason. 1980. Studies on the mechanism of skin tumor promotion: Evidence for several stages of promotion. Proc. Natl. Acad. Sci. USA 77:3659-3663.

15. Mechanisms of Tumor Promotion and Carcinogenesis. T.J. Slaga, A. Sivak, and R.K. Boutwell, eds. 1978. Raven Press: New York. pp. 1-588.

16. Slaga, T.J., S.M. Fischer, C.E. Weeks, and A.J.P. Klein-Szanto. 1981. Cellular and biochemical mechanisms of mouse skin tumor promoters. In: Reviews in Biochemical Toxicology, Vol. 3. E. Hodgson, J. Bend, and R.M. Philpot, eds. Elsevier North-Holland, Inc.: New York. pp. 231-281.

17. Raick A.N. 1973. Ultrastructural, histological, and biochemical alterations induced by 12-O-tetradecanoyl-phorbol-13-acetate on mouse epidermis and their relevance to skin tumor promotion. Cancer Res. 33:269-286.

18. Raick, A.N. 1974. Cell differentiation and tumor-promoting action in skin carcinogenesis. Cancer Res. 34:2915-2925.

19. Slaga, T.J., J.P. Klein-Szanto, S.M. Fischer, C.E. Weeks, K. Nelson, and S. Major. 1980. Studies on mechanism of action of anti-tumor-promoting agents: Their specificity in two-stage promotion. Proc. Natl. Acad. Sci. USA 77:2251-2254.

20. DiGiovanni, J., T.J. Slaga, and R.K. Boutwell. 1980. Comparison of the tumor-initiating activity of 7,12-dimethylbenz[a]anthracene and benzo[a]pyrene in female SENCAR and CD-1 mice. Carcinogenesis 1:381-389.

21. Boutwell, R.K. 1964. Some biological aspects of skin carcinogenesis. Progr. Exptl. Tumor Res. 4:207-250.

22. Slaga, T.J., S.M. Fischer, C.E. Weeks, and A.J.P. Klein-Szanto. 1980. Multistage chemical carcinogenesis in mouse skin. In: Biochemistry of Normal and Abnormal Epidermal Differentiation. I.A. Bernstein and M. Seiji, eds. University of Tokyo Press: Tokyo. pp. 193-218.

23. Phillips, D.H., P.L. Grover, and P. Sims. 1979. A quantitative determination of the covalent binding of a series of polycyclic hydrocarbons to DNA in mouse skin. Int. J. Cancer 23:201-208.

24. Phillips, D.H., P.L. Grover, and P. Sims. 1978. The covalent binding of polycyclic hydrocarbons to DNA in the skin of mice of different strains. Int. J. Cancer 22:487-494.

25. Legraverend, C., B. Mansour, D.W. Nebert, and J.M. Holland. 1980. Genetic differences in benzo[a]pyrene initiated tumorigenesis in mouse skin. Pharmacology 20:242-255.

26. Levin, W., A.W. Wood, P.G. Wislocki, J. Kapitulnik, H. Yagi, D.M. Jerina, and A.H. Conney. 1977. Carcinogenicity of benzo-ring derivatives of benzo[a]pyrene on mouse skin. Cancer Res. 37:3356-3361.

27. Kinoshita, N., and H.V. Gelboin. 1972. The role of aryl hydrocarbon hydroxylase in 7,12-dimethylbenz[a]anthracene skin tumorigenesis: On the mechanism of 7,8-benzoflavone inhibition of tumorigenesis. Cancer Res. 32:1329-1339.

28. Stenback, F. 1980. Skin carcinogenesis as a model system; observations on species, strain, and tissue sensitivity to 7,12-dimethylbenz[a]anthracene with and without promotion from croton oil. Acta Pharmacol. et Toxicol. 46:89-97.

29. Delclos, K.B., D.S. Nagle, and P.M. Blumberg. 1980. Specific binding of phorbol ester tumor promoters to mouse skin. Cell 19:1025-1032.

30. Trainin, N. 1963. Adrenal imbalance in mouse skin carcinogenesis. Cancer Res. 23:415-419.

31. Sisskin, E.E., and J.C. Barrett. 1981. Hyperplasia of Syrian hamster epidermis induced by single but not multiple treatments with 12-O-tetradecanoylphorbol-13-acetate. Cancer Res. 41:346-350.

DISCUSSION

Q.: I think the demonstration of multiple stages and multiple potentials for various agents involved in promotion are going to make the regulatory agencies cringe. In trying to think about ways of regulating tumor promoters, we have to remember how complex this process is. It's going to be awfully hard just to identify them because there are multiple criteria for various stages of promoters. So let's keep that in mind and try not to regulate things without a good, sound scientific basis.

Q.: I know that you've done a fairly detailed biochemical analysis of changes produced by the second-stage-only promoter, mezerein; have you done an equivalent study of the calcium ionophore A23187, which appears to be a pure first-stage promoter? You said it induced the dark cells. What else does it do?

A.: It also is an excellent inducer of hyperplasia. We haven't looked at a lot of the other criteria but definitely it induces hyperplasia as well as TPA does.

Q.: What biochemical changes?

A.: It increases ODC activity and prostaglandin levels.

Q.: I'd like to know what your evidence is that the difference in sensitivity of C57BL and SENCAR isn't due to differences in sensitivity to initiation, rather than promotion.

A.: Admittedly, sensitivity to initiation in the C57 Black and SENCAR are different. But at least in the complete carcinogenic model, where there's no promotional phase, the two are relatively similar. The C57 Black does respond to complete carcinogenesis, so I assume that initiation is occurring.

Q.: Is the TPA-induced first stage of promotion reversible or irreversible and does the induction of dark cells correlate with the reversibility?

A.: There are two ways to look at the reversibility with TPA. The first has to do with the phenomenon of how many papillomas one gets. If you treat a SENCAR mouse with TPA for several weeks, you will get papillomas. If you cease the treatment, the papillomas will regress. If you continue the treatment the papillomas will become permanent and eventually some of them will evolve into carcinomas.

Another way of looking at the reversibility has to do with how long the effect of a single application of TPA will persist. Eight weeks after TPA application, essentially none of its promoting effects persist, but if one gives a single application of TPA, waits four weeks and then uses mezerein as a second-stage promoter, one obtains very good promotion. So it appears that there is at least a period of four weeks during which the effects of TPA persist.

Now, dark cells are induced within six to twelve hours after application of a promoter; there is still fairly high level after two to three days, but virtually all disappear within a week.

Q.: In multistage promotion one tends to think that mezerein, because it can't do everything that TPA does, lacks something that TPA has. I don't think that is necessarily so. I think it's conceivable that mezerein has something that TPA doesn't have; perhaps it's the ability to kill initiated cells. This has been shown for some mustard compounds. It is known that when you give mezerein and TPA simultaneously, mezerein actually inhibits TPA. So it's a good inhibitor of promotion as well as a second-stage agent.

So until the proper experiments are done, I think we have to keep an open mind on how mezerein works as a second-stage agent.

A.: I agree.

THE ROLE OF PHORBOL ESTER RECEPTOR BINDING IN RESPONSES TO PROMOTERS BY MOUSE AND HUMAN CELLS

N. H. Colburn[1], T. D. Gindhart[2], B. Dalal[2], and G. A. Hegamyer[1]

[1]Laboratory of Viral Carcinogenesis, National Cancer Institute, Frederick, Maryland 21701. [2]Laboratory of Chemical Pharmacology, National Cancer Institute, Bethesda, Maryland 20205

INTRODUCTION

One of the major unanswered questions in carcinogenesis today concerns the rate-limiting steps that determine premalignant progression during the long latent period from the onset of carcinogen exposure until tumor appearance. Since tumor promoters apparently act to increase both the probability of occurrence and the rate of traversing events leading to malignancy, attempts to counter these promoter-induced events might offer a promising means of cancer prevention. In this connection, an understanding of the basis for resistance to tumor promoters could lead to an exploitable strategy. Our laboratory has developed the JB6 mouse epidermal cell model system for studying late-stage irreversible promotion of transformation by phorbol esters and other tumor promoters. We have recently described the isolation of promotion-resistant variants of JB6 cells which permit us to study the molecular and cellular basis for resistance (1,2). Since phorbol esters bind to specific cellular receptors and since resistance to a variety of hormones that also bind to specific receptors is associated with receptor deficiency (3), we have investigated whether the resistance of phorbol ester-resistant JB6 mouse cells can be attributed to a lack of phorbol diester receptors. This inquiry has been extended to phorbol ester-resistant variants of human hematopoietic cells.

MATERIALS AND METHODS

Materials

[^{3}H]Phorbol dibutyrate ([^{3}H]PDBu) (7.2 Ci/mM) was obtained from Chemicals for Cancer Research (Edenprairie, MN) and [^{3}H]PDBu (5.0 Ci/mM) from Dr. Mohammed Shoyab, Laboratory of Viral Carcinogenesis, NCI. Transformed cells used in this study were: K562, a human chronic myeloid leukemia in blast crisis (4); HL60, a human acute promyelocytic leukemia line (5); and TG20, a variant of HL60 resistant to induction of differentiation by 12-O-tetradecanoylphorbol-13-acetate (TPA) from Dr. T. Breitman, NIH, Bethesda, MD.

Derivation of TPA-Resistant Variants of Mouse JB6 Cells

The derivation of TPA mitogen-resistant variants of JB6 mouse epidermal cells has been described elsewhere (2). The promotable JB6 Clone 41 (Cl41) was exposed after reaching plateau density to TPA and colchicine in a selection procedure analogous to that described by Pruss and Herschman (6) for producing epidermal growth factor (EGF)-resistant variants of 3T3 cells. The cells that showed a mitogenic response to TPA at plateau density were trapped in mitosis by colchicine, detached, and washed off. The resistant cells remaining were carried through a total of two to six selection cycles and cloned. The TPA promotion-resistant variants of JB6, Cl25 and Cl30, were derived by nonselective cloning of the JB6 parent line, which was promotable to anchorage independence by phorbol diesters and other tumor promoters (1).

Assay for Mitogenic Response

Clonal derivatives of JB6 cells were allowed to reach plateau density in 5% serum. The cells were then exposed to TPA (1 to 100 ng/ml; 1.6×10^{-9} to 1.6×10^{-7} M), conditions that lead to an approximate doubling of JB6 Cl41 cells (2), and were enumerated by hemocytometer or Royco counter.

Assay for Promotion of Anchorage Independence

JB6 cell lines were exposed to TPA in 0.33% agar medium. At 14 days, TPA-dependent colony induction was determined as described (7,8).

Assay for Specific [^{3}H]PDBu Binding to Mouse JB6 Cells in Monolayer Culture

Twenty-four to forty-eight hours after plating in six well dishes, cells at a density $\geq$ 600,000 cells/35-mm well were washed twice with binding medium containing 1.0 mg/ml bovine serum albumin (BSA) (SIGMA). They were then incubated for 30 min at 37°C in a 5% carbon dioxide (CO_2) incubator with [^{3}H]PDBu in binding medium at concentrations ranging from 1 x 10^{-9} to 100 x 10^{-9} M. After removing aliquots of supernatants to determine the concentration of unbound [^{3}H]PDBu, plates were washed twice with ice-cold binding medium and the cell layer was lysed with 1.0 ml 0.5 N NaOH. Radioactivity was determined in a Beckman LS-350 scintillation counter with an efficiency of 40%. Nonspecific binding in the presence of 25 µM unlabeled PDBu was measured in parallel plates. Binding affinities and number of binding sites per cells were determined by Scatchard analysis. All points are the means of duplicates. [^{3}H]PDBu binding is expressed as amount specifically bound per 10^6 cells.

[^{3}H]TPA Binding Assay

Equal volumes of cell suspension and serial [^{3}H]TPA dilutions ranging from 10^{-12} to 10^{-7} M with or without 1.6 x 10^{-6} M unlabeled TPA were incubated in 12- x 75-mm borosilicate glass disposable culture tubes in a final volume of 300 µl for 60 min at 37°C in a metabolic water bath maintaining a 5% CO_2 atmosphere. Each data point is the mean of triplicate determinations.

Each cell type was assayed at a final cell concentration which bound 30 to 50% of input when incubated with a concentration of [^{3}H]TPA approximately equal to the Kd. Kd is defined as the negative of the slope of a Scatchard plot of the binding data according to the equation:

$$Kd = \frac{\text{amount bound}}{-\text{ amount bound/amount free}}$$

A time course of uptake was performed for each cell line and time point for the system equilibrium determined.

At the end of incubation, the tubes were put on ice and then centrifuged at 2000 x g for 10 min at 0°C. Two hundred microliters of supernatant were aspirated and counted. Cells were resuspended in 4 ml binding medium and spun at 2000 x g for 3 min. The supernatant was discarded and tubes inverted in a test-tube rack on absorbent paper to dry overnight. Each tube was cut approximately 1 in from the bottom with a glass tubing cutter. Two hundred microliters absolute ethanol were added to extract TPA, bottoms were counted in polyethylene scintillation vials, and radioactivity was determined by liquid scintillation spectrometry on a Packard Tricarb 460 CD at 60% efficiency using external standard ratio for automatic quench correction. Samples with less than 75% label recovery were discarded. Less than 0.4% of input [^{3}H]TPA remained bound to tubes after this procedure.

Analysis of Binding Data

Data obtained from equilibrium binding were analyzed by: (1) calculating linear regression parameters of the Scatchard plot (when the points were on a straight line) and (2) using nonlinear curve-fitting computer facilities of the Division of Computer Research and Technology at the National Institutes of Health. The M-Lab software of our computer facility employs a modification of Marquardt-Levenberg's iterative curve-fitting routine (9). Programs were developed in M-Lab incorporating one or more of the classical equilibrium models.

RESULTS

Table 1 summarizes the properties of the phorbol ester-resistant cell lines that have been derived from the BALB/c mouse epidermal cell line JB6 (7). Some of the cell lines were obtained by nonselective cloning (JB6 C125, 30, 41) (1) and others by cloning after selection for resistance to plateau density mitogenic stimulation by TPA (all the "R" lines) (2). The 11 TPA mitogen-resistant (M-) variants showed no plateau density mitogen response to 1 to 100 ng/ml (1.6×10^{-9} to 1.6×10^{-7} M) TPA. The four variants that were resistant to promotion of anchorage independence by TPA (P-) were resistant at the same TPA concentrations. As already reported, the identification of the M- P+ class of variants permits dissociation of TPA-dependent mitogenesis from promotion of transformation (2). The M- P+ and M+ P- variants are useful tools for separately investigating the basis for each type of resistance to phorbol ester promoters.

Specifically we asked whether either type of resistance could be attributed to a phorbol ester receptor deficiency. Table 2 shows that the number of phorbol diester binding sites per cell ranged from about 2×10^5 to 1.3×10^6. The resistant variants were indistinguishable from their sensitive counterparts in receptor number. In fact the most receptor-rich cell line (C130) was nonpromotable. Nor did comparison of binding affinities reveal any receptor defect in the resistant lines. The Kd ranged from about 10 to 35 nM for both sensitive and resistant variants. Development of the transformed phenotype in response to TPA (cell

Table 1. Characterization of TPA-Resistant Variants Derived from Mouse JB6 Cells

Phenotype	Cell Line[a]	Plateau Density Mitogenic Response (% Increase in No. of Cells)[b]	Anchorage Independence Promotion Response (% CFE)[c]
M+ P+	JB6C141	102	25.5
	JB6C122	125	24.0
M+ P-[d]	JB6C125	109	0.0
	JB6C130	140	0.1
M-[e] P+	R219	0	12.6
	R6141	7	21.8
	R23	0	12.7
M- P-	R28	0	1.1
	R631	6	0.6
M- Tx[f]	R24	4	52.3 without TPA

[a]Derivation of JB6C141, C125, C130: Nonselectively cloned from JB6 parent cells (1).
[b]Values for mitogenic response and promotion of anchorage independence response to 10 ng/ml TPA are expressed as the mean value for 2 to 3 experiments run in duplicate which varied by $\leq$ 10% from the mean.
[c]Colony-forming efficiency (CFE) in agar medium containing 10% serum minus background (< 0.5% CFE).
[d]Less than 2.0% CFE is considered negative for promotion response (P-).
[e]An increase of 10% or less is considered negative for mitogenic response (M-).
[f]Tx is anchorange-independent transformant.

line R24 in Table 2) does not require a change in receptor number or affinity.

Down-modulation of phorbol ester receptors has been found to occur in mouse JB6 cells as well as in human HL60 leukemic cells (10) following phorbol ester binding. Whether this decrease in available binding sites reflects receptor internalization, externalization, or neither is unknown. Nor is it known what role, if any, receptor down-modulation plays in the biological activity

Table 2. Sensitive and Resistant Variants of Mouse JB6 Cells Showing Similar Numbers and Affinities of Phorbol Diester Binding Sites

Phenotype	Cell Line[a]	No. BS[b]/Cell $x 10^{-3}$	Kd in nM
M+ P+	JB6C141	392	25
	JB6C122	770	19
M+ P-	JB6C125	339	20
	JB6C130	1333	35
M- P+	R219	329	8
	R6141	396	20
	R23	623	31
M- P-	R28	453	31
	R631	175	10
M- Tx	R24	163	10

[a]Cell lines susceptible or resistant to the mitogenic or promoting effects of TPA were assayed in monolayer culture for [^{3}H]PDBu binding sites by Scatchard analysis as described in Materials and Methods.
[b]BS = binding sites. Results are given as the mean for two experiments which varied by 5 to 15% from the mean.

of phorbol esters. In any case, we have observed that both TPA-sensitive and TPA-resistant variants show down-modulation of phorbol ester receptors (11).

We next turned our attention to the significance of phorbol ester binding in some TPA-responsive human hematopoietic cells. Listed in Table 3 are some biologic responses to TPA for peripheral blood mononuclear cells (PBMC), polymorphonuclear leukocytes (PMN), and three human leukemic cell lines (K562, HL60 and TG20). TPA blocks natural killer (NK) cell-mediated cytotoxicity by acting on a subpopulation of mononuclear cells that mediate the response. TPA stimulates reactive oxygen generation in monocytes and PMN, induces resistance to NK cells in K562, and induces adhesion in HL60 and TG20 cell lines. Scatchard analysis of PBMC and PMN indicated Kd for [^{3}H]TPA binding of 1 and 2 nM, respectively (not shown). The ED_{50} for TPA biologic effects are sufficiently close

Table 3. Biologic Effects of TPA on Human Hematopoietic Cells

Cell Type	Biologic Effect	ED_{50}
PBMC[a]	Suppression of NK cell-mediated cytotoxicity	8 nM (18)
PMN[b]	Reactive oxygen generation	10 nM (19)
K562[c]	Induction of resistance to NK cells	48 pM
HL60[d]	Increased adhesion	5 nM
TG20[e]	Increased adhesion	50 nM

[a]Peripheral blood mononuclear cells.
[b]Polymorphonuclear leukocytes.
[c]A myeloid leukemic cell line.
[d]A promyelocytic leukemic cell line.
[e]A variant of HL60 resistant to TPA-induced adhesion.

to the Kd to suggest that these biologic effects are receptor mediated.

Although Scatchard analysis of phorbol diester binding to a variety of cells described to date has revealed only a single binding site (12,13,14), it turned out that cells of the myeloid series (PMN, HL60, and K562) showed a second high-affinity binding site. Figure 1 shows the Scatchard analysis of [^{3}H]TPA binding to K562 cells. The curvilinear plot can be resolved into two components, a low-affinity binding site with a Kd of 6 nM and a high-affinity binding site with a Kd of 70 pM. The 48 pM ED_{50} for TPA induction of resistance to NK cells suggests that this effect is mediated by binding to the high-affinity receptor.

A similar curvilinear plot for HL60 cells indicated for the low-affinity binding site a Kd of 2.5 nM and 10^6 sites/cell and for the high-affinity binding site a Kd of 20 pM and 4×10^4 sites/cell. As shown in Table 3, the TPA induction of adhesion occurs with an ED_{50} of 5 nM for HL60 cells, suggesting that this effect may be mediated by binding to the low-affinity binding site.

A thioguanine-resistant variant of HL60 cells, TG20, was resistant to TPA at 5 nM but required 50 nM TPA for induced adhesion. Once again the basis for TPA resistance appears not to be at the receptor level. Scatchard analysis of phorbol diester

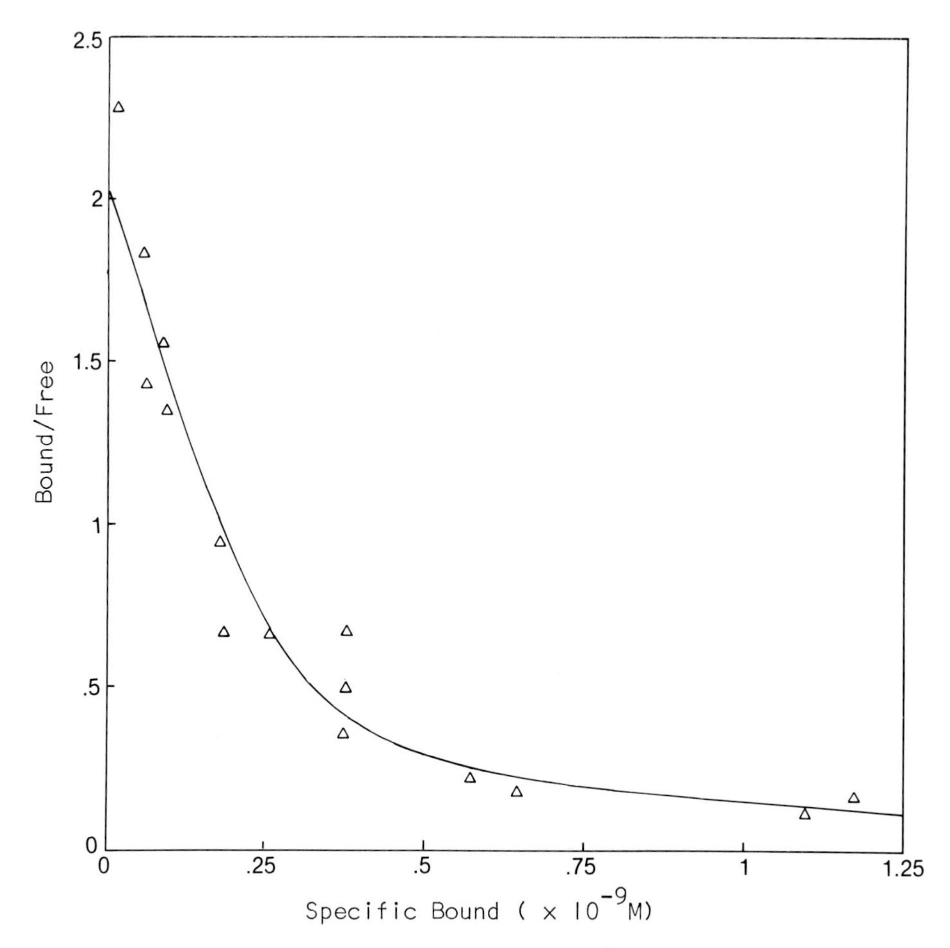

Figure 1. Scatchard analysis of specific [^{3}H]TPA binding sites on human K562 cells. [^{3}H]TPA binding and Scatchard analysis were carried out as described in Materials and Methods.

binding to TG20 (see Figure 2) showed 9 x 10^5 low-affinity sites and 3 x 10^4 high-affinity sites/cell, indicating no deficiency of either type of binding site. Nor could resistance be attributed to reduced affinity since TG20 showed Kds for [^{3}H]TPA of 2.3 nM and 20 pM for the low- and high-affinity binding sites, respectively.

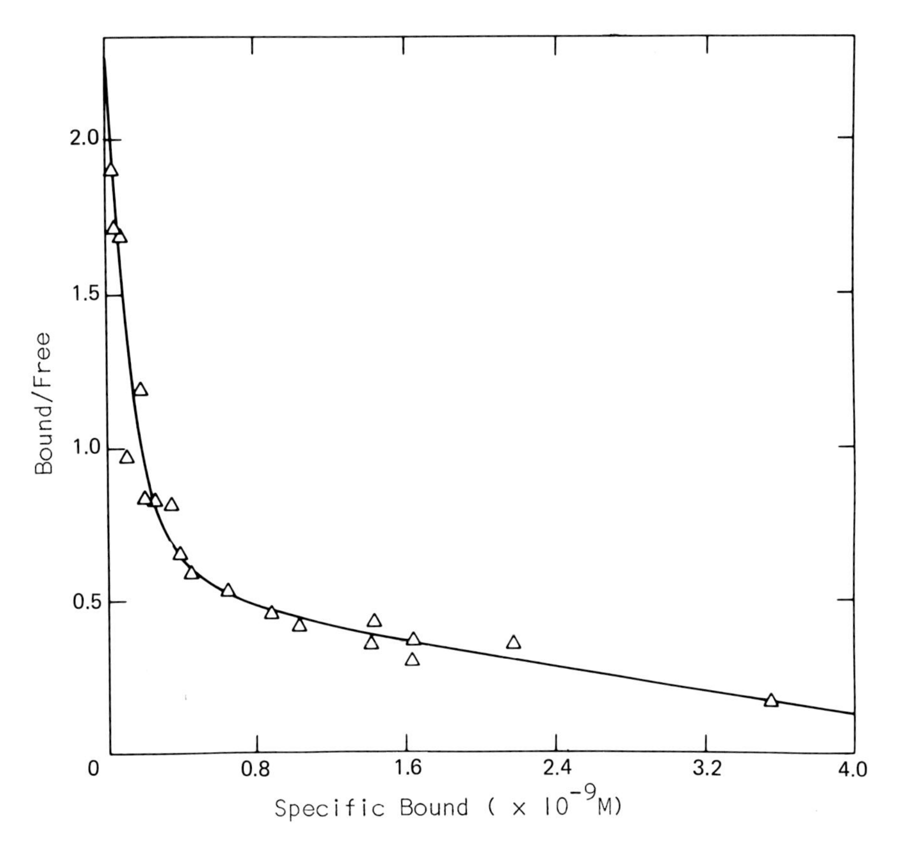

Figure 2. Scatchard analysis of [^{3}H]TPA binding of human TG20 cells.

DISCUSSION

These studies have shown that TPA resistance cannot be attributed to phorbol diester receptor deficiency in several resistant mouse and human cell lines. This generalization is based on studying both promotion of transformation and other biologic responses to TPA. A similar observation has been reported by Fisher et al. (15) and by Solanki et al. (10) who described the existence of normal levels and affinities of phorbol diester receptors on variants of Friend erythroleukemia cells and HL60 cells which are resistant to TPA regulation of differentiation.

Selection for resistance has yielded receptorless variants in the case of epidermal growth factor (6). Since virtually all mammalian cells except erythrocytes have phorbol diester receptors including variants deliberately selected for resistance to TPA (12,13,14), it appears likely that phorbol diester receptors may be essential to life in mammalian cells. If this is the case, attempts to prevent cancer by blocking the phorbol ester receptor might produce serious side effects in the host.

Whether phorbol esters or other ligands that bind to the same receptor can function as promoters of human carcinogenesis _in vivo_ or in human cells in culture is not as yet known. If it is true that phorbol ester receptors serve a basic function in the maintenance of life and if certain ligands that bind to this receptor can function as promoters of human carcinogenesis, then one would expect any heterogeneity in the human population for susceptibility to these promoters to occur at a level distal to receptor binding.

The existence of high- and low-affinity classes of phorbol diester receptors on human myeloid leukemic cell lines appears to be a new finding. A curvilinear Scatchard plot has also been reported by Horowitz et al. (17) for [^{3}H]PDBu binding to rat embryo fibroblasts. The Kd was calculated for the two binding sites to be 7.6 nM and 710 nM, respectively. That HL60 cells might have two or more classes of receptors was suggested by an earlier report of Mendelsohn et al. (16) who found that some responses of HL60 cells to TPA were maturation independent and others, such as TPA activation of membrane-bound NADPH oxidase, maturation dependent. These authors interpreted this observation as suggesting that induction of a new class of receptors accompanied maturation. Although cells of the myeloid series display a second binding site for [^{3}H]TPA which appears biologically active in the case of K562, it appears that cellular variation in [^{3}H]TPA binding is influenced only by direction of differentiation (myeloid versus mononuclear) but not by degree of differentiation or malignant transformation.

REFERENCES

1. Colburn, N.H., B. Koehler, and K.A. Nelson. 1980. A cell culture assay for tumor promoter dependent progression toward neoplastic phenotype: Detection of tumor promoters and promotion inhibitors. Teratogen. Carcinogen. Mutagen. 1:87-96.

2. Colburn, N.H., E.J. Wendel, and G. Abruzzo. 1981. Dissociation of mitogenesis and late-stage promotion of tumor cell phenotype by phorbol esters: Mitogen resistant variants are sensitive to promotion. Proc. Natl. Acad. Sci. USA 78::6912-6916.

3. Pollet, R.J., and G.S. Levey. 1980. Principles of membrane receptor physiology and their application to clinical medicine. Ann. Int. Med. 92:663-680.

4. Lozzio, C.B., and B.B. Lozzio. 1975. Human chronic myelogenous leukemia cell line with positive Philadelphia chromosome. Blood 45:321-334.

5. Collins, S.J., R.C. Gallo, and R.E. Gallagher. 1977. Continuous growth and differentiation of human myeloid leukemic cells in a suspension culture. Nature (London) 270:347-349.

6. Pruss, R.M., and H.R. Herschman. 1977. Variants of 3T3 cells lacking mitogenic response to epidermal growth factor. Proc. Natl. Acad. Sci. USA 74:3918-3921.

7. Colburn, N.H., W.F. Vorderbruegge, J.R. Bates, R.H. Gray, J.D. Rossen, W.H. Kelsey, and T. Shimada. 1978. Correlation of anchorage-independent growth with tumorigenicity of chemically transformed mouse epidermal cells. Cancer Res. 38:624-634.

8. Colburn, N.H., B.F. Former, K.A. Nelson, and S.H. Yuspa. 1979. Tumor promoter induces anchorage independence irreversibly. Nature 281:589-591.

9. Knott, G.D., and D.K. Reece. 1972. M-LAB: A civilized curve-fitting system. Proc. Int. Conf. on Online Interactive Computing, Vol 1. Online Computer Systems, Oxbridge, England. pp. 497-526.

10. Solanki, T.J., M. Slaga, R. Callahan, and E. Huberman. 1981. Down regulation of specific binding of [20-^{3}H]phorbol 12,13-dibutyrate and phorbol ester induced differentiation of human promyelocytic leukemia cells. Proc. Natl. Acad. Sci. USA 78:1722-1725.

11. Colburn, N.H., T.D. Gindhart, G.A. Hegamyer, P.M. Blumberg, B. Delclos, B.E. Magun, and J. Lockyer. (in press). The role of phorbol diester and EGF receptors in determining sensitivity to TPA. Cancer Res.

12. Driedger, P.E., and P.M. Blumberg. 1980. Specific binding of phorbol ester tumor promoters. Proc. Natl. Acad. Sci. USA 77:567-571.

13. Dunphy, W.G., K.B. Delclos, and P.M. Blumberg. 1980. Characterization of specific binding of [^{3}H]phorbol 12,13-dibutyrate and [^{3}H]phorbol-12-myristate 13-acetate to mouse brain. Cancer Res. 40:3635-3641.

14. Delclos, K.B., D.S. Nagle, and P.M. Blumberg. 1980. Specific binding of phorbol ester tumor promoters to mouse skin. Cell 19:1025-1032.

15. Fisher, P.B., H. Cogan, A.D. Horowitz, D. Schachter, and I.B. Weinstein. 1981. TPA resistance in Friend erythroleukemia cells: Role of membrane lipid fluidity. Biochem. Biophys. Res. Comm. 100:370-376.

16. Mendelsohn, N., H.S. Gilbert, J.K. Christman, and G. Acs. 1980. Effect of maturation on the response of human promyelocytic leukemia cells (HL-60) to the tumor promoter 12-O-tetradecanoylphorbol-13-acetate. Cancer Res. 40:1469-1474.

17. Horowitz, A.D., E. Greenbaum, and I.B. Weinstein. 1981. Identification of receptors for phorbol ester tumor promoters in intact mammalian cells and of an inhibitor of receptor binding in biologic fluids. Proc. Natl. Acad. Sci. USA 78:2315-2319.

18. Seaman, W.S., T.D. Gindhart, M.A. Blackman, B. Dalal, N. Talal, and Z. Werb. 1981. Natural killing of tumor cells by human peripheral blood cells: Suppression of killing *in vitro* by tumor promoting phorbol diesters. J. Clin. Invest. 67:1324-1333.

19. Kensler, J.W., and M.A. Trush. 1981. Inhibition of phorbol ester-stimulated chemiluminescence in human polymorphonuclear leukocytes by retinoic acid and 5,6-epoxyretinoic acid. Cancer Res. 41:216-222.

TISSUE AND SPECIES SPECIFICITY FOR PHORBOL ESTER RECEPTORS

Peter M. Blumberg, K. Barry Delclos, and Susan Jaken

Department of Pharmacology, Harvard Medical School, 250 Longwood Avenue, Boston, Massachusetts 02115

INTRODUCTION

Tumor promoters are agents that, although not themselves carcinogenic, induce tumors in animals previously treated with a subthreshold dose of a carcinogen (1-3). Although tumor promotion has been characterized in greatest detail for mouse skin, it has also been demonstrated for the liver, bladder, colon, trachea, and mammary gland (4,5). The potential importance of tumor promotion in human cancer etiology is suggested by a growing body of epidemiological evidence (6-8).

Phorbol esters comprise the most potent class of tumor promoters for mouse skin (9,10). Initially they were thought to be a promoter only for this tissue, but accumulating evidence now suggests that phorbol esters are active promoters for other tissues in the mouse, such as forestomach (11) or vagina (12), as well as for other species (13). *In vitro*, nanomolar concentrations of phorbol esters have dramatic effects on a variety of cell types from a variety of species, including the human (14-17). Prominent among these effects are partial induction of the transformed phenotype in normal cells (18,19), modulation of differentiation and differentiated activities (20), synergy with growth factors and other agents (21,22), and perturbation of membrane functions (23).

As part of the effort to elucidate the mechanism of action of phorbol esters, this laboratory has developed an assay for specific phorbol ester binding (24,31). Specific binding of 12-O-tetra-decanoylphorbol-13-acetate (TPA), the most potent phorbol ester, is largely obscured by the nonspecific partitioning of this compound into membranes (32), a consequence of the high lipophilicity of the tetradecanoic acid side chain (33). To circumvent this difficulty, we synthesized and radioactively labeled phorbol 12,13-dibutyrate (PDBu), a derivative that is somewhat less active biologically than TPA (34,35), and much less lipophilic (36).

This article summarizes three aspects of our studies on the PDBu receptor. First, evidence that the phorbol ester receptor identified in fact modulates biological responses to these agents is reviewed. Second, the tissue, strain, and species distribution of phorbol ester receptors and their pharmacological characteristics are presented. The results suggest that the phorbol ester receptor is a major, highly-conserved membrane protein. Third, the modulation of phorbol ester binding by the phorbol esters and by other agents is described.

MATERIALS AND METHODS

Newly hatched adult Drosophila melanogaster were provided by S.C.R. Elgin, Harvard Biological Laboratories, Cambridge, MA. Eggs of the sea urchin Lytechinus pictus were provided by J.V. Ruderman, Harvard Medical School, Boston, MA. These were fertilized and incubated in sea water for 65 h at 18°C to permit them to reach the pluteus stage before being harvested. Sources of mouse strains were as follows: CD-1, CFW, C57BL/6, and CF1 from Charles River Breeding Laboratories, Wilmington, MA; C3H/Anf, ICR/Ha, 101, CBA, BALB/c, DBA/2, and AKR from Cumberland View Farms, Clinton, TN. Except as noted, mice were 5- to 6-week-old females.

[20-^{3}H]phorbol 12,13-dibutyrate ([^{3}H]PDBu), 1.38 Ci/mmol and 3.42 Ci/mmol, was synthesized as described by Kreibich and Hecker (37). [^{3}H]PDBu, 14.8 Ci/mmol, was provided by New England Nuclear, Boston, MA. Phorbol esters were either synthesized or else purchased from Chemicals for Cancer Research, Eden Prairie, MN, Sigma Chemical Co., St. Louis, MO, or Consolidated Midland, Brewster, NY. Batches of mezerein were obtained from Chemicals for Cancer Research and as a generous gift from J. Douros, National Cancer Institute, Bethesda, MD.

For analysis of binding, cultured cells and invertebrates were routinely homogenized in a Potter-Elvehjem homogenizer. Tissues other than brain were usually homogenized in a Polytron PT-10 homogenizer. Assays of [^{3}H]PDBu binding were routinely done using a centrifugation binding assay (24,25). Briefly, [^{3}H]PDBu was incubated with 75-300 μg of particulate protein for 30 min at 37°C in 0.05 M Tris-Cl (pH 7.4), containing 4 mg/ml of bovine serum albumin. The membranes were pelleted by centrifugation for 45 min at 13,000 rpm in the HB4 rotor of a Sorvall centrifuge. Free [^{3}H]PDBu was determined from the radioactivity in an aliquot of the supernatant. Total bound radioactivity was determined for the pellet. Nonspecific binding was measured in the presence of a large excess (30 μM) of nonradioactive PDBu. Specific binding represents the difference between total and nonspecific binding. In some instances, a filtration assay (28) or a whole cell binding assay (29) was used instead of the centrifugation assay.

RESULTS

Relationship Between Phorbol Ester Binding and Biological Response

Using [^{3}H]PDBu, we were able to demonstrate high affinity, saturable, reversible binding to both whole cells and to particulate preparations from cultured cells and from various tissues. A critical question concerned the specificity of binding: Does the PDBu receptor detected by the binding measurements in fact mediate biological responses to the phorbol esters? We had previously analyzed the structure-activity requirements for loss of fibronectin, a major transformation-sensitive surface protein, using chicken embryo fibroblasts (38-40). We, therefore, compared the half-maximally effective doses (ED_{50}) of various phorbol esters for decreasing the level of fibronectin on chicken embryo fibroblasts with the dissociation constants (K_i) determined for inhibition of [^{3}H]PDBu binding to particulate preparations of chicken embryo fibroblasts (26). Very good agreement was found (see Figure 1).

A related but distinct issue was whether the PDBu receptor mediates tumor promotion. Unfortunately, the available data on the relative tumor promoting activities of phorbol esters are both limited and imprecise. Nonetheless, to the degree that the data permit quantitative comparison, binding affinities to mouse skin and tumor-promoting activities agreed (see Table 1).

Further support for the relationship between PDBu binding activity and tumor promotion came from analyzing representatives of several subclasses of phorbol derivatives that are highly inflammatory but non-promoting (25-27). Although resiniferatoxin is more than 100 times as inflammatory as TPA and 12-deoxyphorbol 13-isobutyrate 20-acetate is within 2-fold of TPA in inflammatory potency, both lack promoting activity. Likewise, both had an affinity for the PDBu receptor several orders of magnitude lower than that of TPA. The results with mezerein supported this same conclusion. Whereas mezerein is 50 times weaker than TPA as a complete promoter, it is comparable in potency to TPA for inflammation and second-stage promotion. The binding affinity of mezerein for the PDBu receptor corresponded to its complete promoting activity.

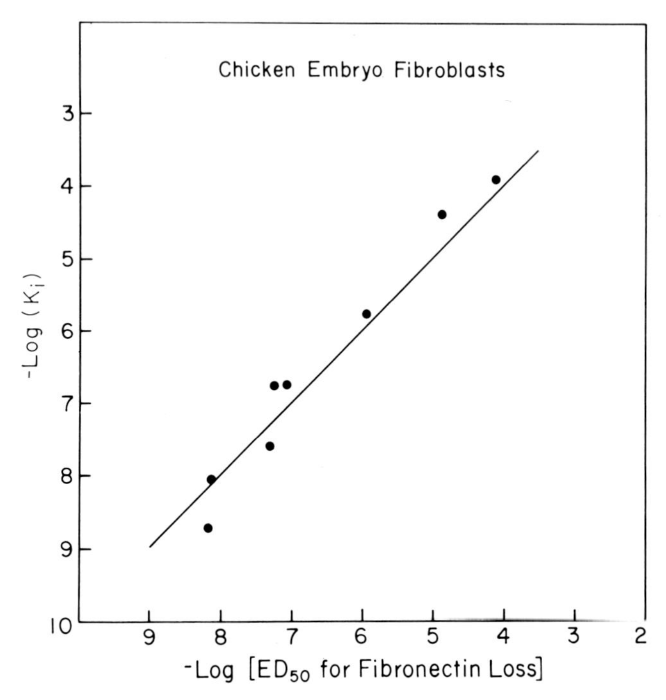

Figure 1. Correlation between phorbol ester binding affinity and biological activity on chicken embryo fibroblasts. The solid line indicates the predicted relationship assuming identical values in the two assays.

Tissue Distribution of Phorbol Ester Binding

Evidence for the promoting activity of the phorbol esters in tissues other than skin together with the variety of cell types for which biological responses to phorbol esters have been found suggests a widespread tissue distribution for the phorbol ester receptor. In agreement with this expectation, [^{3}H]PDBu bound specifically to particulate preparations from all tissues examined except for red blood cells (see Table 2). For the data in Table 2, binding was measured at approximately 40 nM [^{3}H]PDBu to reduce nonspecific binding. At saturating [^{3}H]PDBu concentrations, binding is predicted to be 20 to 60% greater, depending on the dissociation constant (K_d).

Table 1. Comparison of the Tumor-Promoting Activity and Binding Affinity of the Phorbol-Related Diterpene Esters for Mouse Skin

Derivative	Relative Tumor-Promoting Activity[a]	Potencies in Binding Assay[b] (K_i relative to TPA)
12-O-Tetradecanoylphorbol-13-acetate	1	1
Phorbol 12,13-didecanoate	1.5	<7[c]
Mezerein	49	132
Phorbol 12,13-dibutyrate	180-72	32
Phorbol 12,13-dibenzoate	20-100	100
Phorbol 12,13-diacetate	>50	4,000
Phorbol 12,13,20-triacetate	>200	7,600
Phorbol 13-acetate	NT[d]	86,000

[a]See reference 27 for original citations.
[b]See reference 25; K_i for TPA = 0.74 nM.
[c]Upper limits determined by assuming that phorbol 12,13-didecanoate and TPA nonspecifically partition into the particulate preparations to an equal extent.
[d]NT = not tested.

A striking and unpredicted aspect of the tissue distribution of the PDBu receptor was its very high level in the brain (28 pmol/mg at saturation). By markedly enhancing the proportion of total binding which is specific, this high binding level has greatly facilitated quantitation. Among the questions investigated using brain preparations are the following: We have assayed TPA binding directly and demonstrated that PDBu and TPA detect the same receptors (27). We have analyzed the kinetics and thermodynamics of PDBu binding (28). We have shown that the receptor is sensitive to heat and protease (27), and that it is exclusively membrane bound (28). In addition, we have demonstrated the developmental control of the receptor and the regional localization of receptors within the brain (31).

The level of PDBu binding in the brain is much higher than that of receptors either for neurotransmitters or peptide hormones. Instead, the level resembles that of the Na^+-K^+-ATPase (41) or the Ca^{++}-ATPase (42) in the brain. It is somewhat lower than that of calmodulin (43) and somewhat higher than that of the voltage-dependent Na^+ channel (44). Therefore, we have argued that the PDBu receptor is more analogous to a drug receptor than a hormone

Table 2. Tissue Distribution of [^{3}H]PDBu Binding

Tissue	[^{3}H]PDBu Bound (pmol/mg)[a]	No. of Tissue Preparations
Mouse		
Skeletal muscle	.33 ± .08	4
Heart	.57 ± .07	4
Small intestine	.67 ± .30	4
Vagina	.71 ± .11	4
Colon	.87 ± .27	4
Adrenal gland	1.00 ± .34	4
Lung	1.18 ± .37	4
Ovary	1.29 ± .19	4
Skin	2.40 ± .11[b]	3
Spleen	3.56 ± .42	4
Brain	24.00 ± .08[b]	3
Human		
Red blood cells	0.1 ± 0.2	1

[a]Specific binding to particulate preparations was determined using [^{3}H]PDBu at a sub-saturating concentration, approximately 40 nM, to increase the ratio of specific to nonspecific binding. Since partial degradation of [^{3}H]PDBu occurred in some tissues, these values are only approximate. Values represent the mean ± S.E.
[b]Calculated for 40 nM [^{3}H]PDBu, based on the K_d and the level of binding at saturation.

receptor and have proposed that the PDBu receptor normally functions as a transport protein, enzyme, or structural protein (27,31).

Comparison of Phorbol Ester Receptors in Different Mouse Strains

The central purpose of this conference is to identify mechanisms responsible for organ and species specificity in chemical carcinogenesis. The structure-activity relations for the PDBu receptor strongly suggest that this receptor mediates the tumor-promotion response. The question arises, can variations in PDBu receptor levels or affinity account for differences in strain or species responsiveness to promotion by the phorbol esters?

We did an initial survey of the levels of PDBu receptors in the skin of different commercially available mouse strains (see

Figure 2). In addition to CD-1 mice, for which data have been reported previously (25), ten strains were examined. Particulate preparations from whole mouse skin were prepared and specific [^{3}H]PDBu binding was measured (25). The concentration of [^{3}H]PDBu was 97 ± 9 nM (±.S.D.). Binding activities for CD-1, newborn CD-1, and AKR are the mean ± S.E. for 3, 3, and 4 skin preparations, respectively. For the other strains, values are the average of duplicate determinations/assay for one or two assays on a single preparation of skin. CF1, ICR, and CFW were reported to give 25 to 50% of the yield of papillomas obtained for CD-1, and for the two latter strains, a longer latent period was found as well (1). DBA/2N mice were more sensitive to promotion and to phorbol ester-induced inflammation than were C57BL/6N mice (45). C57BL/6J mice were more sensitive to the toxicity from intraperitoneal injection of croton oil than were AKR/J mice (46).

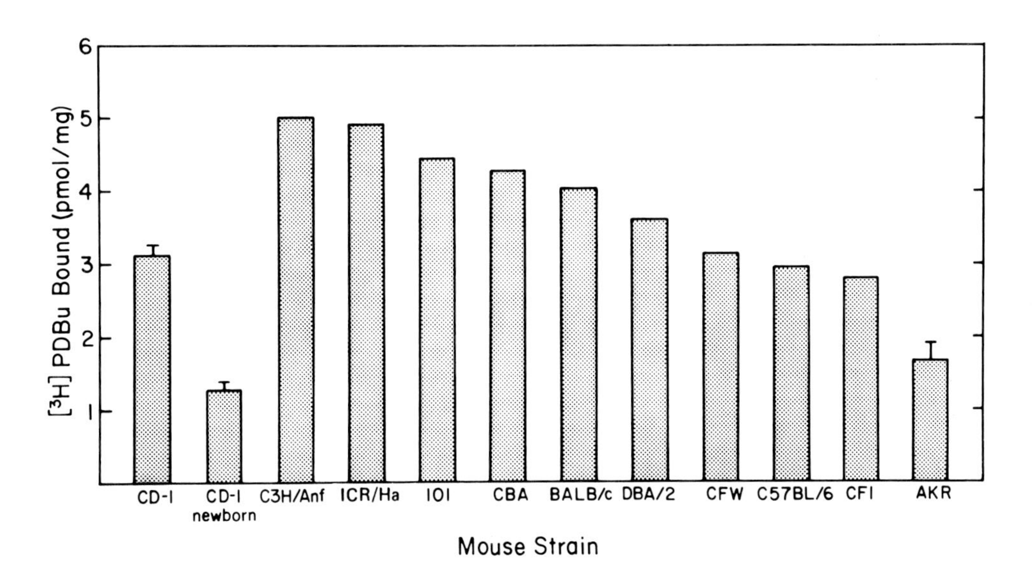

Figure 2. Specific binding of [^{3}H]PDBu to skin preparations from various mouse strains.

Although variation in receptor levels was observed, the values ranged only from 60% greater to 50% less than that for CD-1 mice. Moreover, part of this difference may represent experimental variation, since in most cases only single preparations of mouse skin from each strain were analyzed. The results contrast to those for aryl hydrocarbon hydroxylase activity, for which marked differences were found between strains in inducibility of enzymatic activity (47). While more extensive comparative studies of phorbol ester binding are required, it seems probable that factors other than variations in absolute receptor level predominate in determining sensitivity to tumor promotion. The high degree of conservation of PDBu receptors over the course of evolution discussed later in this paper suggests this same conclusion.

Species Distribution in Vertebrates

Cells or tissues from 11 vertebrate species were examined for specific phorbol ester binding: human (A.I. Tauber, E. Kennington, and P.M. Blumberg, unpublished observations) (48), bovine (31), mouse (25), rat (29), hamster (P.M. Blumberg and J.C. Barrett, unpublished observations), chicken (26), mink (49), bat (49), cat (49), dog (49), and monkey (49). Not only do all contain PDBu receptors, but to the degree data are available, the receptors closely resemble one another in their pharmacological parameters. Thus, for particulate brain preparations from mouse, cow, hamster, and chicken, the measured K_d values for [^{3}H]PDBu binding ranged only between 5.9 and 8.1 nM (see Table 3). Likewise, for receptors from rat, chicken, and mouse, very similar structure-activity relationships were obtained (see Figure 3). To compare structure-activity relationships, the K_i's of various phorbol derivatives were determined from inhibition of specific [^{3}H]PDBu binding. The data for the GH_4C_1 rat pituitary cell line were determined using a whole cell binding assay (29). The values for Caenorhabditis elegans (30), chicken embryo fibroblasts (26), mouse skin (25), and mouse brain (27) were determined using particulate preparations. The values for TPA are corrected for nonspecific partitioning of the ligand into the membranes. The values for phorbol 12,13-didecanoate are upper limits, based on the assumption that phorbol 12,13-didecanoate partitions into membranes at least to the same extent as does TPA.

The binding results are in accord with earlier biological studies. Cells from most of the species examined have been shown to be responsive to nanomolar concentrations of TPA (14,15,17). In addition, for phorbol esters ranging in potency from that of TPA to that of phorbol 13-acetate, ED_{50} values for stimulation of 2-deoxyglucose uptake in chicken embryo fibroblasts and mouse 3T3 cells differed by no more than a factor of 4 (50).

Table 3. Binding of [^{3}H]PDBu to Brain

Species	K_d (nM)	[^{3}H]PDBu Binding Activity (pmol/mg)
Mouse[a]	7.4	28
Bovine[b]	8.1	27
Hamster[c]	5.9	30
Chicken	6.7	20

[a]See reference 39.
[b]See reference 25.
[c]P.M. Blumberg and J.C. Barrett (unpublished observations).

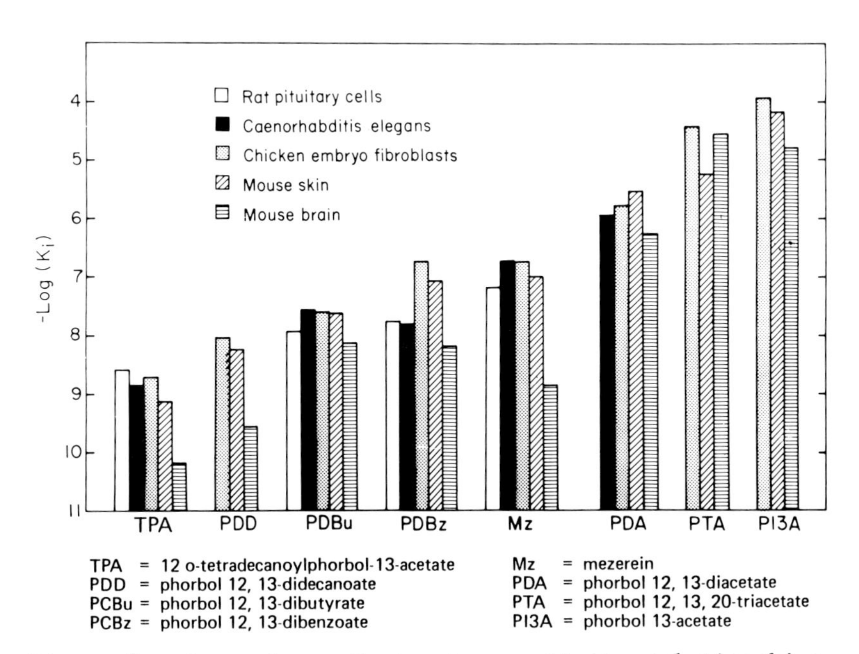

Figure 3. Comparison of structure-activity relationships.

Species Distribution in Invertebrates

Little information is available concerning possible phorbol ester activity on invertebrates. Bresch and Arendt (51) reported that nanomolar concentrations of TPA cause developmental abnormalities in the pluteus stage of the sea urchin *Sphaerechinus granularis*. As in higher systems, 4-O-methyl TPA is at least 100 times less active than TPA, consistent with the activity of TPA being mediated through a receptor similar to that in vertebrates. In addition, "euphorbium," the phorbol ester containing sap of *Euphorbia resinfera*, has traditionally been used in North Africa as an anti-fouling compound on ship bottoms (52). *Croton flavens*, which contains derivatives of 16-hydroxyphorbol and 4-deoxy-16-hydroxyphorbol (53), is reputed to act as an insect repellent (54); and the sap of *Euphorbia tirucalli* is cited as being insecticidal (55). On the negative side, biological effects were observed on the protozoan *Tetrahymena pyriformis* only at the equivalent of 50 μM TPA (56) and on the brine shrimp *Artemia salina* only at 6 μM TPA (57). In bacteria, there is only one report, of a minor effect (58). We therefore wished to determine if phorbol ester receptors occur in invertebrates. If so, how highly conserved are their binding properties, and how primitive are the phyla in which they can be identified?

[^{3}H]PDBu showed specific, saturable binding to the sea urchin *L. pictus* (see Figures 4a and b), the fruit fly *D. melanogaster* (see Figures 4c and d), and the nematode *C. elegans* (30). Specific binding, (●), points are the average of triplicate determinations in a single experiment; bars, ± S.E.; nonspecific binding, (Δ) points are from single determinations. Each experiment was repeated an additional two times on the same particulate preparation with similar results. Specific binding affinities were 9.8 ± 1.2 nM, 43 ± 10 nM, and 27 ± 4 nM, respectively. The corresponding specific binding activities were 0.9 ± 0.1, 1.7 ± 0.4, and 5.7 ± 1.4 pmol/mg protein.

L. pictus, *D. melanogaster*, and *C. elegans* belong to the phyla *Echinodermata*, *Arthropoda*, and *Nematoda*, respectively, and represent three major sub-branches of metazoan evolution: the enterocoelomates, the schizocoelomates, and the pseudocoelomates (59). The K_d values for these three invertebrates all fall within a factor of 2.5 of that for mouse skin. This range agrees with that found for different vertebrate cell types. Likewise, the absolute levels of receptors are similar to those observed for different mouse tissues. We have concluded that phorbol ester receptors appear to have been highly conserved during metazoan evolution.

The high degree of conservation of the PDBu receptor over evolution is further demonstrated by comparing structure-activity

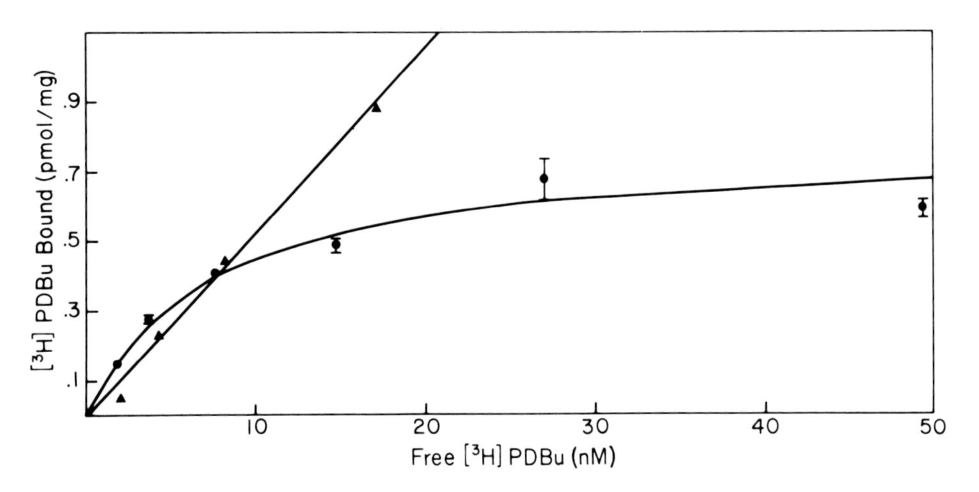

Figure 4a. Specific binding of [^{3}H]PDBu to a particulate preparation from the pluteus stage (68 h after fertilization) of the sea urchin _L. pictus_ (see [27] for methodology).

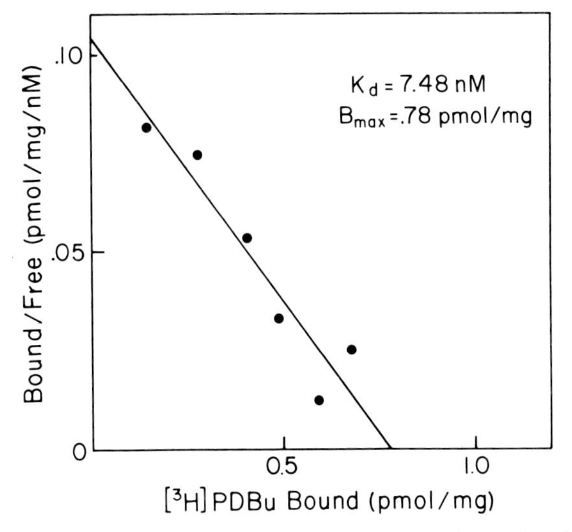

Figure 4b. Scatchard plot of the data in 4a.

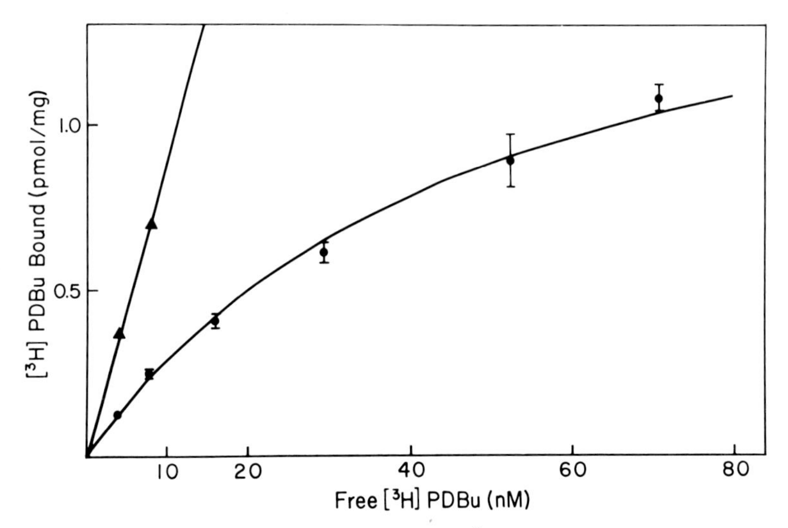

Figure 4c. Specific binding of [^{3}H]PDBu to a particulate preparation from adult _D. melanogaster_.

requirements. Those of the nematode _C. elegans_ and of the vertebrate systems that we have examined are virtually indistinguishable (see Figure 3).

Modulation of PDBu Binding

The analysis of factors modulating the PDBu receptor may lead to new insights regarding the mechanism of the receptor or its regulation. Considerable data indicate an interrelationship, albeit ill-defined, between the actions of TPA and of Ca^{++} (28). Upon chelation of Ca^{++} from brain particulate preparations, the K_d of the receptors for PDBu decreased 2.4 ± 0.4-fold (mean ± S.E. for four experiments) (28). Similar decreases in affinity were observed for TPA, mezerein, and phorbol 12,13-dibenzoate. The concentration of Ca^{++} able to modulate the binding affinity of PDBu was determined using a Ca^{++}-ethylene glycol-bis-(β-aminoethyl)ether N,N'-tetraacetic acid (EGTA) buffer system. An ED_{50} for Ca^{++} of $3.5 \pm 0.5 \times 10^{-7}$ M (mean ± S.E. for three experiments) was obtained (28). This value is similar to the values determined by Potter and coworkers of 2×10^{-7} M for binding of Ca^{++} to the

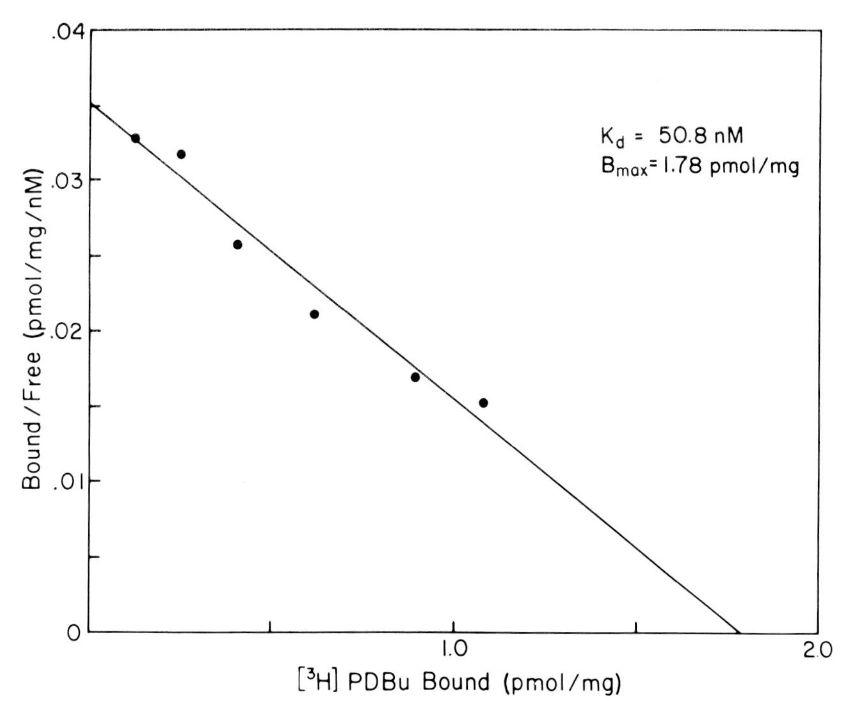

Figure 4d. Scatchard plot of the data in Figure 4c.

Ca^{++}-specific binding sites on purified troponin (60) and of 3×10^{-7} M for calmodulin-activated phosphodiesterase (61). Typically, the concentration of Ca^{++} in the cytosol is 10^{-8} to 10^{-6} M, whereas the concentration in extracellular fluid is 10^{-3} M (62).

The ability of PDBu to down-modulate its own receptors was examined using the GH_4C_1 rat pituitary cell line (29). Incubation of cells in the presence of PDBu decreased PDBu receptors to 54% of control by 6 h and to 19% of control at 24 h. This decrease reflected a change in receptor number with no alteration in binding affinity. The activities of three other phorbol derivatives were compared with that of PDBu. TPA, phorbol 12,13-dibenzoate, and mezerein all induced the same level of down-modulation as did PDBu; their ED_{50} values for inducing down-modulation reflected their respective K_i values for receptor binding. Following removal of PDBu from the cells, receptor levels slowly returned to control values; 75% of the control value was attained by 24 h and 100% of the control value by 48 h.

The GH_4C_1 cell strain was chosen for analyzing PDBu receptor down-modulation because these cells have receptors for several polypeptide hormones, namely, epidermal growth factor (EGF), thyrotropin-releasing hormone (TRH), and somatostatin. The modulation of these hormones by TPA has previously been characterized (63). We wished to examine the converse relationship: Was the PDBu receptor affected by binding of any of these hormones? EGF had no effect. In contrast, TRH caused a decrease in PDBu receptor numbers similar to that induced by PDBu (29). The time course of the decrease, likewise, was similar.

Although the mechanism of the heterologous down-modulation of the PDBu receptor by TRH remains under investigation, it provided a powerful tool to explore the relationship between receptor down-modulation and response. Phorbol esters cause a rapid decrease in high-affinity EGF binding in GH_4C_1 cells as in other cell lines (64,65). This decrease returns to normal over the subsequent 48 h. The dose-response curve for the decrease in EGF binding as a function of PDBu concentration was compared for control cells and for cells pre-incubated for 24 h with TRH (see Figure 5). Experimental details were as follows: GH_4C_1 cells were pretreated for 24 h with 2×10^{-7} M TRH or 10 ng/ml of PDBu. The cultures were rinsed twice with serum-containing medium, then incubated at 37°C for 1 h in serum-containing medium to remove residual TRH or PDBu. Fresh medium was added and the cells were returned to the incubator for 2 h. At the end of this pretreatment period, fresh medium was added, the cells were exposed to PDBu for 5 min, and then [^{125}I]EGF was added for a 1-h incubation at 37°C. [^{3}H]PDBu binding using a 45- to 60-min incubation was estimated in cultures treated the same way. The decreased PDBu receptor number resulting from TRH-pretreatment neither reduced the magnitude of EGF binding loss nor shifted the PDBu dose-response curve to higher concentrations. The same result was obtained if PDBu receptors were down-modulated with PDBu. Therefore, down-modulation does not affect the response to phorbol esters, at least for the parameter of EGF binding. Mechanistically, these findings imply either that the EGF response is mediated by a subpopulation of the phorbol ester receptors that are not down-modulated or that the EGF response depends on the fraction, rather than the absolute number, of phorbol ester receptors that are occupied.

The presence of a high-affinity, highly conserved binding site for phorbol esters strongly suggests the existence of an endogenous ligand. Unless a natural ligand were present to impose an evolutionary constraint on the binding site, this site would be expected to have been lost through genetic drift. Furthermore, since high-affinity binding sites are energetically and entropically unfavorable, they probably would not be present unless serving a function. Consistent with such reasoning, endogenous

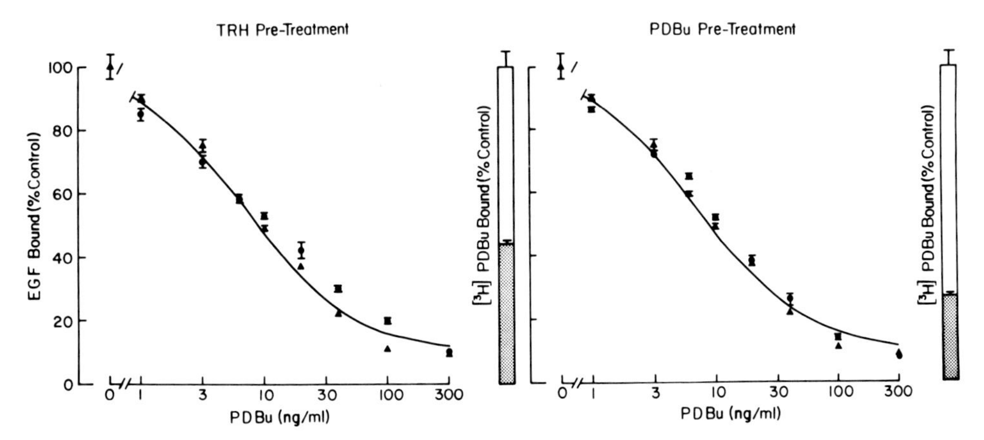

Figure 5. Lack of effect of receptor down-modulation on phorbol ester responsiveness in GH_4C_1 cells. The solid lines are drawn according to the equation $\Delta = (\Delta_{max})(S)/(K_D + S)$ where $K_D = 14$ nM, S = concentration of PDBu, and Δ_{max} = 90% decrease in EGF binding. Δ = EGF binding in control cultures, ● = EGF binding in down-modulated cultures. Open bars indicate PDBu binding in control cultures; cross-hatched bars indicate PDBu binding in down-modulated cultures.

ligands have been reported for a variety of drugs. The identification of the enkephalins as endogenous opiates is one of the more often cited examples.

Inhibition of [^{3}H]PDBu binding provides an efficient means of screening for endogenous compounds affecting the PDBu receptor. Since an endogenous ligand probably would be associated in part with its receptor, we examined whole brain preparations denatured by heat or acidification for inhibitory activity; Inhibition was observed. The boiled brain extracts were fractionated by gel filtration on Bio-Gel P2, revealing a single peak of inhibitory activity (see Figure 6). Experimental details were as follows: The elution position of the inhibitor activity on the Bio-Gel P2 column was consistent with a molecular weight of a few hundred. Inhibition of PDBu binding occurred slowly, requiring 2 h for maximal expression. Calf cortex was homogenized at 4°C in twice its weight of distilled water with a Polytron PT-10 at a setting of 7. The homogenate was incubated in a boiling-water bath for approximately 7.5 min, frozen overnight at -20°C, then thawed and centrifuged at 25,500 g for 1 h. The 25,500 g supernatant was collected and centrifuged at 100,000 g for 75 min. We lyophilized 26 ml of the 100,000 g supernatant, which we then resuspended in 1.5 ml 0.1 M NaCl, applied to a Bio-Gel P2 column (9 mm x 41 cm) and eluted with 0.1 M NaCl at a flow rate of 12 ml/h/cm^2. We assayed 20-μl aliquots of each 0.57-ml fraction for inhibitory activity by incubating for 2 h at 37°C in a final volume of 250 μl containing 0.05 M Tris-Cl (pH 7.4 at room temperature), 100 μg calf cingulate cortex particulate protein, 0.15% dimethyl sulfoxide (DMSO), and 35 nM [^{3}H]PDBu. The amount of [^{3}H]PDBu bound in tubes containing 30 μM nonradioactive PDBu was defined as nonspecific binding. The peak inhibitory fractions were diluted when necessary to quantitate inhibition. Dilution of the inhibitor yielded a dose-response curve. It was thus possible to quantitate the activity. At a maximal inhibitor concentration, approximately 20% of the [^{3}H]PDBu binding activity remained. The nature of the inhibition was determined by Scatchard analysis (see Figure 7). The inhibition was not competitive with PDBu, indicating that the inhibitor did not interact directly at the PDBu binding site on the receptor, and thus, is probably not the desired endogenous ligand. Nonetheless, since the inhibitor may provide information about the PDBu receptor and its regulation, we are pursuing the identification and purification of the inhibitor.

DISCUSSION

The major conclusion from the comparison of PDBu receptors of different strains and species is that the receptor is highly conserved. This finding has several implications. At the *in vivo* level, it supports emerging evidence that two-stage carcinogenesis, as characterized for mouse skin, is applicable to other mouse tissues and to other species, including man. It argues for the validity of the variety of *in vitro* systems currently being used to develop insights into the mode of action of the phorbol esters. Likewise, it suggests that the unique advantages of specific invertebrate systems can be utilized to analyze aspects of phorbol ester action.

An important objective is to obtain genetic confirmation of the conclusions derived from the biochemical and pharmacological studies of the phorbol ester receptor. Isolating phorbol ester unresponsive mammalian cell variants is one approach. Because the high degree of receptor conservation may predict difficulties in obtaining mutants altered in the receptor itself, we are collaborating with Dr. K.K. Lew, a nematode geneticist (Dept. of Neuropathology, Harvard Medical School), in exploring a potentially more manipulable system, that of *C. elegans*.

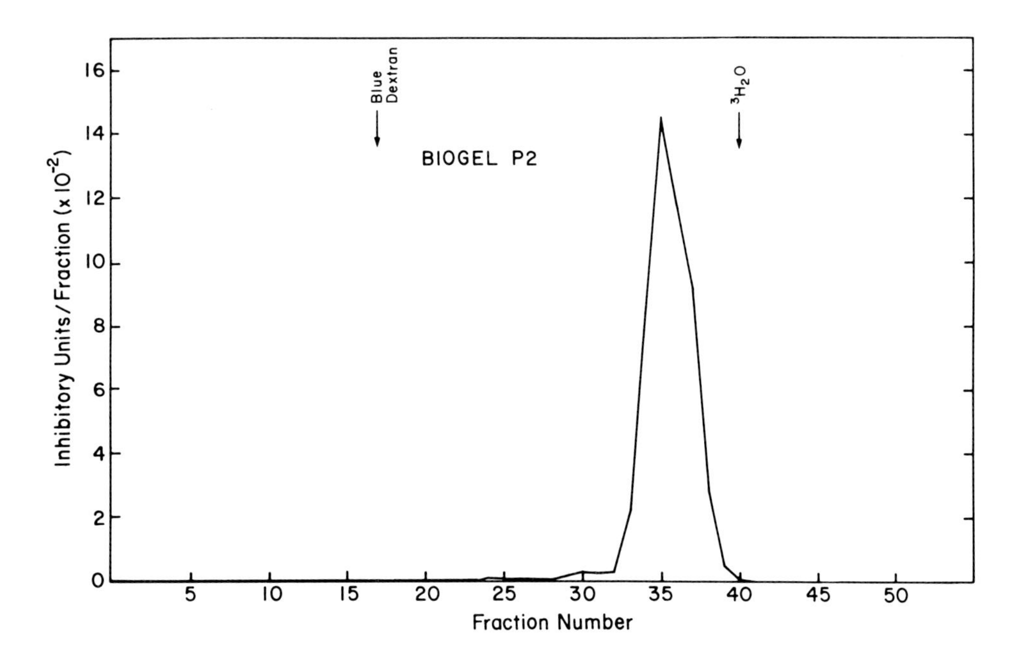

Figure 6. Gel filtration of an inhibitor of [^{3}H]PDBu binding isolated from bovine brain. One inhibitory unit = amount giving 50% of maximal inhibition under usual assay conditions.

C. elegans has been employed extensively for genetic analysis in the areas of developmental biology (66-68), toxicology (69), and neurobiology (70,71). C. elegans is a simple organism, compared to the mouse. The adult contains only 810 somatic cells (72). It has approximately 2000 essential genes, and a total genome size just 20 times that of Escherichia coli (73). Its advantages for genetic analysis include its short generation time (3 days at 25°C) and large brood size (~ 300 progeny). Most importantly, the animal is hermaphroditic, permitting ready isolation of homozygous recessive mutants (70). In addition, the genome of C. elegans has been cloned (74), and techniques are available to identify clones that overlap deletion mutations.

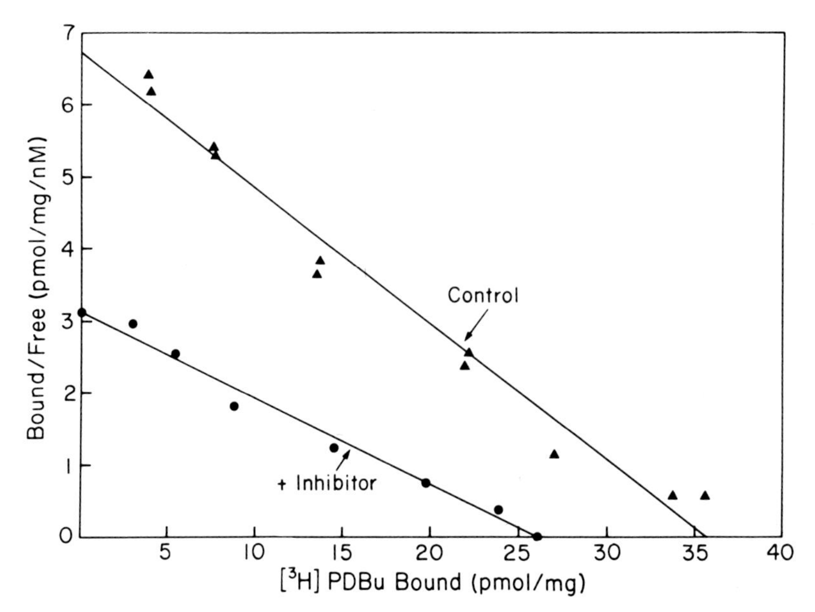

Figure 7. Scatchard analysis of the inhibition of specific [^{3}H]PDBu binding by the pooled Bio-Gel P2 inhibitory peak. Fractions 33 to 49 from the column shown in Figure 6 were pooled, and an aliquot was diluted 30-fold in 0.1 M NaCl. We assayed 30 µl of this dilution at varying concentrations of [^{3}H]PDBu as described.

As described earlier, the PDBu receptor of *C. elegans* is virtually undistinguishable from that of mouse skin. This is the case even for mezerein, which (as in mouse skin) shows much lower binding affinity for the PDBu receptors than does TPA, whereas biologically, it is as active as TPA. With *C. elegans*, it may thus be possible to demonstrate genetically the existence of distinct primary receptors for complete and stage II tumor promoters.

The selection of *C. elegans* variants depends on the expression of suitable biological responses to phorbol esters. In fact, phorbol esters induce a number of changes, including uncoordinated movement and decreases in animal size and in progeny yield (30). Mutants of *C. elegans* altered in their response to phorbol esters have been isolated by Dr. Lew and are currently being analyzed in our laboratory.

Another area of active interest is the existence of multiple classes of phorbol ester receptors. Based initially on comparison of in vitro and in vivo structure-activity relationships, we have postulated distinct receptors for (1) TPA, PDBu and related esters, (2) mezerein, (3) resiniferatoxin, and possibly (4) the short-chain substituted 12-deoxyphorbol derivatives (4,75). These predictions have been partially confirmed. As described earlier, the PDBu receptor shows the pharmacological specificity expected for the first class of agents. Binding showing the structure-activity selectivity for the other classes remains to be demonstrated.

A separate issue is whether there are multiple receptors with similar structure-activity requirements. While the binding of phorbol esters to mouse skin is virtually indistinguishable from that to the nematode, mouse brain binds with significantly higher affinity than does mouse skin. We have suggested two alternative interpretations (27). The receptors in skin and brain may represent the same gene product but be altered in affinity by differences in lipid environment or by modulatory factors such as Ca^{++}, phosphorylation, or proteolysis. Alternately, the receptors reflect different proteins resulting from gene duplication and divergence. Biochemical studies will be required to distinguish these two possibilities.

In the opposite situation, Estensen et al. (48) and Horowitz et al. (76) have reported a second class of receptors present in large numbers ($1.3 - 2.5 \times 10^6$ and 4×10^6 sites/cell) but of low binding affinity (100 nM for TPA; 900 nM for PDBu). Evaluating these results is clouded by difficulties in actually quantitating such binding in the presence of high levels of the phorbol esters taken up into the lipid phase of the membranes. In any case, since drugs commonly bind with low affinity to extraneous sites, the critical question here is that of significance: Does binding to the low affinity sites mediate biological responses?

The highest level of phorbol ester receptors in the mouse is found in the brain. We had previously presented evidence that phorbol esters induce partial mimicry of the transformed phenotype in normal cells (18). It is thus intriguing that the endogenous gene product homologous to the Rous sarcoma virus src gene product is also expressed in the highest level in the brain (preliminary results of J. Brugge using the immune complex protein kinase assay for src kinase activity [personal communication]). Likewise, a normal rat membrane protein believed to be related to the transforming gene product of Kirsten sarcoma virus is found in the greatest amount (20 pmol/mg) in the brain, is present at much lower levels in other tissues, and is absent in erythrocytes (77). Although stimulation of cell division is viewed as an essential response to phorbol esters and to transforming gene products, their normal physiological function may be rather different.

ACKNOWLEDGMENTS

Able technical assistance was provided by D.S. Nagle and E. Kennington. This research was supported by grant CA 22895 from the National Cancer Institute and by grant BC-345 from the American Cancer Society.

REFERENCES

1. Boutwell, R.K. 1964. Some biological aspects of skin carcinogenesis. Prog. Exp. Tumor Res. 4:207-250.

2. Scribner, J.D., and R. Suss. 1978. Tumor initiation and promotion. Int. Rev. Exp. Pathol. 18:137-198.

3. Van Duuren, B.L. 1969. Tumor-promoting agents in two-stage carcinogenesis. Prog. Exp. Tumor Res. 11:31-68.

4. Farber, E., and R. Cameron. 1980. The sequential analysis of cancer development. Adv. Cancer Res. 31:125-226.

5. Sivak, A. 1979. Cocarcinogenesis. Biochim. Biophys. Acta 560:67-89.

6. Cairns, J. 1981. The origin of human cancers. Nature 289:353-357.

7. Day, N.E., and C.C. Brown. 1980. Multistage models and primary prevention of cancer. J. Natl. Cancer Inst. 64:977-989.

8. Higginson, J., and C.S. Muir. 1979. Environmental carcinogenesis: Misconceptions and limitations to cancer controls. J. Natl. Cancer Inst. 63:1291-1298.

9. Evans, F.J., and C.J. Soper. 1978. The tigliane, daphnane, and ingenane diterpenes, their chemistry, distribution, and biological activities: A review. Lloydia 41:193-233.

10. Hecker, E. 1971. Isolation and characterization of the cocarcinogenic principles from croton oil. In: Methods in Cancer Research, Volume 6. H. Busch, ed. Academic Press: New York. pp. 439-484.

11. Goerttler, K., H. Loehrke, J. Schweizer, and B. Hesse. 1979. Systemic two-stage carcinogenesis in the epithelium of the forestomach of mice using 7,12-dimethylbenz[a]anthracene as initiator and the phorbol ester 12-O-tetradecanoylphorbol-13-acetate as promoter. Cancer Res. 39:1293-1297.

12. Goerttler, K., H. Loehrke, and B. Hesse. 1980. Two-stage carcinogenesis in NMRI mice: Intravaginal application of 7,12-dimethylbenz[a]anthracene as initiator followed by the phorbol ester 12-O-tetradecanoylphorbol-13-acetate as promoter. Carcinogenesis 1:707-713.

13. Goerttler, K., H. Loehrke, J. Schweizer, and B. Hesse. 1980. Two-stage tumorigenesis of dermal melanocytes in the back skin of the Syrian golden hamster using systemic initiation with 7,12-dimethylbenz[a]anthracene and topical promotion with 12-O-tetradecanoylphorbol-13-acetate. Cancer Res. 40:155-161.

14. Blumberg, P.M. 1980. In vitro studies on the mode of action of the phorbol esters, potent tumor promoters: Part 1. Crit. Rev. Toxicol. 8:153-197.

15. Blumberg, P.M. 1981. In vitro studies on the mode of action of the phorbol esters, potent tumor promoters: Part 2. Crit. Rev. Toxicol. 8:199-234.

16. Boutwell, R.K. 1974. The function and mechanism of promoters of carcinogenesis. Crit. Rev. Toxicol. 2:419-443.

17. Diamond, L., T.G. O'Brien, and W.M. Baird. 1980. Tumor promoters and the mechanism of tumor promotion. Adv. Cancer Res. 32:1-74.

18. Driedger, P.E., and P.M. Blumberg. 1977. The effect of phorbol diesters on chicken embryo fibroblasts. Cancer Res. 37:3257-3265.

19. Weinstein, I.B., M. Wigler, and C. Pietropaolo. 1977. The action of tumor-promoting agents in cell culture. In: Origins of Human Cancer. H.H. Hiatt, J.D. Watson, and J.A. Winsten, eds. Cold Spring Harbor Laboratory: Cold Spring Harbor, NY. pp. 751-772.

20. Abrahm, J., and G. Rovera. 1980. The effect of tumor-promoting phorbol diesters on terminal differentiation of cells in culture. Molec. Cell. Biochem. 31:165-175.

21. Dicker, P., and E. Rozengurt. 1979. Synergistic stimulation of early events and DNA synthesis by phorbol esters, polypeptide growth factors, and retinoids in cultured fibroblasts. J. Supramol. Struct. 11:79-93.

22. Frantz, C.N., C.D. Stiles, and C.D. Scher. 1979. The tumor promoter 12-O-tetradecanoylphorbol-13-acetate enhances the proliferative response of BALB/c-3T3 cells to hormonal growth factors. J. Cell Phyiol. 100:413-424.

23. Weinstein, I.B., H. Yamasaki, M. Wigler, L.-S. Lee, P.B. Fisher, A. Jeffrey, and D. Grunberger. 1979. Molecular and cellular events associated with the action of initiating carcinogens and tumor promoters. In: Carcinogens: Identification and Mechanisms of Action. A.C. Griffin and C.R. Shaw, eds. Raven Press: New York. pp. 399-418.

24. Blumberg, P.M., K.B. Delclos, W.G. Dunphy, and S. Jaken. (in press). Specific binding of phorbol ester tumor promoters to mouse tissues and cultured cells. In: Cocarcinogenesis and Biological Effects of Tumor Promoters. E. Hecker, ed. Raven Press: New York.

25. Delclos, K.B., D.S. Nagle, and P.M. Blumberg. 1980. Specific binding of phorbol ester tumor promoters to mouse skin. Cell 19:1025-1032.

26. Driedger, P.E., and P.M. Blumberg. 1980. Specific binding of phorbol ester tumor promoters. Proc. Natl. Acad. Sci. USA 77:567-571.

27. Dunphy, W.G., K.B. Delclos, and P.M. Blumberg. 1980. Characterization of specific binding of [^{3}H]phorbol 12,13-dibutyrate and [^{3}H]phorbol 12-myristate 13-acetate to mouse brain. Cancer Res. 40:3635-3641.

28. Dunphy, W.G., R.J. Kochenburger, M. Castagna, and P.M. Blumberg. 1981. Kinetics and subcellular localization of specific [^{3}H]phorbol 12,13-dibutyrate binding by mouse brain. Cancer Res. 41:2640-2647.

29. Jaken, S., A.H. Tashjian, Jr., and P.M. Blumberg. 1981. Characterization of phorbol ester receptors and their down-modulation in GH_4C_1 rat pituitary cells. Cancer Res. 41:2175-2181.

30. Lew, K.K., S. Chritton, and P.M. Blumberg. (in press). Biological responsiveness to the phorbol esters and specific binding of [^{3}H]phorbol 12,13-dibutyrate in the nematode _Caenorhabditis elegans_, a manipulable genetic system. Teratog. Carcinog. Mutag.

31. Nagle, D.S., S. Jaken, M. Castagna, and P.M. Blumberg. 1981. Variation with embryonic development and regional localization of specific [^{3}H]phorbol 12,13-dibutyrate binding to brain. Cancer Res. 41:89-93.

32. Lee, L.-S., and I.B. Weinstein. 1978. Uptake of the tumor-promoting agent 12-O-tetradecanoylphorbol-13-acetate by HeLa cells. J. Env. Pathol. Toxicol. 1:627-639.

33. Jacobson, K., C.E. Wenner, G. Kemp, and D. Papahadjopoulos. 1975. Surface properties of phorbol esters and their interaction with lipid monolayers and bilayers. Cancer Res. 35:2991-2995.

34. Scribner, J.D., and R.K. Boutwell. 1972. Inflammation and tumor promotion: Selective protein induction in mouse skin by tumor promoters. Eur. J. Cancer 8:617-621.

35. Thielmann, H.-W., and E. Hecker. 1969. Beziehungen zwischen der Struktur von Phorbolderivaten und ihren entzündlichen und tumorpromovierenden Eigenschaften. In: Fortschr. d. Krebsforsch., VII. C.G. Schmidt and O. Wetter, eds. Schattauer: New York. pp. 171-179.

36. Kubinyi, H. 1976. Quantitative structure-activity relationships IV. Nonlinear dependence of biological activity on hydrophobic character: A new model. Arzneim.-Forsch. 26:1991-1997.

37. Kreibich, G., and E. Hecker. 1970. On the active principles of croton oil. X: Preparation of tritium-labeled croton oil factor A_1, and other tritium-labeled phorbol derivatives. Z. Krebsforsch. 74:448-456.

38. Blumberg, P.M., P.E. Driedger, and P.W. Rossow. 1976. Effect of a phorbol ester on a transformation-sensitive surface protein of chick fibroblasts. Nature 264:446-447.

39. Driedger, P.E., and P.M. Blumberg. 1979. Quantitative correlation between _in vitro_ and _in vivo_ activities of phorbol esters. Cancer Res. 39:714-719.

40. Driedger, P.E., and P.M. Blumberg. 1980. Structure-activity relationships in chick embryo fibroblasts for phorbol-related diterpene esters showing anomalous activities _in vivo_. Cancer Res. 40:339-346.

41. Akera, T., T.M. Brody, and S.A. Wiest. 1979. Saturable adenosine 5-triphosphate-independent binding of [^{3}H]ouabain to brain and cardiac tissue in vitro. Brit. J. Pharmacol. 65:403-409.

42. Papazian, D., H. Rahamimoff, and S.M. Goldin. 1979. Reconstitution and purification by "transport specificity fractionation" of an ATP-dependent calcium transport component from synaptosome-derived vesicles. Proc. Natl. Acad. Sci. USA 76:3708-3712.

43. Watterson, D.M., W.G. Harrelson, Jr., P.M. Keller, F. Sharief, and T.C. Vanaman. 1976. Structural similarities between the calcium-dependent regulatory proteins of 3':5'-cyclic nucleotide phosphodiesterase and actomyosin ATPase. J. Biol. Chem. 251:4501-4513.

44. Catterall, W.A., C.S. Morrow, and R.P. Hartshorne. 1979. Neurotoxin binding to receptor sites associated with voltage-sensitive sodium channels in intact, lysed, and detergent-solubilized brain membranes. J. Biol. Chem. 254:11379-11387.

45. Nebert, D.W., W.F. Benedict, J.E. Gielen, F. Oesch, and J.W. Daly. 1972. Aryl hydrocarbon hydroxylase, epoxide hydrase, and 7,12-dimethylbenz[a]anthracene-produced skin tumorigenesis in the mouse. Molec. Pharmacol. 8:374-379.

46. Schmid, F.A., M.S. Demetriades, F.M. Schabel, III, and G.S. Tarnowski. 1967. Toxicity of several carcinogenic polycyclic hydrocarbons and other agents in AKR and C57BL/6 mice. Cancer Res. 27:563-567.

47. Nebert, D.W., and N.M. Jensen. 1979. The Ah locus: Genetic regulation of the metabolism of carcinogens, drugs, and other environmental chemicals by cytochrome P-450-mediated monooxygenases. Crit. Rev. Biochem. 6:401-437.

48. Estensen, R.D., D.K. DeHoogh, and C.F. Cole. 1980. Binding of [^{3}H]12-O-tetradecanoylphorbol-13-acetate to intact human peripheral blood lymphocytes. Cancer Res. 40:1119-1124.

49. Shoyab, M., and G.J. Todaro. 1980. Specific high-affinity cell membrane receptors for biologically active phorbol and ingenol esters. Nature 288:451-455.

50. Dunphy, W.G., C.-C. Lau, and P.M. Blumberg. 1980. Phorbol-related diterpene esters have similar structure-activity relationships in Swiss 3T3 cells and chicken embryo fibroblasts. Carcinogenesis 1:347-351.

51. Bresch, H., and U. Arendt. 1978. Disturbances of early sea urchin development by the tumor promoter TPA (phorbol ester). Naturwissenschaften 65:660-662.

52. Pabst, G., ed. 1883. Euphorbia Resinifera. In: Medizinal-Pflanzen, Volume 1. Fr. Eugen. Kohler Verlag. pp. 159.

53. Weber, J., and E. Hecker. 1978. Cocarcinogens of the diterpene ester type from Croton flavens L. and esophageal cancer in Curacao. Experientia 34:679-682.

54. Morton, J.F. 1971. Welensali (Croton flavens): Folk uses and properties. Econ. Bot. 25:457-463.

55. Watt, J.M., and M.G. Breyer-Brandwijk. 1962. The Medicinal and Poisonous Plants of Southern and Eastern Africa. E. & S. Livingstone, Ltd.: Edinburgh and London. p. 415.

56. Calkins, J. 1972. Tobacco smoke, carcinogens, and systems for recovery from DNA injury. Proceedings of the Third Tobacco and Health Workshop, University of Kentucky. pp. 214-231.

57. Kinghorn, A.D., K.K. Harjes, and N.J. Doorenbos. 1977. Screening procedure for phorbol esters using brine shrimp (Artemia salina) larvae. J. Pharmacol. Sci. 66:1362-1363.

58. Soper, C.J., and F.J. Evans. 1977. Investigations into the mode of action of the cocarcinogen 12-O-tetradecanoyl-phorbol-13-acetate using auxotrophic bacteria. Cancer Res. 37:2487-2491.

59. Barnes, R.D. 1980. Invertebrate Zoology. Saunders College: Philadelphia.

60. Potter, J.D., and J. Gergely. 1975. The calcium and magnesium binding sites on troponin and their role in the regulation of myofibrillar adenosine triphosphatase. J. Biol. Chem. 250:4628-4633.

61. Piascik, M.T., P.L. Wisler, C.L. Johnson, and J.D. Potter. 1980. Ca^{++}-dependent regulation of guinea pig brain adenylate cyclase. J. Biol. Chem. 255:4176-4181.

62. Kretsinger, R.H. 1976. Calcium-binding proteins. Ann. Rev. Biochem. 45:239-266.

63. Osborne, R., and A.H. Tashjian, Jr. 1981. Tumor-promoting phorbol esters affect production of prolactin and growth hormone by rat pituitary cells. Endocrinology 108:1164-1170.

64. Lee, L.-S., and I.B. Weinstein. 1978. Tumor-promoting phorbol esters inhibit binding of epidermal growth factor to cellular receptors. Science 202:313-315.

65. Shoyab, M., J.E. DeLarco, and G.J. Todaro. 1979. Biologically active phorbol esters specifically alter affinity of epidermal growth factor membrane receptors. Nature 279:387-391.

66. Hirsh, D. 1975. Patterns of gene expression. In: Microbiology-1975. D. Schlessinger, ed. American Society for Microbiology: Washington, DC. pp. 508-514.

67. Hirsh, D., D. Oppenheim, and M. Klass. 1976. Development of the reproductive system of *Caenorhabditis elegans*. Dev. Biol. 49:200-219.

68. Hirsh, D., and R. Vanderslice. 1976. Temperature-sensitive developmental mutants of *Caenorhabditis elegans*. Develop. Biol. 49:220-235.

69. Lew, K., and A. Kolber. (in press). An *in vitro* assay to screen for mutagens/carcinogens in the nematode *C. elegans*. In: *In Vitro* Toxicity Testing of Environmental Chemicals: Current and Future Possibilities. A. Kolber and T. Wong, eds. Plenum Press: New York.

70. Brenner, S. 1973. The genetics of behaviour. Brit. Med. Bull. 29:269-271.

71. Brenner, S. 1974. The genetics of *Caenorhabditis elegans*. Genetics 77:71-94.

72. Sulston, J., and R. Horvitz. 1977. Post-embryonic cell lineages of the nematode *Caenorhabditis elegans*. Dev. Biol. 56:110-156.

73. Sulston, J., and S. Brenner. 1974. The DNA of *Caenorhabditis elegans*. Genetics 77:95-104.

74. Emmons, S., M. Klass, and D. Hirsh. 1979. Analysis of the constancy of DNA sequences during development and evolution of the nematode *Caenorhabditis elegans*. Proc. Natl. Acad. Sci. USA 79:1333-1337.

75. Driedger, P.E., and P.M. Blumberg. 1980. Different biological targets for resiniferatoxin and phorbol 12-myristate 13-acetate. Cancer Res. 40:1400-1404.

76. Horowitz, A.D., E. Greenebaum, and I.B. Weinstein. 1980. Identification and properties of phorbol ester receptors in rat embryo cells. J. Cell Biol. 87:174a.

77. Scheinberg, D.A., and M. Strand. 1981. A brain membrane protein similar to the rat _src_ gene product. Proc. Natl. Acad. Sci. USA 78:55-59.

DISCUSSION

Q.: Let me propose a crazy idea: that the reason the brain is a preferential target for transplacental carcinogenesis is because the brain contains a lot of endogenous promoters, which is evidenced by the large number of phorbol ester receptors in the brain. Would anyone like to comment on this?

A.: Actually, the idea may be not quite so crazy. There was in the most recent PNAS an article on a normal analogue of the rat src gene (77). It is expressed at much higher levels in brain than anywhere else, and at levels comparable to those we see for the phorbol ester receptor.

The other side of the coin is, why do the endogenous transforming genes, as well as the phorbol ester receptor, tend to be expressed in brain at higher levels?

Q.: Is there a difference between rat and mouse brains in regard to the receptors?

A.: Of course, we have to look. The prediction would be no, because in brains of other species that we have studied the receptor levels are very similar.

Q.: The gerbil brain was also mentioned this morning. Gerbils are completely resistant to carcinogenesis in the nervous system, I believe. I asked Peter at that time if he had looked at gerbil brain and he said he hadn't.

Q.: If the brain has a lot of endogenous ligands then why aren't the phorbol ester receptors occupied by them and therefore not detected by your assay?

A.: Well, it could be that we dilute them out when we're doing the assays because the protein concentrations are lower.

Q.: You mean wash them off?

A.: One of the reasons why we're interested in the endogenous inhibitors is that if they exist, they could act as artifacts that introduce errors when we're trying to measure levels of binding. For example, one could postulate that skin had more receptors than brain but it also had a very high affinity inhibitor, which didn't wash off, so that we only saw the unoccupied receptors.

Also we haven't made too much as yet of the fact that we see a somewhat higher binding affinity in brain than in mouse skin, because the two possibilities are that the receptors are in fact different proteins or alternatively that they are the same protein in a different environment. The only way to answer that is to purify it.

Q.: From your studies, do you know whether these receptors are on the inside or the outside of the cell membrane in brain?

A.: We don't have any data on that. We've done some fractionation which indicates that the receptors are predominantly located in the membrane, but whether they are pointing in or out, we don't know.

LIVER AS A MODEL SYSTEM FOR ANALYZING MECHANISMS OF TUMOR INITIATION AND PROMOTION

Fred J. Stevens and Carl Peraino

Division of Biological and Medical Research, Argonne National Laboratory, Argonne, Illinois 60439

INTRODUCTION

Development of Initiation-Promotion Concept

Evidence that tumorigenesis is a multistage process first emerged from experiments showing that wounding of skin previously treated with coal tar resulted in tumor formation at the wound site (1). Subsequent experiments in which physical trauma was replaced by the application of chemical irritants not intrinsically tumorigenic yielded similar results (2,3). These observations were codified by Rous, who coined the terms "initiation" and "promotion" to denote respectively (a) the production of potentially tumorigenic cells by limited carcinogen treatment and (b) the completion of the neoplastic transformation resulting from subsequent treatment with any of a wide variety of noncarcinogenic irritants and proliferative stimuli (3).

Further major advances in characterizing a multistage skin tumorigenesis system included the discovery of the potent tumor-promoting activity of croton oil (4) and the observation that the initiation stage is irreversible, whereas the promotion stage is reversible (5). Identification of tetradecanoyl phorbol acetate as the active ingredient in croton oil (6) led to the use of this and other phorbol esters in a wide variety of investigations aimed at elucidating the mechanism of tumor promotion (7-10). Such studies disclosed that phorbol esters active as promoters exert a broad range of biological and biochemical effects *in vivo* and *in vitro*. However, a causal relationship between any of these changes and tumor promotion has not yet been demonstrated. The difficulty in identifying such a relationship stems primarily from the paucity of well-defined initiation-promotion systems of tumorigenesis amenable to comparative biological and biochemical analysis. The existence of different systems that could be compared judiciously would permit the identification of biochemical characteristics common to various models and hence potentially relevant to the tumorigenic process.

Demonstration of Initiation and Promotion in Liver Tumorigenesis

Indirect evidence that liver tumorigenesis occurs in stages was obtained several years ago from a number of studies. Cole and Nowell (11) observed that administering the hepatotoxin carbon tetrachloride to previously X-irradiated mice substantially increased tumor incidence. Farber and co-workers examined various types of nodular hepatic lesions occurring during prolonged carcinogen treatment and suggested that malignant liver tumors evolve from cells contained in those lesions termed "hyperplastic nodules," which precede tumor formation in this treatment (12,13). Further evidence indicating that hyperplastic nodules are tumor precursors was obtained by Teebor and Becker (14), who observed that the feeding of 2-acetylaminofluorene (AAF) to rats for 3 separate 3-week intervals, alternating with 1-week intervals on a control diet, produced a high yield of hyperplastic nodules that regressed, with a low subsequent incidence of hepatic tumors. An additional 3-week interval of AAF treatment, however, yielded nodules that persisted after carcinogen withdrawal and a high incidence of hepatic tumors. A later variant of this approach involved administering a single dose of dimethylnitrosamine following the three AAF feeding intervals. This combined treatment produced a high tumor yield, though no tumors were generated by either treatment alone (15). Recent studies by Farber and associates have shown that expression of the tumorigenic potential of hepatocytes exposed to nitrosodiethylamine (DEN) is enhanced by subsequently administering AAF as a cytotoxin combined with proliferative stimulation induced by partial hepatectomy or by administered carbon tetrachloride (16-18).

The studies cited above indicate that limited carcinogen treatment produces preneoplastic hepatocytes that require additional stimuli to complete the transformation into frank tumor cells. However, these investigations suffer from a common methodological problem -- the use of substances with carcinogenic and/or mutagenic activity as additional stimuli. Under such conditions it is not possible to determine whether progressive stages of liver tumorigenesis are qualitatively similar (involving, for example, progressive accumulation of mutations) or dissimilar, as has been demonstrated for skin tumorigenesis.

Definitive evidence that the onset of liver neoplasia proceeds in qualitatively distinct sequential stages first emerged from an investigation of the effect of phenobarbital on AAF-induced hepatocarcinogenesis (19). This study compared the effects of two different types of AAF-phenobarbital exposure modalities on tumor incidence. In the first instance, AAF and phenobarbital were present concurrently in the diet (simultaneous treatment protocol). Under these conditions, hepatic tumor incidence was substantially less than that produced by feeding AAF alone. Phenobarbital exhibited a protective effect when it was administered simultaneously with hepatocarcinogens 4-dimethylaminoazobenzene (20) and DEN (21). Since phenobarbital is a potent inducer of enzymes that actively metabolize these carcinogens (22), it can be concluded that the anticarcinogenic action of phenobarbital in these instances stems from a phenobarbital-mediated shift in the balance of carcinogen metabolism toward detoxification and degradation. The second type of exposure involved prolonged feeding of phenobarbital after a brief interval of AAF feeding (sequential treatment protocol). This regimen produced a markedly greater tumor incidence than that observed in rats receiving only the brief AAF treatment (19).

Contrasting the effects of simultaneous and sequential treatment protocols on tumorigenesis makes it evident that the enhancing effect of phenobarbital cannot be a consequence of increased metabolic activation of the carcinogen. A probable explanation is that phenobarbital given under the sequential treatment protocol facilitates tumorigenic changes previously initiated by exposure to the carcinogen. This interpretation suggests that there are at least two elements of the tumorigenic process that differ in mechanism as well as in temporal sequence. Thus it appears that the intiation-promotion concept of tumorigenesis applies to liver as well as to skin.

During the past several years we have tried to develop a liver tumor initiation-promotion system that can be exploited as effectively as the skin system, thereby providing a basis for cross-system comparisons. The following discussion briefly summarizes what we and others have learned about the characteristics of multistage tumorigenesis in liver.

CHARACTERISTICS OF MULTISTAGE HEPATOCARCINOGENESIS

Agents with Tumor Initiating or Promoting Activity in Liver

After the promotion of AAF hepatocarcinogenesis by phenobarbital (19) was first observed, several reports demonstrated that initiation and promotion in liver can each be produced by a wide variety of agents administered according to the sequential treatment protocol (see Table 1). It is noteworthy that the use of a promoting stimulus has increased liver system sensitivity to the extent that agents previously considered to have no hepatocarcinogenic activity (benzo[*a*]pyrene, 7,12-dimethylbenz[*a*]-anthracene [DMBA], and 2-methyl-4-dimethylaminoazobenzene) are now identified as initiators.

Phenobarbital is clearly not an initiator of hepatocarcinogenesis in mice (21) or rats (23) and, in fact, can protect against hepatic tumorigenesis when administered simultaneously with a known carcinogen. That phenobarbital increased the incidence of liver tumors in mice subject to a spontaneous incidence of such tumors (43-46) suggests that phenobarbital was promoting the phenotypic expression of tumorigenic lesions induced by an unknown initiator. This explanation presumably applies to a similar observation made recently in rats (47). Given this tumorigenic effect by the promotor phenobarbital, it appears reasonable to question the validity of classifying agents such as DDT as carcinogens simply on the basis of their ability to increase liver tumor incidence, when fed at high dietary concentrations for long intervals to mice (48-52) or rats (53,54) susceptible to such tumors. Tumor-promoting activity might also be due to certain plant resins, since prolonged exposure to such substances found in softwood bedding has increased hepatic tumor incidence in susceptible mice (55).

Characteristics of Liver Tumor Promotion by Phenobarbital

In analyzing the characteristics of liver tumor promotion by phenobarbital, we have examined the effects on tumorigenesis of separating carcinogen and phenobarbital treatments by various intervals and varying the duration of phenobarbital exposure and dietary concentration of phenobarbital. We observed that the phenobarbital promoting effect occurred despite a 120-day interval between the termination of the carcinogen treatment and the onset of phenobarbital exposure (56). These findings indicate that carcinogen-modified hepatocytes with tumorigenic potential (initiated hepatocytes) persist long after the initiating event. Such persistence was evident in skin tumorigenesis studies which suggests that the initiation stage of tumorigenesis is irreversible (5,57). In addition, an increase in the duration of phenobarbital treatment following AAF exposure was accompanied by parallel increases in tumor yield (56,58); prolonged exposure to phenobarbital was required for maximum promoting effectiveness (56).

Our most recent investigation (23) compared the promoting effects of different dietary levels of phenobarbital. When fed at

Table 1. Initiation-Promotion Experiments in Liver.

Initiator	Promoter	Reference
2-Acetylaminofluorene (AAF)	Phenobarbital (PB)	19,23-27
Nitrosodiethylamine (DEN)	PB	28-35
Nitrosodimethylamine	PB	36
Benzo[*a*]pyrene	PB	37
7,12-Dimethylbenz[*a*]anthracene	PB	38
4-Dimethylaminoazobenzene	PB	39
3-Methyl-4-dimethylaminoazobenzene	PB	30
2-Methyl-4-dimethylaminoazobenzene	PB	40
AAF	Dichlorodiphenyltrichloroethane (DDT)	34,41
DEN	DDT	34
DEN	Polychlorinated biphenyls	33,34
AAF	Butylated hydroxytoluene	42
DEN	2,3,7,8-Tetrachlorodibenzo-*p*-dioxin	31
DEN	Contraceptive steroids	35
DEN	Choline deficiency	32

dietary concentrations that did not affect body weight gain, phenobarbital elicited dose-dependent increases in the final incidence (plateau level) of hepatic tumors in rats previously fed AAF. However, these phenobarbital treatments did not affect the time of onset or cessation (attainment of the plateau phase) of tumorigenesis. The highest dietary concentration of phenobarbital initially retarded tumor promotion but ultimately had the strongest promoting effect; rats on this regimen also showed a reduction in growth rate. None of the dietary levels of phenobarbital affected the growth rates or the morphological characteristics (degree of differentiation) of the tumors that were produced. The foregoing observations suggest that phenobarbital has no initiating activity, and tumor promotion by phenobarbital primarily involves an increase in the probability that initiated hepatocytes will express the neoplastic phenotype and does not influence the character of this phenotype or the kinetics of its expression.

Organ Specificity of Phenobarbital's Promoting Action

Current experimental evidence suggests that the tumor promoting effect of phenobarbital is specific for the liver. In CF-1 mice, phenobarbital feeding increased the spontaneous incidence of hepatic tumors but had no effect on the spontaneous incidence of other tumors such as lymphomas, lung adenomas, and osteomas (45). Similarly, phenobarbital increased the subsequent incidence of liver tumors in mice treated with DEN at birth but had no effect on DEN-induced lung tumors in these animals (36). Phenobarbital feeding also failed to enhance skin tumorigenesis in mice subjected to prior skin painting with DMBA (59). However, other barbiturate derivatives may be less specific; for example, chronic sodium barbiturate administration promoted intestinal tumorigenesis in rats previously exposed to dimethylhydrazine (60).

The evidence concerning barbiturates' effects on tumorigenesis in liver or other tissue is ambiguous regarding the consequences of human exposure to phenobarbital. In a study of patients receiving long-term treatment with phenobarbital, a slightly greater than expected incidence of liver tumors was observed (61) -- the significance of which has been debated (62,63) -- but no increase occurred in other types of tumors (61). Additional epidemiological studies suggest that chronic barbiturate treatment may increase the risk of brain tumorigenesis in children (64), although this conclusion is also disputed (65,66).

DEVELOPMENT OF MODELS TO SIMULATE MULTISTAGE HEPATOCARCINOGENESIS

Although empirical evidence for initiation and promotion has been obtained from several systems (7-9,67), the liver offers a unique combination of advantages for mechanistic studies. These advantages include

1) the responsiveness of liver to a broader spectrum of initiators and promoters than any other single tissue,
2) the abundance, relative homogeneity, and ready accessibility of the tissue,
3) the vast accumulation of information on hepatic parenchymal cell biochemistry and the relative ease of conducting biochemical studies in liver,
4) the reasonable assurance that the previously mentioned biochemical information has mechanistic relevance, based on the high probability that hepatic parenchymal cells are progenitors of hepatocellular carcinomas,
5) the retention of all cells representing the various stages of tumorigenesis at their sites of origin in contrast to epithelial systems in which some altered cells are lost by sloughing, and
6) the availability of histochemical techniques to identify putative clones of early preneoplastic hepatocytes (18).

Therefore, the liver may be the best available system for characterizing the sequence of events involved in the expression of the neoplastic phenotype. To analyze this sequence of events it is necessary to understand the relationship between data on tumor incidence kinetics, tumor phenotypes, initiator and promoter dose effects, and the numbers, incidence kinetics, sizes, and histochemical phenotypes of the foci of altered hepatocytes that appear in liver prior to tumor formation (18,26,29,68-70). One approach to this problem is to develop models of liver tumor initiation and promotion as the basis for computer simulations of the data generated in our empirical studies. Iterative comparisons of simulated and empirical data permit the mechanistic assumptions upon which the tumorigenesis model is based to be progressively refined and also reveal new questions that can be addressed by appropriate experiments.

Model 1

This model is based on current observations of the characteristics of liver tumor promotion by phenobarbital and is intended to narrow the range of possible mechanisms by which the promoting influence of phenobarbital is exerted. The present form of the model is based on the following assumptions derived from these observations:

1) Initiation occurs randomly; therefore initiated loci are distributed randomly throughout the liver cell population.
2) Tumorigenesis can occur at any time after initiation.

3) All tumors have the same growth rate. The model can be reduced in scope to include only tumors of any particular type in which case this assumption becomes: all tumors of the same type have the same growth rate.
4) A tumor that has not existed for sufficient time to accumulate a mass greater than the minimum required for observation will not be counted.
5) Livers may be differentially vulnerable to initiation.
6) Phenobarbital acts at each initiated locus.

A computer program was developed that incorporated the above points in order to simulate the experimental system of hepatic tumorigenesis by initiation and promotion. This program is briefly described in the flow diagram depicted in Figure 1. The terms used in this discussion are defined as follows:

N	Number of initiated loci in total rat population -- corresponds to AAF dose for whole population.
n_j	Number of initiated loci in liver of rat j.
$P(n_j)$	Probability that rat j with n initiated loci will form a tumor.
α	Probability that an initiated locus will form a tumor in the absence of phenobarbital.
ϕ	Increment in the probability that an initiated locus will form a tumor in the presence of phenobarbital.

The first stage of the program distributes the total N initiated loci throughout the rat population. No assumptions are made regarding the specific nature of the initiation event; one or more events at the molecular level may be involved in the formation of the promotable locus.

The random distribution of initiated loci described above results in a Poisson distribution of these loci throughout the rat population. The program can include heterogeneity of individual liver vulnerability to the action of AAF, in which case a Poisson distribution is not achieved.

The second stage of the program calculates the probability that each rat will form a tumor during the test interval. Since rat j with n_j-initiated loci can form a tumor at any one of these loci

$$P(n_j) = 1 - [1-(\alpha + \phi)]^{n_j}$$

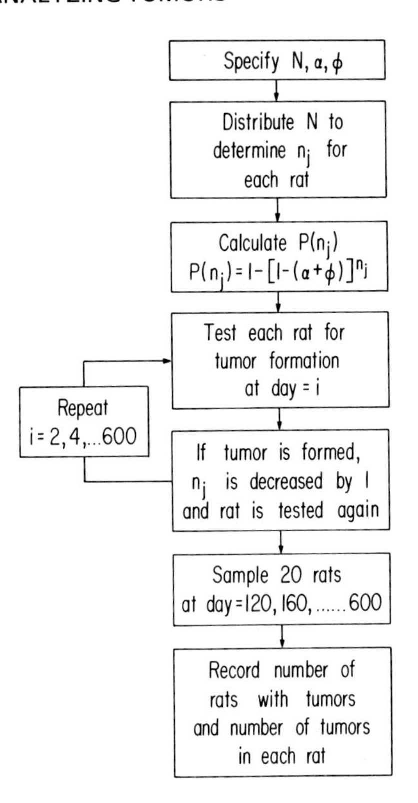

Figure 1. Flow diagram for computer simulation of liver tumor formulation.

where $\alpha + \phi$ represents the total probability that a locus will form a tumor during the 2-day test interval. The values of α and ϕ are small; therefore, the cross product term $\alpha - \phi$ may be neglected.

The third stage of the program begins by testing each rat for tumor formation during the first test interval. A random number is generated and compared to $P(n_j)$. If the number is less than $P(n_j)$, a tumor is formed. Then, N_j is decreased by 1, $P(n_j)$ is recalculated, and the rat is retested for the formation of a second tumor. This process is repeated for each rat and the entire cycle is reiterated at 2-day intervals during the 600-day time course of the experiment (23).

During the simulated experiment, samples were selected from 20 rats and the presence of tumors in these rats 100 days earlier was examined. This interval corresponds to a lag period involving post-initiation processes of transformation and tumor accumulation of sufficient mass to be observed. The number of rats with tumors and the number of tumors in each rat was recorded. The program can also examine the entire rat population at each sampling period.

The product of the current simulation is illustrated in Figure 2 for a rat population equally vulnerable to the initiating effect of AAF. The parameters (see Figure 1) were specified as follows: $N = 500$ and is distributed among 270 rats; $\alpha = 0.00050$. Phenobarbital dosages are given to provide a basis for comparison with the experimental data [(5) Chart 2]. For the zero phenobarbital dosage, ϕ was set at 0.00020; subsequent ϕ values were successively increased by factors of 5. To facilitate comparisons of tumor incidence patterns, the curves were smoothed by averaging the data from 2 adjacent points on the curve and plotting the average at the mean interval between the points (56). The results shown in Figure 2 compare favorably with experimental data presented earlier (23) in terms of maximal percentage of rats with tumors and the suggestion of phenobarbital-dependent plateaus. By introducing a heterogeneity of AAF vulnerability into the rat population, the correspondence of simulated and experimental tumor frequency per liver was improved (not shown).

Although development of the simulation is at a preliminary stage, certain general conclusions can be drawn:

1) The model, derived from simple assumptions including random initiation and random promotion acting through a mechanism that increases the probability of expression of initiated loci, is a reasonable first approximation of the experimental data as currently expressed.
2) Comparison of the experimental data and the model suggests that rats vary in vulnerability to initiation. The possibility of varying susceptibility to phenobarbital also exists.
3) Phenobarbital's promoting effect under experimental conditions is apparently not fully expressed during the early stages of phenobarbital administration, even at dosages that do not affect growth rate (23), which suggests phenobarbital may exert antipromoting as well as promoting activity.
4) The phenobarbital-dependent plateau levels observed experimentally (23) are more defined than the simulated data, suggesting a possible refinement of the elementary probabilistic assumption of promoter action. For instance, the liver's susceptibility to phenobarbital promotion may decrease during the course of the experiment.

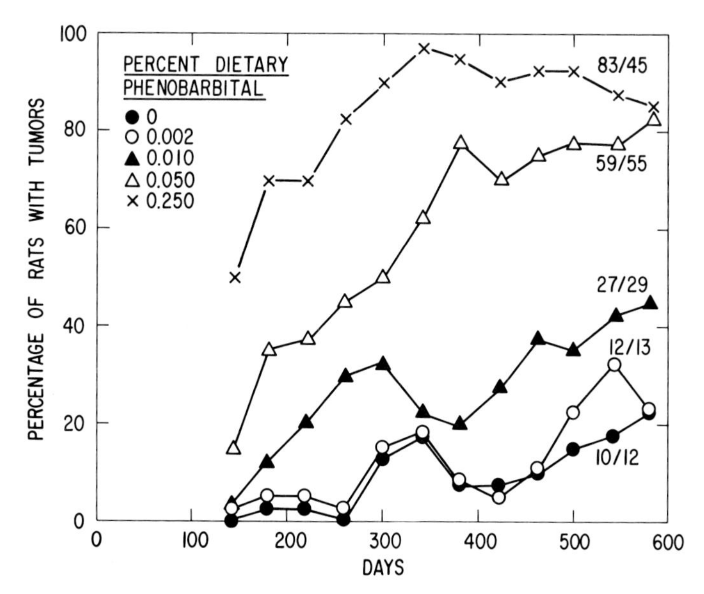

Figure 2. Computer simulation of the effects of varying the dietary concentration of phenobarbital on its enhancement of 2-acetylaminofluorene-induced hepatic tumorigenesis using the initiation-promotion model diagrammed in Figure 1. Each curve represents a separate simulation run. The ratio adjacent to each curve compares the computer-generated overall tumor incidence data in percentage of rats with tumors (numerator) to the empirical data obtained at that phenobarbital dosage (denominator) (23).

Refinement of this model is in progress. Further development of the simulation will be based on more detailed analyses of the kinetics of tumor incidence and occurrences of different tumor types.

Model 2

To understand the mechanism of promotion more fully, a clearer description of initiation is necessary. For instance, as noted above, we and others (70,71) have observed that the tumor multiplicity distribution cannot be attributed to a simple Poisson distribution. Drinkwater and Klotz (72) have employed a generalized Poisson distribution rather than a simple Poisson distribution of tumor development in statistically describing their data. For our purposes, the heterogeneity of tumor expression must be accounted for. In the liver system employed in this laboratory, it could originate from either heterogeneous vulnerability to the initiating agent or heterogeneous susceptibility to the promoter.

To examine the phenomenon of initiation, we are extending our tumorigenesis model to encompass events at the cellular level, and hence, stages in tumor development. Accordingly, it is necessary to develop and frame hypotheses relating to the frequency, kinetics of appearance, and phenotypes of histochemically-altered hepatocyte foci believed to be tumor precursors.

Simplistically stated, the initiation and promotion model postulates that limited exposure to a carcinogen (initiator) results in the formation of potential tumor-forming cells that clonally develop into tumors upon subsequent exposure to the promoter. The frequency of both tumors and altered foci increases in the presence of phenobarbital, and both increases have been described in terms of initiation and promotion (23,29). However, in these experimental systems, the number of foci exceeds the number of tumors by several orders of magnitude. This high ratio of foci to tumors raises two alternative possibilities that are amenable to testing:

1) Most of the foci represent early stages in tumorigenesis but have not yet undergone the full complement of changes necessary for expression of the tumor phenotype.
2) Most of the foci were initially tumor progenitors but have subsequently undergone changes precluding their further development into tumors.

Alternative 1 may be described in a model formulation as the accumulation of appropriate events, perhaps at one or more regulatory loci, resulting in a focus, followed by specific subsequent transitions (stages) that can depend upon additional mutations. If the subsequent transitions require mutations, these mutations are either not dependent upon the presence of the carcinogen, and occur spontaneously during clonal proliferation, or are accumulated during prior exposure to the initiator.

Alternative 2 addresses the possible existence of nontumorigenic foci, as well as the origins of foci with diverse histochemical phenotypes. If initiation results from a genetic lesion at a specific regulatory locus, then observing heterogeneity in focus phenotype implies that the phenotypes are dependent upon additional mutations that may be positive, negative, or neutral with respect to tumorigenesis, since no known histochemical alteration appears in every focus. On the other hand, if the production of a focus is itself only dependent upon the lesion that gives rise to the distinctive phenotype marker, then no separate initiation event need be postulated for focus formation, and initiation in the sense of tumor formation may simply reflect the accumulation of appropriate essential lesions during exposure to the carcinogen.

To formulate a model of initiation and promotion, it is therefore necessary to consider the role of multiple mutations, whether resulting directly from the action of the carcinogen or occurring spontaneously during focus development. The generally accepted working hypothesis, as embodied in Alternative 1 above, is that a tumor results from the accumulation of many mutations, affecting loci specifically involved in the transformation process. According to this scheme, the majority of foci, which did not develop into tumors, represent cells that did not acquire sufficient lesions to complete the transformation process. However, assuming mutation to be a random process and assuming that the loci essential to the transformation process comprise a small fraction of the total genome, it would be expected that many mutations would not contribute to transformation but could, in fact, be detrimental and block the process. Therefore, in developing the hypothetical framework of initiation and promotion in a manner suitable for computer simulation, it is necessary to consider the possibility that some foci that do not develop into tumors may have sustained excess rather than insufficient mutations, and consequently may no longer have tumorigenic potential (Alternative 2).

Alternatives 1 and 2 may be distinguished by the predictions that they generate. Alternative 1 predicts monotonic, though not necessarily linear, responses to increased carcinogen dose. These responses include increases in frequency of foci, proportion of foci with multiple phenotypic changes, tumor frequency, and ratio of tumors to foci. The process predicted by Alternative 2 is biphasic. At low carcinogen dose ranges, increased tumor and focus frequency would be expected with increasing carcinogen levels. At high carcinogen dose ranges, a decreased proportion of foci with multiple phenotypic changes, a decreased ratio of tumors to foci, and a decreased tumor frequency would be expected with increasing levels. (The functional criteria for "low" or "high" dose are undefined. Dosages commonly used experimentally may already approach high levels in the sense used here.) The decline in tumor frequency at high carcinogen dose observed by Scherer and Emmelot (68) and attributed to toxicity is also consistent with the predictions generated by Alternative 2. To test the validity of these inferred predictions clearly requires a mathematical formation supported by computer simulation, in conjunction with the acquisition of empirical data.

ACKNOWLEDGMENTS

This work was supported by the U.S. Department of Energy under contract No. W-31-109-ENG-38.

REFERENCES

1. Deelman, H.T. 1927. The part played by injury and repair in the development of cancer. Brit. Med. J. 1:872.

2. Rous, P., and J.G. Kidd. 1941. Conditional neoplasms and subthreshold neoplastic states. J. Exp. Med. 73:356-389.

3. Friedewald, W.F., and P. Rous. 1944. The initiating and promoting elements in tumor production. J. Exp. Med. 80:101-125.

4. Berenblum, I. 1941. The cocarcinogenic action of croton resin. Cancer Res. 1:41-48.

5. Berenblum, I., and P. Shubik. 1949. The persistence of latent tumor cells induced in the mouse's skin by a single application of 9,10-dimethyl-1-2-benzanthracene. Brit. J. Cancer 3:384-386.

6. Hecker, E. 1967. Phorbol esters from croton oil: Chemical nature and biological activities. Naturwissenschaften 54:282-284.

7. Sivak, A. 1979. Cocarcinogenesis. Biochim. Biophys. Acta 505:67-89.

8. Diamond, L., T.G. O'Brien, and G. Rovera. 1979. Tumor promoters: Effects on proliferation and differentiation of cells in culture. Life Sci. 23:1979-1988.

9. Colburn, N.M. 1980. Tumor promotion and pre-neoplastic progression. In: Carcinogenesis, Volume 5: Modifiers of Chemical Carcinogenesis. T.J. Slaga, ed. Raven Press: New York. pp. 33-56.

10. Slaga, T.J., S.M. Fischer, K. Nelson, and G.L. Gleason. 1980. Studies on the mechanism of skin tumor promotion: Evidence for several stages in promotion. Proc. Natl. Acad. Sci. 77:3659-3663.

11. Cole, L.J., and P.C. Nowell. 1965. Radiation carcinogenesis: The sequence of events. Science 150:1782-1789.

12. Farber, E. 1973. Hyperplastic liver nodules. In: Methods in Cancer Research, Volume 7. H. Busch, ed. Academic Press: New York. pp. 345-375.

13. Farber, E. 1973. Carcinogenesis: Cellular evolution as a unifying thread: Presidential address. Cancer Res. 33:2537-2550.

14. Teebor, G.W., and F.F. Becker. 1971. Expression and persistence of hyperplastic nodules induced by N-2-fluorenylacetamide and their relationship to hepatocarcinogenesis. Cancer Res. 31:1-3.

15. Becker, F.F. 1975. Alteration of hepatocytes by subcarcinogenic exposure to N-2-fluorenylacetamide. Cancer Res. 35:1734-1736.

16. Solt, D., and E. Farber. 1976. New principle for the analysis of chemical carcinogenesis. Nature 263:701-703.

17. Solt, D.B., A. Medline, and E. Farber. 1977. Rapid emergence of carcinogen-induced hyperplastic lesions in a new model for the sequential analysis of liver carcinogenesis. Am. J. Pathol. 88:595-618.

18. Farber, E. 1980. The sequential analysis of liver cancer induction. Biochim. Biophys. Acta 605:149-166.

19. Peraino, C., R.J.M. Fry, and E. Staffeldt. 1971. Reduction and enhancement by phenobarbital of hepatocarcinogenesis induced in the rat by 2-acetylaminofluorene. Cancer Res. 31:1506-1512.

20. Ishidate, M., W. Watanabe, and S. Odashima. 1967. Effect of barbital on carcinogenic action and metabolism of 4-dimethylaminoazobenzene. Gann 58:276-281.

21. Kunz, W., G. Schaude, and C. Thomas. 1969. The effect of phenobarbital and halogenated hydrocarbons on nitrosamine carcinogenesis. Z. Krebsforsch. 72:291-304.

22. Schulte-Hermann, R. 1978. Induction of liver growth by xenobiotic compounds and other stimuli. Crit. Rev. Toxicol. 3:97-158.

23. Peraino, C., E.F. Staffeldt, D.A. Haugen, L.S. Lombard, F.J. Stevens, and R.J.M. Fry. 1980. Effects of varying the dietary concentration of phenobarbital on its enhancement of 2-acetylaminofluorene-induced hepatic tumorigenesis. Cancer Res. 40:3268-3273.

24. Tatematsu, M., K. Nakanishi, G. Murasaki, Y. Myata, M. Horise, and N. Ito. 1979. Enhancing effect of inducers of liver microsomal enzymes on induction of hyperplastic liver nodules by N-2-fluorenylacetamide in rats. 1979. J. Natl. Cancer Inst. 63:1411-1416.

25. Takano, T., M. Tatematsu, R. Hasegawa, K. Imaida, and N. Ito. 1980. Dose-response relationship for the promoting effect of phenobarbital on the induction of liver hyperplastic nodules in rats exposed to 2-fluorenylacetamide and carbon tetrachloride. Gann 71:580-581.

26. Pugh, T.D., and S. Goldfarb. 1978. Quantitative histochemical and autoradiographic studies of hepatocarcinogenesis in rats fed 2-acetylaminofluorene followed by phenobarbital. Cancer Res. 38:4450-4457.

27. Watenabe, K., and G.M. Williams. 1978. Enhancement of rat hepatocellular altered foci by the liver tumor promoter phenobarbital: Evidence that foci are precursors of neoplasms and that the promoter acts on carcinogen-induced lesions. J. Natl. Cancer Inst. 61:1311-1314.

28. Weisburger, J.M., R.M. Madison, J.M. Ward, C. Vignera, and E.F. Weisburger. 1975. Modification of diethylnitrosamine liver carcinogenesis with phenobarbital but not with immunosuppression. J. Natl. Cancer Inst. 54:1185-1188.

29. Pitot, H., L. Barsness, T. Goldsworthy, and T. Kitagawa. 1978. Biochemical characterization of stages of hepatocarcinogenesis after a single dose of diethylnitrosamine. Nature 271:456-458.

30. Kitagawa, T., and H. Sugano. 1978. Enhancing effect of phenobarbital on the development of enzyme-altered islands and hepatocellular carcinomas initiated by 3'methyl-4-(dimethylamino)-azobenzene or diethylnitrosamine. Gann 69:679-687.

31. Pitot, H.C., T. Goldsworthy, H.A. Campbell, and A. Poland. 1980. Quantitative evaluation of the promotion by 2,3,7,8-tetrachlorodibenzo-p-dioxin of hepatocarcinogenesis from diethylnitrosamine. Cancer Res. 40:3616-3620.

32. Shinozuka, H., and B. Lombardi. 1980. Synergistic effect of a choline-devoid diet and phenobarbital in promoting the emergence of foci with γ-glutamyltranspeptidase-positive hepatocytes in the liver of carcinogen-treated rats. Cancer Res. 40:3846-3849.

33. Nishizumi, M. 1976. Enhancement of diethylnitrosamine hepatocarcinogenesis in rats by exposure to polychlorinated biphenyls or phenobarbital. Cancer Lett. 2:11-16.

34. Nishizumi, M. 1979. Effect of phenobarbital, dichlorodiphenyltrichloroethane, and polychlorinated biphenyls on diethylnitrosamine-induced hepatocarcinogenesis. Gann 70:835-837.

35. Yager, J.D., and R. Yager. 1980. Oral contraceptive steroids as promoters of hepatocarcinogenesis in female Sprague-Dawley rats. Cancer Res. 40:3680-3685.

36. Uchida, E., and I. Hirono. 1979. Effects of phenobarbital on induction of liver and lung tumors by dimethylnitrosamine in newborn mice. Gann 70:639-644.

37. Kitagawa, T., T. Hirakawa, T. Ishakawa, N. Nemoto, and S. Takayama. 1980. Induction of hepatocellular carcinomas in rat liver by initial treatment with benzo[a]pyrene after partial hepatectomy and promotion by phenobarbital. Toxicol. Lett. 65:167-171.

38. Pitot, H.C. 1979. Drugs as promoters of carcinogenesis. In: The Induction of Drug Metabolism. R.W. Estabrook, and E. Lindlaub, eds. F.K. Schattauer-Verlag: New York. pp. 471-483.

39. Peraino, C., R.J.M. Fry, and D.D. Grube. 1978. Drug-induced enhancement of hepatic tumorigenesis. In: Carcinogenesis, Volume 2. T.J. Slaga, A. Sivak, and R.K. Boutwell, eds. Raven Press: New York. pp. 421-432.

40. Kitagawa, T., H.C. Pitot, E.C. Miller, and J.A. Miller. 1979. Promotion by dietary phenobarbital of hepatocarcinogenesis by 2-methyl-N,N-dimethyl-4-aminoazobenzene in the rat. Cancer Res. 39:112-115.

41. Peraino, C., R.J.M. Fry, E. Staffeldt, and J.P. Christopher. 1975. Comparative enhancing effects of phenobarbital, amobarbital, diphenylhydantoin and dichlorodiphenyl-trichloroethane on 2-acetylaminofluorene-induced hepatic tumorigenesis in rats. Cancer Res. 35:2884-2890.

42. Peraino, C., R.J.M. Fry, E. Staffeldt, and J.P. Christopher. 1977. Enhancing effects of phenobarbital and butylated hydroxytoluene on 2-acetylaminofluorene-induced hepatic tumorigenesis in the rat. Food Cosmet. Toxicol. 5:93-96.

43. Peraino, C., R.J.M. Fry, and E. Staffeldt. 1973. Enhancement of spontaneous hepatic tumorigenesis in C3H mice by dietary phenobarbital. J. Natl. Cancer Inst. 51:1349-1350.

44. Thorpe, E., and A.T. Walker. 1973. The toxicology of dieldrin (HEOD). II. Comparative long-term oral toxicity studies in mice with dieldrin, DDT, phenobarbitone, B-BC, and 2-BHC. Food Cosmet. Toxicol. 11:433-442.

45. Ponomarkov, V., L. Tomatis, and V. Turosov. 1976. The effect of long-term administration of phenobarbitone in CF-1 mice. Cancer Lett. 1:167-172.

46. Kitagawa, T., K. Watanabe, and H. Sugano. 1980. Induction of γ-glutamyltranspeptidase activity by dietary phenobarbital in "spontaneous" hepatic tumors in C3H mice. Gann 71:537-542.

47. Rossi, L., M. Ravera, G. Repetti, and L. Santi. 1977. Long-term administration of DDT or phenobarbital-Na in Wistar rats. Int. J. Cancer 19:179-185.

48. Innes, J.R.M., B.M. Ulland, M.G. Valerio, L. Petrucelli, L. Fishbein, E.R. Hart, A.J. Pallota, R.R. Bates, H.L. Falk, J.J. Gart, M. Klein, I. Mitchell, and J. Peters. 1979. Bioassay of pesticides and industrial chemicals for tumorigenicity in mice: A preliminary note. J. Natl. Cancer Inst. 42:1101-1114.

49. Tomatis, L., V. Turosov, N. Day, and R.T. Charles. 1972. The effect of long-term exposure to DDT on CF-1 mice. Int. J. Cancer 10:489-506.

50. Turosov, V.S., N.E. Day, L. Tomatis, E. Gati, and R.T. Charles. 1973. Tumors in CF-1 mice exposed for six consecutive generations to DDT. J. Natl. Cancer Inst. 51:983-997.

51. Tomatis, L., C. Partensky, and R. Montesano. 1973. The predictive value of mouse liver tumor induction in carcinogenicity testing: A literature survey. Int. J. Cancer 12:1-20.

52. Terracini, B., M.C. Testa, T.R. Cabral, and N. Day. 1973. The effects of long-term feeding of DDT to BALB/c mice. Int. J. Cancer 11:747-764.

53. Fitzhugh, O.G., and A.A. Nelson. 1947. The chronic oral toxicity of DDT (2,2-bis(p-chlorophenyl)1,1,1-trichloroethane). J. Pharmacol. Exp. Ther. 89:18-30.

54. Deichmann, W.B., M. Keplinge, and F. Sala. 1967. Synergism among oral carcinogens. IV. The simultaneous feeding of four tumorigens to rats. Toxicol. Appl. Pharmacol. 11:88-103.

55. Sabine, J.R., B.J. Horton, and M.B. Wicks. 1973. Spontaneous tumors in C3H-A and C3H-AfB mice: High incidence in the United States and low incidence in Australia. J. Natl. Cancer Inst. 50:1237-1242.

56. Peraino, C., R.J.M. Fry, and E. Staffeldt. 1977. Effects of varying the onset and duration of exposure to phenobarbital on its enhancement of 2-acetylaminofluorene-induced hepatic tumorigenesis. Cancer Res. 37:3623-3627.

57. Boutwell, R.K. 1964. Some biological aspects of skin carcinogenesis. Prog. Exp. Tumor Res. 4:207-250.

58. Peraino, C., R.J.M. Fry, E. Staffeldt, and W.E. Kisieleski. 1973. Effects of varying the exposure to phenobarbital on its enhancement of 2-acetylaminofluorene-induced hepatic tumorigenesis in the rat. Cancer Res. 33:2701-2705.

59. Grube, D.D., C. Peraino, and R.J.M. Fry. 1975. The effects of dietary phenobarbital on the induction of skin tumors in hairless mice with 7,12-dimethylbenz[a]anthracene. J. Invest. Dermatol. 64:258-262.

60. Pollard, M., and P.H. Luckert. 1979. Promotional effect of sodium barbiturate on intestinal tumors induced in rats by dimethylhydrazine. J. Natl. Cancer Inst. 63:1089-1092.

61. Clemmesen, J., V. Fuglsang-Fredricksen, and C.N. Plum. 1974. Are anti-convulsants oncogenic? Lancet 1:705-707.

62. Schneiderman, M.A. 1974. Phenobarbitone and liver tumors. Lancet 2:629-630.

63. Clemmesen, J., and S. Hjalgrim-Jensen. 1978. Is phenobarbital carcinogenic? A follow-up of 8087 epileptics. Ecotoxicol. Environ. Safety 1:457-470.

64. Gold, E., L. Gordis, J. Tonascia, and M. Szklo. 1978. Increased risk of brain tumors in children exposed to barbiturates. J. Natl. Cancer Inst. 61:1031-1034.

65. Annegers, J.F., L.T. Kurland, and W.A. Hauser. 1979. Brain tumors in children exposed to barbiturates. J. Natl. Cancer Inst. 63:3.

66. Gold, E.B., L. Gordis, J.A. Tonascia, and M. Szklo. 1979. Brain tumors in children exposed to barbiturates. J. Natl. Cancer Inst. 63:3-4.

67. Pitot, H.C., and A.E. Sirica. 1980. The stages of initiation and promotion in hepatocarcinogenesis. Biochim. Biophys. Acta 605:191-215.

68. Scherer, E., and P. Emmelot. 1975. Kinetics of induction and growth of precancerous liver-cell foci, and liver tumor formation by diethylnitrosamine in the rat. Eur. J. Cancer 11:689-696.

69. Ogawa, K.D., B. Solt, and E. Farber. 1980. Phenotypic diversity as an early property of putative preneoplastic populations in liver carcinogenesis. Cancer Res. 40:725-733.

70. Pollisar, M.J., and M.B. Shimkin. 1954. A quantitative interpretation of the distribution of induced pulmonary tumors in mice. J. Natl. Cancer Inst. 15:377-403.

71. Falconer, D.S., and J.L. Bloom. 1962. A genetic study of induced lung tumors in mice. Brit. J. Cancer 16:665-685.

72. Drinkwater, N.R., and J.H. Klotz. 1981. Statistical methods for the analysis of tumor multiplicity data. Cancer Res. 41:113-119.

DISCUSSION

Q.: Did the other promoter that you used produce the same morphologic changes?

A.: Yes. DDT and BHT showed a similar picture.

Q.: Do any of the biochemical changes that one sees in mouse skin undergoing promotion, such as increase in ornithine decarboxylase (ODC) activity, occur in liver being treated with phenobarbital?

A.: ODC is not induced by phenobarbital in the liver. That is the point of the introductory remarks that I made. I think we have to start comparing different systems rather than focusing on any one system; then we can start examining the relevance of various responses, beginning with whether they occur in different initiation/promotion systems.

Q.: I'm not sure that what you said today concerning the kinds of tumors you get is consistent with what you published in '75. I'm wondering at what time you looked at the tumors histologically. If you had looked much earlier, would you have seen the adenomas that you reported and, how did that compare to the preneoplastic nodules or the enzyme-altered foci that other groups that are working in this model have reported?

A.: I'm not a pathologist and I have to avoid what I perceive as a very subjective analysis of the proportion of different histological types of tumors. In '75, we were cooperating with a different pathologist than we were when we did the latest experiment, and the description of results was considerably different. What is firm is that phenobarbital does not appear to increase or decrease the degree of differentiation of the tumors. I'm wary of saying whether it increases or decreases the proportion of different sub-types within the spectrum of neoplastic nodules to carcinomas, which I think is very subjective.

Q.: Would you agree with the people who are using enzyme-altered foci as a criterion, that in promotion, the major increase is in the total number of those foci?

A.: We get about a five-fold increase in liver tumors with phenobarbital. We and others have also looked at preneoplastic foci, and we also get about a five-fold increase. Now, there are more preneoplastic foci than tumors by several orders of magnitude. I don't know about the causal relationship between foci and tumors, but the incremental effect of phenobarbital is the same for both types of lesions.

Q.: Would you consider your lowest dose a real threshold? How would an increased level of AAF initiation affect promotion by low levels of phenobarbital?

A.: If you increase the dose of the initiator, you reduce the incremental effect of the promoter. I think even our lowest dose of phenobarbital alone showed a very small effect on tumor incidence. I'm sure there is a threshold for promotion, but I'm not sure we've achieved it yet.

Q.: Of course, everybody talks about thresholds with promoters, so this is of practical relevance.

A.: I would think that there is a threshold. In our slide showing percentage of rats with hepatomas, there was no effect at the 0.002% phenobarbital level. There may have been a slight increase in the number of tumors per animal at the end of the experiment. But it was very marginal, so I would think any incremental effect of phenobarbital below 0.002% would be virtually undetectable.

PROMOTION OF URINARY BLADDER CARCINOGENESIS

Samuel M. Cohen

Department of Pathology, St. Vincent Hospital, Worcester, Massachusetts 01604

INTRODUCTION

The relationship of chemicals to urinary bladder carcinogenesis was initially observed in the species of ultimate concern in cancer research -- the human being. Rehn in 1895 noticed an increased incidence of cancer of the urinary bladder in workers in the German aniline dye industry (1,2). Hueper and his colleagues were able to demonstrate that one of the carcinogens to which these workers were exposed was 2-aminonaphthalene. Hueper's experiments involving dogs also demonstrated the necessity for relatively high doses of the carcinogen and the long periods of time required for the experimental induction of bladder cancer (1,2). Aromatic amines since then have remained of central importance in bladder cancer research in animals and in humans.

A brief description of aromatic amine metabolism as related to organ and species specificity will be reviewed here, but greater detail will be presented by Dr. Charles Irving later in this symposium. The remainder of this presentation describes various animal models of bladder cancer and the mechanism of carcinogenesis with an emphasis on differences and similarities between species.

CHEMICALS CARCINOGENIC FOR THE URINARY BLADDER

Aromatic Amines and Amides

Several aromatic amines and amides have been demonstrated to have carcinogenic activity in a number of species including humans. However, the organ specificity between species differs strikingly.

In man, aromatic amines and amides have a tropism for the urothelial lining of the lower urinary tract extending from the renal pelvis throughout the ureters and the urinary bladder (1,). Thus, 2-aminonaphthalene, benzidine, and 4-aminobiphenyl induce tumors of the urinary bladder, and phenacetin-containing analgesics induce tumors predominantly in the renal pelvis but also of the ureters and urinary bladder (3,4). In the dog, aromatic amines also induce tumors of the urinary bladder (1,2). In rodents, aromatic amines and amides induce tumors predominantly of the liver but also of the urinary bladder, mammary gland, Zymbal's gland, and other organs, depending on species (1,2). Although not entirely clear, these differences appear to be related in large extent to differences in metabolism. Susceptibility of a species to the carcinogenic action of aromatic amines and amides depends on the ability of the species to hydroxylate the amine substituent. Guinea pigs, which are resistant to the carcinogenic action of aromatic amines and amides, are unable to N-hydroxylate to any appreciable extent (1,2). If the N-hydroxylated form, for example N-hydroxy-2-acetylaminofluorene, is administered to guinea pigs, tumors are induced, whereas none arise with the parent compound, 2-acetylaminofluorene (AAF).

N-Hydroxylation appears to be a necessary but insufficient step in the metabolic activation of these aromatic amine and amide compounds (5). As demonstrated by the Millers (5), subsequent formation of an ester is required, resulting in a reactive electrophilic reagent. Apparently, different esters result in variations in organ specificity. Strong evidence has been presented that the sulfate ester of N-hydroxy-2-AAF is important in the induction of liver tumors by these compounds. However, the other target organs of aromatic amines and amides do not have sufficient levels of the sulfotransferase necessary for the generation of this metabolite. Thus, other enzymes must be involved in these other tissues. For the urinary bladder several possible mechanisms might be involved. Dogs are not capable of N-acetylating aromatic amines, while other species, including man, can acetylate amines. In humans, N-acetylation involves a genetically polymorphic enzyme, with people being divided into slow and rapid acetylators (6). This differentiation has pharmacological significance related to a number of drugs, but its significance in bladder carcinogenesis is as yet unknown. Some evidence exists that slow acetylators may be more susceptible to the carcinogenic action of aromatic amines than the rapid acetylators (7).

The role of N-glucuronidation of amines and amides in the liver has also been suggested as important in the generation of bladder cancers, since these are relatively stable compounds that are transported through the urine (8). Recently, the ability of the urinary bladder mucosa to N-hydroxylate aromatic amines and amides has been demonstrated and appears to involve two different enzyme systems: the mixed microsomal drug-metabolizing enzymes similar to those in the liver (9); and a number of peroxidase-type enzymes, including prostaglandin endoperoxide synthetase (10). The relationship of these various enzyme systems to the etiology of bladder cancer is yet to be ascertained.

N-(4-[5-Nitro-2-Furyl]-2-Thiazolyl)Formamide

Although the aromatic amines and amides have proved useful in urinary bladder carcinogenesis, they have not been specific in rodents for the urinary bladder and thus have had shortcomings as a model for this disease. In the 1960s, three bladder-specific carcinogens were discovered in rats that have provided very useful animal models for studies on mechanism, ultrastructure, therapy, etc. Nitroso-n-butylamine was shown to induce tumors of the urinary bladder but also tumors of other tissues, including the esophagus and liver (11). Its metabolite, nitroso-n-butyl-(4-hydroxy-n-butyl)amine (BBN), was shown to be specific for the urinary bladder in a number of species including mouse, rat, hamster, and dog. Similarly, N-(4-[5-nitro-2-furyl]-2-thiazolyl)-formamide (FANFT) was shown to be bladder-specific in a number of species (12), initially in Sprague-Dawley female rats, but subsequently in male and female rats as well as mice, hamsters, and dogs. The guinea pig appears to be resistant to this compound and to other nitrofurans. BBN is administered in the drinking water and FANFT in the diet. Intravesical instillation of nitrosomethylurea (MNU), a direct-acting carcinogen, was also shown to be carcinogenic for the urinary bladder (13). With all three of these carcinogens, the course of the disease appears similar. The urinary bladder epithelium progresses from the normal three layers to a simple hyperplasia followed by a focal nodular and papillary hyperplasia. Subsequently papillomas, non-invasive carcinomas, and eventually invasive carcinomas are formed. These are usually transitional cell in nature in most species, although squamous cell carcinomas are common in mice. Metastases are rare in animal models and blockage of the ureters with resultant hydronephrosis is also uncommon (14). However, all three of these chemicals provide models similar enough to the human disease to provide very useful information.

Organ specificity varies markedly with the different nitrosamines and nitrosamides (11). Similarly, 5-nitrofurans induce a wide variety of tumors depending on the substituent at the 2 position. In rats and mice, FANFT appears strikingly unique as a bladder carcinogen, although some of the other nitrofurans tested have induced tumors of the kidney as well as other types of tissues (12). The deformylated metabolite of FANFT, 2-amino-4-(5-nitro-2-furyl)thiazole (ANFT) is a bladder carcinogen in rats (15). In hamsters, the three nitrofurans tested, including FANFT, are bladder carcinogens; the two nitrofurans tested in dogs have been bladder carcinogens. At present, these differences in organ specificity for the various 5-nitrofurans remain unexplained, but are very likely related to the pharmacodynamics of these compounds. Presumably, the carcinogenicity of 5-nitrofurans involves reduction of the nitro group, possibly to the nitroso or N-hydroxylated form (16). Since urinary bladder carcinogenesis most likely results from exposure to carcinogens in the urine (see below), the nitrofuran must be able to be excreted in the urine without destruction of the nitro group. This process appears to be so for FANFT, since a large percentage of the compound is excreted in the urine as either FANFT or as ANFT, with the nitro group intact (16). However, it is obvious that the retention of the nitro group is not by itself sufficient to cause bladder cancer. Nitrofurantoin is a 5-nitrofuran used for treatment of urinary tract infections, and is effective because it is excreted to an appreciable extent intact through the urine. To date no evidence exists that 5-nitrofurantoin induces tumors of the urinary bladder, or for that matter, tumors of any other tissues (12), despite the demonstrated strong mutagenic activity of nitrofurantoin and of the urine of patients or animals administered nitrofurantoin (17).

We have concentrated our efforts on the induction of bladder cancer in the inbred Fischer F344 male rat by feeding FANFT in the diet (18,19). Female rats appear to be as susceptible as male rats (unpublished observation). Administration of FANFT in the diet at a dose of 0.2% for 20 weeks or more was shown early to be sufficient to induce a 100% incidence of bladder tumors if the rats were allowed to live long enough, generally for a year or more. A dose-response with FANFT has been demonstrated. The incidence of bladder tumors induced is 100% if the dose is 0.2, 0.1, or 0.05%, but the incidence drops to below 10% if the dose is 0.01%, and to 0 at still lower doses (20). The duration of administration of FANFT also appears to be critical, since administration of FANFT at 0.2% for 12 or more weeks induces lesions that progress to carcinoma if the rats are allowed to live sufficiently long (19,21). Rats fed FANFT for 8 to 10 weeks and then given control diet initially show regression of the lesions but these lesions eventually proliferate so that all rats develop hyperplasia of the bladder or carcinoma (19,21). Administration of FANFT for six weeks also leads to initial lesions that regress completely. No tumors are observed if the animals are allowed to live for 18 months (21), but a low incidence is observed if the animals are allowed to live for two years (22).

PROMOTION OF CARCINOGENESIS IN THE URINARY BLADDER

Multistage Carcinogenesis in the Urinary Bladder

Administration of several bladder carcinogens at low doses was shown by Ito and his colleagues to result in an additive or synergistic effect in the induction of bladder tumors (23). Simultaneous administration of BBN, FANFT, AAF, and 3,3'-dichlorobenzidine to rats induced a significant incidence of bladder tumors, whereas the administration of any of the chemicals individually did not. In addition, administration of the same four carcinogens sequentially rather than simultaneously also resulted in a significant incidence of bladder tumors (24). However, it should be kept in mind that these are all bladder carcinogens when administered in sufficiently large dosages.

The relevance of the initiation and promotion model of carcinogenesis to the urinary bladder became evident with experiments using MNU (25), FANFT (22), or BBN (26) as initiators, and sodium saccharin (22,25,26), sodium cyclamate (25), tryptophan (22), or phenacetin (27) as promoters in rats. Administration of any of the promoting chemicals alone, without initiation, resulted in either low incidences or absence of bladder tumors. In experiments in our laboratory (22), FANFT was originally administered for six weeks in the diet at a dose of 0.2%, followed either immediately or after a delay of six weeks with either sodium saccharin at a dose of 5% or D,L-tryptophan at a dose of 2% of the diet. A significant incidence of tumors occurred with both promoting chemicals, while the incidence in the group fed FANFT for six weeks followed by control diet resulted in a much lower incidence of carcinomas plus papillomas (see Table 1). The six-week delay did not have a significant effect on the activity of saccharin or tryptophan, indicating that in this model, as in the original murine skin tumor model, initiation appears to be irreversible. Six weeks after discontinuing FANFT, the chemical was excreted from the bodies of the rats, and the mild hyperplasia had regressed, so that the bladders were normal at the time the saccharin or the tryptophan was administered. However, the critical experiment -- reversing the order of the initiator and promoter -- has not yet been reported, although one such experiment is under way in our laboratory.

The incidence of bladder tumors with six weeks of FANFT followed by control diet for a total of two years was not zero. We repeated the experiment (28) using four weeks of FANFT as initiator followed by either 5% sodium saccharin or 2% of L-tryptophan (rather than the D,L racemic mixture, since the L form became economically available). The results, summarized in Table 2, show that the incidence of tumors, although less than with six weeks of FANFT as initiator, were significant in the group fed 5% sodium

Table 1. Occurrence of Bladder Tumors in Rats Administered FANFT as an Initiator for Six Weeks[a]

Group	No. of Rats Affected	Rats with Bladder Tumors	
		Papilloma	Carcinoma
FANFT → Saccharin	19	0	18
FANFT → Control → Saccharin	18	0	13
Control → Saccharin	20	0	0
FANFT → D,L-tryptophan	19	1	10
FANFT → Control → D,L-tryptophan	20	4	10
Control → D,L-tryptophan	19	0	0
FANFT → Control	20	1	4
FANFT (long-term)	40	0	40
Control	42	0	0

[a]See reference 22.

saccharin after four weeks of FANFT. However, the incidence with L-tryptophan was not quite statistically significant. We believe that the results with L-tryptophan do not negate its role as a promoter, but rather that the dose of initiator was insufficient for a significant result with the relatively small number of animals used in this experiment. FANFT administered for two weeks followed by 5% sodium saccharin appears to be insufficient to induce bladder tumors (unpublished observations). Additional evidence for the promoting activity of tryptophan includes experiments using D,L-tryptophan following 2-aminonaphththalene administered to dogs (29) and L-tryptophan administered after FANFT initiation to mice (30), in which bladder tumors were induced. Tryptophan has not yet been reported as a carcinogen in any species. Promoting activity for the non-nutritive sweeteners has been reported only in rats.

Generally, promoting chemicals have not been found to be mutagenic in various assay systems (31). The same has been found to be true for sodium saccharin (32) and for tryptophan and its various metabolites (33). A property of promoting agents is to induce increased cell proliferation in the target tissues. Originally, sodium saccharin was reported to induce only tumors of the urinary bladder in a few rats, with non-tumor-bearing rats having normal bladders. Examination of the urinary bladders of rats fed sodium saccharin, with more sensitive techniques such as

Table 2. Occurrence of Bladder Lesions in Rats Administered FANFT as an Initiator for Four Weeks[a]

Group	No. of Rats Affected	Rats with Bladder Lesions		
		Nodular Hyperplasia	Papilloma	Carcinoma
FANFT → Saccharin	26	1	2	5
Control → Saccharin	26	0	0	0
FANFT → Control	25	0	1	0
Control	27	0	0	0
FANFT (long-term)	8	0	0	8
FANFT → L-tryptophan	26	2	3	2
Control → L-tryptophan	26	0	0	0

[a]See reference 28.

scanning electron microscopy and autoradiography, indicated that sodium saccharin does increase the rate of proliferation in the bladder mucosa (34) and that the response is related to dose (35). Hyperplasia of the urinary bladder has been reported also following the administration of tryptophan or some of its metabolites (36).

The Role of Urine

Urinary bladder carcinogenesis has long been considered to result from exposure of the urinary bladder epithelium to carcinogens in the urine, the so-called urogenous or carrier theory. The concentrating ability of the urine compared to the blood is one of the reasons given for this mechanism. Scott and Boyd (37) demonstrated that dogs fed 2-aminonaphthalene and having the urine diverted to the sigmoid colon by ureterosigmoidostomies prevented the induction of bladder tumors. McDonald and Lund (38) tied off the top half of dog bladders, preventing exposure to the urine flow but leaving the bottom half exposed to urine. The dogs were fed 2-aminonaphthalene and tumors were found only in the half of the bladder exposed to urine. An indication that urine might be more than a carrier of carcinogens came from the experiments of Chapman et al. (39) in which paraffin wax pellets were inserted into both halves of a bladder which had been tied with a suture around the middle. Again tumors, although benign, were induced in the portion of the bladder exposed to urine but not in the unexposed portion. The presence of calculi greatly increased the incidence of bladder tumors in the portion of the bladder exposed to urine. However, the addition of 3-hydroxyanthranilic acid to the paraffin wax pellets did not enhance the tumor incidence, possibly because of the very slow release of the chemical from the pellets.

In an experiment by Bryan and Springberg (40), subcutaneous injection of the 8-methyl ether of xanthurenic acid, followed by the insertion of a cholesterol pellet into the bladder of mice, resulted in significantly increased incidence of tumors compared to the cholesterol pellet alone, and the subcutaneous injection of the chemical did not induce the tumors, but the administration of the chemical in the cholesterol pellet did. The relationship of the pellet to the carcinogenic process will be discussed further below.

Rowland et al. (41) recently provided additional evidence that urine is more than merely a carrier of carcinogens. FANFT was fed at a dose of 0.2% of the diet for 14 weeks. At that time, half of the rats underwent urinary diversion with bilateral ureterosigmoidostomies, and the other half were sham-operated. Eight of the 19 sham-operated animals developed bladder tumors within six months of the time of operation, compared to only 1 of the 18 rats that had undergone urinary diversion. These data would indicate that urine is acting as a promoting substance, since it was required for the appearance of tumors despite the administration of an apparently carcinogenic dose of FANFT. Oyasu et al. (42) also demonstrated the promoting activity of urine using their heterotopic bladder model. In this model, urinary bladders are transplanted subcutaneously into syngeneic rats attached to an Ommaya reservoir through which substances can be instilled. When BBN was given to rats and their bladders were transplanted as heterotopic bladders instilled with 0.9% sodium chloride, no tumors developed in the heterotopic bladders after 38 weeks and 2 of 13 rats had tumors in the heterotopic bladder after 44 weeks. In comparison, if the BBN was followed by instillation of urine adjusted to equiosmolal with the sodium chloride solution, 8 of 9 animals had bladder tumors in the heterotopic bladder after 38 weeks and 8 of 14 had tumors after 44 weeks. If either sodium chloride solution or urine were instilled without previous BBN administration, no tumors appeared in the heterotopic or host bladder. Oyasu and his colleagues (43) also demonstrated that urine increased ornithine-decarboxylase activity in an *in vitro* assay of rat bladder tumors, but it was not as potent as the phorbol ester, 12-O-tetradecanoylphorbol-13-acetate (TPA). Although increased activity was also induced by the presence of 3-hydroxyanthranilic acid, most of the activity in urine was present in the fraction with a molecular weight greater than 10,000 daltons.

Although these data indicate that urine or some other substance(s) in urine has promoting activity, it must be considerably less potent than exogenous promoting substances such as sodium saccharin. For example, FANFT administered as 0.2% of the diet for six weeks followed by control diet resulted in the induction of bladder tumors in 5 of 20 rats, whereas 18 of 19 rats administered 5% sodium saccharin after the FANFT developed bladder tumors (22). When FANFT was administered for four weeks, only 1 of 26 rats developed a small papilloma, while 7 of the 26 rats fed sodium saccharin after the FANFT developed bladder tumors (28).

In the model of initiation and promotion proposed by Boutwell (44), promotion was divided into at least two phases. The first phase of promotion was called conversion and apparently required something more than mere proliferation of the target tissue after initiation. Thus, croton oil could act as a converting agent, but turpentine, an inducer of cell proliferation on the mouse skin, had considerably weaker activity. The second phase of promotion was referred to as propagation and apparently only a substance that increased cell proliferation had to be administered. Thus, either croton oil or turpentine was active in this phase. Slaga has refined this experiment considerably using the purified active ingredient of croton oil, TPA, as a converting agent and mezerein as the propagating agent (45). The experiments of Slaga also indicate that the period required for conversion is relatively short. The propagation phase appears to be the rate-limiting phase of tumor induction.

Based on this model of promotion, it is likely that urine acts as a propagating agent rather than as a complete promoter. In this model, very brief exposure to an initiating agent and exposure to a converting agent for a somewhat longer period of time would be enough to induce bladder cancer, since urine would always be present as an endogenous agent. Without additional exposure to stronger exogenous promoting substances, a low incidence of bladder tumors would be expected, despite only brief exposure to carcinogens. A similar model can be formulated for most epithelial tissues with some normally present endogenous agent acting as the propagating substance. This activity would help to explain induction of tumors in certain instances involving very short exposures to carcinogens and would also partially explain the relatively long period of time necessary for the induction of mouse tumors.

How does this model relate to species differences? Although urine is present in all mammalian species, the urine is quite different from species to species (46). For example, the osmolality of the urine in rats and mice is considerably higher than what is usually found in man. Also, the pH of the urine in rodents is generally higher than that of humans. Surprisingly, little comparative data are available on constituents of urine in various species and continued investigation is required.

CELL PROLIFERATION AND BLADDER CARCINOGENESIS

The above experiments provide evidence that the model of initiation-promotion is relevant to urinary bladder carcinogenesis. In the MNU model (25), an initiating dose of the MNU is applied as a single instillation of chemical into the urinary bladder, a method similar to the model of initiation in the mouse skin tumor system. With FANFT, however, administration of an initiating dose requires four to six weeks of the chemical in the diet at a level of 0.2% (22,28). Although the promotion phase is long in the animal model, it is similar to the experiments in humans where bladder tumors are generally a disease of the elderly. One of the characteristics for initiating agents in studies in other systems is the necessity for the completion of at least one cell cycle to fix initiation irreversibly (31). The urinary bladder normally has a very low rate of cell turnover; the labeling index is approximately 4 per 10,000 epithelial cells. We postulated that administration of FANFT to an animal with a proliferating bladder mucosa might reduce the required time of administration (47). Although somewhat elaborate (see Table 3), the basic test group is group 1. Marked regenerative hyperplasia of the bladder was induced by Shirai's method of freeze-ulceration (48). In group 1, ulceration was followed immediately by oral administration of FANFT for two weeks, and then promoted by sodium saccharin administered as 5% of the diet for the remaining 102 weeks of the experiment. The appropriate control groups were included as well as a set of groups that used cyclophosphamide as the hyperplasia-inducing agent rather than freeze-ulceration. Although the total microscopic evaluation of all the slides has not yet been completed, the results, based on gross tumor incidences, were quite surprising (Table 3). Bladder tumors occurred in the main test group (group 1) with ulceration followed by FANFT and then sodium saccharin. A similar incidence was induced if the ulcer was followed by 2 weeks of control diet and then sodium saccharin (group 3), or if sodium saccharin immediately followed the ulcer (group 10). Two weeks of FANFT followed by sodium saccharin, without an initial ulcer, resulted in one rat with a small papilloma. Sodium saccharin, FANFT, or ulcer alone did not induce tumors. The results with cyclophosphamide, a mutagen as well as an inducer of hyperplasia of the urinary bladder, were quite similar to the results with the freeze ulcer. Somewhat surprisingly, the group that was given FANFT for two weeks and then ulcerated had only a few bladder tumors, and the incidence was increased if sodium saccharin was fed subsequently. These data indicate that the presence of a mutagen during urinary carcinogenesis is unnecessary and has little effect. Cyclophosphamide was no more effective than ulceration by freezing, and FANFT in the diet for two weeks was no more effective than control diet.

Table 3. Effect of Ulceration on Urinary Bladder Carcinogenesis[a]

Group	Rats	Rats With Bladder Tumors	
		No.	(%)
1. Ulcer → FANFT → Saccharin	22	3	14
2. Ulcer → FANFT → Control	22	0	
3. Ulcer → Control → Saccharin	19	4	21
4. Ulcer → Control	23	0	
5. FANFT → Saccharin	21	1	5
6. FANFT → Control	19	0	
7. Control → Saccharin	17	0	
8. FANFT → Ulcer → Saccharin	22	8	36
9. FANFT → Ulcer → Control	21	2	10
10. Ulcer → Saccharin	21	4	19
11. CP → FANFT → Saccharin	22	7	32
12. CP → FANFT → Control	9	0	
13. CP → Control → Saccharin	16	5	31
14. CP → Control	7	1	14
15. CP → Saccharin	17	6	35
16. Control	32	0	
17. Saccharin	24	0	

[a]FANFT = 0.2% N-[4-(5-nitro-2-furyl)-2-thiazolyl]formamide; Saccharin = 5% sodium saccharin; Ulcer = freeze ulceration; CP = cyclophosphamide-induced ulceration (100 mg/kg i.p.); Control = control diet without added test chemical. See reference 47 for further details.

These results are quite consistent with the results of other experiments with sodium saccharin. Although sodium saccharin administration to a single generation of rats induced a few bladder tumors, the incidence was generally 1% or less. However, if administered to two generations, by administration to mother animals during pregnancy and the suckling period as well as to the offspring after weaning, a considerably greater incidence of bladder tumors was induced (32,49). *In utero*, the urinary bladder is in an active state of proliferation, whereas almost immediately after birth, the bladder attains its adult slow turnover rate. Thus, the *in utero* exposure is similar to the exposure after ulceration with the increased proliferative rate.

Sodium saccharin was shown initially to be carcinogenic for the urinary bladder in experiments in which the chemical was administered in a cholesterol pellet inserted into the urinary bladder (50). We have shown that the surgical procedure involved in the insertion of the pellet induced the same type of proliferation with approximately the same time course as that following freeze ulceration (51). As in the above described model of conversion and propagation, the short exposure of the actively proliferating bladder mucosa to saccharin leached from the pellet provides the conversion necessary for bladder carcinogenesis; the pellet then acts as a propagating agent along with the urine.

These experiments, if applicable to the human situation, suggest possible groups at increased risk of development of bladder carcinoma. It is well known that people exposed to certain chemicals such as 2-aminonaphthalene, benzidine, and 4-aminobiphenyl have an increased risk of developing bladder cancer. It is also well known that males have an increased risk of developing bladder cancer compared to females (1,2). Could this increase be related to the development of prostatism in elderly males with consequent changes in the bladder epithelium? Is exposure to certain chemicals *in utero* and shortly after birth responsible for an increased risk of development of bladder cancer since the epithelium is proliferating during these times? Are people who have recurrent episodes of acute cystitis with its accompanying regenerative hyperplasia at increased risk if exposed to certain chemicals such as sodium saccharin or cigarette smoke? Obviously, we have much to learn about bladder carcinogenesis in humans. Hopefully, the results in these animal models will provide clues for us to evaluate the human situation.

ACKNOWLEDGMENTS

The comments of Dr. R.E. Greenfield and Dr. G.H. Friedell are greatly appreciated. I thank Dorothy Morrissey for her assistance with this manuscript. Work reported in this presentation from this laboratory has been supported in part by U.S. Public Health Service grants CA 15945 and CA 28015 from the National Cancer Institute through the National Bladder Cancer Project.

REFERENCES

1. Clayson, D.B., and E.H. Cooper. 1970. Cancer of the urinary tract. Adv. Cancer Res. 13:271-381.

2. Price, J.M. 1971. Etiology of bladder cancer. In: Benign and Malignant Tumors of the Urinary Bladder. E. Maltry, ed. Medical Examination Publishing Co., Inc.: Flushing, NY. pp. 189-251.

3. Johansson, S., L. Angervall, U. Bengtsson, and L. Wahlquist. 1974. Uroepithelial tumors of the renal pelvis associated with abuse of phenacetin-containing analgesics. Cancer 33:743-753.

4. Lomax-Smith, J., and A.E. Seymour. 1980. Unsuspected analgesic nephropathy in transitional cell carcinoma of the upper tract: A morphological study. Histopathology 4:255-269.

5. Miller, J.A., and E.C. Miller. 1977. Ultimate chemical carcinogens as reactive mutagenic electrophiles. In: Origins of Human Cancer, Cold Spring Harbor Conferences on Cell Proliferation, Volume 4. H.H. Hiatt, J.D. Watson, and J.A. Winsten, eds. Cold Spring Harbor Laboratory: Cold Spring Harbor, NY. pp. 605-627.

6. Glowinski, I.B., H.E. Radtke, and W.W. Weber. 1978. Genetic variation in N-acetylation of carcinogenic arylamines by human and rabbit liver. Molec. Pharmacol. 14:940-949.

7. Lower, G.M., T. Nilsson, C.E. Nelson, H. Wolfe, T.E. Gamsky, and G.T. Bryan. 1979. N-Acetyltransferase phenotype and risk in urinary bladder cancer: Approaches in molecular epidemiology. Environ. Hlth. Perspect. 29:71-79.

8. Kadlubar, F.F., J.A. Miller, and E.C. Miller. 1977. Hepatic microsomal N-hydroxy arylamines in relation to urinary bladder carcinogenesis. Cancer Res. 37:805-814.

9. Radomski, J.L., J.M. Poupko, and W.L. Hearn. 1980. Environmental bladder carcinogens. National Bladder Cancer Project Abstracts, Saratoga, FL. p. 35 (abstract).

10. Cohen, S.M., T.V. Zenser, G. Murasaki, S. Fukushima, M.B. Mattammal, N.S. Rapp, and B.B. Davis. (1981). Aspirin inhibition of N-[4-(5-nitro-2-furyl)-2-thiazolyl]formamide-induced lesions of the urinary bladder correlated with inhibition of metabolism by bladder prostaglandin endoperoxide synthetase. Cancer Res. 41:3355-3359.

11. Druckrey, H., R. Preussmann, D. Schmähl, and S. Ivankovic. 1967. Organotrope carcinogene Wirkungen bei 65 verschiedenen N-Nitroso-Verbindungen an BD-Ratten. Z. Krebsforsch. 69:103-201.

12. Cohen, S.M. 1978. Toxicity and carcinogenicity of nitrofurans. In: Carcinogenesis - A Comprehensive Survey, Volume 4, Nitrofurans. G.T. Bryan, ed. Raven Press: New York. pp. 171-231.

13. Hicks, R.M., and J.St.J. Wakefield. 1972. Rapid induction of bladder cancer in rats with N-methyl-N-nitrosourea. I. Histology. Chem.-Biol. Interact. 5:139-152.

14. Erturk, E., S.M. Cohen, J.M. Price, and G.T. Bryan. 1969. Pathogenesis, histogenesis, histology, and transplantability of urinary bladder carcinoma induced in albino rats by oral administration of N-[4-(5-nitro-2-furyl)-2-thiazolyl] formamide. Cancer Res. 29:2219-2228.

15. Wang, C.Y., and Y. Kamirya. 1978. Carcinogenicity of 2-amino-4-(5-nitro-2-furyl)thiazole in rats and metabolism of this carcinogen by cultured dog urothelial cells. Proc. Am. Assoc. Cancer Res. 19:146 (abstract).

16. Swaminathan, S., and G.M. Lower, Jr. 1978. Biotransformations and excretion of nitrofurans. In: Carcinogenesis - A Comprehensive Survey, Volume 4, Nitrofurans. G.T. Bryan, ed. Raven Press: New York. pp. 59-97.

17. Wang, C.Y., R.C. Benson, Jr., and G.T. Bryan. 1977. Mutagenicity for Salmonella typhimurium of urine obtained from humans receiving nitrofurantoin. J. Natl. Cancer Inst. 58:871-873.

18. Tiltman, A.J., and G.H. Friedell. 1971. The histogenesis of experimental bladder cancer. Invest. Urol. 9:218-226.

19. Cohen, S.M., J.B. Jacobs, M. Arai, S. Johansson, and G.H. Friedell. 1976. Early lesions in experimental bladder cancer: Experimental design and light microscopic findings. Cancer Res. 36:2508-2511.

20. Arai, M., S.M. Cohen, J.B. Jacobs, and G.H. Friedell. 1979. Effect of dose on urinary bladder carcinogenesis induced in F344 rats by N-[4-(5-nitro-2-furyl)-2-thiazolyl]formamide. J. Natl. Cancer Inst. 62:1013-1016.

21. Jacobs, J.B., M. Arai, S.M. Cohen, and G.H. Friedell. 1977. A long-term study of reversible and progressive urinary bladder cancer lesions in rats fed N-[4-(5-nitro-2-furyl)-2-thiazolyl]formamide. Cancer Res. 37:2817-2821.

22. Cohen, S.M., M. Arai, J.B. Jacobs, and G.H. Friedell. 1979. Promoting effect of saccharin and D,L-tryptophan in urinary bladder carcinogenesis. Cancer Res. 39:1207-1217.

23. Tsuda, H., Y. Miyata, G. Murasaki, H. Kinoshita, S. Fukushima, and N. Ito. 1977. Synergistic effect of urinary bladder carcinogenesis in rats treated with N-butyl-N-(4-hydroxy-butyl)nitrosamine, N-[4-(5-nitro-2-furyl)-2-thiazolyl]-formamide, N-2-fluorenylacetamide, and 3,3'-dichlorobenzidine. Gann 68:183-192.

24. Tatematsu, M., Y. Miyata, M. Mizutani, M. Hananouchi, M. Hirose, and N. Ito. 1977. Summation effect of N-butyl-N-(4-hydroxybutyl)nitrosamine, N-[4-(5-nitro-2-furyl)-2-thiazolyl]formamide, N-2-fluorenylacetamide, and 3,3'-dichlorobenzidine on urinary bladder carcinogenesis in rats. Gann 68:193-202.

25. Hicks, R.M., J.St.J. Wakefield, and J. Chowaniec. 1975. Evaluation of a new model to detect bladder carcinogens or cocarcinogens; results obtained with saccharin, cyclamate and cyclophosphamide. Chem.-Biol. Interact. 11:225-233.

26. Nakanishi, K., M. Hirose, T. Ogiso, R. Hasegawa, M. Arai, and N. Ito. 1980. Effects of sodium saccharin and caffeine on the urinary bladder of rats treated with N-butyl-N-(4-hydroxybutyl)nitrosamine. Gann 71:490-500.

27. Nakanishi, K., S. Fukushima, M. Shibata, T. Shirai, T. Ogiso, and N. Ito. 1978. Effect of phenacetin and caffeine on the urinary bladder of rats treated with N-butyl-N-(4-hydroxybutyl)nitrosamine. Gann 69:395-400.

28. Friedell, G.H., S.M. Cohen, D.M. Demers, S. Fukushima, and J.B. Jacobs. 1980. Promoting effects of sodium saccharin (NaS) and L-tryptophan (L-T) in rat urinary bladder carcinogenesis and their effects on urinary constituents. Proc. Am. Assoc. Cancer Res. 21:111 (abstract).

29. Radomski, J.L., T. Radomski, and W.E. MacDonald. 1977. Cocarcinogenic interaction between D,L-tryptophan and 4-aminobiphenyl or 2-naphthylamine in dogs. J. Natl. Cancer Inst. 58:1831-1834.

30. Matsushima, M. 1977. The role of the promoter L-tryptophan on tumorigenesis in the urinary bladder. 2. Urinary bladder carcinogenicity of FANFT (initiating factor) and L-tryptophan (promoting factor) in mice. Jap. J. Urol. 68:731-736.

31. Scribner, J.D., and R. Suss. 1978. Tumor initiation and promotion. Int. Rev. Exp. Path. 18:137-198.

32. Cancer Testing Technology and Saccharin. 1977. Office of Technology Assessment. United States Government Printing Office: Washington, DC.

33. Bowden, J.P., K.T. Chung, and A.W. Andrews. 1976. Mutagenic activity of tryptophan metabolites produced by rat intestinal microflora. J. Natl. Cancer Inst. 57:921-924.

34. Fukushima, S., and S.M. Cohen. 1980. Saccharin-induced hyperplasia of the rat urinary bladder. Cancer Res. 40:734-736.

35. Murasaki, G., and S.M. Cohen. (1981). Effect of dose of sodium saccharin on the induction of rat urinary bladder proliferation. Cancer Res. 41:942-944.

36. Radomski, J.L., E.M. Glass, and W.B. Deichmann. 1971. Transitional cell hyperplasia in the bladders of dogs fed D,L-tryptophan. Cancer Res. 31:1690-1694.

37. Scott, W.W., and H.L. Boyd. 1953. A study of the carcinogenic effect of beta-naphthylamine on the normal and substituted isolated sigmoid loop bladder of dogs. J. Urol. 70:914-925.

38. McDonald, D.F., and R.R. Lund. 1954. The role of the urine in vesical neoplasm. 1. Experimental confirmation of the urogenous theory of pathogenesis. J. Urol. 71:560-570.

39. Chapman, W.H., D. Kirchheim, and J.W. McRoberts. 1973. Effect of the urine and calculus formation on the incidence of bladder tumors in rats implanted with paraffin wax pellets. Cancer Res. 33:1225-1229.

40. Bryan, G.T., and P.D. Springberg. 1966. Role of the vehicle in the genesis of bladder carcinomas in mice by the pellet implantation technique. Cancer Res. 26:105-109.

41. Rowland, R.G., M.O. Henneberry, R. Oyasu, and J.T. Grayback. 1980. Effects of urine and continued exposure to carcinogen on progression of early neoplastic urinary bladder lesions. Cancer Res. 40:4524-4527.

42. Oyasu, R., Y. Hirao, and K. Izumi. 1981. Enhancement by urine of urinary bladder carcinogenesis. Cancer Res. 41:478-481.

43. Izumi, K., Y. Hirao, L. Hopp, and R. Oyasu. 1981. In vitro induction of ornithine decarboxylase in urinary bladder carcinoma cells. Cancer Res. 41:405-409.

44. Boutwell, R.K. 1964. Some biological aspects of skin carcinogenesis. Prog. Exp. Tumor Res. 4:207-250.

45. Slaga, T.J., S.M. Fischer, K. Nelson, and G.L. Gleason. 1980. Studies on the mechanism of skin tumor promotion: Evidence for several stages in promotion. Proc. Natl. Acad. Sci. USA 77:3659-3663.

46. Minsky, B.D., and F.J. Chlapowski. 1978. Morphometric analysis of the translocation of lumenal membrane between cytoplasm and cell surface of transitional epithelial cells during the expansion-contraction cycles of mammalian urinary bladder. J. Cell Biol. 77:685-697.

47. Murasaki, G., S. Fukushima, R.E. Greenfield, and S.M. Cohen. (1981). Effect of ulceration on urinary bladder carcinogenesis induced by N-[4-(5-nitro-2-furyl)-2-thiazolyl]formamide (FANFT) and sodium saccharin (SAC). Proc. Am. Assoc. Cancer Res. (abstract) 22:128.

48. Shirai, T., S.M. Cohen, S. Fukushima, M. Hananouchi, and N. Ito. 1978. Reversible papillary hyperplasia of the rat urinary bladder. Am. J. Path. 91:33-48.

49. Arnold, D.L., C.A. Moodie, H.C. Grice, S.M. Charbonneau, B. Stavric, B.T. Collins, P.F. McGuire, Z.Z. Zawidska, and I.C. Munro. 1980. Long-term toxicity of ortho-toluenesulfonamide and sodium saccharin in the rat. Toxicol. Appl. Pharmacol. 52:113-152.

50. Bryan, G.T., E. Erturk, and O. Yoshida. 1970. Production of urinary bladder carcinomas in mice by sodium saccharin. Science 168:1238-1240.

51. Fukushima, S., S.M. Cohen, M. Arai, J.B. Jacobs, and G.H. Friedell. (1981). Scanning electron microscopy of reversible hyperplasia of the rat urinary bladder. Am. J. Path. 102:373-380.

DISCUSSION

Q.: Are your results compatible with the hypothetical presence of an endogenously synthesized nitrosamine in the urine as an initiator, and that initiation's being promoted by the ulcertaion?

A.: That is certainly possible. However, we have not identified the nitrosamine in the urine.

Q.: I'm still not convinced that you have clearly demonstrated promotion of chemical carcinogenesis in the urinary bladder. It seems to me that one very beautiful experiment, using the heterotopic bladder, clearly demonstrates the need for urine. But if urine is a critical factor, then most of the experiments we've done on the original theory of bladder cancer fall by the wayside, because when urine is diverted from parts of the bladder, you don't get tumors there, and you're back to square 1 again.

A.: I'm not sure I fully agree it's diverted away from the bladder, because in the heterotopic system, the heterotopic bladder is exposed to urine and so is the *in situ* bladder. They're both exposed to urine and they've both been exposed to DBN.

Q.: That's correct. Therefore, as the heterotopic bladder with urine gets tumors, but without it, doesn't, this means that urine is essential to the development of the tumor.

A.: That experiment does say urine is necessary, but it obviously isn't sufficient by itself, because spontaneous bladder tumor incidence is negligible in experimental animals.

Q.: What I am saying is that the carcinogen could have reached it either by the urine, which I think is very likely though not proved, or by the blood. However the carcinogen comes in, you still need the urine there. It is the urine and not the urine-carried carcinogen which you've shown to be essential.

A.: We have to go back, then, to the experiments in the dog.

Q.: Those experiments suffer from the same deficiency.

Q.: Another question: You had a most beautiful proliferative response in bladder urothelium following saccharin. Have you looked at this more than one time or just two or three days after saccharin?

A.: The dose-response was done at only one time, but at the highest dose, we looked at this several times, up to eighteen weeks. We've now looked through two years and it continues.

Q.: Your ulceration procedure looks like a first-stage promoter. Did you try to reverse the order of the saccharin and the ulceration?

A.: We haven't. We still are left without an initiator. It fits very nicely with the two stages of promotion, but we still have to find the initiator in the system. The saccharin certainly has not been shown to be a mutagen.

Q.: In your ulcertation experiment, how did you cool the probe that you created the ulcer with?

A.: It's frozen in dry ice and acetone.

Q.: Are you carrying any acetone over to the bladder?

A.: It's a possibility.

Q.: Would it happen to be an initiator?

A.: I hope not.

Q.: Have you tried using liquid nitrogen to do this?

A.: We tried using liquid nitrogen; it gives the same effect as far as the ulcer goes, and as far as the proliferation goes. We haven't done it in a long-term experiment to see if it also affects tumorigenesis by saccharin, but the proliferation is the same.

SPECIES AND ORGAN DIFFERENCES IN THE BIOTRANSFORMATION OF CHEMICAL CARCINOGENS

Mont R. Juchau

Department of Pharmacology, School of Medicine, University of Washington, Seattle, Washington 98195

INTRODUCTION

Although numerous species and organ differences in the biotransformation of foreign organic chemicals, including chemical carcinogens, have been reported in the literature (for recent reviews see references 1-8), in most instances the studies were not designed for rigorous comparative analyses. Often the differences were noted only as interesting sidelights of a study that did not focus upon precise comparative aspects. Nevertheless, profound differences are known to exist and research on biotransformation in recent years has provided considerable evidence for the existence of numerous species-specific, organ-specific, and cell-specific isozymic forms of the well-known xenobiotic-biotransforming enzymes.

Abundant indirect evidence for species- and organ-specific isozymes has been provided by observations of differential developmental patterns, differential responses to inducers, repressors, inhibitors, activators, and numerous physiologic factors known to affect rates of particular reactions. With advances in the isolation and purification of the pertinent enzymes, more direct evidence for such differences is rapidly accumulating; the differences can be manifested by observations of differential immunologic cross-reactivity, substrate specificity and amino acid sequences of the purified forms. Therefore, whenever rigorous comparative analyses of species, strains, organs, tissues, and cells are performed, it has become the norm to expect that differences in modes and rates of xenobiotic biotransformation will be found, even in different cells from the same clone.

Virtually all research performed to date tends to substantiate such an expectation, particularly with respect to rates.

While such differences in modes and rates of xenobiotic biotransformation tend to be frustrating because they inhibit inter- and and intraspecies extrapolations, the apparent lack of any phylogenetic (or other) basis for observed species/strain differences is even more dissatisfying. In his review of species differences in hepatic microsomal monooxygenase activities, C.H. Walker (2) found that a general, inverse correlation between mammalian body weights and hepatic monooxygenase activities appeared to exist. The exceptions to this overall general trend, however, are so numerous and frequent that accurate predictions are rendered virtually impracticable, at least in terms of current knowledge. Nevertheless, room for encouragement has been provided by increasing evidence that despite the qualitative differences in studied isozymes, differences in generated metabolites are largely quantitative rather than qualitative. Hopefully investigations of the regulation of the relevant xenobiotic biotransforming enzymes and of the rates of reactions that they catalyze eventually will lead to generalizations that will allow reasonable predictions to be made.

At present, the still fragmentary knowledge of carcinogen biotransformation at target sites precludes reliable predictions of even general trends. Innumerable examples illustrate the current unpredictability. For example, the human fetal adrenal gland was observed to be remarkably active in terms of the monooxygenation of several procarcinogens (9-14). However, the human fetal kidney (borderline activity in most investigations) exhibited far higher activity than the fetal adrenal gland when 7,12-dimethylbenz[a]-anthracene (DMBA) was used as substrate for monooxygenation and bioactivation reactions (15-17). Meanwhile, the fetal brain tissues from rats (but not mice) effectively converted DMBA to mutagenic intermediates in the Ames test as well as to a variety of hydroxylated metabolites (18).

Some particularly surprising and interesting observations pertaining to species and organ differences in carcinogen biotransformation recently have been made in our laboratory. During investigations of the characteristics of rabbit aortic monooxygenases (19), we observed that micromolar quantities of hematin added to reaction vessels increased reaction rates approximately 30-fold. Subsequent investigations (20-23) revealed that this effect could be observed in a variety of extrahepatic -- but not hepatic -- tissues and was most pronounced in the rabbit. Increases as high as 70-fold were observed with brain tissues from rabbits. All observations thus far are in harmony with the postulate that extrahepatic tissues contain quantities of free P-450 apoprotein(s), which possess a relatively low affinity for the heme prosthetic group. Interaction of a reaction product (e.g., 3-hydroxybenzo[a]pyrene) with the apoprotein appears to result in a conformational change in the apoprotein. The change in conformation increases the affinity for heme and results in the formation of active holocytochrome(s) with a high substrate turnover number. A very striking substrate and position-specificity of the hematin-mediated monooxygenation reactions (24-26) as well as the observed inhibition by P-450 inhibitors provide additional indirect evidence for the postulated mechanism. If confirmed, a potentially extremely important mode of short-term regulation of rates of monooxygenation reactions in target tissues is provided.

FUTURE RESEARCH AREAS

These observations indicate the incompleteness of our knowledge concerning modes of regulation of rates of highly important carcinogen biotransforming reactions in target cells. Such understanding is prerequisite if the role of biotransformation of carcinogens as a determinant of species/organ susceptibility is to be established. Future research should emphasize two important areas:

(1) Biotransformation seems to play a role principally in the initiation of tumorigenesis. Thus, the most intensive investigations should focus first on the relationships between capacity for tumor initiation per se (rather than on complete carcinogenesis) and the bioactivation/bioinactivation of the initiating agent in target cells. Encountered difficulties could be expected due to a variety of reasons: (a) lack of knowledge concerning the mechanism of the initiating event; (b) lack of well-defined two-stage (initiation-promotion) or multiple-stage systems for many organs of interest (The mouse skin represents the most intensively investigated system but, until fairly recently, was the only definitive system.); (c) observations suggesting that initiating agents also may function in the transition from benign to malignant tumors during studies of carcinogenesis by single agents (Most initiating agents also appear to possess promoting properties.); (d) lack of knowledge concerning precise mechanisms whereby tumor initiation can be prevented, repaired, or otherwise obscured from scientific observation; and (e) the fact that species, strain, organ, tissue, and cell differences in susceptibility to tumor initiation have not been systematically and rigorously investigated. Species differences expressed in terms of dose-response relationships, for example, are extremely rare. More pertinent would be studies in which concentration-effect relationships at the target sites could be expressed in terms of concentrations of reactive intermediates and a marker event for initiation. Only very recently have beginnings in this direction

been initiated. Measurement of steady-state levels of the pertinent causative reactive intermediates represent an even more difficult problem, but significant advances toward this goal have been made for benzo[a]pyrene, nitrosodimethylamine, aflatoxin B_1, and others.

Despite the difficulties and problems enumerated, focus on these aspects is still feasible. Studies from our own (27-32) and numerous other laboratories suggest strongly that perturbation of carcinogen biotransformation can exert an extremely powerful influence on the initiating capacity of chemical agents. At present, however, such evidence is based on correlations rather than strong, direct verification and is complicated by the possibility that those substances capable of altering biotransformation also may be capable of affecting numerous other processes involved in the eventual appearance of tumors (e.g., repair, balance between cellular proliferation and differentiation, promotion, and immunologic factors).

(2) The second major area of research should focus on the biotransformation of chemical carcinogens in relation to their biologic effects. In this case, different considerations are required as compared to most biologically active substances. Evidence suggests that relatively short-lived reactive intermediate metabolites rather than the parent compounds per se are responsible for the observed tumorigenic effects. The usual kinds of pharmacokinetic approaches are therefore much less meaningful. Steady-state levels of reactive intermediates at the target sites (as opposed to plasma levels of parent compounds) appear to be far more pertinent. Thus, identification of the pertinent reactive intermediates and their critical targets is essential for continued progress in this area. Measurement of steady-state levels of the appropriate adducts then becomes feasible, and the relationships between species/organ differences in biotransformation and species/organ differences in tumor initiation susceptibility could be approached with a far higher degree of confidence. Considerable progress toward these goals is currently being made.

REFERENCES

1. Parke, D.V., and R.L. Smith, eds. 1976. In: Drug Metabolism from Microbe to Man. Taylor and Francis: London. pp. 1-435.

2. Walker, C.H. 1978. Species differences in microsomal monooxygenase activity and their relationship to biological half lives. Drug Metab. Rev. 7:295-324.

3. Kato, R. 1979. Characteristics and differences in the hepatic mixed function oxidases of different species. Pharmac. Ther. 6:41-98.

4. Thorgeirsson, S.S., S.A. Atlas, A.R. Boobis, and J.S. Felton. 1979. Species differences in the substrate specificity of hepatic cytochrome P-448 from polycyclic hydrocarbon-treated animals. Biochem. Pharmacol. 28:217-226.

5. Caldwell, J. 1980. Comparative aspects of detoxication in mammals. In: Enzymatic Basis of Detoxication, Volume 1. W.B. Jakoby, ed. Academic Press: New York. pp. 85-116.

6. Gram, T.E., ed. 1980. Extrahepatic Metabolism of Drugs and Other Foreign Compounds. Spectrum Publications: Jamaica, New York. 601 pp.

7. Lu, A.Y.H., and S.B. West. 1980. Multiplicity of mammalian microsomal cytochromes P-450. Pharmacol. Rev. 31:277-295.

8. Vainio, H.V. 1980. Role of extrahepatic metabolism. In: Concepts in Drug Metabolism, Part A. P. Jenner and B. Testa, eds. Marcel Dekker, Inc.: New York. pp. 251-285.

9. Juchau, M.R., M.G. Pedersen, and K.G. Symms. 1972. Hydroxylation of benzo[a]pyrene in human fetal tissue homogenates. Biochem. Pharmacol. 21:2269-2272.

10. Juchau, M.R., and M.G. Pedersen. 1973. Drug biotransformation reactions in the human fetal adrenal gland. Life Sci. 12:193-204.

11. Juchau, M.R., M.J. Namkung, D.L. Berry, and P.K. Zachariah. 1975. Oxidative biotransformation of 2-acetylaminofluorene in fetal and placental tissues of humans and monkey: Correlations with aryl hydrocarbon hydroxylase activities. Drug Metab. Disp. 3:494-502.

12. Zachariah, P.K., and M.R. Juchau. 1975. Spectral characteristics of human fetal adrenal microsomes. Life Sci. 16:55-63.

13. Berry, D.L., P.K. Zachariah, T.J. Slaga, and M.R. Juchau. 1977. Analysis of the biotransformation of benzo[a]pyrene in human fetal and placental tissues with high pressure liquid chromatography. Eur. J. Cancer 13:667-675.

14. Namkung, M.J., P.K. Zachariah, and M.R. Juchau. 1977. O-Sulfonation of N-hydroxy-2-fluorenylacetamide and 7-hydroxy-N-2-fluorenylacetamide in fetal and placental tissues of humans and guinea pigs. Drug Metab. Disp. 5:288-294.

15. Jones, A.H., A.G. Fantel, R.M. Kocan, and M.R. Juchau. 1977. Bioactivation of procarcinogens to mutagens in human fetal and placental tissues. Life Sci. 21:1831-1837.

16. Juchau, M.R., M.J. Namkung, A.H.Jones, and J. DiGiovanni. 1978. Biotransformation and bioactivation of 7,12-dimethylbenz[a]anthracene in human fetal and placental tissues. Drug Metab. Disp. 6:273-281.

17. Juchau, M.R., A.H. Jones, M.J. Namkung, and J. DiGiovanni. 1978. Extrahepatic bioactivation of 7,12-dimethylbenz[a]-anthracene and benzo[a]pyrene in human fetal tissues. In: Carcinogenesis, Volume 3, Polynuclear Aromatic Hydrocarbons. R. Freudenthal and P.W. Jones, eds. Raven Press: New York. pp. 361-370.

18. Juchau, M.R., J. DiGiovanni, M.J. Namkung, and A.H. Jones. 1979. A comparison of the capacity of fetal and adult liver, lung, and brain to convert polycyclic aromatic hydrocarbons to mutagenic and cytotoxic metabolites in mice and rats. Toxicol. Appl. Pharmacol. 49:171-178.

19. Bond, J.A. C.J. Omiecinski, and M.R. Juchau. 1979. Kinetics, activation, and induction of aortic monooxygenases: Analyses of the mixed-function oxidation of benzo[a]pyrene with high-pressure liquid chromatography. Biochem. Pharmacol. 28:305-312.

20. Omiecinski, C.J., J.A. Bond, and M.R. Juchau. 1978. Stimulation by hematin of monooxygenase activity in extrahepatic tissues from rats, rabbits, and chickens. Biochem. Biophys. Res. Comm. 83:1004-1011.

21. Omiecinski, C.J., S.J. Chao, and M.R. Juchau. 1980. Modulation of monooxygenase activities by hematin and 7,8-benzoflavone in fetal tissues of rats, rabbits, and humans. Dev. Pharmacol. Therap. 1:90-100.

22. Omiecinski, C.J., and M.R. Juchau. 1980. Augmentation by hematin of rates of benzo[a]pyrene hydroxylation: The possible involvement of cytochrome P-450. In: Microsomes, Drug Oxidations, and Chemical Carcinogenesis. M.J. Coon, A.H. Conney, R.W. Estabrook, H.V. Gelboin, J.R. Gillette, and P.J. O'Brien, eds. Academic Press: New York. pp. 969-972.

23. Omiecinski, C.J., M.J. Namkung, and M.R. Juchau. 1980. Mechanistic aspects of the hematin-mediated increases in brain monooxygenase activities. Molec. Pharm. 17:225-232.

24. Chao, S.T., C.J. Omiecinski, M.J. Namkung, S.D. Nelson, B.H. Dvorchik, and M.R. Juchau. 1981. Catechol estrogen formation in placental and fetal tissues of humans, macaques, rats, and rabbits. Dev. Pharmacol. Therap. 2:1-17.

25. Omiecinski, C.J., and M.R. Juchau. 1981. Hematin-dependent monooxygenation of benzo[a]pyrene: Positional specificity and DNA binding in vitro. In: Polynuclear Aromatic Hydrocarbons. W.M. Cooke, and A.J. Dennis, eds. Battelle Press: Columbus, Ohio. pp. 697-705.

26. Omiecinski, C.J., M.J. Namkung, and M.R. Juchau. (in press). Substrate and position specificity of hematin-activated monooxygenation reactions. Biochem. Pharmacol.

27. DiGiovanni, J., T.J. Slaga, A. Viaje, D.L. Berry, R.G. Harvey, and M.R. Juchau. 1978. The effects of 7,8-benzoflavone on skin tumor initiating activities of various 7- and 12-substituted derivatives of 7,12-dimethylbenz[a]anthracene. J. Natl. Cancer Inst. 61:135-140.

28. Berry, D.L., T.J. Slaga, J. DiGiovanni, and M.R. Juchau. 1979. Studies with chlorinated dibenzo-p-dioxins, polybrominated biphenyls, and polychlorinated biphenyls in a two-stage system of mouse skin carcinogenesis: Potent anticarcinogenic effects. Ann. NY Acad. Sci. 320:405-415.

29. DiGiovanni, J., D.L. Berry, M.R. Juchau, and T.J. Slaga. 1979. 2,3,7,8-tetrachlorodibenzo-p-dioxin: Potent anticarcinogenic activity. Biochem. Biophys. Res. Comm. 86:577-584.

30. DiGiovanni, J., D.L. Berry, T.J. Slaga, A.H. Jones, and M.R. Juchau. 1979. Effects of pretreatment with 2,3,7,8-tetrachlorodibenzo-p-dioxin on the capacity of hepatic and extrahepatic mouse tissues to convert procarcinogens to mutagens for Salmonella typhimurium auxotrophs. Toxicol. Appl. Pharmacol. 50:229-239.

31. DiGiovanni, J., D.L. Berry, T.J. Slaga, and M.R. Juchau. 1979. Studies on the relationships between induction of biotransformation and tumor-initiating activity of 7-12-dimethylbenz[a]anthracene in mouse skin. In: Polynuclear Aromatic Hydrocarbons. P.W. Jones, and P. Leber, eds. Ann Arbor Science Publishers: Ann Arbor, MI. pp. 553-568.

32. DiGiovanni, J., T.J. Slaga, D.L. Berry, and M.R. Juchau. 1980. Inhibitory effects of environmental chemicals in polycyclic aromatic hydrocarbon carcinogenesis. In: Modifiers of Chemical Carcinogenesis. T.J. Slaga, ed. Raven Press: New York. pp. 145-157.

33. Juchau, M.R., and K.G. Symms. 1972. Aniline hydroxylation in the human placenta--Mechanistic aspects. Biochem. Parmacol. 21:2053-2065.

34. Symms, K.G., and M.R. Juchau. 1974. The aniline hydroxylase and nitro-reductase activities of partially purified cytochromes P-450, P-420 and cytochrome b_5 solubilized from rabbit hepatic microsomes. Drug Metab. Disp. 2:194-201.

DISCUSSION

Q.: Do I understand you correctly in saying that in the presence of hematin the metabolism of benzo[a]pyrene was altered? If that is the case, is it possible that this is due to a peroxidation mechanism rather than a hematin incorporated into a P-450?

A.: Yes, we've considered that possibility. The peroxidation of the benzo[a]pyrene primarily results in the formation of quinones. The most reactive position on benzo[a]pyrene is at the 6-position, not at the 3-position. The only way we can explain increased hydroxylation at the 3-position is via some mechanism which, presumably would be cytochrome P-450-mediated.

Q.: Have you run the controlled experiment where you would have hematin and benzo[a]pyrene and your electron donor without the enzyme present?

A.: Yes.

Q.: Did you observe anything?

A.: No, there's nothing at all.

Q.: The reason I ask this question is that several years ago we reported an interesting anomaly in which you could metabolize benzo[a]pyrene in the presence of an electron acceptor such as 1,2-naphthoquinone and NADPH without any microsomal enzymes. We isolated 9-hydroxy, 2 quinones and 4 or 5 --

A.: No. That was our first concern, that this kind of thing may be going on. And in fact, several years before, we discovered the capacity of the hemoglobin to catalyze aniline hydroxylation (33,34). We simply had to add hemoglobin and aniline and an electron donor and obtained a very nice reaction in which aniline is parahydroxylated. That was the first thing that came to my mind, that something like this may be going on. But any one of a number of controls that we have utilized indicated there was no such thing.

SPECIES HETEROGENEITY IN THE METABOLIC PROCESSING OF BENZO[a]PYRENE

James K. Selkirk, Michael C. MacLeod, Betty K. Mansfield, Patsy A. Nikbakht, and Kris C. Dearstone

Biology Division, Oak Ridge National Laboratory, Oak Ridge, Tennessee 37830

INTRODUCTION

The detoxification response of the organism toward chemical carcinogens is to transform these potentially toxic compounds into more polar, less lipid soluble substances that are readily excretable and therefore harmless. However, it would appear that nature has made a serious mistake in the case of chemical carcinogens. This concept can be stylized by superimposing the steps in metabolic activation upon a chemical energy activation diagram (see Figure 1). It is generally assumed that the parent molecules of an environmentally prevalent chemical carcinogen are structurally stable and relatively inactive metabolically. This assumption is not unreasonable from a teleological point of view since one would expect labile chemical substances to be rapidly degraded or oxidized, due to sunlight and weather, if released in the open environment. Synthetically prepared activated carcinogens, such as polyaromatic epoxides and nitrosamines, have been shown to possess very short half-lives under physiological conditions. Therefore, the parent compound undergoes a decrease in entropy to increase its potential energy for subsequent metabolic degradation. This change requires enzymatic transformation into a reactive intermediate antecedent to further catabolism. Current evidence shows that all known carcinogenic chemicals are electrophilic reagents that seek out nucleophilic sites inside the cells (1). The peak of the curve in Figure 1 is the zone where the electron-deficient reactive metabolite is thought to interact with nucleophilic target sites hypothesized to begin the process of malignant transformation. If no such interaction takes place, the most common reaction is hydroxylation to form a metabolically inactive polar structure that is more hydrophilic and can be readily excreted. Therefore, the major thrust of the detoxification process is to render the parent compound into a structure of greater entropy and consequently less potential to exert a toxic effect.

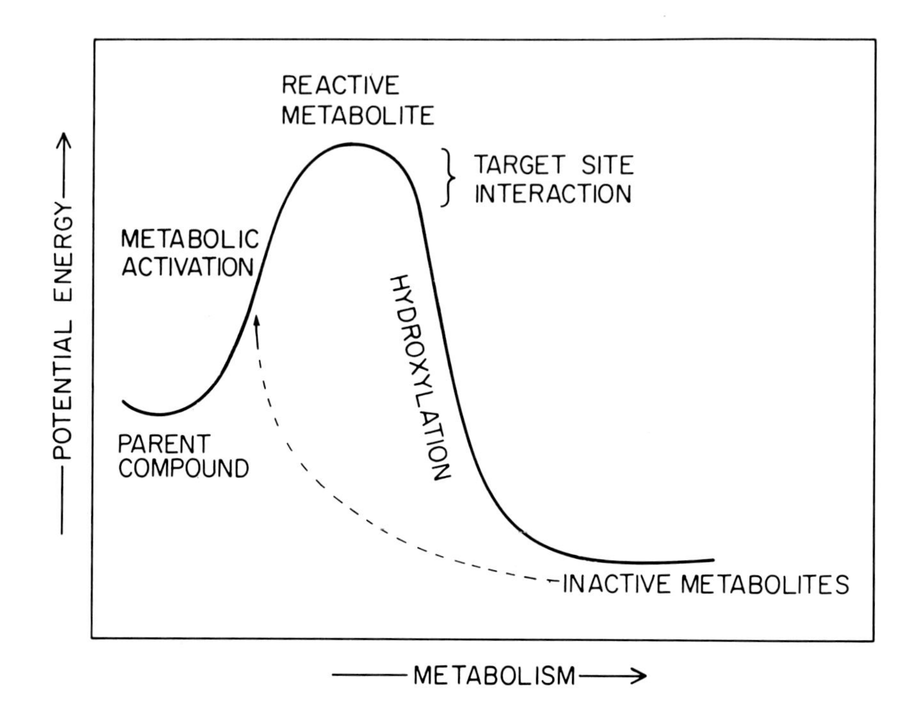

Figure 1. Hypothetical orientation of metabolic activation of xenobiotics superimposed on activation-energy curve. The parent compound requires input energy to become reduced to an inactive metabolite. During this active state the reactive intermediate presumably imparts its carcinogenic effect.

All of the major carcinogen chemicals, including polyaromatic hydrocarbons, aflatoxins, aromatic amines, and nitrosamines, follow the same biochemical scheme and must pass through this highly reactive state during metabolism. Presumably, all types of chemical carcinogens possess some common physical-chemical relationship that provokes the same type of disruption to cellular homeostasis that transforms it from a normal cell into a cancer cell. Burgeoning research in all these classes of carcinogens has produced a host of new biochemical data that more clearly describes the mode of activation, the sites of interaction, and the various types of detoxification products formed. Yet, the complete mechanism of malignant transformation, for any of these carcinogens, remains obscure. Possibly, the problem of carcinogenesis must now be approached through a kinetic mechanism that exploits the knowledge of resistant and susceptible species, strains, and cells that has accumulated from the numerous model systems developed in recent years. The rationale behind relative resistance and susceptibility may be viewed through a hypothesis that deals with the net accumulation and spatial orientation of the reactive carcinogenic intermediate within the cell. If one assumes that the qualitative nature of the carcinogen metabolite profile is common to both susceptible and resistant cells, then it may be possible that a susceptible cell is producing an active metabolite at a rate faster than the hydroxylating and conjugating enzymes can remove it. Similarly, this same cell may produce the reactive metabolites at a rate equivalent to a resistant cell, but possess a reduced capacity to hydroxylate or conjugate carcinogenic intermediates. In either case, the net result would be a longer half-life for the reactive intermediate with a concomitant increase in the probability that the activated intermediate will interact with a critical target site for malignant transformation.

Benzo[a]pyrene (BP) is metabolized to a series of oxygenated derivatives. The structures seen in Figure 2 represent the major known metabolites found in all eukaryotic systems. They are isolated in their free-oxygenated, non-conjugated forms in cell-free systems. However, intact cells that contain a total complement of metabolic machinery will further metabolize them to their conjugated excretion products (below the line (2). Most of these derivatives have been tested for carcinogenic and mutagenic activity in both *in vivo* (3) and *in vitro* (4,5,6) systems. It is currently felt that the pathway critical for carcinogenesis and mutagenesis is that seen in the lower right-hand corner of the figure where BP forms the intermediate 7,8-epoxide which becomes hydrated by microsomal epoxide hydrase and then is reactivated by the mixed-function oxidases to form the 7,8-diol-9,10-epoxide (7). This result is seen more clearly in Figure 3 in which BP is acted on by aryl hydrocarbon hydroxylase (AHH) twice to form the unstable diol-epoxide that opens to form a trihydroxy-carbonium as the major alkylating species of BP.

Extensive research has been performed on the stereochemistry of BP dihydrodiol-epoxides which can form two stereo-isomers (see Figure 4) named according to the position of the 7-OH group in relation to the oxide. At left is the syn-isomer (4-7,t-8-dihydroxy-c-9,10-oxy-7,8,9,10-tetrahydrobenzo[a]pyrene, and at the right is the anti-isomer (4-7,t-8-dihydroxy-t-9,10-oxy-7,8,9,10-tetrahydro-benzo[a]pyrene).

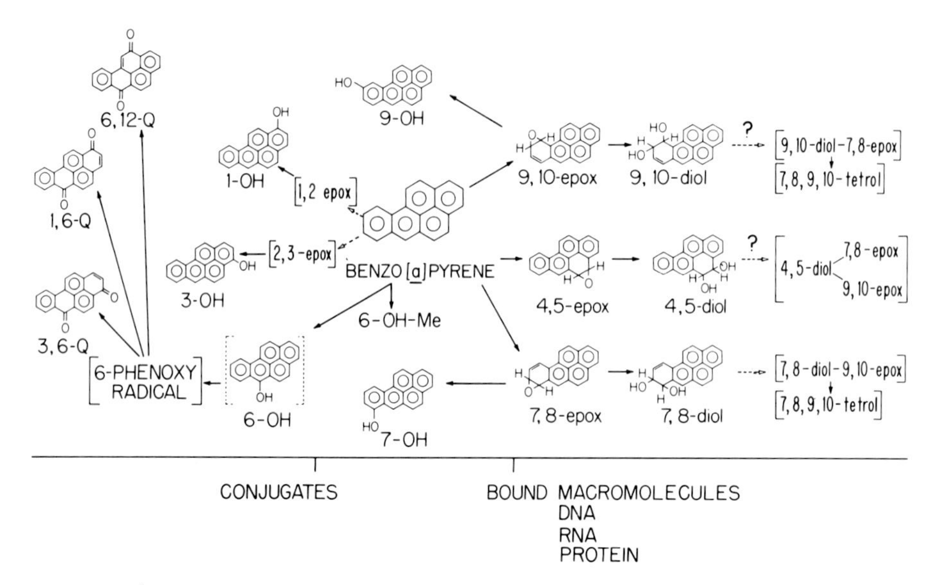

Figure 2. Composite of BP metabolism in *in vivo* and *in vitro* systems.

Similarity of metabolic products in both susceptible and resistant cells in conjunction with an identical alkylation pattern for DNA suggests a dynamic model for susceptibility to carcinogenesis by polycyclic hydrocarbons. Figure 5 exhibits some possible processing pathways for BP. The heavy line depicts activation via an epoxide and onto a reactive dihydrodiol-epoxide followed by alkylation of macromolecules leading to tumorigenesis. The lightweight line shows all ancillary pathways where a cell can channel away various reactive intermediates into conjugated excretable forms. Constants K_1 through K_{10} are hypothetical rate constants that could be used to describe and compare metabolic processing of a carcinogen in susceptible and resistant cells. Possibly, a critical step in determining relative susceptibility of a given cell to malignant transformation by BP is determined by how much carcinogen entering the cells is processed toward alkylation of DNA as compared to how efficient the cell is in removing metabolic intermediates out of the putative tumorigenic pathway.

Qualitative similarity of BP metabolism is seen for several species using liver microsomes in Figure 6. The predominant metabolite in cell-free systems in which cytoplasmic transferases have been removed is 3-OH-BP (8). The ratio between 9-OH-BP and 3-OH-BP is quite variable; 9-OH-BP is a significant metabolite for

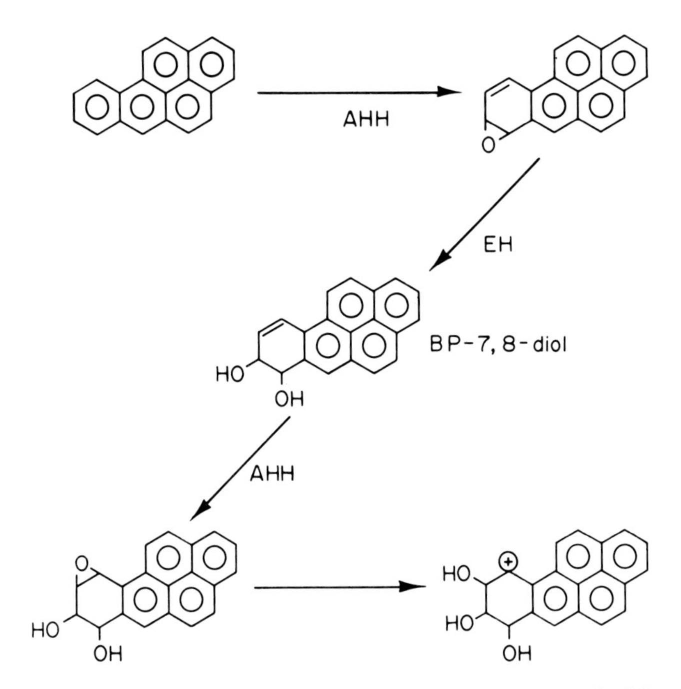

Figure 3. Formation of reactive BP-7,8-dihydrodiol-9,10-epoxide by the microsomal mixed-function oxidase.

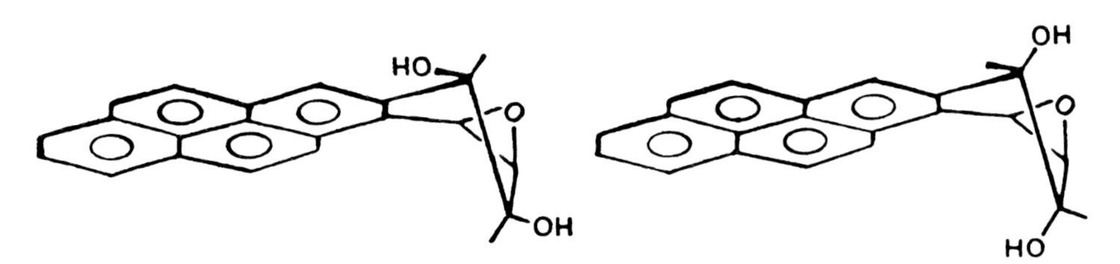

Figure 4. Benzo[a]pyrene-dihydrodiol epoxide diastereomers. Syn-configuration is at left and anti-configuration at right.

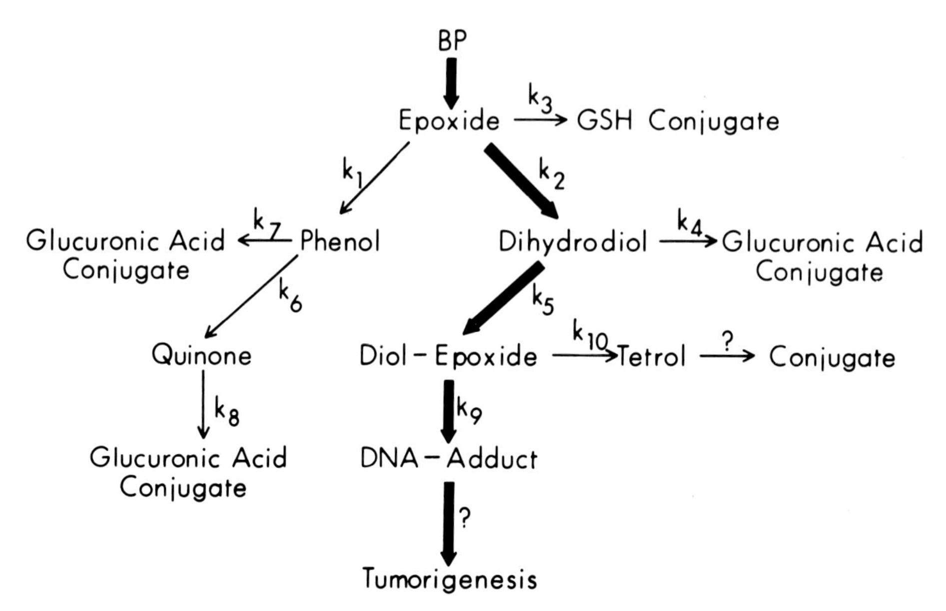

Figure 5. Suppositional kinetic scheme outlining competing tumorigenic (heavy line) and nontumorigenic (light line) pathways.

the mouse and relatively absent for the hamster, while rat and human liver microsomes show measurable quantities. Also ratios of the three metabolic dihydrodiols are species variable, with the predominant dihydrodiol for the hamster being at the 4,5-position while the 9,10-dihydrodiol is the major metabolite for the rat. The lower panel showing human hepatic microsomal metabolism is presented to show the relatively weak metabolism of BP in noninduced human liver as compared to rodent liver.

Intact cell metabolism is significantly different from cell-free (see Figure 7). Fibroblast metabolism utilizes cytoplasmic transferase to remove toxic phenols and quinones. All species studied show dihydrodiols as less active substrates for conjugation. Dihydrodiol accumulation allows a greater probability for remetabolism by the mixed-function oxidases to more reactive electrophiles. The lower panel shows the insignificant metabolic activity of human foreskin fibroblasts. Clearly, a qualitative identity exists in microsomally-catalyzed formation of metabolites from BP, and it is assumed that binding to DNA is a critical step for formation of malignant transformation.

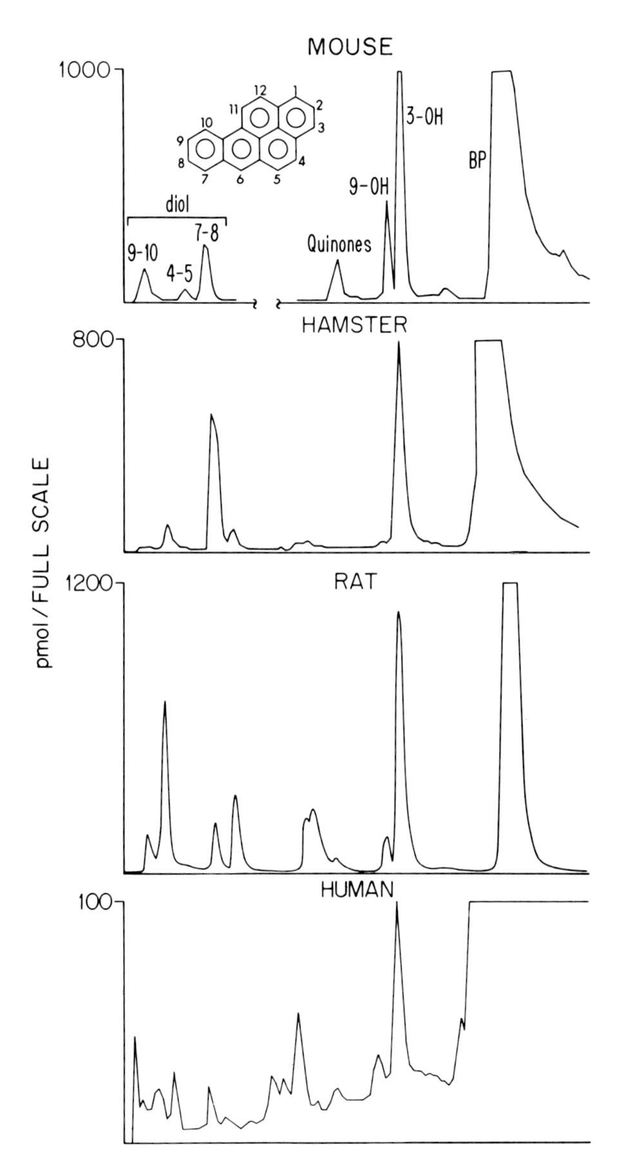

Figure 6. Species comparison of hepatic microsomal metabolism of BP using high-pressure liquid chromatographic assay of organic solvent soluble metabolites. Note qualitative similarity and quantitative variance between species.

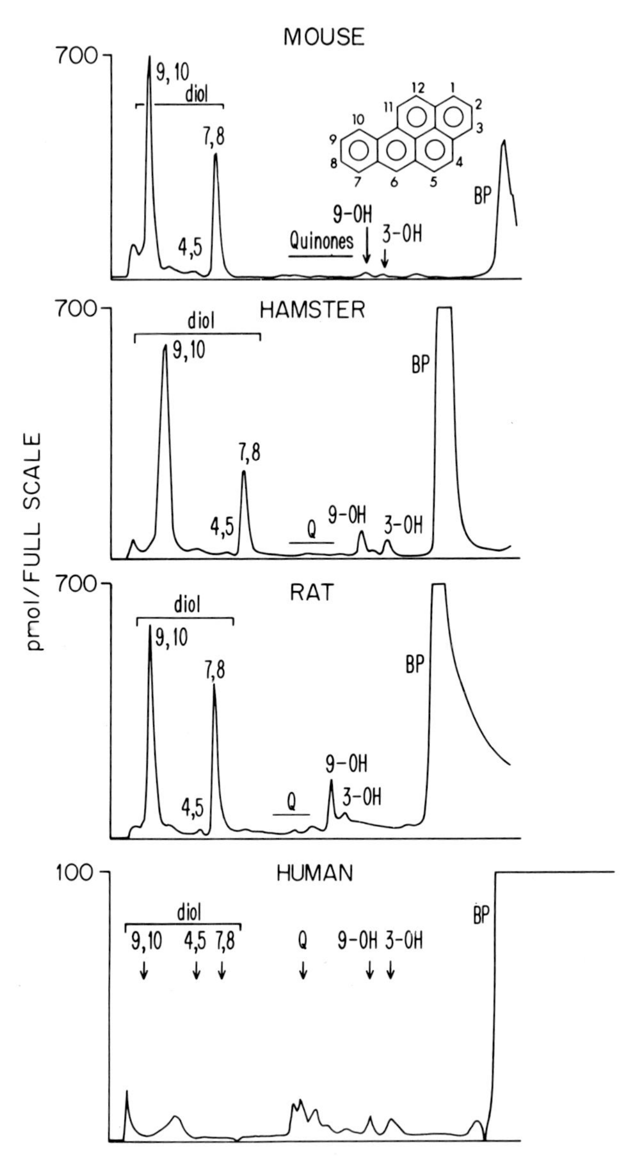

Figure 7. Species comparison of fibroblast metabolism of BP using high-pressure liquid chromatographic assay of organic solvent soluble metabolites. Note absence of phenols and quinones due to removal of conjugates by cytoplasmic transferases.

All studies to date would implicate the anti-isomer as being more important in mutagenesis (9) and carcinogenesis (10). It has been clearly demonstrated that the anti-isomer is the major DNA-binding species with a high affinity for the exocyclic amino group of guanine. However, the mechanism by which this or any other base alkylation precipitates the process to malignant transformation is unknown. Therefore, determining the pattern of nuclear processing of the carcinogen and its interaction with all nuclear macromolecules in chromatin can aid in following the metabolic pathway toward or away from the transforming agent.

Figure 8 shows the SDS-polyacrylamide gel separation of nuclear proteins from confluent cultures of hamster embryo fibroblasts (HEF) incubated with [^{3}H]BP and [^{3}H]BP-7,8-dihydrodiol and [^{3}H]BP-9,10-dihydrodiol. [^{3}H]-7,8-diol-9,10-epoxide was incubated with nuclei. The extreme left lane (protein stain) represents nuclear proteins isolated from HEF and stained with Coomassie-blue. In the second lane ([^{3}H]BP), of the four subunits associated with nucleosome core proteins, H3 and H2A were heavily labeled with little or no radioactivity associated with H2B and H4. A strong band of radioactivity was found in the H1 region of the gel and many nonhistone proteins were also labeled. The basis for this biochemical selectivity remains unknown. Analysis of proteins from cells incubated with [^{3}H]BP-7,8-dihydrodiol revealed the same selectivity for core histones H3 and H2A with a marked decrease in labeling associated with the H1 regions and with nonhistones. Similar results were seen for binding of BP-7,8-diol-9,10-epoxide ([^{3}H]BPDE) which was coincident with the fact that the BP-7,8-dihydrodiol is the precursor to the 7,8-diol-9,10-epoxide. The most dramatic finding was seen with BP-9,10-diol ([^{3}H]BP-9,10-diol) incubated with cells. Almost no binding was seen for nucleosomal core histones while the vast majority of radioactivity was associated with a heavy band in the H1 region of the gel. Figure 9 shows a reconstruction of BP incubation (lane 1) by overlapping nuclear incubations of BP-9,10-diol (lane 2) and BP-7,8-diol (lane 3). By superimposing lanes 2 and 3, an identical pattern is seen to lane 1, strongly suggesting BP metabolism in the nucleus generates both 7,8-dihydrodiol-9,10-epoxide and 9,10-dihydrodiol-7,8-epoxide, followed by a highly specific partitioning between alkylation sites.

These results clearly show a marked specificity occurring at the nuclear level that is not readily apparent when measuring overall metabolism. The 9,10-dihydrodiol is a major dihydrodiol metabolite in cell-free metabolite studies (8). During cellular incubation of BP in tissue culture, this dihydrodiol is rapidly removed from the cytoplasm and unlike phenols and quinones is excreted into the surrounding medium as a free dihydrodiol. Since this dihydrodiol is a major nuclear protein alkylator, it is possible that this "reverse" dihydrodiol-epoxide is generated by

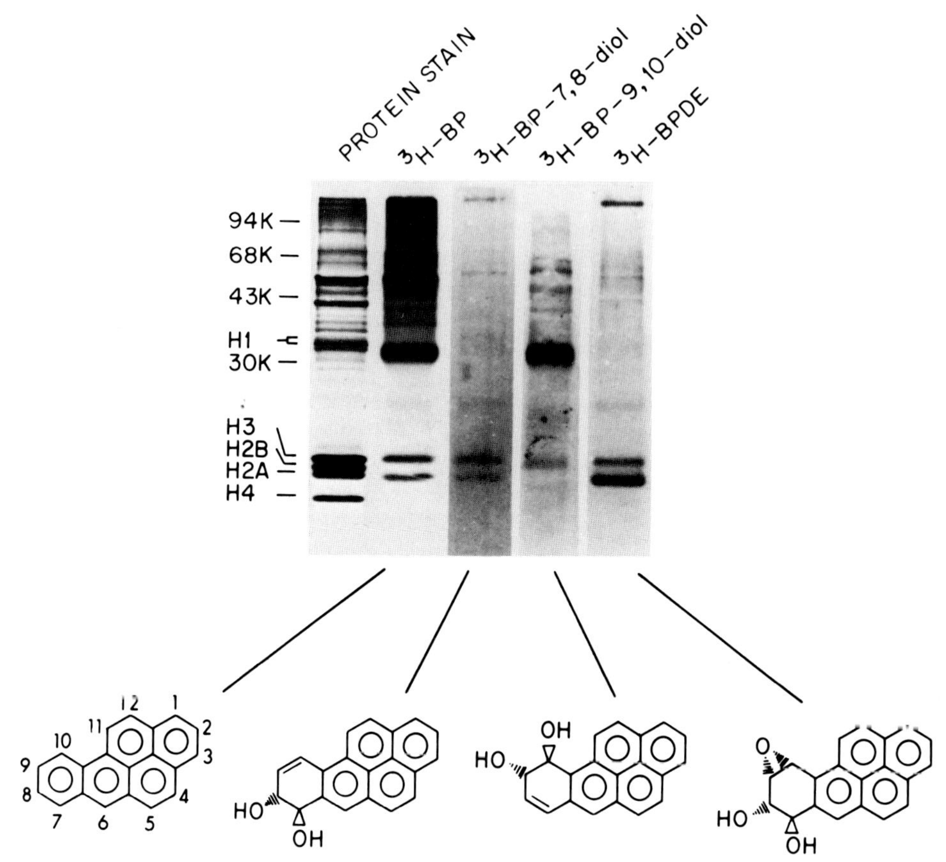

Figure 8. Nuclear protein separation by SDS-polyacrylamide gel. Hamster cells or nuclei (see text) were incubated with BP, two dihydrodiols, and the diol-epoxide. The left lane was stained with Coomassie-blue while the remaining four lanes are fluorograms of the incorporated tritium label.

nuclear reactivation of dihydrodiol within the nucleus (11). The role of this site-specific nuclear protein alkylation in disruption of homeostatic control of transcription or translation remains obscure.

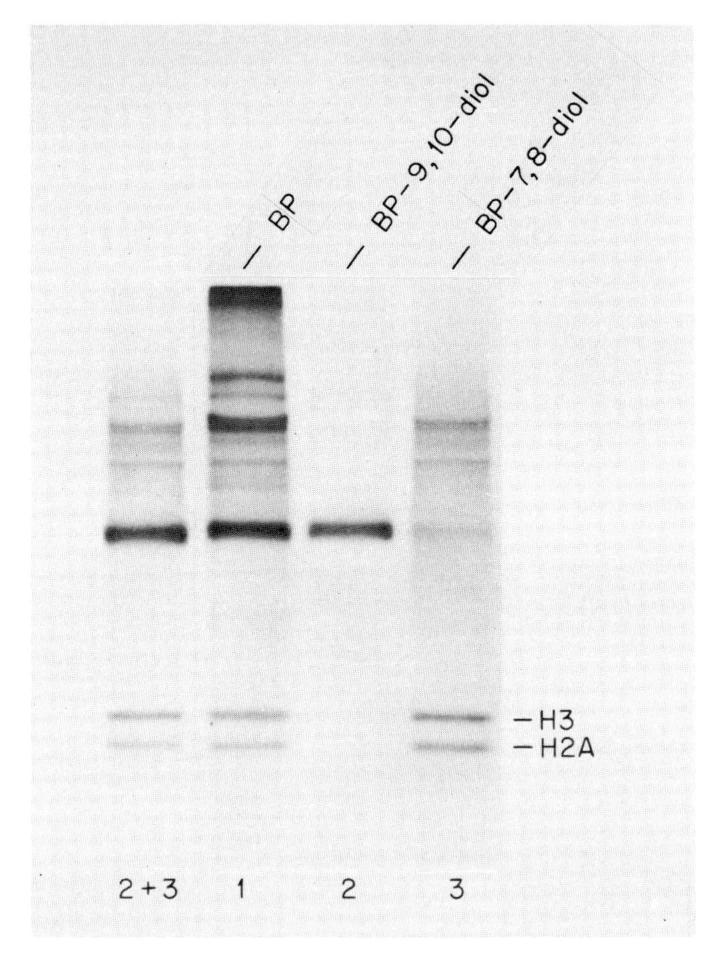

Figure 9. Superimposition of lanes from incubation of the two dihydrodiols (2 and 3) compared to the lanes from the parent BP incubation. Left lanes (2 and 3) are almost identical to lane 1, suggesting a major nuclear protein binding of the "reverse" diol-epoxide.

REFERENCES

1. Miller, J.A., and E.C. Miller. 1977. Ultimate chemical carcinogens as reactive mutagenic electrophiles. In: Origins of Human Cancer, Volume B. H.H. Hiatt, J.D. Watson, and J.A. Winsten, eds. Cold Spring Harbor Laboratory: New York. pp. 605-627.

2. Paulson, G.D. 1980. Conjugation of foreign chemicals by animals. Residue Review 76:31-72.

3. Public Health Service Document no. 149. 1978. Survey of compounds have been tested for carcinogenic activity. U.S. Government Printing Office.

4. Mager, R., E. Huberman, S.K. Yang, H.V. Gelboin, and L. Sachs. 1977. Transformation of normal hamster cells by benzo[a]pyrene diol-epoxide. Int. J. Cancer 19:814-817.

5. Marquardt, H., P.L. Grover, and P. Sims. 1976. In vitro malignant transformation of mouse fibroblasts by non-K-region dihydrodiols derived from 7-methylbenz[a]anthracene, 7,12-dimethylbenz[a]anthracene and benzo[a]pyrene. Cancer Res. 36:2059-2064.

6. Levin, W., A.W. Wood, P.G. Wislocki, R.L. Chang, J. Kapitulnik, H.D. Mah, H. Yagi, D.M. Jerina, and A.H. Conney. 1978. Mutagenicity and carcinogenicity of benzo[a]pyrene and benzo[a]pyrene derivatives. In: Polycyclic Hydrocarbons and Cancer, Volume 1. H.V. Gelboin and P.O.P. Ts'o, eds. Academic Press, Inc.: New York. pp. 189-204.

7. Sims, P., and P.L. Grover. 1974. Oxides in polycyclic aromatic hydrocarbon metabolism and carcinogenesis. Adv. Cancer Res. 20:165-274.

8. Selkirk, J.K., R.G. Croy, P.P. Roller, and H.V. Gelboin. 1974. High-pressure liquid chromatographic analysis of benzo[a]pyrene metabolism and covalent binding and the mechanism of action of 7,8-benzoflavone and 1,2-epoxy-3,3,3-trichloropropane. Cancer Res. 34:3474-3480.

9. Huberman, E., L. Sachs, S.K. Yang, and H.V. Gelboin. 1976. Identification of mutagenic metabolites of benzo[a]pyrene in mammalian cells. Proc. Natl. Acad. Sci. USA 73:607-611.

10. Slaga, T.J., A. Viaje, W.M. Bracken, D.L. Berry, S.M. Fisher, D.R. Miller, and S.M. LeClerc. 1977. Skin-tumor-initiating ability of benzo[a]pyrene-7,8-diol-9,10-epoxide (anti) when applied topically in tetrahydrofuran. Cancer Lett. 3:23-30.

11. MacLeod, M.C., A. Kootstra, B.K. Mansfield, T.J. Slaga, and J.K. Selkirk. 1980. Specificity in interaction of benzo[a]pyrene with nuclear macromolecules: Implication of derivatives of two dihydrodiols in protein binding. Proc. Natl. Acad. Sci. USA 77:6396-6400.

ENDOCRINE REGULATION OF XENOBIOTIC CONJUGATION ENZYMES

Coral A. Lamartiniere and George W. Lucier

Laboratory of Organ Function and Toxicology, National Institute of Environmental Health Sciences, Research Triangle Park, North Carolina 27709

INTRODUCTION

The balance of events involved in the activation/deactivation of xenobiotics is enormously complex. The metabolic activation of non-toxic chemicals to compounds that are reactive intermediates has been implicated in a wide variety of toxic reactions including carcinogenesis, teratogenesis, and toxicity (1-3). Figure 1 illustrates the enzymatic transformation of benzo[a]pyrene (BP) to reactive intermediates, primarily BP-epoxides. These electrophilic compounds can bind to DNA or to other cellular macromolecules to initiate toxicity. Toxic metabolites of polycyclic aromatic hydrocarbons can be enzymatically deactivated by a number of enzyme systems, such as the glutathione S-transferases, glucuronyltransferases, and sulfotransferases.

Our laboratory has been studying the ontogeny and endocrine regulation of two of these xenobiotic conjugative enzyme systems, the hepatic glutathione S-transferases and UDP-glucuronyltransferases. Their postpubertal developmental patterns result in higher activities in adult male rats than in adult females, while no sex difference is seen in immature rats. Figure 2 shows the postnatal developmental pattern of hepatic glutathione S-transferase conjugation with 1,2-dichloro-4-nitrobenzene as substrate. While sex differences in hepatic metabolism of adult animals can be explained partly by "activational effects" (i.e., induction, repression, activation, or inhibition due to the direct presence or absence of an effector), considerable evidence has accumulated to link the perinatal period of development in the rat as a critical period for "organizational effects" to program for and eventually account for sex

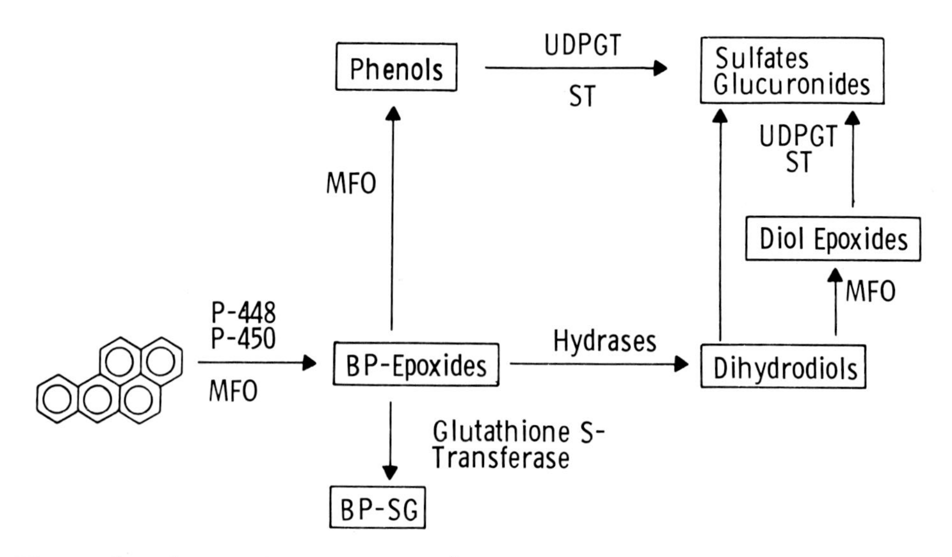

Figure 1. Enzymatic activation/deactivation scheme of benzo[a]-pyrene (BP). BP is activated by the mixed-function oxygenases (MFO) to electrophilic intermediates. Reactive intermediates may be deactivated by conjugating with glutathione (GS-) via the glutathione S-transferases or glucuronides via UDP-glucuronyltransferase (UDPGT) or by the action of sulfotransferases (ST).

differentiation (4-9). According to this mechanism, testosterone secreted from the immature testes reaches the target cells in the developing brain; this testosterone is converted into estrogen that in turn programs the nerve endings for a male type of metabolism and behavior. These sex-differentiated parameters are not expressed until sexual maturation and are mediated via the hypothalamic-pituitary-gonadal axis. We report here on the complex interplay of events leading to the postnatal expression of these hepatic xenobiotic conjugative enzymes.

Endocrine Regulation of Glutathione S-Transferases

The glutathione S-transferases are a group of cytosolic proteins that catalyze many reactions in which glutathione participates as a nucleophile. These enzymes bind a large number of hydrophobic compounds and act as a storage facility prior to

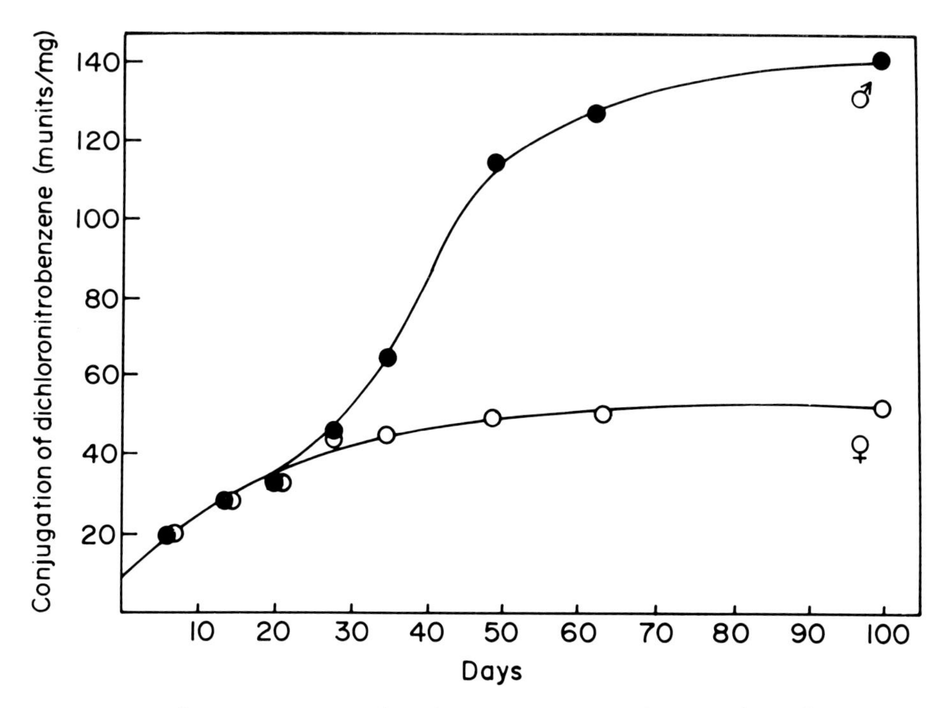

Figure 2. Postnatal development of rat liver glutathione S-transferase.

metabolism or excretion of the ligand (10) and undergo covalent-bond formation with reactive electrophilic carbons (11). The glutathione S-transferases have been separated on the basis of differences in physical properties. While individual proteins have been found to catalyze reactions with more than one class of substrate, each protein displays preferred specificity (12). In our studies, we measured glutathione S-transferase activities as a function of reduced glutathione conjugation towards the substrates 1-chloro-2,4-dinitrobenzene and 1,2-dichloro-4-nitrobenzene (12).

Glutathione conjugation toward these two substrates indicates that glutathione S-transferase activities are low in the livers of prepubertal male and female rats (13,14). While activities continue to rise in animals of both sexes, conjugation towards 1-chloro-2,4-dinitrobenzene is slightly higher in adult males than in adult females and two- to threefold higher towards 1,2-dichloro-4-nitrobenzene in males than in females (see Figure 2). Sex steroids in the adult animal do not seem to play a role in the postpubertal sex differentiation of the glutathione S-transferases. Gonadectomy of adult male or female rats with or without appropriate hormone replacement produces no significant change in enzyme activities (15). On the other hand, the pituitary is responsible for negative modulation of the glutathione S-transferase activities. Hypophysectomy results in increases in glutathione S-transferase activities. Figure 3 demonstrates the effect of the pituitary on glutathione S-transferase activities towards 1,2-dichloro-4-nitrobenzene in the male rat. To gain insight into the nature of this hypophyseal regulation, we implanted a pituitary from an adult age-matched donor or four pituitaries from 21-day-old males (equivalent weight) to hypophysectomized animals. These ectopic pituitary treatments were capable of reversing the effect of hypophysectomy on glutathione S-transferase activities (15). Similar results were obtained in female rats.

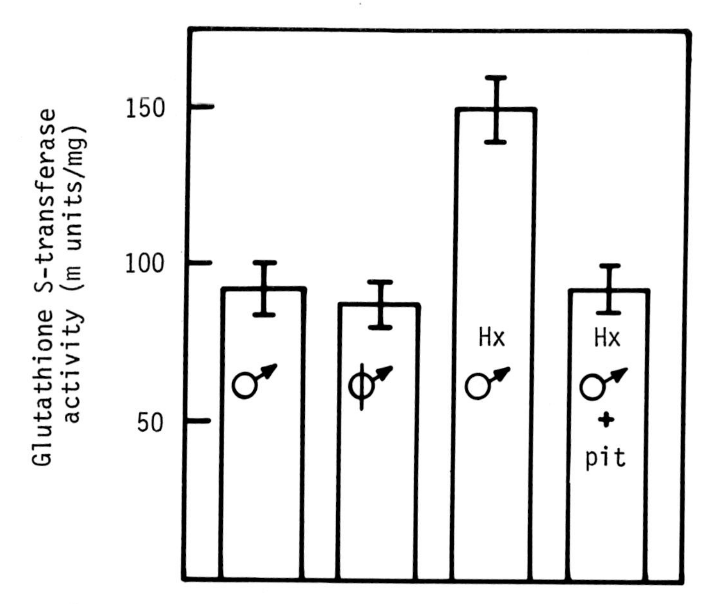

Figure 3. Pituitary-gonadal regulation of glutathione S-transferase activity. Gonadectomy (ɸ♂) or hypophysectomy (Hx) was carried out on day 42 and ectopic pituitaries (pit) were transplanted under the kidney capsule on day 56. Animals were sacrificed eight days later.

The increase in glutathione S-transferase activities in hypophysectomized animals was followed by a decrease in serum prolactin concentrations and the reverse was found in those hypophysectomized animals receiving ectopic pituitaries, i.e., a decrease in enzyme activity and an increase in prolactin. This discovery led us to investigate the possibility of prolactin mediating the regulation of the glutathione S-transferases. Rat prolactin (NIAMDD-Rat Prolactin-B-1, 7 units/mg) was given by subcutaneous injections in saline to hypophysectomized rats at concentrations of 780 μg/kg BW twice daily for eight days. This prolactin treatment was not capable of altering glutathione S-transferase activities but was capable of stimulating accessory sex organ weights. A similar experiment with growth hormone as a possible hypophyseal effector was carried out. Bovine growth hormone (NIH GH-B-18, 0.83 units/mg) administered under the same schedule as prolactin at a concentration of 5 mg/kg BW was able to reverse the effect of hypophysectomy on glutathione S-transferase activities (15). This action demonstrates an inverse relationship between glutathione S-transferase activities and growth hormone.

In an effort to gain further insight into the mechanisms of the hypothalamic-hypophyseal regulation of glutathione S-transferases, arcuate nucleus lesions of the hypothalamus were induced by injecting neonatal rats with pharmacological doses of monosodium-L-glutamate according to the methods of Nemeroff et al. (16). Light microscopic examination of Nissl-stained sections of the medial basal hypothalamus of neonatal rats shortly after monosodium-L-glutamate injections revealed considerable damage in the region of the arcuate nucleus (16). Glutathione conjugation towards 1,2-dichloro-4-nitrobenzene in adult males treated neonatally with monosodium-L-glutamate was reduced to activities comparable to control females, whereas activity in females was only slightly reduced. Glutathione conjugation towards 1-chloro-2,4-nitrobenzene was not significantly altered in males or females. Serum growth hormone concentrations in control male and female rats were 56 ± 12 ng/ml and 54 ± ng/ml, respectively, while the monosodium-L-glutamate-treated male and female rats had 4.0 ± 0.2 ng/ml and 4.0 ± 0.1 ng/ml, respectively (15). Neonatal administration of monosodium-L-glutamate to male rats produced more definitive results; we observed a decrease in growth hormone concentrations and a decrease in glutathione S-transferase activity towards 1,2-dichloro-4-nitrobenzene.

The results from the growth hormone replacement experiments in hypophysectomized rats, and the results from the monosodium-L-glutamate rats, taken together, argue that growth hormone alone does not regulate adult levels of glutathione S-transferase. The possibility remains, however, that growth hormone may act by concerted action with other hormones or act indirectly via another hormone (15).

Endocrine Regulation of UDP-Glucuronyltransferase

The UDP-glucuronyltransferases are located in the membrane of the endoplasmic reticulum and catabolize the conjugation of glucuronic acid to compounds containing hydroxyl, carboxyl, amino, imino, and sulfhydryl groups, consequently rendering these products more hydrophilic and more readily excretable. Considerable evidence has accumulated in the literature to demonstrate multiple forms of UDP-glucuronyltransferases. One class has been characterized as belonging to the "late-fetal group" (17) and conjugates mostly non-steroidal compounds (18), while the other class is of the "neonatal group" (17) and conjugates mostly steroids (18). This report deals with the former group due to the ease and sensitivity of measuring enzyme activity with p-nitrophenol as substrate.

While prepubertal UDP-glucuronyltransferase activity is similar in male and female rats, postpubertal sexual differentiation results in male activities that are nearly twice that of females (19). Postpubertal castration of male rats results in reduced enzyme activity (see Figure 4), whereas ovariectomy of females causes no significant alteration in activity levels. Testosterone propionate administered to castrate males is capable of restoring UDP-glucuronyltransferase activity to normal levels. Hypophysectomy of male rats results in a decrease in enzyme activity, whereas hypophysectomy has no effect on female UDP-glucuronyltransferase. Hypophysectomy therefore abolishes postpubertal sex differences of this enzyme activity. A pituitary transplant under the kidney capsule with or without exogenous testosterone treatment is not capable of reversing the effect of hypophysectomy on UDP-glucuronyltransferase activity (19). These experiments demonstrate that testosterone and the pituitary are positive modulators of UDP-glucuronyltransferase activity, but an *in situ* pituitary is obligatory for androgen action. Furthermore, it would appear from the pituitary transplant experiments that the positive modulation by the pituitary is under the control of a hypothalamic "releasing factor." Exogenously administered prolactin or growth hormone to the hypophysectomized rats was not capable of reversing the effect of hypophysectomy on enzyme activity.

Neonatal Imprinting

During the early period of development in the rat, critical organizational events take place in the brain. These developmental events can determine many of the sex-differentiated characteristics of the adult animal. Adult patterns of sexual behavior, hepatic enzyme metabolism, and endocrine secretions are determined in part during the perinatal period (4-9). These laboratories have shown

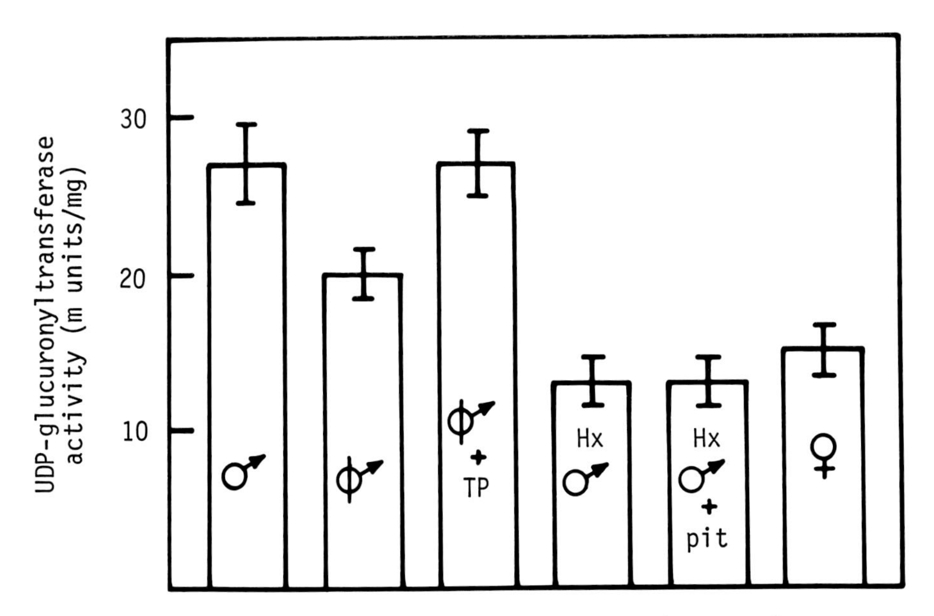

Figure 4. Pituitary-gonadal regulation of UDP-glucuronyltransferase activity. Gonadectomy (♂̸) or hypophysectomy (Hx) was carried out on day 42. Testosterone propionate (TP) was injected (sc) at a concentration of 2 mg/kg BW daily for one week and the animals sacrificed 18 h after the last injection. Ectopic pituitaries (pit) were transplanted under the kidney capsule eight days prior to sacrificing.

that adult male-type hepatic metabolism is dependent on neonatal androgen exposure. In the newborn male rat, testicular androgen reaches the brain and is aromatized to estrogen (20); this estrogen then binds the estrogen receptor (21). The estrogen receptor-ligand complex is subsequently translocated to the nucleus where transcription, translation, and post-translation processes take place to program for a male type of metabolism, sex behavior, or or endocrine secretion in subsequent adult rats (4-9).

It has been demonstrated for several enzymes that neonatal androgen deprivation via castration on day 1 causes a feminization of adult male enzyme activities (5,8,9). The administration of testosterone to neonatal castrates on day 2, however, prevents this feminization (8,9). For these reasons, we investigated the effects of castration and hormone administration on hepatic glutathione S-transferase and UDP-glucuronyltransferase activities. Neonatal castration (day 1) resulted in feminization (a decrease) of glutathione S-transferase and UDP-glucuronyltransferase activities, activities that are intermediate to those found in control males and females (15,19). A group of neonatally castrated males was treated with 1.45 μmol testosterone propionate on day 2 (the treatment regime shown to be successful in reversing the feminization of the steroid metabolizing enzymes [8] and monoamine oxidase [9]), but this failed to restore activity levels to those of control males. Testosterone propionate (2 mg/kg BW) administered in adulthood to these animals was also not capable of reconstituting the system. However, these gonadectomized animals have additional altered endocrine secretions other than the lack of testosterone, as this surgical manipulation causes other hormone-dependent functions that are dependent on the hypothalamic-hypophyseal-gonadal axis. The influence of such factors on hepatic enzyme development must still be elucidated.

Altered Ontogeny

We subsequently investigated the effect that neonatal hormone exposure on intact rats would have on hepatic sex-differentiated enzymes in the adult animal. Newborns were treated on days 2, 4, and 6 postpartum with 1.45 μmol testosterone propionate, diethylstilbestrol, or 20 μl propylene glycol (vehicle). Adult males that had received the hormones neonatally had significantly lower UDP-glucuronyltransferase activities than the controls (see Table 1). Neonatal testosterone propionate or diethylstilbestrol treatment had no effect on UDP-glucuronyltransferase activity in prepubertal males or females or in adult females. Glutathione S-transferase activities were unaltered in these treatment groups. Neonatal treatment with testosterone propionate and diethylstilbestrol resulted in reduced reproductive organ weights in adult male and female rats, but only neonatal diethylstilbestrol had an adverse effect on spermatogenesis and on circulating testosterone levels (19). It would appear that the feminization of UDP-glucuronyltransferase activities in those neonatally treated males must reflect more than a reduction in androgen levels. Apparently, other alterations from this treatment are responsible for reduced enzyme activity in diethylstilbestrol- and testosterone-propionate-treated animals.

Numerous environmental chemicals have been demonstrated to possess hormone activity. Estrogenic substances have been used extensively in a variety of drugs and environmental chemicals. Diethylstilbestrol (22), polychlorinated biphenyls (PCBs) (23), zearalanone (24), tetrahydrocannabinol (25), DDT and methoxychlor (23), all have estrogenic activity. Using two pure polychlorinated biphenyl congeners, we investigated the effects of perinatal exposure of the 3,4-3',4' tetrachlorobiphenyl (4-CB) and

Table 1. UDP-Glucuronyltransferase Activity in Adult Male Rats Neonatally Exposed to Propylene Glycol, Testosterone Propionate, or Diethylstilbestrol

Treatment	UDP-glucuronyltransferase (m units/mg)	Testosterone (ng/ml)
Propylene glycol	27 ± 2	2.5 ± 0.3
Testosterone propionate	22 ± 2	3.2 ± 0.3
Diethylstilbestrol	22 ± 2	0.5 ± 0.1

the 2,4,5-2',4',5' hexachlorobiphenyl (6-CB) on these xenobiotic conjugative enzymes (26,27). Date-bred rats were treated orally on alternate days from the 8th through the 18th day of gestation, with either 3 mg/kg 4-CB or 30 mg/kg 6-CB. These doses did not cause fetotoxicity or decreased survival rate. Neonatal, prepubertal, and adult male and female rats exposed perinatally to 6-CB had higher glutathione S-transferase activities than the controls (26). In contrast, perinatal 6-CB exposure does not alter prepubertal and adult female UDP-glucuronyltransferase, but it does decrease adult male enzyme activities (27). The metabolism and disposition of pure PCB congeners differ according to the degree and position of chlorination. The 6-CB does not have the configuration required for rapid hydroxylation but has a long biological half-life. While this characteristic may account for the ability of 6-CB to stimulate glutathione S-transferase activities in all ages investigated, it may be through another mechanism that perinatal 6-CB causes feminization of adult male UDP-glucuronyltransferase. One possibility is that neonatal exposure to PCBs alters activity of steroid-metabolizing enzymes during the critical period of early development when organizational effects are taking place. This effect could cause alterations in the hormonal milieu during the period of early development, resulting in altered sex differentiation of hepatic enzymes. Reports in the literature indicate that PCBs do alter activities of steroid-metabolizing enzymes in adult rats (28,29).

Effects of Neonatal Hormones on the Hepatic Monooxygenase System

In addition to effects on conjugative enzymes, neonatal hormones can alter sex differentiation of the hepatic monooxygenase system. Several components of the monooxygenase system do undergo sex differentiation (30-36). Sex-related differences in the hepatic microsomal ethylmorphine N-demethylation activities are observed in mature rats; specific activities in male are four times higher than in females (34,36). Administration of testosterone propionate or diethylstilbestrol to neonates results in the "feminization" (depression) of hepatic ethylmorphine N-demethylation activities of adult male rats without significantly altering the enzyme activities in either the mature female rats or immature rats of either sex. Furthermore, kinetic studies reveal neonatal "feminization" of Km values for the N-demethylation in adult males that have received neonatal diethylstilbestrol (36). Reduction in serum androgen levels of adult male rats was associated with the treatment of neonates with diethylstilbestrol but not with testosterone. Reduction of hepatic ethylmorphine N-demethylation activity and cytochrome P-450 content following cadmium (Cd) treatment (2.0 mg/kg, i.p.) was also age- and sex-dependent in the rat; marked reduction in enzyme activity was observed only in adult male rats (36-40). Adult male rats that had received testosterone or diethylstilbestrol treatments during the neonatal period exhibited decreased sensitivity towards the hepatotoxic effects of Cd; responses in the treated groups were similar to those of females (Figure 5).

Recent evidence suggests hypophyseal regulation of certain sex-dependent characteristics of the hepatic monooxygenase system in the rat (35). Changes in the hepatic monooxygenase system following hypophysectomy include an increase in the magnitude of the Cd-mediated depression of hepatic monooxygenase system in both male and female rats (41). These data suggest that Cd does not exert its hepatotoxic effects by direct pituitary action. However, the presence of the pituitary influences the liver to reduce the hepatic response to Cd. Since the hepatic monooxygenase system of immature rats of either sex is not altered by acute Cd treatment, the effect of hypophysectomy of rats at 20 days of age on the hepatic response to Cd in the subsequent 80-day-old male and female rats was also investigated (41). Cadmium treatment did not alter the hepatic monooxygenase system activities of these animals. These observations suggest that the development of susceptibility of the hepatic monooxygenase system to Cd requires pituitary action during the period of hepatic sex differentiation (between 20 and 50 days of age). Effects on enzyme activity correlated well with histological changes in livers of the various groups of animals exposed to Cd (41).

The turnover characteristics of hepatic P-450 (based on time-course disappearance of labeled heme) and SDS-polyacrylamide gel electrophoretic profiles of hepatic microsomes have been used to investigate the nature of the responsiveness of P-450 to Cd in intact and hypophysectomized rats (41,42). There were no significant sex differences in total P-450 levels in microsomes isolated from adult rats; however, the concentrations of the

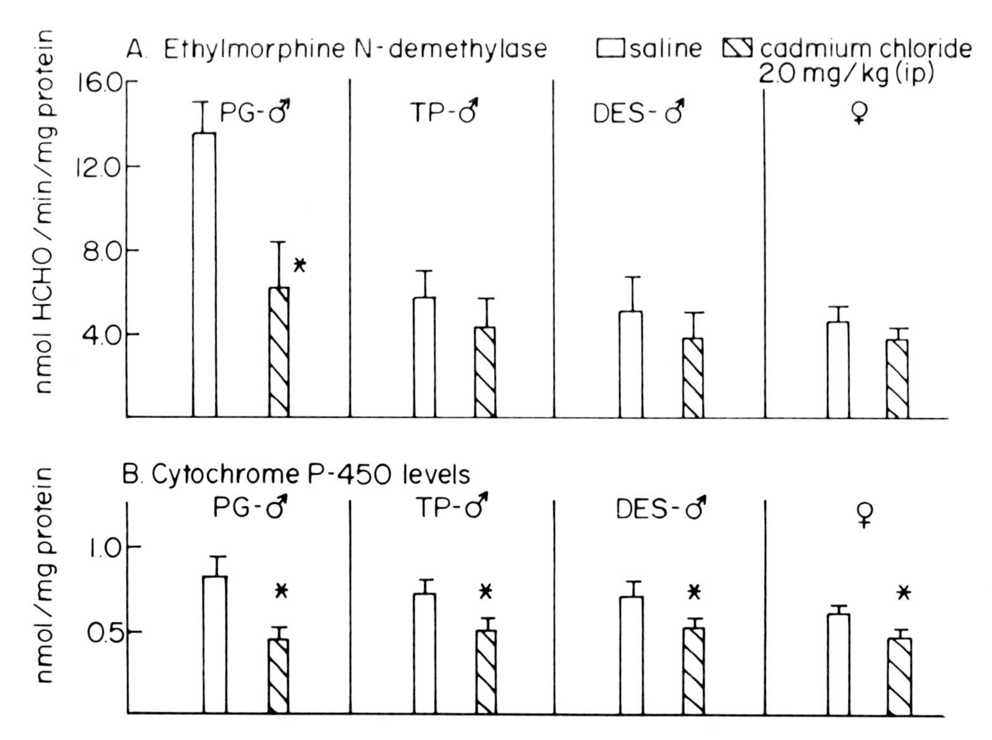

Figure 5. Influence of neonatal testosterone propionate (TP) or diethylstilbestrol (DES) treatment on Cd-induced repression of hepatic ethylmorphine N-demethylase activities (a) and cytochrome P-450 content (b) in 63-day-old male rats. The hepatic response to Cd in adult female rats was included for comparison. TP and DES (1.45 μmol) were administered on days 2, 4, and 6 postpartum. Animals received a single injection of cadmium chloride (2.0 mg/kg i.p.) or comparable volumes of saline before sacrifice. The values represent the mean enzyme activities or the mean hemoprotein contents. The lines represent the standard derivation of the mean from four to five individual rats. The asterisk (*) signifies statistically significant differences from control values at $P < 0.05$.

slow-phase components were clearly sex-related (male > female). This sex difference appears to be imprinted by neonatal androgens (34,43). The concentrations of total cytochrome P-450 contents and slow-phase components were elevated in both male and female rats by prior hypophysectomy. Acute Cd treatment resulted in a significant reduction of microsomal P-450 content (total and slow-phase components) in intact males and hypophysectomized males and females, but not in intact females. Polyacrylamide gel electrophoresis studies revealed at least one Cd-sensitive microsomal protein band (m.w. ≅ 60,000) (44). The intensity of this protein band was sex-related (male > female) and was elevated by prior hypophysectomy. In all experiments, the amount of Cd-sensitive protein was correlated with Cd-mediated decreases in P-450 content. These data suggest that sexual dimorphism for the Cd-induced reduction of hepatic P-450 in adult rats is related to the sex differences in the levels of specific form(s) of Cd-sensitive P-450. The levels of Cd-sensitive forms appear to be imprinted at the pituitary-hypothalamic level during a critical period of neonatal development by androgens (44).

Administration of methadone to male neonates results in female-type Km values for the hepatic monooxygenase system in the subsequent adult animal whereas V_{max} values are unchanged (45). This feminization of kinetic values appears to be related to a methadone-mediated depression of testosterone levels in neonates suggesting that methadone prevents the imprinting of the monooxygenase system. This idea was reinforced by the finding that simultaneous administration of testosterone and methadone to neonates results in normal sex differentiation of enzyme activity and kinetic constants.

CONCLUDING REMARKS

The fetus and newborn are particularly susceptible to numerous factors that can have deleterious effects on the developing organism. Perinatal exposure of the brain or target organ to chemicals during this critical period of development can exert permanent irreversible manifestations that can cause alterations in the offspring's postnatal development. These alterations may be expressed overtly as teratogenesis or a disease state, or subtly as alterations in reproductive capacity, sex behavior, endocrine secretion, or the capacity to metabolize xenobiotics.

For example, Miller et al. (46) reported that the liver of male rats is more susceptible to carcinogenic aromatic amine derivatives than the liver of female rats. Weisburger et al. (47) treated female rats on the day of parturition with estrogen and shortly after weaning with the carcinogen N-hydroxy-acetylamino-fluorene. Autopsies 26 weeks later showed a higher incidence of liver cancer in the estrogen- and carcinogen-treated animals than in control animals. The authors suggested that endocrine and possibly central nervous-system factors may play a role in formation of liver tumors. It has also been reported that neonatal exposure to pharmacologic doses of phenobarbital produces a permanent and irreversible modification of the adult hepatic monooxygenase system and the rate of formation of DNA adducts to aflatoxin metabolites (48). These researchers theorized that phenobarbital altered the hormonal environment during the critical period of early development and thereby affected brain differentiation in a way that permanently altered pituitary regulation of the hepatic monooxygenase system.

Neonatal imprinting is a metabolic alteration that takes place early in life, is permanent and irreversible. Steroid hormones or hormonally-active xenobiotics may well exert such an effect on the metabolic activation/deactivation systems of the liver, reducing its capacity to metabolize chemicals. Such alterations may predispose the individual to cancer or some other biochemical insult.

REFERENCES

1. Conney, A.H. 1967. Pharmacological implications of microsomal enzyme induction. Pharmacol. Rev. 19:317-366.

2. Short, C.R., D.A. Kinden, and R. Stith. 1976. Fetal and neonatal development of the microsomal monooxygenase system. Drug Metab. Rev. 5:1-42.

3. Lucier, G.W., E.M.K. Lui, and C.A. Lamartiniere. 1979. Metabolic activation/deactivation reactions during perinatal development. Environ. Hlth. Perspect. 29:7-16.

4. Harris, G.W. 1964. Sex hormones, brain development, and brain function. Endocrinology 75:627-648.

5. DeMoor, P., and C. Denef. 1968. The "puberty" of the rat liver. Feminine patterns of cortisol metabolism in male rats castrated at birth. Endocrinology 82:480-492.

6. McEwen, B.S. 1976. Interactions between hormones and nerve tissue. Sci. Am. 235:48-58.

7. Gorski, R.A., R.E. Harlan, and L.W. Christensen. 1977. Perinatal hormonal exposure and the development of neuroendocrine regulatory processes. J. Toxicol. Environ. Hlth. 3:97-121.

8. Gustafsson, J.A., A. Mode, G. Norstedt, T. Hohfelt, C. Sonnenschein, P. Eneroth, and P. Skett. 1980. The hypothalamo-pituitary-liver axis, a new hormonal system in control of hepatic steroid and drug metabolism. In: Biochemical Actions of Hormones, Volume 7. G. Litwack, ed. Academic Press: New York. pp. 47-90.

9. Illsley, N.P., and C.A. Lamartiniere. 1980. The imprinting of adult hepatic monoamine oxidase levels and androgen responsiveness by neonatal androgen. Endocrinology 107:551-556.

10. Jakoby, W.B., and J.H. Keen. 1977. A triple-threat in detoxification: The glutathione S-transferases. Trends in Biomed. Sci. 2:229-231.

11. Keen, J.H., and W.B. Jakoby. 1978. Glutathione transferases. Catalysis of nucleophilic reactions of glutathione. J. Biol. Chem. 253:5654-5657.

12. Habig, W.H., M.J. Pabst, and W.B. Jakoby. 1974. Glutathione S-transferase. The first enzymatic step in mercapturic acid formation. J. Biol. Chem. 249:7130-7139.

13. Hales, B.F., and A.H. Neims. 1976. A sex difference in hepatic glutathione S-transferase B and the effect of hypophysectomy. Biochem. J. 160:223-229.

14. Hales, B.F., and A.H. Neims. 1976. Developmental aspects of glutathione S-transferase B (Ligandin) in rat liver. Biochem. J. 160:231-236.

15. Lamartiniere, C.A. 1981. The hypothalamic-hypophyseal-gonadal regulation of hepatic glutathione S-transferases in the rat. Biochem. J. 198:211-217.

16. Nemeroff, C.B., R.J. Konkel, G. Bissette, W. Youngblood, J.B. Martin, P. Brazeau, M.S. Rone, A.J. Prange, Jr., G.R. Breeze, and J.S. Kizer. 1977. Analysis of the disruption in hypothalamic-pituitary regulation in rats treated neonatally with monosodium-L-glutamate (MSG): Evidence for the involvement of tuberoinfundibular cholinergic and dopaminergic systems in neuroendocrine regulation. Endocrinology 101:613-622.

17. Wishart, G.J. 1978. Functional heterogeneity of UDP-glucuronyltransferase as indicated by its differential development and inducibility by glucocorticoids. Demonstration of two groups within the enzyme's activity towards twelve substrates. Biochem. J. 174:485-489.

18. Lucier, G.W., and O.S. McDaniel. 1977. Steroid and non-steroid UDP-glucuronyltransferase: Glucuronidation of synthetic estrogens as steroids. J. Ster. Biochem. 8:867-872.

19. Lamartiniere, C.A., C.S. Dieringer, E. Kita, and G.W. Lucier. 1979. Altered sexual differentiation of hepatic uridine diphosphate glucuronyltransferase by neonatal hormone treatment in rats. Biochem. J. 180:313-318.

20. Naftolin, F., R.J. Ryan, I.J. Davies, V.V. Reedy, F. Flores, M. Kuhn, R.J. White, Y. Takaoha, and L. Wolin. 1975. The formation of estogrens by central neuroendocrine tissues. Recent Prog. Horm. Res. 31:295-315.

21. McEwen, B.S., L. Plapinger, C. Chaptal, J. Gerlack, and G. Wallack. 1975. Role of fetoneonatal estrogen-binding proteins in the association of estrogen with neonatal brain cell receptors. Brain Res. 96:400-406.

22. Dodds, E.C. 1938. Oestrogenic activity of certain synthetic compounds (letter to the editor). Nature 141:247-248.

23. Bitman, J., and H.C. Cecil. 1970. Estrogenic activity of DDT analogs and polychlorinated biphenyls. J. Agr. Food Chem. 8:1108-1112.

24. Mirocha, C.J., and C.M. Christensen. 1974. Oestregenic mycotoxins synthesized by Fusarium. In: Mycotoxins. I.F.H. Purchase, ed. Elsevier: Amsterdam. pp. 129-148.

25. Okey, A.B., and G.P. Bondy. 1977. Is delta-9-tetrahydrocannabinol estrogenic? Science 195:904-905.

26. Lamartiniere, C.A., C.S. Dieringer, and G.W. Lucier. 1979. Altered ontogeny of glutathione S-transferases by 2,4,5-2',4'5'-hexachlorobiphenyl. Toxicol. Appl. Pharmacol. 51:233-238.

27. Lucier, G.W., and O.S. McDaniel. 1979. Developmental toxicology of the halogenated aromatics: Effects on enzyme development. Ann. NY Acad. Sci. 320:449-457.

28. Norwicki, H.G., and A.W. Norman. 1972. Enhanced hepatic metabolism of testosterone, 4-androstene-3,17-deone, and estradiol-17β in chickens pretreated with DDT or PCB. Steroids 19:85-97.

29. Dieringer, C.S., C.A. Lamartiniere, C.M. Schiller, and G.W. Lucier. 1979. Altered ontogeny of hepatic steroid-metabolizing enzymes by pure PCB congeners. Biochem. Pharmacol. 28:2511-2513.

30. Kato, R., E. Chiesara, and G. Frontino. 1962. Influence of sex difference on the pharmacological action and metabolism of some drugs. Biochem. Pharmacol. 11:221-227.

31. Kato, R., and K. Onoda. 1970. Studies on the regulation of the activity of drug oxidation in rat liver microsomes by androgen and estrogen. Biochem. Pharmacol. 19:1649-1660.

32. El Defrawy El Masry, S., G.M. Cohen, and G.J. Mannering. 1974. Sex-dependent differences in drug metabolism in the rat. I. Temporal changes in the microsomal drug-metabolizing system of the liver during sexual maturation. Drug Metab. Dispos. 2:267-278.

33. El Defrawy El Masry, S., and G.J. Mannering. Sex-dependent differences in drug metabolism in the rat. II. Qualitative changes produced by castration and the administration of steroid hormones and phenobarbital. Drug Metab. Dispos. 2:279-284.

34. Chung, L.W.K. 1977. Characteristics of neonatal androgen-induced imprinting of rat hepatic microsomal monooxygenases. Biochem. Pharmacol. 26:1979-1984.

35. Kramer, R.E., J.W. Greiner, R.C. Rumbaugh, T.D. Sweeney, and H.D. Colby. 1979. Requirement of the pituitary gland for gonadal hormone effects on hepatic drug metabolism in rats. J. Pharmacol. Exp. Ther. 208:19-23.

36. Lui, E.M.K., and G.W. Lucier. 1980. Neonatal feminization of hepatic monooxygenase in adult male rats: Altered sexual dimorphic response to cadmium. J. Pharmacol. Exp. Ther. 212:211-216.

37. Pence, D.H., T.S. Miya, and R.C. Schnell. 1977. Cadmium alteration of hexobarbital action: Sex-related differences in the rat. Toxicol. Appl. Pharmacol. 39:89-96.

38. Means, J.R., G.P. Carlson, and R.G. Schnell. 1979. Studies on the mechanism of cadmium-induced inhibition of the hepatic microsomal monooxygenase of the male rat. Toxicol. Appl. Pharmacol. 48:293-304.

39. Means, J.R., and R.G. Schnell. 1979. Cadmium-induced alteration of the microsomal monooxygenase system in male rat liver: Effects on hemoprotein turnover and phospholipid content. Toxicol. Lett. 3:177-184.

40. Schnell, R.C., J.R. Means, S.A. Roberts, and D.H. Pence. 1979. Studies on cadmium-induced inhibition of hepatic microsomal drug biotransformation in the rat. Environ. Hlth. Perspect. 28:273-279.

41. Lui, E.M.K., and G.W. Lucier. 1981. Hypophyseal regulation of cadmium-induced depression of the hepatic monooxygenase system in the rat. Molec. Pharmacol. 20:165-171.

42. Levin, W., and D. Ryan. 1975. In: Basic and Therapeutic Aspects of Perinatal Pharmacology. Raven Press: New York. pp. 265-275.

43. Favino, A., A.H. Baille, and K. Griffith. 1966. Androgen synthesis by the testes and adrenal glands of rats poisoned with cadmium chloride. J. Endocrinol. 35:185-192.

44. Lui, E.M.K., R.S. Slaughter, R.M. Philpot, and G.W. Lucier. 1980. Cadmium sensitive cytochrome P-450 in rat liver. Fed. Proc. 39:865.

45. Lui, E.M.K., J. Gregson, and G.W. Lucier. 1981. Altered sex differentiation of hepatic ethylmorphine N-demethylation in the male rat following neonatal methadone exposure. Ped. Pharmacol. 1:187-196.

46. Miller, E.C., J.A. Miller, and H.A. Hartmann. 1961. N-hydroxy-2-acetylaminofluorene; a metabolite of 2-acetylaminofluorene with increased carcinogenic activity in the rat. Cancer Res. 21:815-824.

47. Weisburger, J.H., R.S. Yamamoto, J. Korzis, and E.K. Weisburger. 1966. Liver cancer; neonatal estrogen enhances induction by a carcinogen. Science 154:673-674.

48. Faris, R.A., and T.C. Campbell. 1981. Exposure of newborn rats to pharmacologically active compounds may permanently alter carcinogen metabolism. Science 211:719-721.

DISCUSSION

Q.: In your work, you've shown differences in the levels of the enzymes of the different sexes. Are there any differences in the substrates for the glucuronyltransferases and glutathione transferases between the two sexes?

This might be an important factor in how the enzymes actually operated *in vivo*.

A.: In this presentatiion, I referred mostly to 1,2-dichloro-4-nitrobenzene as a substrate for glutathione S-transferase since it shows a large sex differences. Another glutathione S-transferase substrate that we use in our laboratory is 1-chloro-2,4-dinitrobenzene. These are conveniently measured by spectrophotometric method. Activity towards this substrate is only slightly higher in males than in females. Other substrates that demonstrate sex differences are styrene oxide and benzo[*a*]pyrene 4,5-oxide. We have not measured these because they are time-consuming assays.

For the glucuronyltransferases, we are aware of two main classes of substrates, steroidal and nonsteroidal. The substrate, p-nitrophenyl, is an example of a nonsteroidal substrate.

As to your second comment, I am reluctant to speculate since we measure selected substrates and, therefore, don't have enough information at this time. What I hope to point out, was how these enzyme levels can be altered by hormones and hormonally active xenobiotics.

Q.: Have you looked at the sex differences in more than one strain of rat to see if it's really a characteristic of the particular strain of animals that you're working with?

A.: We just recently looked at the Fischer rat and found higher hepatic glutathione S-transferse and UDP-glucuronyltransferase activities in male rats and in female rats, but higher hepatic histadase activity in adult females than in adult males. Enzyme sex differences are also found in mice ARK-J and BALB/cJ).

MULTIPLE EFFECTS AND METABOLISM OF α-NAPHTHOFLAVONE IN INDUCED AND UNINDUCED HEPATIC MICROSOMES

Stephen Nesnow

Carcinogenesis and Metabolism Branch, Genetic Toxicology Division, Health Effects Research Laboratory, U.S. Environmental Protection Agency, Research Triangle Park, North Carolina 27711

INTRODUCTION

α-Naphthoflavone (7,8-benzoflavone [ANF]) (see Figure 1) has been reported to elicit multiple effects with regard to the mixed-function oxidase enzymes that metabolize drugs, steroids, and xenobiotics (1). These effects -- enzyme induction, enzyme inhibition, and enzyme activation -- seem to occur by different mechanisms in the mammalian species studied. ANF has been reported to be a less effective inducer of cytochrome P-448-mediated hepatic mixed-function oxidases in rats than its isomer β-naphthoflavone (BNF) (2). ANF is a potent inhibitor of 3-methylcholanthrene (3-MC)-induced or BNF-induced rat liver microsomes (cytochrome P-448) and was first described by Diamond and Gelboin (3) and Wiebel et al. (2). In addition, ANF is found to have no inhibitory effect on the mixed-function oxidases from phenobarbital (PB)-induced rat liver (cytochrome P-450) (2,4). In fact, ANF stimulates or activates these enzymes (2,4). This activation phenomenon is also observed in hepatic preparations from untreated rats, mice, rabbits, and humans (1). The mechanisms by which ANF activates or inhibits the mixed-function oxidases were of interest to us, and we began a series of investigations to try to elucidate them. This paper reviews these previous and present investigations and presents new findings that may help to explain the multiple effects of ANF observed in mammalian hepatic tissues.

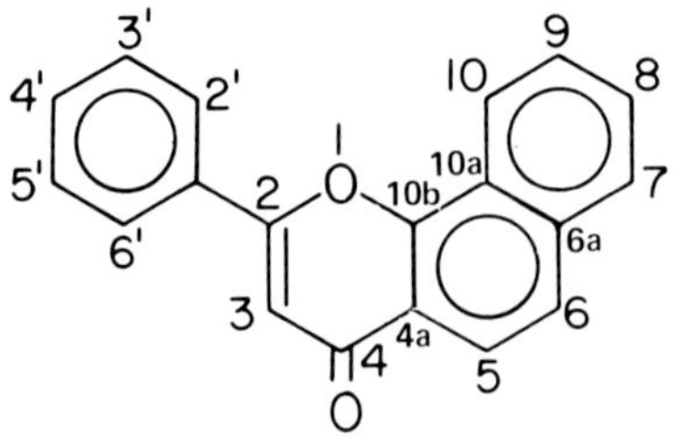

-NAPHTHOFLAVONE
2-PHENYL-4H-NAPHTHO(1,2-b) PYRAN-4-ONE
7,8-BENZOFLAVONE

Figure 1. Chemical structure and numbering system of ANF.

MATERIALS AND METHODS

Chemicals and Radiochemicals

[^{3}H]ANF was prepared by Amersham (Arlington Heights, IL), using ANF obtained from Aldrich Chemical Co. (Milwaukee, WI). It was purified by high pressure liquid chromatography (HPLC), using a DuPont Instruments (Wilmington, DE) Model 848 chromatograph fitted with a 4.6-mm i.d. x 25-cm Zorbax-ODS column. An isocratic solvent system of methanol was employed at a flow rate of 2.0 ml/min, and under these conditions ANF exhibited a retention time of 5.0 min. Radiochemical purity was estimated to be > 99% using this system. Authentic metabolite standards of 6-hydroxy-ANF, 7-hydroxy-ANF, and 9-hydroxy-ANF were synthesized by Dr. Robert Roth (Midwest Research Institute) by modifying the method of Mahal and Venkataraman (5), using the appropriately substituted methoxy-2-acetyl-1-naphthols. The analytic and spectroscopic data of these synthetic phenols were fully consistent with their structure.

Preparation of Microsomes

Male Charles River CD rats (60 days old), male CD-1 mice (30 days old), male Syrian golden hamsters (60 days old), and male New Zealand white rabbits (4 months old) were maintained on lab chow and water *ad libitum*. Groups of at least four rats were induced with either PB (Mallinckrodt Chemical Co., St. Louis, MO) at 80 mg/kg in 0.5 ml sodium chloride solution (0.85%), or with BNF or 3-MC (Aldrich Chemical Co., Milwaukee, WI) at 20 mg/kg in 0.5 ml corn oil. Both substances were injected i.p. on each of four successive days. Animals were starved for 24 h after the last treatment, and microsomes prepared according to van der Hoeven et al. (6). Microsomes from livers of untreated mice, rats, rabbits, and hamsters were prepared from each individual animal. Protein concentrations were determined by the method of Lowry et al. (7), using bovine serum albumin as the protein standard (Sigma Chemical Co., St. Louis, MO).

Metabolism of [^{3}H]ANF

[^{3}H]ANF was incubated with microsomes and an NADPH-generating system according to the following procedure (8). A 5.0-ml incubation mixture contained 0.005 mmol $NADP^+$, 0.0225 mmol glucose 6-phosphate, 9 units glucose 6-phosphate dehydrogenase, 0.015 mmol magnesium chloride, 0.25 mmol potassium phosphate buffer (pH 7.50), 0.025 mM [^{3}H]ANF (specific activity 1 to 2 mCi/mmol), and 2.0 mg microsomal protein. Reaction was begun at 37°C with agitation and addition of substrate. The reaction was terminated upon the addition of 15 ml ethyl acetate-acetone (2:1). After thorough mixing and centrifugation at 800 g, a 12-ml aliquot of the organic layer was removed and evaporated under dry nitrogen. The samples were reconstituted in 0.075 ml methanol and chromatographed by HPLC on a 6.2-mm i.d. x 22.5-cm Zorbax-ODS column, using a mixture of methanol-water (85:15) at a flow rate of 1.8 ml/min. Fractions (12-s) were collected directly into liquid scintillation vials for subsequent radiochemical analysis.

Binding of [^{3}H]ANF to Microsomal Protein

Radioactivity bound to microsomal protein after incubation with [^{3}H]ANF and extraction was determined by adding trichloroacetic acid to the aqueous layer to a final concentration of 5%. The precipitated protein was pelleted by centrifugation at 800 g and washed with 5% trichloroacetic acid. The protein was resuspended in 0.1 M tris buffer (pH 7.4) and washed repeatedly with ether until the unbound radioactivity was removed. The protein was then centrifuged and digested with Protosol (New England Nuclear, Boston, MA), neutralized, and counted. Overall recovery was greater than 90% of radioactivity.

Inhibition of Benzo[a]pyrene Monooxygenase by Flavones

Benzo[*a*]pyrene (BP) monooxygenase was assayed by the method of Nesnow et *al*. (9) as follows. A 1.0-ml incubation mixture contained microsomal protein, 0.001 mmol NADP, 0.0045 mmol glucose 6-phosphate, 1.80 units glucose 6-phosphate dehydrogenase, 0.003 mmol magnesium chloride, 0.05 mmol potassium phosphate buffer (pH 7.50), and 60 nmol [^{3}H]BP (specific activity 12 to 25 mCi/mmol), with and without flavone inhibitor as appropriate. Inhibitor was dissolved in 0.025 ml acetone. Reaction was begun after adding substrate dissolved in 0.05 ml acetone-methanol (1:2) and, after 15 min of incubation at 37°C, was terminated by adding 1.0 ml of 0.5 N sodium hydroxide in 80% aqueous ethanol. Each sample was vortexed, 3.0 ml spectrograde hexane was added, and the sample was vortexed again for 1.5 min. After centrifugation for 10 min at 2500 rpm, an aliquot (0.3 ml) of the lower phase was removed, neutralized with 0.5 N hydrochloric acid, and the radioactivity was determined by liquid scintillation spectrometry. Each sample was corrected for background by subtracting the activity obtained using ethanolic sodium hydroxide-treated microsomes in the incubation mixture. Control incubations contained microsomes, NADPH-generating system, buffer, [^{3}H]BP, and 0.025 ml solvent in which the inhibitor was dissolved. Microsomal protein concentration was 0.4 mg/ml using PB-induced microsomes and 0.2 mg/ml with BNF- or 3-MC-induced microsomes. The concentration of flavone inhibitor that causes a 50% reduction in enzymatic activity (I_{50}) was determined for each inhibitor by constructing a dose-response relationship between log concentration of inhibitor and percent enzyme activity. At least four concentrations of inhibitor were examined for each agent.

RESULTS AND DISCUSSION

Using the metabolism of BP as an indicator of microsomal mixed-function oxidase activity, the inhibitory activity of a series of flavones and related derivatives was examined (4). In these studies two specific types of cytochromes were employed: cytochrome P-450 from PB-induced rats and cytochrome P-448 from 3-MC- or BNF-induced rats. Both 3-MC and BNF induce the similar hepatic enzymes and were used interchangeably. The inhibition curves of ANF with BP metabolism from induced microsomes are shown in Figure 2 using the BP monooxygenase assay, a procedure that measures the overall metabolism of BP (9). ANF exhibits an I_{50} of 10 μM with cytochrome P-448 microsomes and has no inhibitory effect up to 100 μM with cytochrome P-450 microsomes (4).

Our previous work has shown that substitution on the exocyclic phenyl ring at position 4' with chlorine has virtually no effect on the inhibitory activity of the flavone in cytochrome P-448 containing microsomes from rat livers (see Table 1) (4). However, substitution at position 4' with either a methoxy or nitro group causes a significant loss in inhibitory activity. Substitution at position 3' with a methoxy group has no effect, while nitro

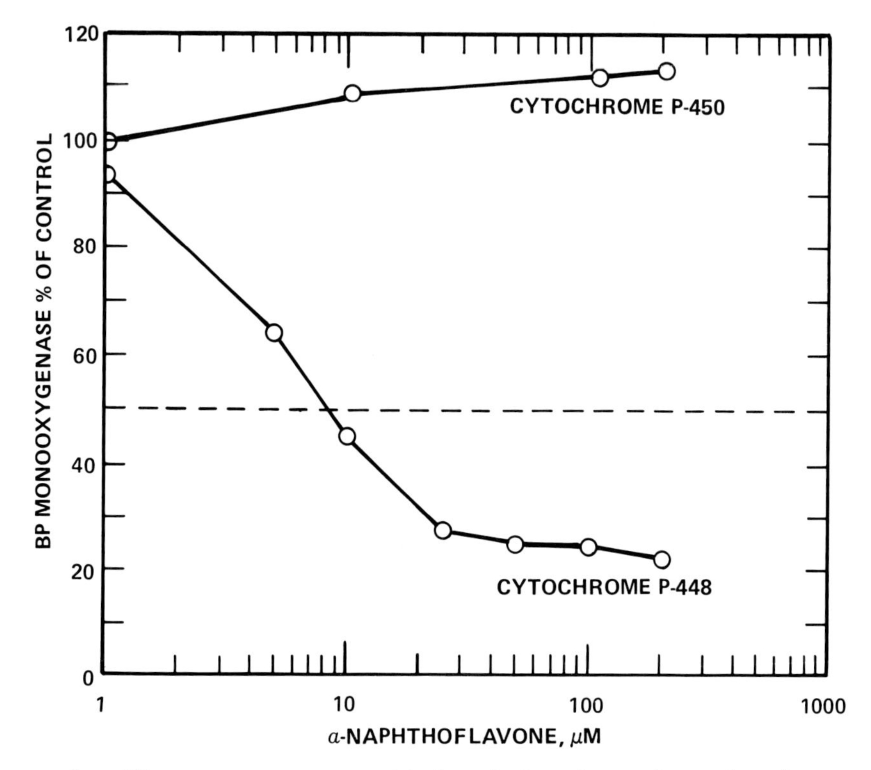

Figure 2. BP monooxygenase activity induced rat hepatic microsomes in the presence of increasing concentrations of ANF.

substitution markedly reduces activity. Substitution at position 2' with a methoxy group or replacement of phenyl with a naphthyl group does not affect inhibitory activity. The marked differences observed with the three methoxy-ANFs lead to the conclusion that the portion of the cytochrome P-448 that binds the phenyl ring seems to have rigid spatial requirements (4).

Substitution at position 6 on the naphthalene ring also results in a complete loss of activity of the flavone when these substituents are nonoxidizable. With an amino group at position 6, inhibitory activity is moderately reduced in cytochrome P-448 microsomes and, surprisingly, is observed in cytochrome P-450 microsomes, the first reported sample of an ANF inhibiting that type of induced microsome. Finally, contraction of the pyran-4-one

Table 1. Inhibition of BP Monooxygenase in Induced Hepatic Microsomes from Rats by ANF Derivatives and Related Agents[a]

Inhibitor	I_{50} (μM)[b] Microsomes Cytochrome P-448	Cytochrome P-450
7,8-Benzoflavone	10	> 100
3'-Methoxy-7,8-benzoflavone	11	> 98
2-(2-Naphthyl)-4H-naphtho-[1,2-b]pyran-4-one	11	> 100
2'-Methoxy-7,8-benzoflavone	13	> 100
4'-Chloro-7,8-benzoflavone	13	> 99
6-Amino-7,8-benzoflavone	31	82
6-Bromo-7,8-benzoflavone	> 97	> 97
4'-Nitro-7,8-benzoflavone	> 99	> 99
7,8-Benzoisoflavone	> 100	> 100
3'-Nitro-7,8-benzoflavone	> 100	> 100
4'-Methoxy-7,8-benzoflavone	> 100	> 100
2-Phenyl-4H-naphtho-[1,2-b]furan	> 104	> 104
6-Nitro-7,8-benzoflavone	> 200	> 200

[a]BP monooxygenase activity was determined by the method of Nesnow et al. (9). The data for Table 1 were taken from Nesnow (4).
[b]I_{50} is the concentration of inhibitor that inhibits the enzymatic reaction by 50% and is expressed in micromolar (μM) as the mean of three replicate samples: BP concentration (60 μM); the specific activity of untreated controls in cytochrome P-448 microsomes (2.1 to 3.5 nmol BP oxidized/min/mg protein); cytochrome P-450 microsomes (0.80 to 1.02 nmol BP oxidized/min/ mg protein). Protein concentrations in the assay were 0.2 mg/ml for cytochrome P-448 microsomes, and 0.4 mg/ml for cytochrome P-450. Inhibitors were dissolved in acetone.

ring to a furan (loss of the carbonyl group) or substitution of the phenyl ring on the 3 position results in complete loss of inhibitory activity (4).

The interesting observations that 6-position blockage with a nonoxidizable substituent causes complete loss of inhibitory activity prompted us to investigate the interaction of ANF with

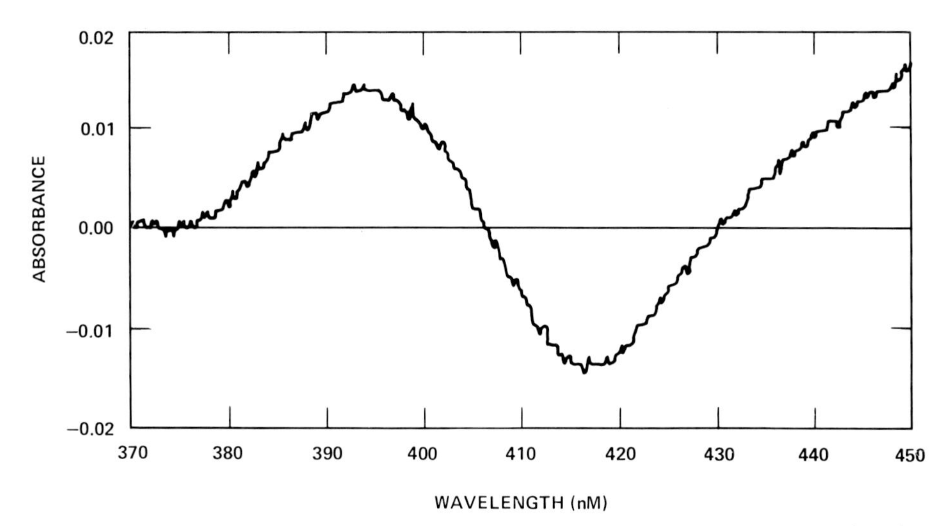

Figure 3. Binding spectra of ANF with cytochrome P-450 rat liver microsomes (data from Nesnow and Bergman [8]). Cytochrome P-448 microsomes gave the same result.

induced rat liver microsomes. We found that ANF gives a classical Type I binding spectrum with either cytochrome P-448 or cytochrome P-450 (see Figure 3), indicating no significant effects in the type or magnitude of the binding response of ANF to either cytochrome type (8).

Metabolism studies of radiolabeled ANF by both types of induced microsomes were undertaken and gave qualitatively similar but quantitatively dissimilar results (8). HPLC analyses of the organic-soluble metabolites formed after 15 min of incubation of 25 μM ANF are shown in Figure 4. The major difference observed is the greater amount of peak 1b, formed by the cytochrome P-448 microsomes, compared to the cytochrome P-450 microsome.

Structural identification of peaks 1b, 2, 3, and 4 was carried out using a combination of low- and high-resolution mass spectrometry, cochromatography with authentic synthesized standards, ultraviolet spectrometry, and chemical or enzymatic conversion to authentic standards. Metabolites were isolated by

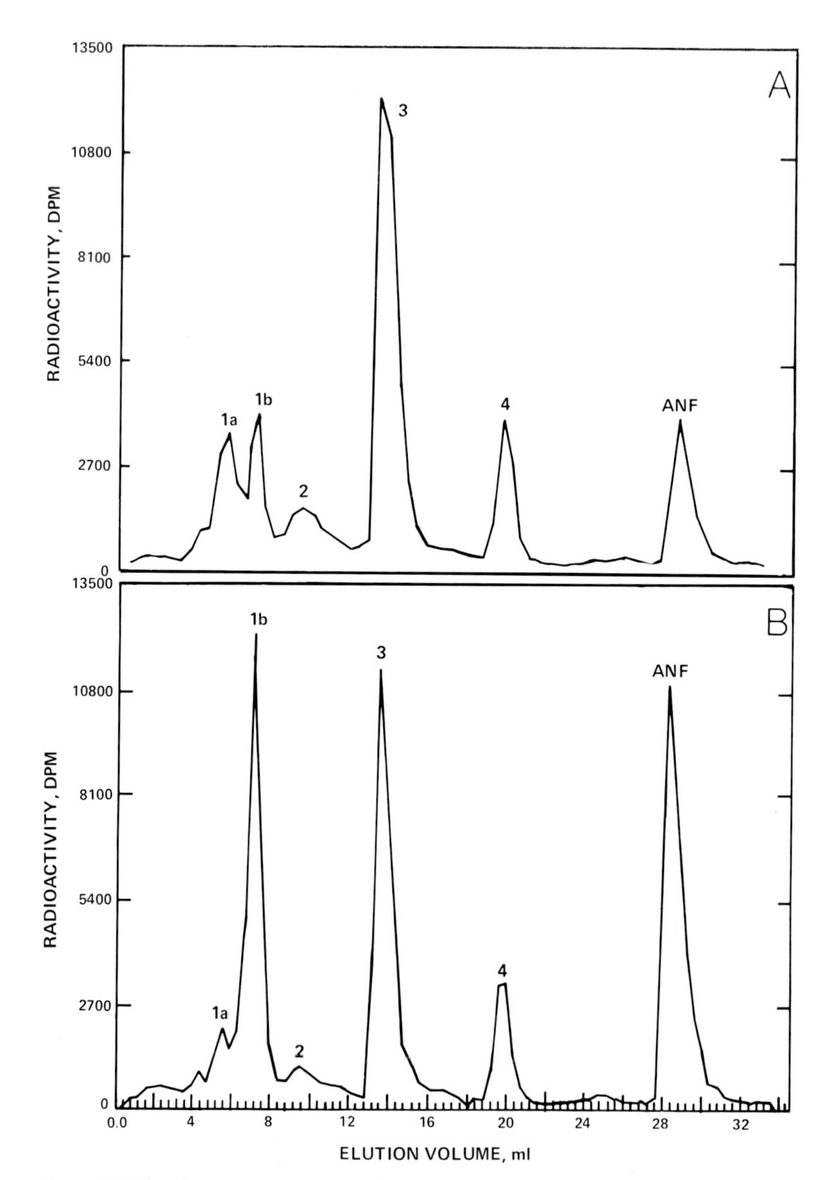

Figure 4. HPLC chromatograms of ANF metabolites produced after 15 min incubations of [^{3}H]ANF (25 μM) with cytochrome P-450 hepatic microsomes (A) and cytochrome P-448 hepatic microsomes (B). Peak 1a is a mixture of unknown metabolites; 1b is 5,6-dihydro-5,6-dihydroxy-ANF; 2 is 9-hydroxy-ANF; 3 is ANF-5,6-oxide; and 4 is 6-hydroxy-ANF (data from Nesnow and Bergman [8]).

preparative HPLC and purified by repetitive HPLC chromatography. During the course of this work, we isolated another peak (peak 3a) that migrated between peaks 3 and 4. This material cochromatographed with an authentic standard of 7-hydroxy-ANF.

A major part of the structural analysis was the use of mass spectral fragmentation patterns observed in ANF and its metabolites. The mass spectra of ANF reveal a major fragmentation loss of m/e 102 or C_8H_6 (see Figure 5). Fragmentation of ANF to a neutral species (m/e 102) and a charged species (m/e 170) can occur by either of two routes (see Figure 6). Using synthetic flavones 6-bromo-ANF, 6-nitro-ANF, 4'-methoxy-ANF, 3'-methoxy-ANF, and 2-methoxy-ANF, it was concluded that pathway a predominates (8).

Since all isolated metabolites exhibited mass spectra with increases in the charged fragment (m/e 170), we concluded that the metabolites arose from oxidation on positions 5 to 10 (see Figure 1). The results of our structural identification studies are presented in Figure 7. ANF is metabolized at the 5,6-bond to form ANF-5,6-oxide, which is stable and isolated as peak 3. Hydration of ANF-5,6-oxide gives 5,6-dihydro-5,6-dihydroxy-ANF, isolated as peak 1b. Rearrangement of ANF-5,6-oxide gives 6-hydroxy-ANF (peak 4). We propose that ANF is metabolized at its 7,8 and 9,10 bonds to give the corresponding arene oxides that are not isolated but rearranged to form the isolated 7-hydroxy-ANF (peak 3a) and 9-hydroxy ANF (peak 2), respectively (8).

The metabolism of ANF is inhibited by carbon monoxide, SKF-525A, and phenanthrene-9,10-quinone and requires NADPH for activity (see Table 2). These results strongly suggest that ANF is metabolized by the NADPH requiring cytochrome P-450 mixed-function oxidases (8).

Examining some of the ANF metabolites' ability to inhibit or enhance microsomal oxidative processes was of interest to us as their activities might explain the differential effects observed with ANF in cytochrome P-450 and cytochrome P-448 microsomes. Using BP oxidation as a measure of oxidative metabolism, we determined the microsomal inhibition constants of three chemically synthesized flavone metabolites, 6-hydroxy-ANF, 7-hydroxy-ANF, and 9-hydroxy-ANF (see Table 3). None of the ANF metabolites were active against BP metabolism in cytochrome P-450 microsomes. Also, no stimulation of enzymatic activity was observed, indicating that these metabolites were not involved in the stimulation of microsomal enzyme activity by ANF. However, different results were obtained with cytochrome P-448 microsomes. 7-Hydroxy-ANF had no inhibitory effect while 6-hydroxy-ANF had the same I_{50} as ANF. 9-Hydroxy-ANF inhibited 50% of the metabolism of BP at 1/4 the concentration of ANF itself. This observation makes 9-hydroxy-ANF the most potent ANF derivative yet tested and provides a major

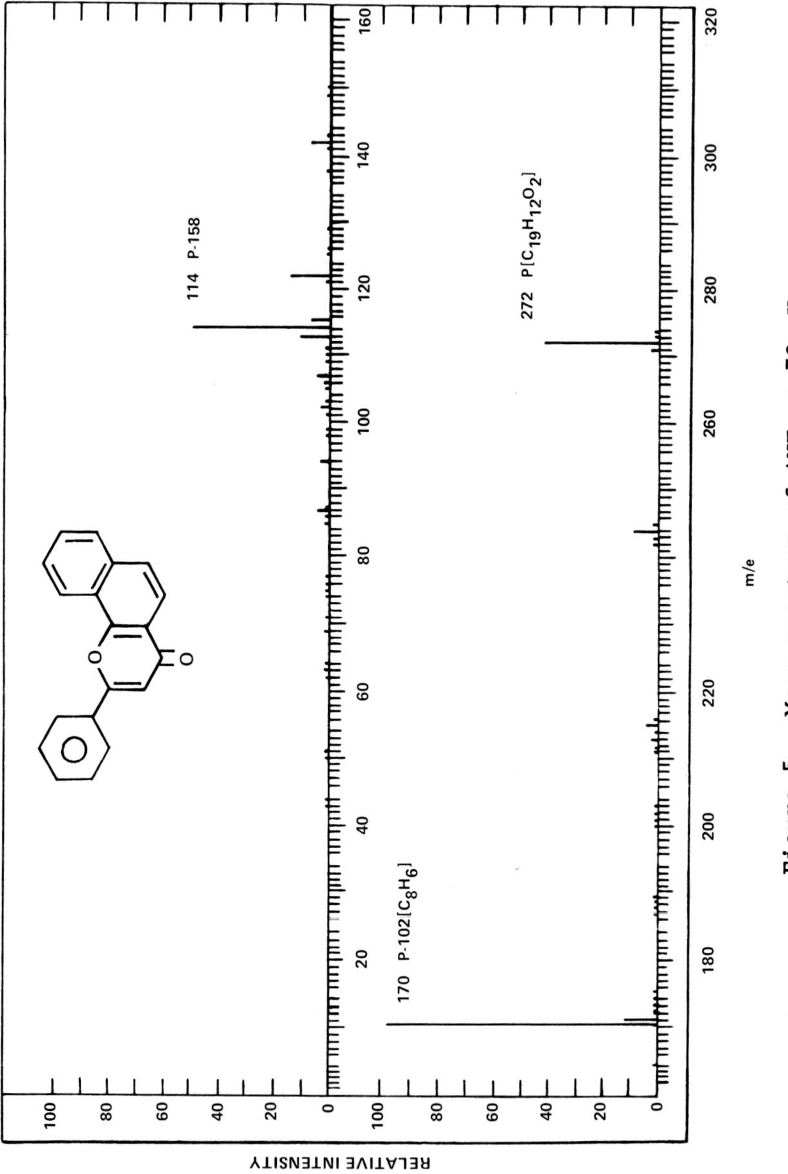

Figure 5. Mass spectrum of ANF at 70 eV.

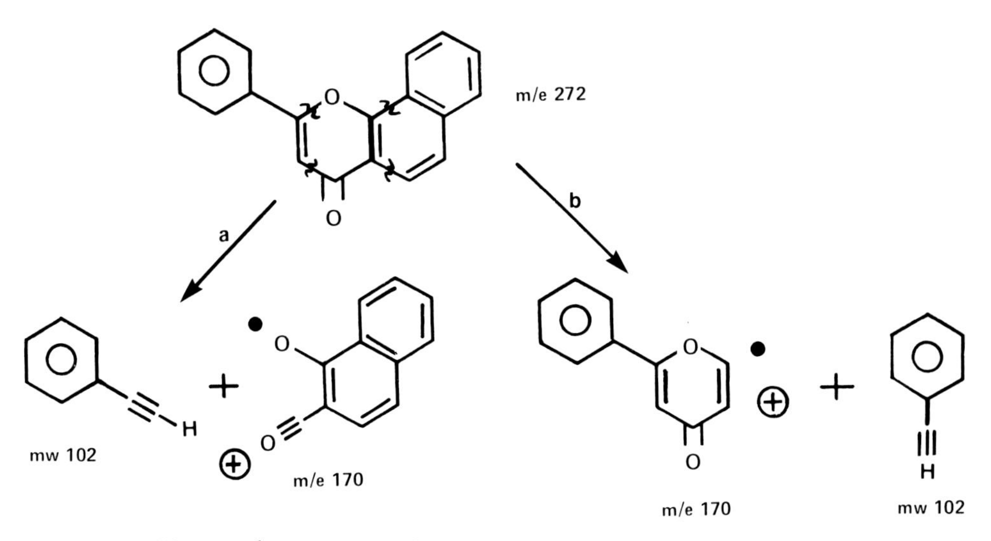

Figure 6. Proposed fragmentation schemes of ANF.

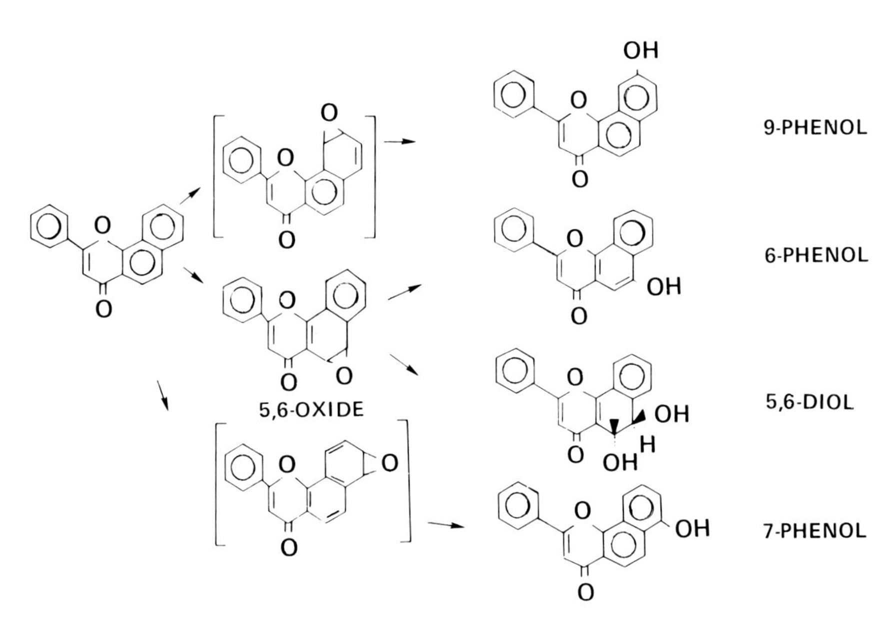

Figure 7. Identification of ANF metabolites and their proposed routes of formation.

Table 2. Effect of Cofactors and Inhibitors on the Metabolism of ANF[a]

Incubation Condition[b]	Microsomes[c]	
	Cytochrome P-450	Cytochrome P-448
Complete mixture	35.3 (100)	36.9 (100)
-NADP	0 (0)	0 (0)
+Carbon monoxide	2.84 (8)	2.75 (7)
+SKF-525A (500 μM)	13.7 (39)	ND[d]
+Phenanthrene-9,10-quinone (25 μM)	ND[d]	2.06 (6)

[a]Values are mean total organic-soluble ANF metabolites formed per milligram microsomal protein. The coefficient of variation was 15%. (Data from Nesnow and Bergman [8]).
[b]Incubation mixtures of [^{3}H]ANF (50 μM) with microsomes (0.4 mg/ml) were carried out for 15 min under the various conditions listed. See Materials and Methods.
[c]Numbers in parentheses represent the percent of activity compared to the complete mixture.
[d]Not determined.

piece of evidence supporting the concept that ANF requires metabolic activation, in part, for its inhibitory activity in cytochrome P-448-induced rat hepatic microsomes. Wiebel and Gelboin (10) have suggested, using a kinetic analysis of the inhibition of BP hydroxylation by ANF, that at concentrations below 3.3 μM, ANF is a competitive inhibitor, while at higher concentrations ANF inhibits the oxygenation reaction by a more complex mechanism. Our results are in agreement with these observations in that at high concentrations both ANF and 9-hydroxy-ANF inhibit BP oxidation while at low ANF concentration little 9-hydroxy-ANF is present, and ANF can act as the sole competitive inhibitor.

We have observed that ANF is converted to forms that bind to the microsomal protein, and this conversion is time dependent (see Table 4). Cytochrome P-448 microsomes bind statistically greater amounts of ANF to microsomal protein than do cytochrome P-450 microsomes. The magnitude of the binding, a small part of the overall metabolic rate of ANF, is significant, however, in terms of the amount bound per molecule of the cytochrome. A greater than

Table 3. Inhibition Constants of ANF Metabolites in Hepatic Microsomes From Induced Rats[a]

	I_{50}[c] (μM)	
ANF Metabolite[b]	Cytochrome P-448	Cytochrome P-450
6-Hydroxy-ANF	4.54 ± 0.86	>50[d]
7-Hydroxy-ANF	>50[d]	>50[d]
9-Hydroxy-ANF	1.47 ± 0.37	>50[d]
ANF	5.98 ± 0.72	ND[e]

[a]BP monooxygenase activity was determined by the method of Nesnow et al. (9).
[b]Agents dissolved in acetone.
[c]BP monooxygenase assay was performed for 15 min using 60 μM BP. Values are mean ± SD for six replicate determinations.
[d]No stimulation was observed at the stated concentration.
[e]Not determined.

Table 4. Conversion of [^{3}H]ANF to Protein Bound Forms[a]

	nmol [^{3}H]ANF bound/nmol P-450[b]			
Cytochrome	7.5 min	12.5 min	15 min	20 min
P-450[c]	0.587 ± 0.082	0.850 ± 0.024	0.967 ± 0.101	0.953 ± 0.070
P-448[d]	0.722 ± 0.030	1.16 ± 0.07[e]	1.27 ± 0.05[e]	1.47 ± 0.10[e]

[a]Radioactivity bound to microsomal protein was determined according to Materials and Methods using various incubation times. None of the values have been adjusted for the activity found in boiled enzyme controls, which did not vary with incubation time and was less than 0.112 nmol [^{3}H]ANF bound/nmol P-450. Cytochrome P-450 determinations were by the method of Omura and Sato (11).
[b]Values are mean ± SD for three replicate samples.
[c]Cytochrome P-450 level was 2.10 ± 0.05 nmol/mg protein.
[d]Cytochrome P-450 level was 1.58 ± 0.13 nmol/mg protein.
[e]Significantly different than cytochrome P-450 value by Student's t-test, $p < 0.01$.

equimolar amount of ANF is bound per molecule cytochrome in cytochrome P-448 microsomal protein after 15 min of incubation. At this time, whether the flavone is bound to or near the active site of the hemoprotein is unknown, although ANF does give a Type I difference spectra, indicating that the parent hydrocarbon does interact with cytochrome P-450. Various chemicals are shown to destroy cytochrome P-450, including vinyl chloride and barbiturates (1); however, the importance of the binding of ANF (or its metabolites) to microsomal protein in the mechanism by which ANF inhibits microsomal enzyme activity is unknown.

The phenomenon of enzyme activation observed in PB-induced rat hepatic microsomes has also been reported in hepatic microsomes from untreated rats, mice, rabbits, and humans (1). Enzyme activation has also been observed (data not shown) in uninduced hamster liver microsomes. A comparative study was undertaken to examine the metabolism of ANF in hepatic microsomes from untreated rats, mice, hamsters, and rabbits to ascertain if any similarity existed between the tissues that were susceptible to enzyme activation and specific ANF metabolites.

The metabolism of ANF by hepatic microsomes from the four mammalian species was determined from incubations after 15 min with a 50 μM substrate and an NADPH-generating system. The chromatographic system used to separate the metabolites is shown in Figure 8. All four species produced ANF-5,6-oxide, 5,6-dihydro-5,6-dihydroxy-ANF, 6-hydroxy-ANF, and 7-hydroxy-ANF. 9-Hydroxy-ANF was produced approximately equally by all species studied except hamster liver (see Table 5). Within experimental error all species produced equivalent amounts of 6-hydroxy-ANF, and rat, mouse, and rabbit produced the same amount of 7-hydroxy-ANF. Hamster liver metabolized more ANF to 7-hydroxy-ANF than rat, mouse, or rabbit. Both mouse and hamster produced significantly more 5,6-dihydro-5,6-dihydroxy-ANF than rat or rabbit.

The data make it difficult to identify one metabolite that might account for the stimulation effect of ANF, since all preparations produced similar metabolites. Studies with the synthetic metabolites 6-hydroxy-ANF, 7-hydroxy-ANF, and 9-hydroxy-ANF (see Table 3) indicate that they do not stimulate BP metabolism. Studies are in progress to examine ANF-5,6-oxide, 5,6-dihydro-5,6-dihydroxy-ANF, and polyhydroxylated ANF metabolites for their potential to stimulate mixed function oxidase activity.

ANF, an inhibitor of chemical carcinogenesis *in vivo* and *in vitro* (1), inhibits mixed-function oxidases induced by polycyclics. This specificity may be due in part to the ability of these enzymes to metabolize ANF to 9-hydroxy-ANF, a species considerably more active than ANF itself, and in part to the sensitivity of these

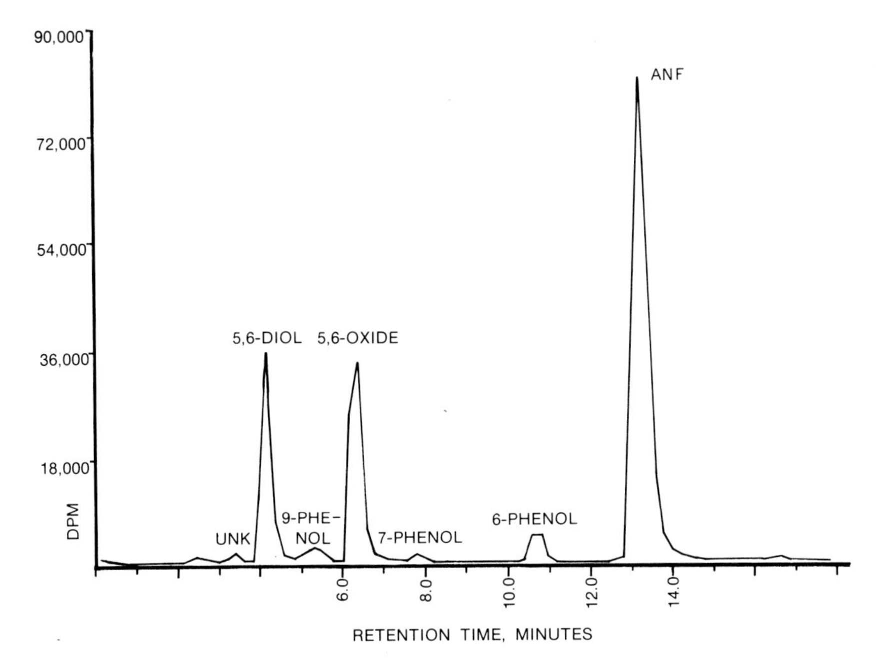

Figure 8. HPLC chromatographic system used to determine ANF metabolites. See Materials and Methods for details.

induced enzymes towards that metabolite. The observation that ANF covalently binds to microsomal protein also needs to be considered.

ANF stimulates microsomal enzyme activity in uninduced or PB-induced liver microsomes. ANF is metabolized simultaneously with BP in PB-induced microsomes, and each substrate has little effect on the other's metabolic rate (Nesnow, unpublished data). This result indicates that within the group of PB-induced cytochromes certain hemoproteins metabolize mainly BP, while others metabolize mainly ANF. If this is the case, then the stimulation of BP metabolism by ANF could be explained by the following argument: Assume, for example, that BP has a low K_m and V_{max} for cytochrome 1, while it has a high K_m and V_{max} for cytochrome 2. If ANF is metabolized by and competitively inhibits cytochrome 1 but has no effect on cytochrome 2, it will in effect increase the rate of BP metabolism and act as an enzyme activator.

Other hypotheses exist that could be put forth to explain enzyme activation. These hypotheses are currently under study in our laboratory.

Table 5. Microsomal Metabolism of ANF[a]

Species	5,6-Bond Oxidation[b]	9,10-Bond Oxidation[c]	7,8-Bond Oxidation[d]	Total Organic-Soluble[e]	Polyhydroxylated (Aqueous-Soluble)
Rat[f]	19.3	1.2	1.5	22.3	6.93
Mouse[f]	26.7	1.9	1.2	31.6	7.16
Rabbit[g]	18.2	2.4	1.2	22.9	6.30
Hamster[f]	20.9	0	4.8	27.9	11.7
PB-Induced rat[h]	27.6	2.0	ND	34.9	5.01

[a]Values are mean for n replicates in nmoles ANF metabolite per milligram protein. The coefficient of variation did not exceed 20%.
[b]5,6-Bond oxidation is the total metabolite formation at the 5,6-bond (ANF-5,6-oxide, 5,6-dihydro-5,6-dihydroxy-ANF, and 6-hydroxy-ANF).
[c]9,10-Bond oxidation is the total metabolite formation at the 9,10-bond (9-hydroxy-ANF).
[d]7,8-Bond oxidation is the total metabolite formation at the 7,8-bond (7-hydroxy-ANF).
[e]Total of 5,6, 9,10, 7,8 bond oxidation products and unidentified organic-soluble metabolites.
[f]n = 10.
[g]n = 9.
[h]n = 3 (data from Nesnow and Bergman [8]).

ACKNOWLEDGMENTS

The author thanks Ms. Hinda Bergman and Mr. Robert Easterling, and Drs. Wayne Sovacool and David Millington for the mass spectra.

REFERENCES

1. Wiebel, F.J. 1980. Activation and inactivation of carcinogens by microsomal monooxygenase: Modification by benzoflavones and polycyclic aromatic hydrocarbons. In: Carcinogenesis, A Comprehensive Survey, Volume 5. T.J. Slaga, ed. Raven Press: New York. pp. 57-84.

2. Wiebel, F.J., J.C. Leutz, L. Diamond, and H.V. Gelboin. 1971. Aryl hydrocarbon benzo[a]pyrene hydroxylase in microsomes from rat tissues differential inhibition and stimulation by benzoflavones and organic solvents. Arch. Biochem. Biophys. 144:78-86.

3. Diamond, L., and H.V. Gelboin. 1969. Alpha-naphthoflavone: An inhibitor of hydrocarbon cytoxicity and microsomal hydroxylase. Science 166:1023-1025.

4. Nesnow, S. 1979. A preliminary structure activity study of the mixed-function oxidase inhibitor 7,8-benzoflavone. J. Med. Chem. 22:1244-1247.

5. Mahal, H.S., and K. Venkataraman. 1934. Synthetical experiments in the chromone group part XIV. The action of sodamide on 1-acyloxy-2-acenaphthones. J. Chem. Soc. 1767-1769.

6. van der Hoeven, T.A., D.A. Haugen, and M.J. Coon. 1974. Preparation and properties of partially purified cytochrome P-450 and reduced nicotinamide adenine dinucleotide phosphate-cytochrome P-450 reductase from rabbit liver microsomes. J. Biol. Chem. 249:6302-6310.

7. Lowry, O.H., N.J. Rosebrough, A.L. Farr, and R.J. Randall. 1951. Protein measurement with the Folin phenol reagent. J. Biol. Chem. 193:265-275.

8. Nesnow, S., and H. Bergman. 1981. Metabolism of α-naphthoflavone by rat liver microsomes. Cancer Res. 41:2621-2626.

9. Nesnow, S., W.E. Fahl, and C.K. Jefcoate. 1977. An improved radiochemical assay for benzo[a]pyrene monooxygenase. Anal. Biochem. 80:258-266.

10. Wiebel, F.J., and H.V. Gelboin. 1975. Aryl hydrocarbon (benzo[a]pyrene) hydroxylases in liver from rats of different age, sex, and nutritional status. Biochem. Pharmacol. 24:1511-1515.

11. Omura, T., and R. Sato. 1964. The carbon monoxide binding pigment of liver microsomes 1. Evidence for its hemoprotein nature. J. Biol. Chem. 239:2370-2378.

SPECIES DIFFERENCES IN THE ACTIVATION OF BENZO[a]PYRENE IN THE TRACHEAL EPITHELIUM OF RATS AND HAMSTERS

Marc J. Mass and David G. Kaufman

Department of Pathology, School of Medicine, University of North Carolina, Chapel Hill, North Carolina 27514

INTRODUCTION

Model systems have been developed to study bronchogenic carcinoma in laboratory animals in order to better understand the pathogenesis and etiology of this disease in humans (1). By extrapolating the characteristics of experimental models for respiratory carcinogenesis, some risk factors for human lung cancer may ultimately be elucidated.

A broad dose-response relationship has been demonstrated between the incidence of lung cancer in humans and the number of cigarettes smoked (2). Nonetheless, it is not possible at the present time to predict which individuals in the population of smokers will eventually develop lung cancer. Recent studies have shown that the capacity to metabolize and activate chemical carcinogens in human bronchial and other target tissues varies widely between individuals (3-6). At present no correlation has been established between the capacity to metabolize a given chemical carcinogen in a specific tissue of an individual and susceptibility to a particular cancer in that tissue (7). The difficulty in establishing such a relationship may stem from the fact that the human population is genetically heterogeneous and individuals are exposed to numerous and varied environmental factors that could modify the development of clinical cancer. For this reason, the relationship between carcinogen metabolism and cancer susceptibility might best be studied with species of more homogeneous genetic constitution under the controlled conditions of the laboratory.

Cancers of the tracheobronchial epithelial lining account for 90% of lung cancers in humans (8); hence, many species have been tested as possible models for induction of such epidermoid cancers by polynuclear hydrocarbons (PNH). Respiratory tract cancers of chemical etiology that resemble histologically those associated with cigarette smoking in humans have been induced with regularity in Syrian golden hamsters and Fischer strain 344 rats. The intratracheal instillation technique using benzo[a]pyrene (BP)-ferric oxide particles produced this spectrum of tumors in hamsters (9). When this technique was applied to rats, no tracheobronchial epidermoid carcinomas were produced. Instead, bronchiolo-alveolar cancers of the peripheral lung resulted from intratracheal administration of BP-ferric oxide (10,11), 7,12-dimethylbenz[a]anthracene-ferric oxide (12), or 3-methylcholanthrene (3-MC) without carrier particles (13) to rats. A spectrum of tumors resembling human lung cancers can be produced in rat tracheas when they are treated with carcinogens as heterotopic tracheal grafts. Similarly, 3-MC will elicit tracheal cancers in grafted hamster tracheas but, apparently, at a much lower dose (14).

Studies of rates of clearance of BP-ferric oxide from the respiratory tracts of rats and hamsters given identical doses of BP indicate that the tracheas of both species are exposed to equivalent doses of BP over time (11). Differences in exposure of the target tissue, therefore, cannot explain the discrepancies in tumor incidence. Data from the tracheal graft model, which minimize any effects due to clearance, also suggest that hamster tracheas are more sensitive to PNH-induced carcinogenesis than are rat tracheas.

In this study we considered whether differences in the activation of BP in the tracheas of rats and hamsters could explain the marked differences in sensitivity of the tracheal epithelium of these two species to PNH-induced neoplasia. Rats and hamsters were compared with respect to the kinetic properties of benzo[a]pyrene monooxygenase in tracheal cells, to the BP metabolites produced in tracheal microsomes and organ cultures, and to the specific binding activities of BP to DNA in epithelial cells of tracheas maintained in organ culture.

METHODS

Tissue Preparation

Random-bred Syrian golden male hamsters (80 to 100 g) or Fischer strain 344 male rats (100 to 200 g) obtained from A.R. Schmidt (Madison, WI) were used in these experiments. Animals were anesthetized with ether and exsanguinated by severing the abdominal aorta. Tracheas were excised and freed of connective tissue by blunt dissection, and then a longitudinal cut was made along the trachealis muscle. Tracheas were placed in Ham's F-10 medium (Grand Island Biological Company [GIBCO], Grand Island, NY) containing 10% calf serum (GIBCO), buffered to pH 7.4 with 0.25 M HEPES and sodium bicarbonate, and held at 0°C until they could be transferred to an incubator. This preparation was always accomplished within a 30-min period.

Exposure to BP for Monooxygenase Induction

Benzo[a]pyrene (Eastman Organic Chemicals, Rochester, NY) dissolved in dimethyl sulfoxide (DMSO) was added to calf serum, and the serum was diluted with nine volumes of Ham's F-10. Media containing 5 μM BP were routinely used for BP monooxygenase induction. Groups of three tracheas were maintained in 60-mm plastic tissue culture dishes in a humidified incubator at 37°C in an atmosphere of 95% air and 5% carbon dioxide (CO_2). Tissues placed in the culture medium but lacking BP served as uninduced controls. At the end of the 18-h induction period, tracheas were removed from the medium containing BP, blotted to remove adherent fluid, transferred to new dishes containing medium without BP, and incubated for an additional 4 h.

Preparation of Tracheal Cell Homogenates and Microsomes

Tracheas were blotted free of adherent culture fluid, placed on a wax board with the mucosal side up and immobilized at one end by a flat weighing spatula. A 100-μl aliquot of 0.25 M sucrose solution containing 0.05 M Tris-HCl, at 4°C and pH 7.4, was applied to the trachea. The surface was scraped 20 times with the edge of a scalpel blade held perpendicular to the surface (15). The resulting suspension of tracheal epithelial cells was aspirated, and a second aliquot of fluid was applied and aspirated. Suspensions containing cells pooled from groups of 10 tracheas were diluted with an equal volume of the sucrose/Tris-HCl buffer and homogenized in a Dounce homogenizer with 50 strokes of the pestle. The homogenate, which was free of intact cells as determined by phase contrast microscopy, was centrifuged at 10,000 g at 4°C to produce the 10,000 g supernatant. Microsomes were prepared by centrifuging the 10,000 g supernatant at 100,000 g for 1 h. The pellet containing microsomes was barely visible and was suspended in 0.1 ml of 0.05 M Tris-HCl at pH 7.4. The protein contents of the above fractions were determined by the sensitive method described by Schaffner and Weissman (16); bovine serum albumin was used as the protein standard.

[^{3}H]BP Purification

Generally labeled [^{3}H]BP obtained from the radiochemical manufacturer (Amersham, Arlington Heights, IL) was visibly contaminated with BP quinones, as evidenced by the yellow-orange tint which colored solutions of [^{3}H]BP. The [^{3}H]BP was always purified 24 h prior to its use to minimize background radioactivity from oxidation products and thereby maximize the detection of metabolites. The purification procedure attributed to Yang et al. (17) was used with modifications. The [^{3}H]BP was purified by chromatography on a silica gel column with hexane as the eluent. Purity of the [^{3}H]BP was always greater than 99% as determined by high pressure liquid chromatography (HPLC). All manipulations involving [^{3}H]BP were performed under subdued or yellow fluorescent lights.

Benzo[a]pyrene Monooxygenase Assay

The method of DePierre et al. (18) was modified to increase sensitivity and was scaled down in accord with the minute quantities of microsomal protein available, often 4 to 8 μg per assay tube. The standard reaction mixture contained 0.2 ml including microsomal protein, 0.36 μmol of NADPH, and 3 μmol of $MgCl_2$. The reaction tubes were kept in an ice bath and [^{3}H]BP was added. The [^{3}H]BP was used at the specific activity obtained when purchased and was never diluted with unlabeled BP; the specific activities ranged from 16 Ci/mmol to 40 Ci/mmol. After appropriate incubation periods, tubes were removed from the shaker bath, placed in an ice bath, and the reaction was quenched with 1.8 ml of 0.27N NaOH dissolved in 44% ethanol. Addition of this reagent resulted in the concentrations of NaOH and ethanol as described originally by DePierre et al. (18). Calculation of metabolism was based upon the quantity of tritium remaining in the polar phase after hexane extraction. Aliquots of the polar phase were neutralized with an equal volume of 0.25N HCl and were counted in 10 ml of Biofluor (New England Nuclear Corp., Boston, MA) with a liquid scintillation counter; counting efficiency was about 40% as determined by internal standards.

Isolation and Purification of DNA

Suspensions of epithelial cells scraped from tracheas were incubated with an equal volume of Proteinase K (1 mg/ml; Merck, Darmstadt, Germany) containing 2% sarcosyl (Bio-Rad Laboratories, Richmond, CA) at 45°C for 30 min. The samples were homogenized with two volumes of water-saturated phenol to further deproteinize the DNA and to remove unreacted, unbound [^{3}H]BP. After centrifugation at 10,000 g for 2 min, the aqueous layer was removed and again homogenized with phenol and centrifuged. Two volumes of absolute ethanol were added to the aqueous phase of each sample; the samples were refrigerated at -20°C overnight. The resulting precipite was sedimented at 10,000 g for 2 min and the supernatant discarded. The pellet was resuspended in 0.5 ml of 0.1 M Tris-HCl, pH 7.4. Extraction with diethyl ether was performed until no radioactivity could be detected in the volatile phase; this stage was usually achieved after eight extractions. The ether was evaporated in a stream of nitrogen gas. RNA was removed by hydrolysis with 200 μg/ml RNAse (Worthington, Freehold, NJ) for 1 h at 37°C. Samples were then dialyzed against three 2-liter volumes of 0.05 M Tris-HCl containing 0.05 M EDTA, pH 7.4. All samples were adjusted to a refractive index of 1.3996 with cesium chloride and isopyknic gradients were formed by ultracentrifugation for 66 h at 35,000 rpm in a Beckman Type 65 rotor, or for 18 h at 42,000 rpm in a Dupont 865B vertical rotor. The resulting density gradients were fractionated through punctures made in the bottoms of the ultracentrifuge tubes. Absorbance of each fraction was determined at 257 nm, and radioactivity was determined by scintillation counting.

Metabolite Analysis

Metabolites produced by tracheal microsomes. Tracheal microsomes (80 μg) were incubated for 30 min with optimum levels of cofactors and with either 2 μM [^{3}H]BP for hamster tracheal microsomes or 5 μM [^{3}H]BP for rat tracheal microsomes. The [^{3}H]BP was delivered in 10 μl of methanol. The reaction was terminated with 1 ml of acetone and then 2 ml of ethylacetate, containing 0.8% butylated hydroxytoluene (Aldrich Chemical Company, Milwaukee, WI), was added to reduce the likelihood of spontaneous conversion of BP phenols to BP quinones during the extraction period (19). Metabolites were extracted by vortexing for 2 min, after which the phases were separated by centrifugation at 900 rpm for 5 min. The extraction was repeated two more times, and the acetone/ethylacetate phases were pooled. The acetone/ethylacetate phase was dried over anhydrous magnesium sulfate to remove water. The acetone/ethylacetate containing metabolites was evaporated with nitrogen gas.

Metabolites produced by tracheal organ cultures. Rat and hamster tracheas in tissue culture were incubated with 1 μM [^{3}H]BP for 18 h. A culture dish containing no tissue but containing 5 ml of medium with 1 μM [^{3}H]BP was used as a control. After the incubation period, the tracheas were removed and the media was divided into two aliquots. The first was subjected to acetone/ethylacetate extraction as described above. The second was adjusted to pH 5 by the addition of an equal volume of 0.2 M sodium acetate buffer. Aryl sulfatase (11 units) and β-glucuronidase (1000 units) (Sigma Chemical Company, St. Louis, MO) were added and incubated for 2 h at 37°C to release BP metabolites conjugated with sulfate and glucuronic acid. Extraction with acetone/ethylacetate followed as above.

The quantity and proportion of water-soluble or acetone/ethylacetate-soluble metabolites were determined by measuring the volumes of each phase and their respective tritium contents. The quantity and proportion of the metabolites were also determined by a modification of a thin-layer chromatography (TLC) technique described by Sims (20). Three volumes of methanol were added to the culture medium containing metabolites to precipitate serum proteins. After refrigeration at -20°C for 3 h and subsequent centrifugation at 900 rpm, an aliquot of the supernatant was applied to a silica gel G plate (Eastman). An aliquot of an acetone/ethylacetate extract of the same sample of medium was applied to another track on the plate. A few microliters of a 2-mM solution of unlabeled BP in acetone was applied over the spots containing the metabolites to serve as a marker for the migration of BP. The plate was developed in solution of equal amounts of hexane and benzene. After drying, the TLC plate was examined under ultraviolet light and the position of the BP noted. In this solvent system, only BP migrates; the polar metabolites remain at the origin. Sections of the TLC plate containing BP and its metabolites were cut out, and the radioactivity in the individual spots was measured. For these measurements, the ratios of BP to its metabolites were calculated for the culture medium and for the sample of organic-soluble materials applied to the plate.

HPLC Analysis of Metabolites. The residue obtained from acetone/ethylacetate extracts was dried under nitrogen and measured by HPLC. Samples were dissolved in absolute methanol containing authentic BP metabolites obtained from the Carcinogenesis Program of the National Cancer Institute. BP tetrols were synthesized by the method of Yang and Gelboin (21). A 10-μl aliquot was injected into a custom-made high pressure liquid chromatograph fitted with a CO:PELL ODS guard column (Whatman, Englewood Cliffs, NJ), and a μBondapak C_{18} column (Waters Associates, Milford, MA). Metabolites were eluted at ambient temperature at an initial flow rate of 0.8 ml/min using a linear gradient of methanol/water (60% methanol to 80% methanol) until BP was eluted from the column. Fractions were collected at 30-sec intervals and tritium counts were measured by liquid scintillation. All metabolites were identified solely by chromatographic retention times; therefore, it is quite possible that other unidentified metabolites were also present within the radioactively-labeled peaks of identified metabolites.

RESULTS

Kinetic Analysis of BP Monooxygenase in Tracheal Epithelial Microsomes

Microsomes isolated from epithelial cells of tracheas were incubated for 5 min with [^{3}H]BP at substrate concentrations ranging from 0.25 to 20 μM. Because of the short incubation period and low microsomal protein concentrations, the maximum quantity of substrate that was converted to oxygenated products was measured to be less than 2% of the initial substrate added. This low conversion rate yielded signal-to-noise ratios of 0.3 to 10, that were directly proportional to BP monooxygenase activity and inversely related to the substrate concentration.

Microsomes from hamster tracheas that were cultured for 24 h in the presence of unlabeled BP demonstrated a substrate-inducible BP monooxygenase activity. The apparent K_m values from both control tracheas and BP-pretreated tracheas were between 1 and 2 μM and were considered equal ($p > 0.1$). The apparent V_{max} values, which differed by a factor of three ($p < 0.001$), were 30.2 pmol/mg microsomal protein/min for the constitutive BP monooxygenase and 97 pmol/mg microsomal protein/min for the induced BP monooxygenase. Lineweaver-Burk plots illustrating the K_m and V_{max} determinations are shown in Figure 1.

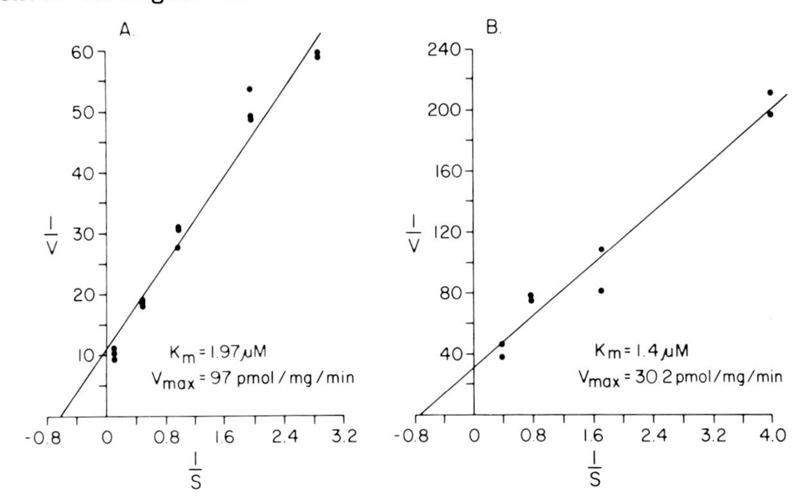

Figure 1. Lineweaver-Burk plot for BP monooxygenase activity: A, constitutive BP monooxygenase in hamster tracheal epithelial microsomes; B, microsomes from BP-pretreated hamster tracheas. Vertical axis is expressed as min/pmol; horizontal axis is inverse substrate concentration expressed as 1/μM.

The activity of BP monooxygenase in microsomes from epithelial cells of rat tracheas could not be measured, i.e., the activity was below the limit of detection for this assay at the small protein concentrations used. Instead, 10,000 g supernatants from rat tracheal cell homogenates were used. The activity was still undetectable in 10,000 g supernatants from homogenates of control rat tracheas, but was detectable if the rat tracheas were exposed to 5 μM BP for 24 h in culture. To aid in comparison with BP monooxygenase in hamster tracheas, a Lineweaver-Burk plot of BP monooxygenase from 10,000 g supernatants from epithelial cells of hamster tracheas incubated for 24 h in the presence of 5 μM BP is shown in Figure 2. The K_m values are equivalent. The V_{max} is 6.3 pmol/mg protein/min for BP monooxygenase in rat tracheas and 13.5 pmol/mg protein/min for BP monooxygenase in hamster tracheas; these values are significantly different at a level of $p < 0.05$.

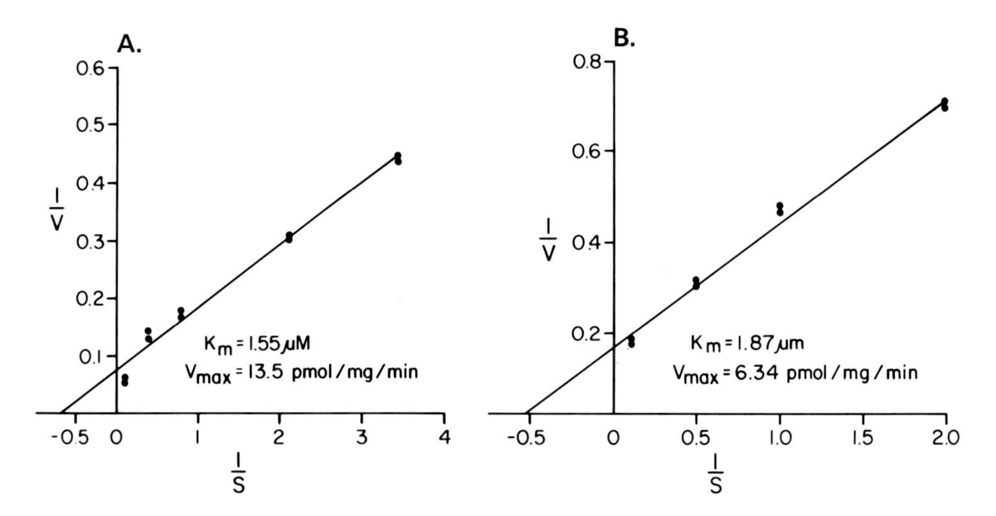

Figure 2. Lineweaver-Burk plot for BP monooxygenase activity in supernatants of tracheal epithelial cell homogenates centrifuged at 10,000 g: A, BP-pretreated hamster tracheas; B, BP-pretreated rat tracheas.

High Pressure Liquid Chromatography Analysis

Hamster tracheal microsomes were incubated with 2 μM [^{3}H]BP for 30 min in a reaction mixture similar to that used for the BP monooxygenase assay but containing 80 μg of microsomal protein. The acetone/ethylacetate-extractable metabolites produced during this incubation cochromatographed with the 9,10-dihydro-9-10-dihydroxybenzo[a]pyrene (9,10-diol), 4,5-dihydro-4,5-dihydroxybenzo[a]pyrene (4,5-diol), 7,8-dihydro-7,8-dihydroxybenzo[a]pyrene (7,8-diol), BP-quinones, 3-hydroxy BP and 9-hydroxybenzo[a]pyrene (9-hydroxy BP) (Figure 3). Greater than half of the radioactivity cochromatographed with BP quinones and BP phenols. Since butylated hydroxytoluene was present during the acetone/ethylacetate extractions, it is not likely that the BP quinones arose from spontaneous oxidation of BP phenols during the extraction steps.

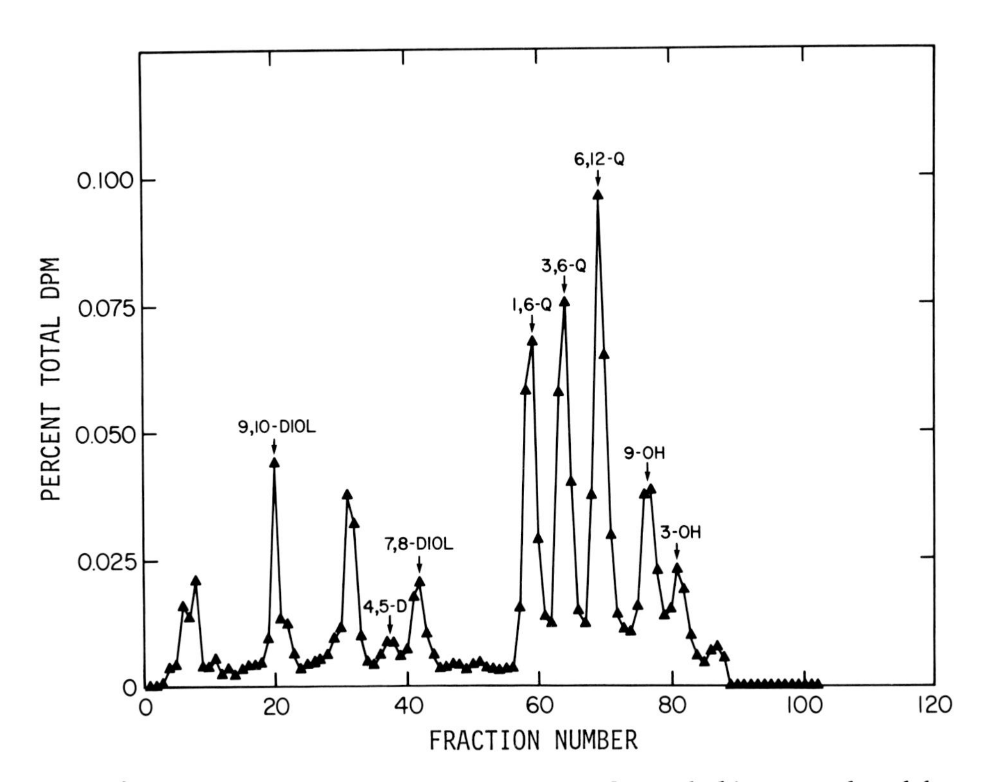

Figure 3. Reverse-phase HPLC separation of metabolites produced by microsomes from BP-pretreated hamster tracheas after 30-min incubation with [^{3}H]BP and cofactors at 37°C.

Rat tracheal microsomes incubated with [^{3}H]BP for 30 min produced entirely different quantities and proportions of acetone/ethylacetate-soluble metabolites (Figure 4). Most of the radioactivity cochromatographed with 3-hydroxy BP. Small peaks corresponding to BP quinones and the 9,10-diol were also observed. Other secondary metabolic processes chemically modify microsomal metabolites so that their presence is not detected in the intact tissues. In the presence of appropriate substrates, this secondary metabolism can be observed by incubating [^{3}H]BP with whole tracheas in culture. Since conjugation with glucuronic acid and sulfate reduces the apparent quantity of acetone/ethylacetate-soluble metabolites, HPLC profiles were constructed by plotting the quantity of radioactivity present in the medium that was initially acetone/ethylacetate-extractable. These were superimposed over the chromatogram profiles obtained from acetone/ethylacetate extractions of the culture medium after treatment with β-glucuronidase and aryl sulfatase.

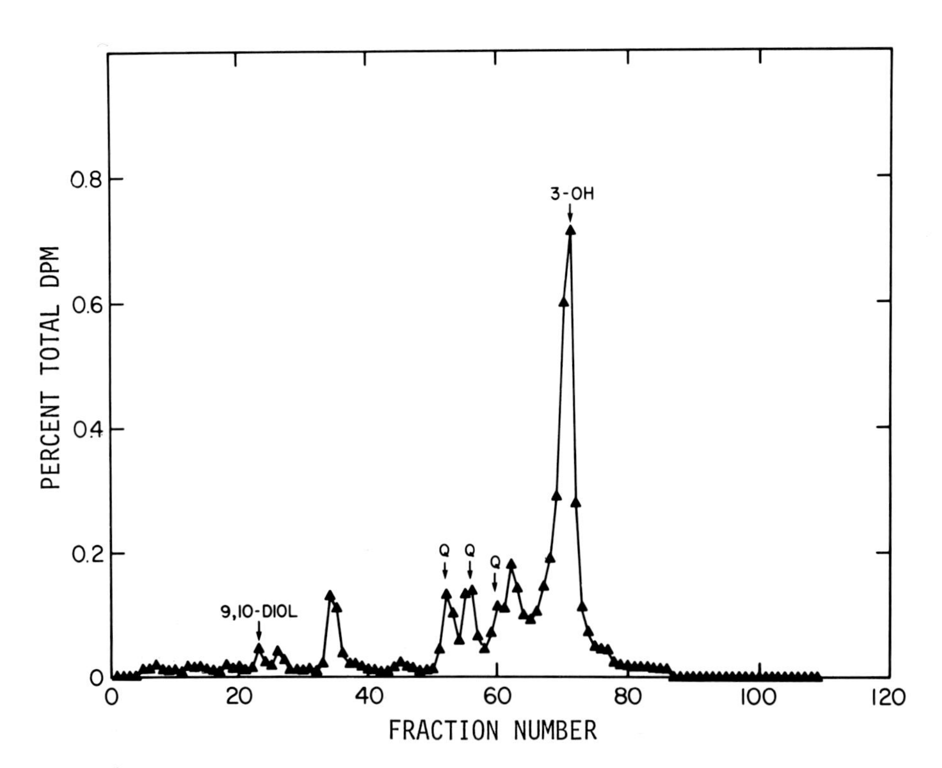

Figure 4. Reverse-phase HPLC separation of metabolites produced by rat tracheal microsomes isolated from BP-pretreated tracheas. Microsomes were incubated for 30 min with [^{3}H]BP and cofactors at 37°C.

Figure 5 is an HPLC profile obtained from tissue cultures of hamster tracheas that were incubated with 1 μM [^{3}H]BP for 18 h. The acetone/ethylacetate-soluble products comprise 35% of the total products released into the culture medium. Exposure of this medium to β-glucuronidase and aryl sulfatase released another 30% of the products. The major metabolite was the 9,10-diol, which was not conjugated with glucuronic acid or sulfate. BP phenols accounted for the next most abundant class of metabolites, and they served as good substrates for conjugation. The 7,8-diol and BP quinones were present largely as glucuronide or sulfate esters (22). BP tetrols were produced in small amounts that did not increase after exposure to β-glucuronidase and aryl sulfatase. Metabolites more polar than BP tetrols comprised about 20% of the metabolites present after exposure to the deconjugating enzymes.

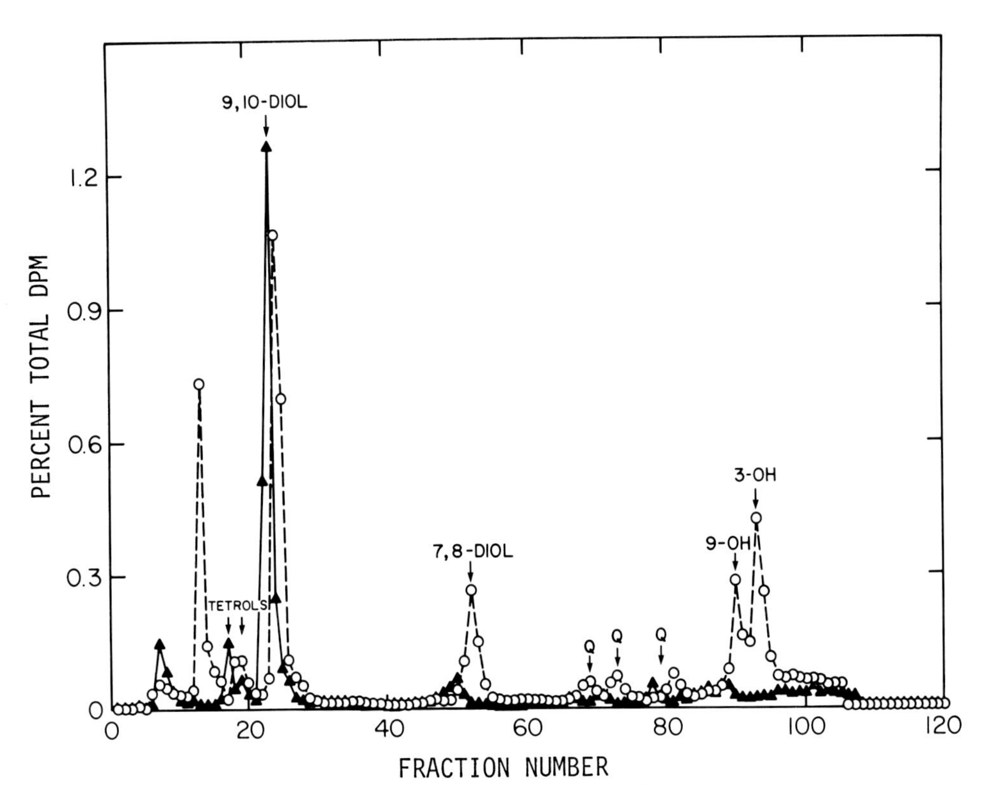

Figure 5. High pressure liquid chromatograms of culture media for hamster tracheas incubated for 24 h with 1 μM [^{3}H]BP. Metabolites were extracted from the media by acetone/ethylacetate (▲ --- ▲), or exposed to 11 units of aryl sulfatase and 1000 units of β-glucuronidase at pH 5 for 2 h prior to acetone/ethylacetate extraction (O - O).

Rat tracheas in organ culture (Figure 6) produced less acetone/ethylacetate- and water-soluble metabolites per unit mass of tracheal tissue than did cultures of hamster tracheas. The total quantity of these metabolites produced during the 24-h incubation were 3.7 pmol/mg tissue for rat tracheas and 7.8 pmol/mg tissue for hamster tracheas. Although the major acetone/ethylacetate-extractable metabolite appears to be the 9,10-diol, β-glucuronidase and aryl sulfatase treatment of the rat tracheal organ culture medium released a large quantity of BP phenols into the acetone/ethylacetate phase of the medium; the BP phenols represented 40% of the total metabolites identified. In contrast,

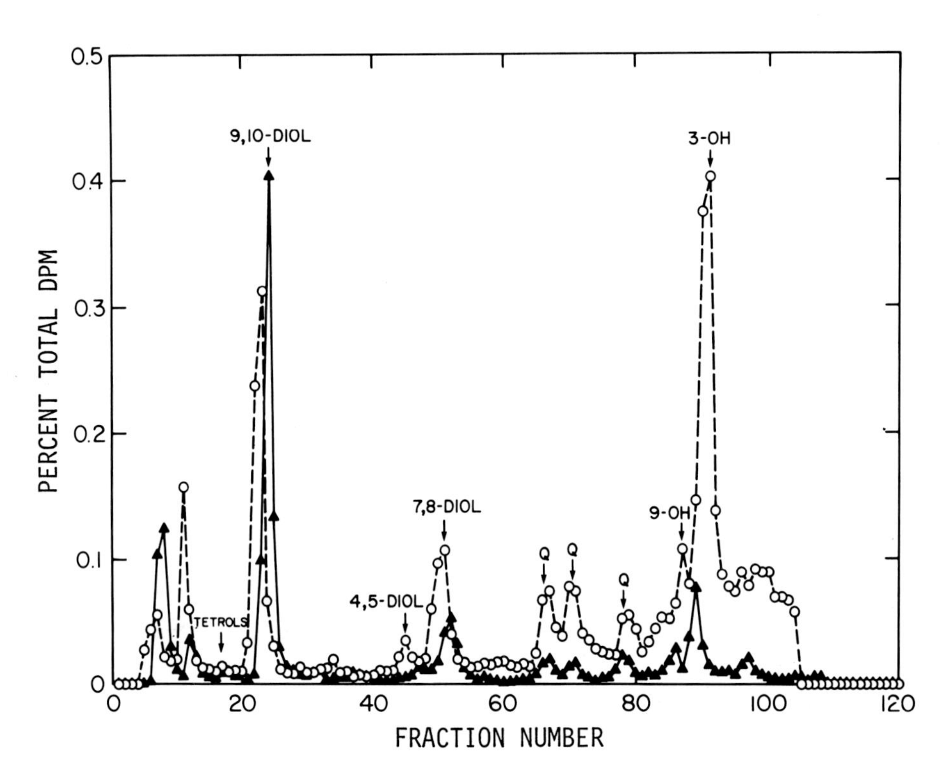

Figure 6. High pressure liquid chromatograms of culture media for rat tracheas incubated for 24 h with 1 μM [^{3}H]BP. Metabolites were extracted from the media by acetone/ethylacetate (▲ --- ▲), or exposed to 11 units of aryl sulfatase and 1000 units of β-glucuronidase at pH 5 for 2 h prior to acetone/ethylacetate extraction (O - O).

BP phenols made up approximately 25% of the acetone/ethylacetate-soluble metabolites before treatment of the medium with β-glucuronidase and aryl sulfatase. BP quinones, the 7,8-diol, and the 4,5-diol comprised the remaining metabolites in the culture medium in which rat tracheas were incubated. The quantity of BP tetrols did not differ before or after β-glucuronidase and aryl sulfatase treatment of the medium. BP tetrols represented only about 1% of the total products identified. The quantities of acetone/ethylacetate-soluble metabolites recovered from the rat and hamster trachea culture medium after incubation with β-glucuronidase and aryl sulfatase are shown in Table 1. This information is shown graphically in Figure 7. The ratio of the quantity of products produced by hamster and rat tracheas varies from 1.1 to 22. The greatest discrepancy in ratios is that of BP tetrol formation: hamster tracheas produce 22-fold more BP tetrols than do rat tracheas.

Table 1. Comparison of Metabolites Produced by Rat and Hamster Tracheal Organ Cultures

Metabolite	Hamster (pmole metabolite/ mg tissue/24 h)	Rat (pmole metabolite/ mg tissue/24 h)	Ratio (Hamster/Rat)
Pre-tetrols	0.86	0.18	4.78
Tetrols	0.22	0.01	22.0
9,10-Diol	1.41	0.30	4.70
4,5-Diol	0.05	0.04	1.26
7,8-Diol	0.46	0.15	3.07
Quinones	0.45	0.30	1.50
9-OH	0.48	0.11	4.36
3-OH	0.61	0.56	1.09

Binding of [^{3}H]BP to DNA in Epithelial Cells of Rat and Hamster Tracheas

To determine the quantity of metabolites that bound to DNA of tracheas in culture, tracheas were incubated for 24 h in the presence of 1 μM [^{3}H]BP. Epithelial cells were scraped from tracheas and the cellular DNA was isolated by phenol extraction. The DNA was enzymatically freed of contaminating proteins and RNA, and non-covalently-bound radioactivity was removed by exhaustive ether etraction. The DNA was further purified on isopyknic cesium

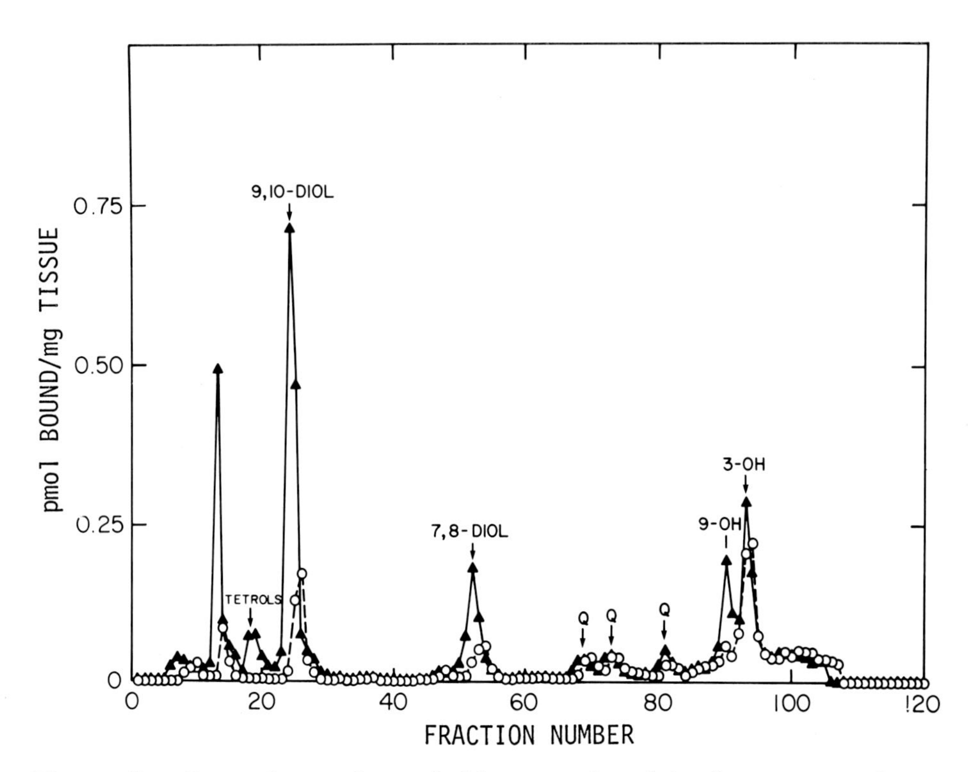

Figure 7. Comparison of metabolites produced by hamster tracheas (▲ --- ▲) or rat tracheas (0 --- 0) after exposure of tissue culture fluid to β-glucuronidase and aryl sulfatase. The results have been normalized for the weight of tissue utilized in the incubation.

chloride gradients. Table 2 summarizes the results of several experiments with rat and hamster tracheas. The [^{3}H]BP binding determinations in rat tracheas are the accumulation of five experiments that provided nine separate observations. A total of 48 rats was used. The mean binding level was 1.55 x 10^{-4} pmol [^{3}H]BP/ μg DNA/24 h. Two observations were from an experiment to determine the effect of a 24-h pretreatment with 20 μM BP. A level of 1.23 x 10^{-4} pmol/ μg DNA/24 h was observed in the BP-pretreated trachea and a level of 0.91 x 10^{-4} pmol/ μg DNA/24 h was found in DNA from control rat tracheas. BP-pretreatment of hamster tracheas resulted in greater than twofold increases in binding (i.e., from 16.9 x 10^{-4} to 42.6 x 10^{-4} pmol/ μg DNA/24 h). The level of binding of [^{3}H]BP had a mean of 26.7 x 10^{-4} pmol/µg DNA/24 h (26 hamsters were used in total). A t-test of the null hypothesis, that the mean binding levels were equal, was rejected at a value of $p = 0.003$. The mean value for [^{3}H]BP binding to DNA in hamster tracheas was 17-fold greater than for rat tracheas.

Table 2. Specific Activity of Binding of [^{3}H]BP to DNA in Rat and Hamster Tracheas

Rat		Hamster	
No. of Tracheas	Specific Activity (pmole/µg DNA)	No. of Tracheas	Specific Activity (pmole/µg DNA)
6	1.12	6	13.8
6	0.92	6	20.9
6	0.66	5	36.1
6	0.90	5	30.1
6	0.68	3	16.9[a]
5	3.19	3	42.6[a]
5	4.30		
3	0.91[a]		
3	1.24[a]		
Mean ± S.D.	1.55 ± 1.29[b]		26.6 ± 11.4[b]
	Ratio (Hamster/Rat) = 17.5		

[a]Paired experiment for control tracheas and tracheas exposed to 20 µM BP for 24 h, respectively.
[b]These values differ significantly at a level of $p = 0.003$.

DISCUSSION

Hamster tracheal epithelium is extremely sensitive to tumor induction by intratracheal instillation of BP-ferric oxide (1); further, heterotopically-grafted hamster tracheas are so sensitive to these agents that microgram doses of PNH delivered in beeswax pellets are lethal (P. Nettesheim, personal communication, National Institute of Environmental Health Sciences, Research Triangle Park, NC). Presumably, this effect is due to the high metabolic capacity for BP of the hamster tracheal epithelium: 9 µg of 3-MC released slowly by Lycra fibers is sufficient to induce epidermoid carcinoma in grafted hamster tracheas (14). Nettesheim et al. (23)

could not induce epidermoid carcinoma in grafted rat tracheas with any less than 300 μg of BP. Consistent with this observation of lesser susceptibility of rat tracheas to BP carcinogenesis, intratracheal instillations of BP-ferric oxide have never produced a tumor in the tracheal epithelium of rats. The success of the heterotopic tracheal graft model is undoubtedly due to the delayed release of BP from the beeswax pellets, the localized and prolonged contact of BP with the epithelium, and the subsequent metabolism of BP to active forms. In contrast, intratracheal instillations of BP-ferric oxide, though comprising a greater total dose, are probably removed from the respiratory tract comparatively rapidly.

The results described within this study demonstrate the necessity of the use of the target tissue in evaluations of carcinogen susceptibility. The tumor incidences elicited in the tracheas of rats and hamsters from an intratracheal dose of BP-ferric oxide could not have been extrapolated from studies of carcinogen activation in whole lung microsomes or in lung organ cultures. In direct contrast to the effects of BP-ferric oxide in the tracheas of rats and hamsters, epidermoid carcinomas of the peripheral lung are easily inducible in rats (13), whereas hamster lungs are relatively refractory to carcinogenesis by BP-ferric oxide (13). In fact, this difference might be predicted from lung microsomal BP monooxygenase studies: BP monooxygenase levels, though equal in microsomes from rat and hamster lungs, are two- to threefold greater in microsomes from lungs of 3-MC-pretreated rats than in identical preparations from hamster lungs (24). This biochemical assessment well reflects the tumor incidence data for rat and hamster lungs, but it is the direct opposite of those for the tracheas.

The V_{max} values obtained for BP monooxygenase in hamster tracheal microsomes with BP-pretreatment are very low (25). They are approximately 50-fold less active than BP monooxygenase in microsomes from livers of rats pretreated with 3-MC. The constitutive BP monooxygenase in rat tracheal cells was undetectable. Using microsomes isolated from whole homogenized rat trachea, Simberg and Uotila (26) demonstrated aryl hydrocarbon hydroxylase (AHH) activity by fluorometric assay. The AHH activity they observed corresponds to approximately 2 pmol/mg microsomal protein/min. Although these investigators used a 30-min incubation, a time which probably was not in the linear range for the reaction (24), the low activity observed by Simberg and Uotila (26) is thoroughly consistent with results of measurements made in our studies with rat trachea. Our results are in excellent qualitative agreement with results of previous chromatographic studies of Cohen et al. (27-29) in hamster and rat tracheal organ cultures, despite differences in culture media and substrate concentrations.

The formation of 7,8-dihydroxy-7,8-dihydro-9,10 epoxybenzo[a]pyrene, a bay-region diol-epoxide of BP and its binding to DNA are presumed to be significant events in the initiation of neoplasia. The presence in the culture medium of BP tetrols, spontaneous hydrolysis products of the bay-region diol-epoxide of BP, should be a measure of the production of this ultimate carcinogen and should bear some relationship to the tumor incidences in this tissue. Since the identifications were based only on chromatographic retention times, we cannot be absolutely certain that the peaks designated as BP tetrols consist only of BP tetrols; however, the BP-DNA binding data exhibit ratios between rats and hamsters (22.0, see Table 1) that are of equal magnitude to the ratios for BP-tetrols (17.5, see Table 2). Autrup et al. (30) have examined BP metabolism, BP-DNA binding, and BP-deoxynucleoside adducts in the respiratory epithelia of several species including rats and hamsters. In agreement with the results presented here, the epithelium of hamsters was found to metabolize BP at a rate higher than in rats. Autrup et al. (30) also found that the BP-deoxynucleoside adducts in the tracheal epithelium of rats and hamsters are different (see also Autrup et al. in this volume).

In summary, the existing body of consistent evidence demonstrates that the tracheal epithelium of rats is less susceptible to the carcinogenic effects of PNH than is the tracheal epithelium of hamsters. Previous investigations have noted no clear anatomic, histologic, or physiologic difference in the respiratory tracts of these animals that can account for this marked sensitivity of hamsters and the relative resistance of rats. Consequently, the 10- to 20-fold difference in conversion of BP to metabolites that bind to DNA in rat and hamster tracheas appears to be a significant factor contributing to the vast difference in susceptibility to carcinogenesis in this tissue observed between these species.

REFERENCES

1. Nettesheim, P., and R.A. Griesemer. 1978. Experimental models for studies of respiratory tract carcinogenesis. In: Pathogenesis and Therapy of Lung Cancer. C.C. Harris, ed. Marcel Dekker: New York. pp. 75-188.

2. Doll, R. 1978. An epidemiologic perspective of the biology of cancer. Cancer Res. 38:3573-3583.

3. Harris, C.C., H. Autrup, G.D. Stoner, S.K. Yang, J.C. Leutz, H.V. Gelboin, J.K. Selkirk, R.J. Conner, L.A. Barrett, R.T. Jones, E.M. McDowell, and B.F. Trump. 1977. Metabolism of benzo[a]pyrene and 7,12-dimethylbenz[a] anthracene in cultured human bronchus and pancreatic duct. Cancer Res. 37:3349-3355.

4. Harris, C.C., H. Autrup, G.D. Stoner, B.F. Trump, E. Hillman, P.W. Schaefer, and A.M. Jeffrey. 1979. Metabolism of benzo[a]pyrene, N-nitrosodimethylamine, and N-nitrosopyrrolidine and identification of major carcinogen-DNA adducts formed in human esophagus. Cancer Res. 39:4401-4406.

5. Autrup, H., C.C. Harris, B.F. Trump, and A.M. Jeffrey. 1978. Metabolism of benzo[a]pyrene and identification of major benzo[a]pyrene-DNA adducts in cultured human colon. Cancer Res. 38:3689-3696.

6. Mass, M.J., N.T. Rodgers, and D.G. Kaufman. 1981. Benzo[a]pyrene metabolism in organ cultures of human endometrium. Chem.-Biol. Interact. 33:195-205.

7. Harris, C.C., H. Autrup, R. Conner, L.A. Barrett, E.M. McDowell, and B.F. Trump. 1976. Interindividual variation in binding of benzo[a]pyrene to DNA in cultured human bronchi. Science 194:1067-1069.

8. Galofre, M.L., S.W. Payne, L.B. Woolner, O.T. Clagett, and R.P. Gage. 1964. Pathologic classification and surgical treatment of bronchogenic carcinoma. Surg. Gynecol. Obstet. 119:51-61.

9. Saffiotti, U., F. Cefis, and L.H. Kolb. 1968. A method for the experimental induction of bronchogenic carcinoma. Cancer Res. 28:104-124.

10. Blair, W.H. 1974. Chemical induction of lung carcinomas in rats. In: Experimental Lung Cancer: Carcinogenesis and Bioassays. E. Karbe, and J.F. Parks, eds. Springer-Verlag: Berlin. pp. 199-206.

11. Schreiber, H., D.H. Martin, and N. Pazmino. 1975. Species differences in the effect of benzo[a]pyrene-ferric oxide on the respiratory tract of rats and hamsters. Cancer Res. 35:1654-1661.

12. Blair, W.H., N. Otero, and H. Rao. 1973. Development of lung neoplasms in rats treated with 7,12-dimethylbenz[a]anthracene. Proc. Am. Assoc. Cancer Res. 14:497.

13. Schreiber, H., P. Nettesheim, and D.H. Martin. 1972. Rapid development of bronchiolo-alveolar squamous cell tumors in rats after intratracheal injection of 3-methylcholanthrene. J. Natl. Cancer Inst. 49:541-546.

14. Mossman, B.T., and J.E. Craighead. 1978. Induction of neoplasms in hamster tracheal grafts with 3-methylcholanthrene-coated Lycra fibers. Cancer Res. 38:3717-3722.

15. Smith, J.M., M.B. Sporn, D.A. Berkowitz, T. Kakefuda, E. Callan, and U. Saffiotti. 1971. Isolation of enzymatically active nuclei from epithelial cells of the trachea. Cancer Res. 31:199-202.

16. Schaffner, W., and C. Weissman. 1973. A rapid, sensitive, and specific method for the determination of protein in dilute solution. Anal. Biochem. 56:502-515.

17. Yang, S.K., H.V. Gelboin, H. Autrup, and C.C. Harris. 1977. Metabolic activation of benzo[a]pyrene and binding to DNA in cultured human bronchus. Cancer Res. 37:1210-1215.

18. DePierre, J.W., M.S. Moron, K.A.M. Johannesen, and L. Ernster. 1975. A reliable, sensitive, and convenient radioactive assay for benzpyrene monooxygenase. Anal. Biochem. 63:470-484.

19. Burke, M.D., H. Vadi, B. Jernstrom, and S. Orrenius. 1977. Metabolism of benzo[a]pyrene and degradation of DNA-binding derivatives. J. Biol. Chem. 18:6424-6431.

20. Sims, P. 1967. The metabolism of benzo[a]pyrene by rat liver homogenates. Biochem. Pharmacol. 16:613-618.

21. Yang, S.K., and H.V. Gelboin. 1976. Nonenzymatic reduction of benzo[a]pyrene diol-epoxides to trihydroxypentahydrobenzo[a]pyrenes by reduced nicotinamide adenine dinucleotide phosphate. Cancer Res. 36:4185-4189.

22. Mass, M.J., and D.G. Kaufman. 1979. Benzo[a]pyrene quinone metabolism in tracheal organ cultures. Biochem. Biophys. Res. Comm. 89:885-892.

23. Nettesheim, P., R.A. Griesemer, D.H. Martin, and J.E. Caton. 1977. Induction of preneoplastic and neoplastic lesions in grafted hamster tracheas continuously exposed to benzo[a]pyrene. Cancer Res. 37:1272-1278.

24. Prough, R.A., V.W. Patrizi, R.T. Okita, B.S.S. Masters, and S.W. Jakobsson. 1979. Characteristics of benzo[a]pyrene metabolism by kidney, liver, and lung microsomal fractions from rodents and humans. Cancer Res. 39:1199-1206.

25. Mass, M.J., and D.G. Kaufman. 1978. [^{3}H]Benzo[a]pyrene metabolism in tracheal epithelial cell microsomes and tracheal organ cultures. Cancer Res. 38:3861-3866.

26. Simberg, N., and P. Uotila. 1978. Stimulatory effect of cigarette smoke on the metabolism and covalent binding of benzo[a]pyrene in the trachea of the rat. Int. J. Cancer 22:28-31.

27. Cohen, G.M., and B.P. Moore. 1976. Metabolism of benzo[a]-pyrene by different portions of the respiratory tract. Biochem. Pharmacol. 25:1623-1629.

28. Cohen, G.M., A.C. Marchok, P. Nettesheim, V.E. Steele, F. Nelson, S. Huang, and J.K. Selkirk. 1979. Comparative metabolism of benzo[a]pyrene in organ and cell cultures derived from rat tracheas. Cancer Res. 39:1980-1984.

29. Moore, B.P., and G.M. Cohen. 1978. Metabolism of [^{3}H]BP and its major metabolites to ethyl-acetate-soluble and water-soluble metabolites by cultured rodent trachea. Cancer Res. 38:3066-3075.

30. Autrup, H., F.C. Wefald, A.M. Jeffrey, H. Tate, R.D. Schwartz, B.F. Trump, and C.C. Harris. 1980. Metabolism of benzo[a]-pyrene by cultured tracheobronchial tissues from mice, rats, hamsters, bovines, and humans. Int. J. Cancer 25:293-300.

DISCUSSION

Q.: Have you found any benzo[a]pyrene sulfate conjugates in the rats?

A.: We did not analyze our water-soluble metabolites separately for sulfate conjugates, but analyzed the water-soluble metabolites simultaneously for sulfate together with glucuronide conjugates.

SUBCELLULAR METABOLIC ACTIVATION SYSTEMS: THEIR UTILITY AND LIMITATIONS IN PREDICTING ORGAN AND SPECIES SPECIFIC CARCINOGENESIS OF CHEMICALS

Helmut Bartsch, Christian Malaveille, and Anne-Marie Camus

Division of Environmental Carcinogenesis, International Agency for Research on Cancer, 150 cours Albert-Thomas, 69008 Lyons, France

INTRODUCTION

Extensive studies evaluating short-term tests for the detection of genotoxic agents as reliable predictors of the potential carcinogenic hazard of chemicals (1-5) have revealed that, apart from the indicator organism or the end points scored, the metabolic activation system used is of critical importance. Because of the widespread use of subcellular metabolic activation systems for the detection of DNA-damaging agents in short-term tests, a data base has become available that helps determine to what extent species and organ specific carcinogenesis of chemicals can be attributed to metabolic activation (or detoxification) reactions.

The detection of electrophilic intermediates in short-term tests produced from active precarcinogens (premutagens) by metabolism (6) is a complex problem. Electrophilic ultimate carcinogenic/mutagenic metabolites are formed either directly or through one or more intermediates (proximate carcinogens) from the precarcinogens. Once formed, the ultimate carcinogen may react with target molecules such as DNA in genetic indicator organisms, or it may be deactivated by binding with other cellular nucleophiles, spontaneous breakdown, or enzymatic detoxification. Similarly, pre- and proximate carcinogens may be subject to enzymic and non-enzymic detoxification reactions. Thus, the carcinogenicity/mutagenicity of many chemicals is largely determined by competition between activation and detoxification reactions. The specificity of some chemical carcinogens/mutagens that are not active in certain animal species and organs seems to be partly determined by the concentration of reactive metabolites in the target organ or cells.

The utility and limitations of subcellular metabolic activation systems in predicting such specific chemical carcinogenesis is illustrated by results obtained with N-nitrosamines, polycyclic aromatic hydrocarbons (PAHs), phenacetin, haloethylenes, 3,3-dimethyl-1-phenyltriazene, and other carcinogens with known organ/species specific action. The results are discussed with reference to review articles, rather than the original publications. A general review of the subject has appeared elsewhere (7).

MATERIALS AND METHODS

Chemicals

Test compounds were selected either because of their socio-economic importance and the lack of data on carcinogenicity or because of interest in studying their mechanism of action in chemical carcinogenesis or mutagenesis.

Mutagenicity assays in bacterial cells in the presence of microsome-, cell-, or host-mediated metabolic activation systems are commonly used for the detection of carcinogens. The following procedures were applied.

Plate Incorporation Assay in the Presence of Salmonella typhimurium Tester Strains

The test compound, dissolved in dimethyl sulfoxide (DMSO), was combined with 0.5 ml of a mixture of various amounts of tissue S9 (normally up to 150 µl), cofactors, Sorensen phosphate buffer, pH 7.4 (S9 mix), a suspension of 1 to 2 x 10^8 bacteria, and 2 ml histidine-poor soft agar (see references 1,5). The agar mixture (with a final volume of 2.7 ml) was poured onto plates of minimal agar; these were incubated at 37°C. The number of his^+ revertant colonies was determined, usually after incubation for 48 h.

Pre-Incubation Assay

The bacteria was pre-incubated with S9 mix and the test compound at 37°C for 5 to 30 min prior to the addition of soft agar (see reference 8).

Gaseous Exposure Assay

Mutagenicity tests with compounds that are volatile or gaseous at room temperature were performed by exposing inverted petri dishes containing bacteria and the same ingredients used in the plate assay (except for DMSO and the test compound), to various concentrations of the test compound in air in 10-litre desiccators for various times at 37°C in the dark (see reference 5). The desired concentration of a gaseous compound in air was achieved by evacuating the desiccator, introducing a known volume of the gas to be tested, and allowing air to enter until atmospheric pressure was reached. Mutants were scored after a total of 48 h incubation time. Quantitation of the test compound dissolved in the aqueous phase was achieved by gas-liquid chromatography.

Liquid Incubation

The incubation medium (with a final volume of 220 µl) may contain 60 µl liver S9 cofactors, Sorensen phosphate buffer (pH 7.4), a bacterial suspension averaging 4×10^7 cells, and the test compound dissolved in saline or DMSO solution. The incubation was carried out at 37°C for 30 min under oxygen and stopped by dilution with ice-cold saline. The number of mutants and survivors was determined by plating on selective medium after the appropriate dilution.

Cell-mediated Bacterial Mutagenesis

Freshly isolated rat hepatocytes were obtained by perfusion of liver with collagenase, 10^5 to 2×10^7 viable hepatocytes, determined by the Trypan blue exclusion test, and 5 to 15×10^8 bacteria (*S. typhimurium* his^- strains) were suspended in 4 ml Williams E or Hank's medium buffered with 20 mM HEPES to pH 7.4. Hepatocytes and bacteria were co-incubated in suspension at 37°C for up to 3 h in the absence or presence of varying concentrations of the test compound. At the end of incubation, bacteria were recovered by centrifugation and plated on a minimal agar plate.

Host-mediated Assay

The host-mediated assay, described previously for mice (9), was adapted for rats. In the first procedure, groups of 4 to 6 rats received a single oral application of N-nitrosodiethylamine (0.2 g/kg bw) dissolved in 0.5 ml DMSO/oral intubation. Control animals received the same volume of solvent. After 10 min, 1 ml of the S. typhimurium TA1530 strain bacterial suspension in saline (3 to 5 x 10^9 bacteria) was injected i.p. into each rat. After 1, 3, and 6 h, the rats were killed, the bacteria were removed from the peritoneal cavity, and the number of his^+ revertants and survivors were scored after the appropriate dilution by the addition of aliquots to histidine-poor (or histidine-containing) soft agar and plating. Colonies were counted after 48-h incubation at 37°C.

In the second procedure, rats were treated with a single oral dose of 0.2 g/kg bw N-nitrosodiethylamine and 10 min later were injected with TA1530 cells, as described above. After 1, 3, and 6 h, the intraperitoneal liquid, liver, kidneys, and lungs were isolated from the decapitated animals. The organs were washed and gently homogenized in a Potter Elvejhem-type homogenizer. After centrifugation (200g for 10 min), the supernatant fraction of the organ homogenate was centrifuged (1900g for 15 min). The sedimented bacteria was then resuspended in saline, and the number of his^+ revertants determined as in the first procedure. Mutation frequencies were expressed as the number of revertants/10^6 surviving cells.

RESULTS AND DISCUSSION

Variation in Hepatic Metabolic Activation Reactions of Chemicals

Pronounced species differences are seen in the activity of many of the enzymes associated with xenobiotic metabolism (10). Accordingly, large differences between species in their capacity for activation were observed when liver tissues from different experimental animal species were used to activate precarcinogens.

The importance of the animal species from which the liver postmitochondrial tissue supernatant (PMS) is derived for the efficient detection of carcinogens/mutagens is illustrated in Table 1, based on results from the Salmonella/microsome mutagenicity assays. Hamster liver PMS was much more efficient in showing the mutagenicity of a series of N-nitrosamines and of 2-acetylaminofluorene than were rat and mouse liver. Vinylidene chloride was three times as mutagenic in the presence of mouse than in the presence of rat liver PMS (11). Aflatoxin B_1 was activated into its presumed 2,3-oxide most efficiently by duck and rat liver PMS, followed by monkey and mouse liver PMS (12).

In routine screening tests for the detection of potential chemical carcinogens, the use of mixtures of liver homogenates from different animal species is recommended to circumvent some of the possible metabolic limitations of using those from only one species (e.g., rat).

Table 1. Species Variations in the Capacity of Liver Tissue Fractions from Experimental Animals to Activate Selected Pre-Carcinogens[a]

Test Compound	Inducer Treatment For Rodent[b]	Species Activation Capacity[c]
N-nitrosodimethylamine	none, PCB or PB	H>M>R
	PCB	H>M>R>GP
N-nitrosodiethylamine	none	H>R
	PB	R>H
Benzo[*a*]pyrene	none	M>GP
	none	GP>M>H>R
	PCB	R>M>GP>H
2-Acetylaminofluorene	none	H>GP>M>R
	PCB	H>GP>M>R
	none	GP>RB>R>M
Aflatoxin B_1	none	D>R>MK>M

[a]Measured by the *Salmonella* mutagenicity assay (adapted from reference 7).
[b]PCB: polychlorinated biphenyls; PB: phenobarbitone.
[c]M: mouse; H: hamster; R: rat; GP: guinea pig; RB: rabbit; D: duck; MK: monkey.

This procedure seems to be particularly pertinent in the case of phenacetin, a drug that is consumed by human subjects in analgesic and antipyretic formulations. Although it was not initially found to be mutagenic in *S. typhimurium* in the presence of rat liver fractions (2), further independent studies (13) have shown that it was mutagenic in *S. typhimurium* TA100 when liver fractions from Aroclor-pretreated hamsters, instead of rats, were used (5,14). We have investigated in more detail the pathways by which phenacetin is converted to mutagenic metabolites in hamster tissues and *in vivo* by testing known or synthetic putative metabolites (see Figure 1). N-Hydroxyphenacetin and N-acetoxyphenacetin were found to be mutagenic in *S. typhimurium* TA100 in liquid assays, as reported previously (13,15). Both required activation by liver fractions from Aroclor-pretreated hamsters. The metabolites 2-hydroxyphenacetin and 2-acetoxyphenacetin were inactive. N-Hydroxyphenetidine (the deacetylated metabolite of N-hydroxyphenacetin) and p-nitrosophenetol were the only metabolites (products) found to be strongly mutagenic in Salmonella strains when assayed under N_2.

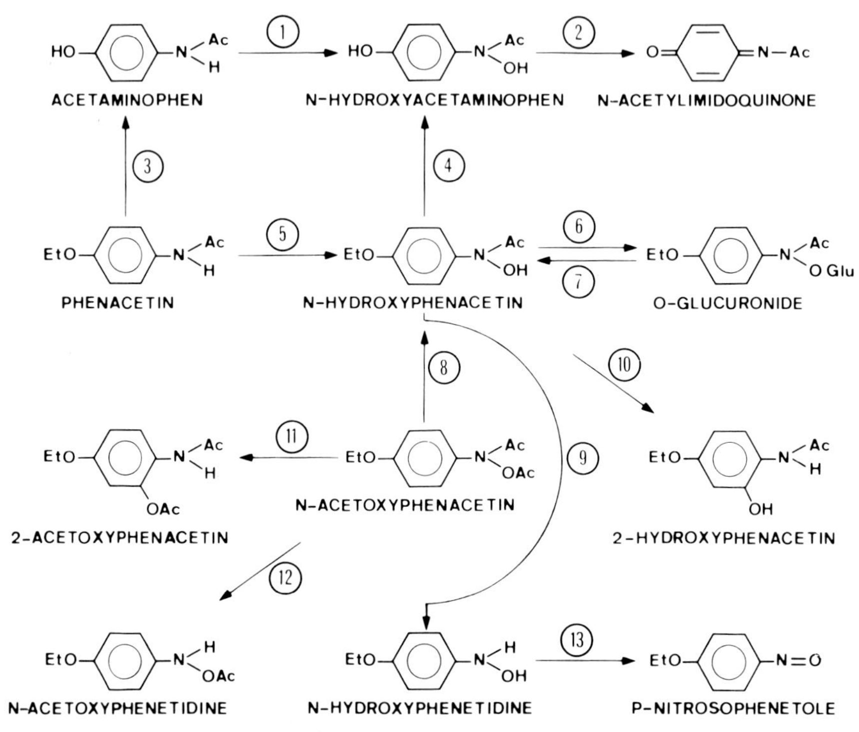

Figure 1. Metabolic pathways of phenacetin in the hamster leading to non-mutagenic and mutagenic intermediates, based on results from our studies and those of Wirth et al. (13).

These results, which confirm independent studies by Wirth et al. (13), indicate that activation of phenacetin into bacterial mutagens proceeds via N-hydroxyphenacetin → N-hydroxyphenetidine (→ p-nitrosophenetol in the presence of O_2). An analogous sequence of steps has been shown to occur for N-hydroxy-2-acetylaminofluorene (16).

Phenacetin was also administered to BDVI rats and male Syrian golden hamsters, and the urinary metabolites were concentrated on XAD-2 resin (17); the concentrate was then deconjugated with β-glucuronidase/arylsulfatase and reactivated by hamster liver fractions. Mutagenicity was demonstrated in S. typhimurium TA100 with urine from phenacetin-treated hamsters, but not with urine from the rats. N-Hydroxyphenacetin was isolated by thin-layer and high performance liquid chromatography from hamster urine after treatment by deconjugating enzymes, and it was identified by mass spectral analysis. The data suggest that N-hydroxyphenacetin is a proximate mutagenic metabolite of phenacetin that is responsible for the mutagenicity observed in vitro and in the urine of hamsters (in collaboration with Drs. M. Friesen, International Agency for Research on Cancer (IARC) Lyons, France, and A. Croisy, Institut du Radium, Orsay, France).

Our observation that rats were unable to catalyze efficiently the N-hydroxylation of phenacetin in vitro and in vivo explains why this compound had not previously been detected as a mutagen. The data, however, strongly support the hypothesis that the adverse biological effects of phenacetin involve the formation of electrophiles, as has been noted for many other carcinogenic chemicals (6).

Apart from the use of cell-free activation systems in a variety of short-term tests for systematic prescreening of compounds, there is an increasing interest in studying the differences in activation capacity, with the aim of elucidating the extent to which species variation in carcinogenic response to chemicals can be attributed to metabolic activation (or detoxification) reactions.

The results obtained with 2-acetylaminofluorene and N,N-dimethyl-4-aminoazobenzene were the first to strongly support the theory that the activity of liver enzymes involved in N-hydroxylation and subsequent esterification with sulfate by hepatic sulfotransferase(s) closely correlates with the susceptibility of different rodent species, sex, or strains to these hepatocarcinogens (6). Because these pathways do not lead to mutagens for Salmonella in vitro, such a parallelism is not observed when liver PMS-mediated mutagenicity assays are used (16,18).

Other examples of compounds in which the hepatic capacity of different animal species to activate this compound into mutagens paralleled the susceptibility of each species included aflatoxin B_1 (see Table 1) (12). Similarly vinylidene chloride produced tumors in mice (but not in rats), in keeping with the higher efficiency of mouse liver to activate this halo-olefin into mutagens (11).

From data available so far on tissue-mediated mutagenicity experiments, the susceptibility to chemically induced tumors of an animal species did not always parallel the activation capacity of subcellular fractions of its liver, possibly because of the following:

1) Assays using subcellular fractions (e.g., PMS plus an NADPH-generating system) favor activation pathways and thus do not mimic the entire metabolic capacity of the intact cell.

2) The pathways leading to mutagenic metabolites *in vitro* (and thus their relative concentrations) may be different from those that are relevant for the induction of tumors *in vivo*. Such discrepancies have become apparent for 2-acetylaminofluorene (16) and for certain PAHs such as benzo[*a*]pyrene (BP) (19-21).

3) Tumors may arise in an organ from one specific cell type. The use of organ homogenates may obscure their metabolic competence by dilution with other existing cell populations.

4) *In vitro* assays do not account for pharmaco-kinetic parameters of absorption, distribution, and excretion.

5) Other factors (not related to pharmaco-kinetics and metabolism) can determine the species (organ and cell) specificity of a chemical carcinogen. Such factors could account for the difficulty in predicting target organs within an animal species, which is discussed later in the paper.

Carcinogen/Mutagen Activation by Human Liver (or Other Tissue) Enzymes

In vitro short-term assays are also useful in studies on species differences in pathways or rates of carcinogen metabolism using tissue fractions or cells from various human organs (in most cases, surgical liver biopsy specimens or autopsy material). Such data may be helpful in extrapolating from animal species to man when human tissues or cells are qualitatively or quantitatively compared with those from experimental animals. An increasing number of results (7) obtained with different classes of carcinogens (such as N-nitrosamines, aromatic amino and nitro compounds, PAHs, halogenated olefins, naturally occurring carcinogens and miscellaneous compounds, including drugs and cigarette smoke condensate) in the presence of various human liver microsomes or liver PMS have been shown to be converted into electrophilic metabolites that can react with DNA of the indicator organism (in many cases, S. typhimurium strains or V79 Chinese hamster cells). Other studies identified mutagenic metabolites in the urine of carcinogen- or mutagen-exposed human subjects, following incubation of the urinary metabolites in the presence or absence of deconjugating enzymes with or without metabolic activation (mostly liver PMS).

Some of our results are listed in Table 2. The enzymic capacities of liver PMS samples from different human subjects to convert 10 chemical carcinogens/mutagens into electrophiles are compared with that of rat and mouse liver. Results obtained with four heterocyclic N-nitrosamines, which are carcinogenic in animals (although to a variable extent) and to which humans may be exposed (22), and with vinyl chloride, indicated that all the human subjects were able to convert these carcinogens into alkylating and mutagenic intermediates. Although interindividual variations were observed, the average activity of the human samples was generally close to that of rat liver, with the exception of one compound: N-nitroso-N'-methylpiperazine.

The capacity of human liver specimens to activate metabolically N-nitrosamines and the other halo-olefins listed in Table 2, similar to that of the rodents, strengthens our suspicion that classes of carcinogens such as N-nitrosamines are possible carcinogenic hazards to man. Although great caution must be exercised when trying to extrapolate from data obtained in vitro to mechanisms in the intact organism, the validity of studies using human material in vitro for predicting susceptibility to carcinogens is, in fact, supported by the example of vinyl chloride. As can be seen in Table 2, the average activation capacity of all the human liver samples was close to that of rat liver, the principal target organ for vinyl chloride carcinogenicity (23).

Comparative studies on carcinogen metabolism with tissues from humans and from experimental animals have already revealed both interindividual and species differences. (For a review, see reference 10.) In our studies, a notable example was N-nitroso-N'-methylpiperazine, a weak carcinogen in rats, which was activated into mutagens seven times more efficiently by human liver mixed function oxidase (monooxygenase) system (MFO) (in some individuals up to 40 times) than by rat liver (see Table 2). In contrast, the metabolic capacity of human liver MFO to convert aflatoxin B_1 into its presumed mutagenic 2,3-oxide was <10% of rat liver, in keeping with other published results (24-26). Because the efficiency with which the liver of each animal species activates aflatoxin B_1 into mutagens corresponds to that species' susceptibility to the hepatocarcinogenic effect of these mycotoxins (12), such data may be useful in human risk assessment.

Table 2. Enzymic Capacities of Liver Samples from Humans to Convert Chemicals to Electrophilic Mutagens[a].

Compound	Type of Assay[b]	Source of Liver[c]	No. of Samples Tested	Mutagenic in Strain		Mutagenic Activity[d]			
						Revertants/μmol		Relative Activity (%)	
				TA1530	TA100	Range	Mean	Range	Mean
2-Chloro-1,3-butadiene	G	M			+		36		100
	G	Hu	3		+	0-8.4	2.8	0-20	7
1,4-Dichlorobutene-2	P	M			+		310		100
	P	Hu	3		+	52-260	110	12-84	46
Vinyl bromide	G	M			+		12		100
	G	Hu	3		+	2.7-4.3	3.6	22-36	30
Vinyl chloride	G	R		+			2.4		100
	G	Hu	18	+		0.5-5	2	20-220	84
Vinylidine chloride	G	M			+		9.3		100
	G	Hu	4		+	1-3.5	1.8	11-38	21
Aflatoxin B_1	P	R			+		8×10^6		100
	P	Hu	2		+	$(8-40) \times 10^4$	24×10^4	1-5	3
N-Nitroso-N'-methylpiperazine	P	R		+			3		100
	P	Hu	10	+		2-110	23	65-3660	754
N-Nitrosomorpholine	P	R		+			63		100
	P	Hu	13	+		2-84	27	5-110	43
	L	R		+			52		100
	L	Hu	8	+		0-93	43	0-180	83
N-Nitrosopiperidine	P	R		+			6		100
	P	Hu	3	+		5-13	10	80-210	156
N-Nitrosopyrrolidine	P	R		+			12		100
	P	Hu	3	+		6-14	10	50-115	85

[a]Samples were taken for diagnostic purposes or were surgical specimens (5).
[b]P: plate incorporation assay; G: plate assay to test volatile compounds or gases; L: liquid incubation assay.
[c]Samples from untreated rats (R), mice (M), or humans (Hu).
[d]Expressed as revertants/μmol for plate assays (P), as revertants/μmol/h of exposure for assays for gaseous compounds (G), or as revertants/μmol/ml/30 min of incubation for liquid assay (L). The number of revertants in each experiment is used to calculate % relative activity, with rodent liver as 100%.

Metabolic Activation of Carcinogens by Rodent Extrahepatic Tissue Fractions

Because of the widespread use of liver PMS in screening tests, two interrelated questions are often raised: What is the justification for using liver fractions in particular as the unique source of activation of chemical carcinogens, since all of these carcinogens by no means produce liver tumors in animals (or humans)? Can such assays using homogenates from different organs predict the target organ(s) of the carcinogen in a given animal species?

Studies aimed at investigating the possible relation between organ specificity of carcinogens and metabolic activation reactions *in situ* have revealed the versatility of mutagenicity assays as a research tool. Thus, studies have been made with subcellular fractions derived from numerous extrahepatic rodent tissues, many of which displayed a metabolic activation capacity for various carcinogens that could be detected in sensitive mutagenicity assays (see Table 3).

Mutagenicity studies on various carcinogens support the use of PMS from liver rather than from extrahepatic tissues as a first approximation of carcinogen metabolism *in vivo* by microsomal MFO and other enzymes. Although there are some exceptions, rodent extrahepatic tissue fractions did not produce higher mutagenic activity than did rodent liver fractions (when compared on a wet-weight organ basis) when different classes of precarcinogens such as N-nitrosamines, PAHs, and halo-olefins (see Table 4) were assayed. In addition, no evidence exists that the pathways whereby most carcinogens activated metabolically in rodent liver differ qualitatively from those in extrahepatic tissues. These comparative data, together with the common knowledge that liver enzymes are the most active in metabolizing foreign compounds, may explain why PMS-mediated mutagenicity tests using liver fractions are reliable in predicting that a chemical can be converted into electrophiles in the organism (and thus, in predicting its carcinogenic potential).

However, in many cases, such tests give no indication of the target organ(s) for carcinogenicity as exemplified by the class of PAH or some β-oxidized N-nitrosodipropyl derivatives (carcinogens that produce a spectrum of extrahepatic tumors in rodents, the type of tumor depending on the structure of the alkyl chain of the nitrosamine).

In vitro mutagenicity tests, using different organ homogenates from rats and hamsters for activation of the precarcinogens (27), gave little or no indication of extrahepatic target organs for carcinogenicity. With one exception (see Table 4), the relative

Table 3. Metabolic Activation of Carcinogens/Mutagens by Extrahepatic Tissue Fractions from Rats, Mice or Hamsters[a]

Subcellular Tissue Fraction[b]	Test Compounds
Lung	Benzo[a]pyrene 7,12-Dimethylbenz[a]anthracene 2-Acetylaminofluorene N-Nitrosodimethylamine N-Nitroso-di-n-propylamine; N-nitroso-propyl(2-hydroxypropyl)amine
Kidney	N-Nitrosodimethylamine Benzo[a]pyrene 7,12-Dimethylbenz[a]anthracene 2-Acetylaminofluorene N-Nitrosomethyl(acetoxymethyl)amine N-Nitroso-bis(2-acetoxypropyl)amine
Small intestine (mucosa)	N-Nitrosomethyl(acetoxymethyl)amine
Colon (mucosa)	Benzo[a]pyrene 2-Aminoanthracene 2-Aminofluorene
Pancreas	N-Nitrosodimethylamine N-Nitroso-bis(2-oxopropyl)amine
Placenta	7,12-Dimethylbenz[a]anthracene 2-Acetylaminofluorene
Skin	Benzo[a]pyrene 7,8-dihydrodiol
Brain	Benzo[a]pyrene 7,12-Dimethylbenz[a]anthracene 2-Acetylaminofluorene
Spleen	N-Nitrosomethyl(acetoxymethyl)amine

[a]Using the *Salmonella* mutagenicity assay (adapted from reference 7).
[b]Either postmitochondrial tissue supernatant or purified microsomes.

Table 4. Activation of Chemicals into Bacterial Mutagens by Hepatic and Extrahepatic Tissue Fractions

Chemical	Relative Mutagenicities with Liver:Kidney:Lung S9[a]		
	Hamster	Rat	Mouse
N-Nitroso-di-n-propylamine and β-oxidized derivatives	100:0:$\leq$3[b]	100:0:0[b]	n.a.
N-nitroso-di(2-acetoxypropyl)amine	100:7:95	100:0:0	n.a.
Vinyl chloride	n.a.	100:10:$\leq$9	100:20:$\leq$7[b]
Vinylidene chloride	n.a.	100:17:10[c]	100:20:6[c]

[a]Compared as revertants/μmol/mg wet organ weight (liver = 100).
[b]Strain TA1530 (phenobarbitone-treated animals) (27,28).
[c]Strain TA100 (untreated animals) (11).

carcinogen-activating capacity, when expressed on a wet-weight organ basis, was always highest with liver fractions, although the tissue was often not affected by tumor growth.

PAHs are another example of carcinogens that, in general, do not affect rodent liver as a target organ, yet they are easily activated by liver PMS to mutagenic metabolites such as BP (see Table 5). In some of our recent studies (29), mouse epidermal microsomal preparations apparently converted BP 7,8-diol into mutagens in a manner similar to rat liver, even though the BP hydroxylase (AHH) activity of the rat liver preparations was 40-fold higher than that of similar mouse epidermal fractions (see Table 5). The precise reasons for this high efficiency are not clear; the relative amounts of cytochromes P450 and P448 may vary between liver and epidermis, and the enzymes in the two tissues may differ qualitatively. These may be in the susceptibility of mouse skin and the comparative resistance of rat liver to the carcinogenic effects of PAH. Thus, it appears that results from _in vitro_ assays using subcellular tissue fractions for activation of precarcinogens do not reliably predict the extrahepatic organ-specific action of carcinogens. Their predictive value may be limited by the same factors that determine whether a tissue will develop in a particular animal species. Some of the difficulties can be circumvented by the use of intact mammalian cells (or

Table 5. Microsome-Mediated Mutagenicity of BP 7,8-Diol in *S. typhimurium* TA100[a] and Comparative Aryl Hydrocarbon BP Hydroxylase Activities[b].

Source of Microsomes[c]	Hydrocarbon Treatment (nmol/Animal[d])	AAH Activity[e]	Microsome-Mediated Mutagenicity[f]	Relative Activity[g]
Rat liver	none	3730	2160	100
Mouse skin	none	90	1700	79
	7,12-dimethylbenz[a]anthracene (50)	250	2830	131
	Benz[a]anthracene (50)	180	3000	140

[a]In the presence of microsomes from rat liver or mouse skin.
[b]Adapted from reference 29.
[c]Prepared either from untreated or from PAH-treated rodents.
[d]Applied to the shaved dorsal skin as a solution in acetone (100 μl).
[e]pmol of 3-hydroxybenzo[a]pyrene/mg microsomal protein/10 min.
[f]His^+ revertants/μM of BP 7,8-diol/mg microsomal protein; the values were calculated from the dose-response curves at a substrate concentration of 2.5 μM or from results obtained in assays that were performed in the presence of 0.14-0.28 mg of rat liver or of 0.15-0.18 mg of mouse-skin microsomal protein. The number of revertants occurring in the absence of an NADPH-generating system, but in the presence of the microsomes, have been subtracted from each value listed.
[g]Relative mutagenicity with results obtained with rat liver as 100.

host-mediated assays) as a source of activation that allows easier investigation of the cell or tissue specificity of chemical carcinogens (30,31). But even by including these more sophisticated techniques, it seems unlikely that they would have predicted the neurotropic carcinogenic action of 3,3-dimethyl-1-phenyltriazene (see below).

Multiple-Step Metabolic Activation Processes

For many of the carcinogens (mentioned earlier in the paper) requiring metabolic activation, the site of their tumorigenic action appears to be partly determined by the final concentration of ultimate metabolites available for reaction with cellular macromolecules *in situ*, resulting from the critical balance between activation and detoxification of the chemical *in vivo*. Thus, the chemico-physical properties of these ultimate metabolites (i.e., their half-lives, their ability to react either by uni- or bi-molecular nucleophilic substitution, and the partition coefficients between biological fluids and cell compartments where they are generated) are parameters that influence binding reactions with cellular macromolecules, and are thus expected to govern the species- and organ-specific carcinogenicity (32).

An alternative mechanism by which some chemical carcinogens may exert their organ-specific action is metabolic activation by multi-step processes involving the formation of proximate carcinogenic metabolites (free or conjugated) in the liver. These relatively stable compounds could be transported to remote tissues and eventually, by deconjugation and reactivation or by non-enzymic reaction, could yield ultimate carcinogens. Such a mechanism is supported by experimental data for 3,3-dimethyl-1-phenyltriazene. This carcinogen induces tumors in extrahepatic tissues, preferentially in the central and peripheral nervous systems or kidneys (33-35). Previous studies have shown that this compound is metabolically activated by oxidative N-demethylation in the liver (36-38), a non-target organ, to yield 3-methyl-1-phenyltriazene, which is a direct-acting, alkylating, mutagenic and carcinogenic agent that is unstable in aqueous media (36,39,40). No such similar reaction was observed with brain slices (P. Kleihues, personal communication, University of Freiburg, Federal Republic of Germany) and brain homogenates (37). Consequently, 3-methyl-1-phenyltriazene has been proposed, but not equivocally confirmed, as the active metabolite of 3,3-dimethyl-1-phenyltriazene. Activation of the parent compound in the liver and migration of an intermediate (3-methyl-1-phenyltriazene) to distant organs was supported by the following data from work done in collaboration with G. Kolar (German Cancer Research Center, Heidelberg, Federal Republic of Germany):

1) After incubation of 3,3-dimethyl-1-phenyltriazene with rat liver microsomes, a mutagen intermediate previously shown to be the monomethyl derivative was released (36,37).

2) The synthetic monomethyl was shown to be mutagenic in *Salmonella* strains in the absence of any metabolic activation system and was not enzymatically inactivated by rat liver PMS.

3) The monomethyl triazene had a half-life of 1.13 min at neutrality (32). This would be long enough to allow such a compound, formed in the liver, to be transported by the bloodstream to the brain.

4) Finally, strong support for the theory that monomethyltriazene can alkylate brain tissue was obtained in a study in which (C^{14}-monomethyl)1-phenyltriazene was injected subcutaneously into rats (41).

Many tissues, including brain and liver, were alkylated, thus demonstrating that the half-life *in vivo* of monomethyltriazene is sufficiently long to allow its distribution throughout the organism. In addition, the ratio of DNA:RNA alkylation in liver was similar to that found 8 h after administration of the parent 3,3-dimethyl-1-phenyltriazene (42). In DNA, 3-methyladenine and N7- and O^6-methylguanine were found. The latter products were also found by Kleihues et al. (42) after administration of the 3,3-dimethyl-1-phenyltriazene. Most important, the O^6- and N7-methylguanine ratio found 8 h after injection of the labeled monomethyltriazene was lowest in the liver (0.08), indicating a higher rate of O^6-methylguanine removal; the ratio was highest in the brain (0.15), the principal target organ of the parent triazene, indicating a lower capacity of removal of this miscoding DNA lesion. Although only one time interval was investigated, it appears that 3-methyl-1-phenyltriazene is the alkylating species released in the body from parent dimethyl compound. These findings with 3-methyl-1-phenyltriazene are in agreement with earlier results on the persistence of alkylated mucleic acid bases in rat tissues after administration of nitrosomethyl- or nitrosoethylurea, for example, for which the brain is also a major target organ (43,44).

Thus, the organ specificity of the closely related carcinogens N-dimethylnitrosamine and 3,3-dimethyl-1-phenyltriazene (both are believed to yield a methylating agent as ultimate carcinogen) is partly determined by the half-lives of the proximate carcinogenic metabolites released, which prevent their distribution in the body by covalent reactions with organs or cells in which they are generated. In the case of the nitrosamine, a half-life of ⩽5 sec has been estimated (45). In contrast, for the closely related compound 3,3-dimethyl-1-phenyltriazene, metabolic activation in the liver leads to 3-methyl-1-phenyltriazene, whose half-life (1.13 min) appears long enough to permit its distribution in the body and to the brain. Persistence of certain alkylated bases in DNA may finally determine which organ is affected by tumor growth.

Carcinogens Detected as Mutagens Using Cell- and Host-Mediated but Not Liver PMS-Mediated Assays

Validation studies of the liver PMS-mediated mutagenicity assays for the detection of chemical carcinogens have shown that certain carcinogens are not revealed as mutagens (false-negative compounds). This inability to predict the carcinogenic potential of certain compounds may arise from the use of liver 9000*g* supernatant. This metabolic activation system may be inefficient in producing mutagenic metabolites from precarcinogens at concentrations high enough to be detected. In our own and published studies, three such carcinogenic chemicals, N-nitrosodiethylamine (46), 1,2-dimethylhydrazine (1), and procarbazine (47), were not detected as bacterial mutagens with rodent liver PMS-mediated mutagenicity assays in *Salmonella*. Nitramine was shown to be mutagenic in host-mediated assays (46) and 1,2-dimethylhydrazine and procarbazine were shown to be mutagenic in rat hepatocyte-mediated assays. These results support the view that these carcinogens are DNA-damaging agents. The 1,2-dimethylhydrazine and procarbazine were previously found to be mutagenic in host-mediated assays in rodents and to induce recessive lethal mutations in *Drosophila melanogaster* (48,49).

These data demonstrate the need to use mammalian cells or the intact organism for activation of chemicals as complementary systems to detect genotoxic carcinogens affecting the liver or extrahepatic organs as well as to predict their species- or site-specific action.

ACKNOWLEDGMENTS

Research activities were partially supported by contract NO1 CP 55630 with the National Cancer Institute, USA. The authors are grateful to Ms. M.M. Courcier for her skilled secretarial assistance.

REFERENCES

1. McCann, J., E. Choi, E. Yamasaki, and B.N. Ames. 1975. Detection of carcinogens as mutagens in the Salmonella/microsome test: Assay of 300 chemicals. Proc. Natl. Acad. Sci. USA 72:5135-5139.

2. Sugimura, T., S. Sato, M. Nagao, T. Yahagi, T. Matsushima, Y. Seino, M. Takeuchi, and T. Kawachi. 1976. Overlapping of carcinogens and mutagens. In: Fundamentals in Cancer Prevention. P.N. Magee, ed. University of Tokyo Press/University Park Press: Tokyo/Baltimore. pp. 191-215.

3. Purchase, I.F.H., E. Longstaff, J. Ashby, J.A. Styles, D. Anderson, P.A. Lefevre, and F.R. Westwood. 1978. An evaluation of 6 short-term tests for detecting organic chemical carcinogens. Brit. J. Cancer 37:873-959.

4. Hollstein, M., J. McCann, F.A. Angelosanto, and W.W. Nichols. 1979. Short-term tests for carcinogens and mutagens. Mutat. Res. 65:132-226.

5. Bartsch, H., C. Malaveille, A.M. Camus, G. Martel-Planche, G. Brun, A. Hautefeuille, N. Sabadie, A. Barbin, T. Kuroki, C. Drevon, G. Piccoli, and R. Montesano. 1980. Validation and comparative studies on 180 chemicals with S. typhimurium strains and V79 Chinese hamster cells in the presence of various metabolizing systems. Mutat. Res. 76:1-50.

6. Miller, E.C. 1978. Some current perspectives on chemical carcinogenesis in humans and experimental animals. Cancer Res. 38:1479-1496.

7. Bartsch, H., T. Kuroki, M. Roberfroid, and C. Malaveille. (in press). Metabolic activation systems in vitro for carcinogen/mutagen screening tests. In: Chemical Mutagens - Principles and Methods for Their Detection, Volume 7. Plenum Press: New York & London.

8. Nagao, M., T. Yahagi, Y. Seino, T. Sugimura, and N. Ito. 1977. Mutagenicities of quinoline and its derivatives. Mutat. Res. 42:335-342.

9. Legator, M.S., and H.V. Malling. 1971. The host-mediated assay, a practical procedure for evaluating potential mutagenic agents in mammals. In: Chemical Mutagens, Volume 2. A. Hollaender, ed. Plenum Press: New York & London. pp. 569-588.

10. Conney, A.H., and W. Levin. 1974. Carcinogen metabolism in experimental animals and man. In: Chemical Carcinogenesis Essays, IARC Scientific Publications No. 10. R. Montesano, and L. Tomatis, eds. International Agency for Research on Cancer: Lyons, France. pp. 3-24.

11. Bartsch, H., C. Malaveille, R. Montesano, and L. Tomatis. 1975. Tissue-mediated mutagenicity of vinylidene chloride and 2-chlorobutadiene in Salmonella typhimurium. Nature 255:641-643.

12. Hsieh, D.P.H., J.J. Wong, Z.A. Wong, C. Michas, and B.H. Ruebner. 1977. Hepatic transformation of aflatoxin and its carcinogenicity. In: Origins of Human Cancer. H.H. Hiatt, J.D. Watson & J.A. Winsten, eds. Cold Spring Harbor Laboratory: Cold Spring Harbor, NY. pp. 697-707.

13. Wirth, P.J., E. Dybing, C. von Bahr, and S.S. Thorgeirsson. 1980. Mechanism of N-hydroxyacetylarylamine mutagenicity in the Salmonella test system: Metabolic activation of N-hydroxyphenacetin by liver and kidney fractions from rat, mouse, hamster, and man. Molec. Pharmacol. 18:117-127.

14. Matsushima, T., T. Yahagi, Y. Takamoato, M. Nagao, and T. Sugimura. 1980. Species differences in microsomal activation of mutagens and carcinogens, with special reference to new potent mutagens from pyrolysates of amino acids and proteins. In: Microsomes, Drug Oxidations and Chemical Carcinogenesis. M.J. Coon, A.H. Conney, R.W. Estabrook, H.V. Gelboin, J.R. Gillette, and J. O'Brien, eds. Academic Press: New York. pp. 1093-1102.

15. Shudo, K., T. Ohta, Y. Orihara, T. Okamoto, M. Nagaa, Y. Takahashi, and T. Sugimura. 1978. Mutgenicities of phenacetin and its metabolites. Mutat. Res. 58:367-370.

16. Weeks, C.E., W.T. Allaben, N.M. Tresp, S.C. Louie, E.J. Lazear, and C.M. King. 1980. Effects of structure of N-acyl-N-2-fluorenylhydroxylamines on arylhydroxamic acid acyltransferase, sulfotransferase, and deacylase activities and on mutations in Salmonella typhimurium TA1538. Cancer Res. 40:1204-1211.

17. Ames, B.N., J. McCann, and E. Yamasaki. 1975. Methods for detecting carcinogens and mutagens with the Salmonella/mammalian-microsome mutagenicity test. Mutat. Res. 31:347-364.

18. McGregor, D. 1975. The relationship of 2-acetamidofluorene mutagenicity in plate tests with its in vivo liver cell component distribution and its carcinogenic potential. Mutat. Res. 30:305-316.

19. Selkirk, J.K. 1977. Divergence of metabolic activation systems for short-term mutagenesis assays. Nature 270:604-607.

20. Bigger, C.A.H., J.E. Thomaszewski, and A. Dipple. 1978. Differences between products of binding of 7,12-dimethylbenz[a]anthracene to DNA in mouse skin and in rat liver microsomal system. Biochem. Biophys. Res. Comm. 80:229-235.

21. Bartsch, H., C. Malaveille, B. Tierney, P.L. Grover, and P. Sims. 1979. The association of bacterial mutagenicity of hydrocarbon-derived 'bay-region' dihydrodiols with the Iball indices for carcinogenicity and with the extents of DNA-binding on mouse skin of the parent hydrocarbons. Chem.-Biol. Interact. 26:185-196.

22. IARC. 1978. Some N-nitroso compounds. In: IARC Monographs on the Evaluation of Carcinogenic Risk of Chemicals to Humans, Volume 17. International Agency for Research on Cancer: Lyons, France.

23. IARC. 1979. Some monomers, plastics and synthetic elastomers and acrolein. In: IARC Monographs on the Evaluation of Carcinogenic Risk of Chemicals to Humans, Volume 19. International Agency for Research on Cancer: Lyons, France.

24. Buening, M.K., J.G. Fortner, A. Kappas, and A.H. Conney. 1978. 7,8-Benzoflavone stimulates the metabolic activation of aflatoxin B_1 to mutagens by human liver. Biochem. Biophys. Res. Comm. 82:348-355.

25. Tang, T., and M.A. Friedman. 1977. Carcinogen activation by human liver enzymes in the Ames mutagenicity test. Mutat. Res. 46:387-394.

26. Sabadie, N., C. Malaveille, A.M. Camus, and H. Bartsch. 1980. Comparison of the hydroxylation of benzo[a]pyrene with the metabolism of vinyl chloride N-nitrosomorpholine and N-nitroso-N'-methylpiperazine to mutagens by human and rat liver microsomal fractions. Cancer Res. 40:119-126.

27. Camus, A., B. Bertram, F.W. Kruger, C. Malaveille, and H. Bartsch. 1976. Mutagenicity of β-oxidized N,N-di-n-propylnitrosamine derivatives in S. typhimurium mediated by rat and hamster tissues. Z. Krebsforsch. 86:293-302.

28. Bartsch, H., C. Malaveille, and R. Montesano. 1975. Human, rat and mouse liver-mediated mutagenicity of vinyl chloride in S. typhimurium strains. Int. J. Cancer 15:429-437.

29. Camus, A.M., W.G. Pyerin, P.L. Grover, P. Sims, C. Malaveille, and H. Bartsch. 1980. Mutagenicity of benzo[a]pyrene 7,8-dihydrodiol, and 7,12-dimethylbenz[a]anthracene 3,4-dihydrodiol in S. typhimurium mediated by microsomes from rat liver and mouse skin. Chem.-Biol. Interact. 32:257-265.

30. Langenbach, R., H.J. Freed, and E. Huberman. 1978. Liver cell-mediated mutagenesis of mammalian cells by liver carcinogens. Proc. Nat. Acad. Sci. USA 75:2864-2867.

31. Langenbach, R., H.J. Freed, D. Raveh, and E. Huberman. 1978. Cell specificity in metabolic activation of aflatoxin B_1 and benzo[a]pyrene to mutagens for mammalian cells. Nature 276:277-280.

32. Bartsch, H., G.P. Margison, C. Malaveille, A.M. Camus, G. Brun, J.M. Margison, G.F. Kolar, and M. Wiessler. 1977. Some aspects of metabolic activation of chemical carcinogens in relation to their organ specificity. Arch. Toxicol. 39:51-63.

33. Druckrey, H.S., S. Ivankovic, and R. Preussman. 1967. Neurotrope carcinogene Wirkung von Phenyl-dimethyltriazen an Ratten. Naturwissenschaften 54:171.

34. Preussmann, R., H. Druckrey, S. Ivankovic, and A. von Hodenberg. 1969. Chemical structure and carcinogenicity of aliphatic hydrazo, azo, and azoxy compounds, and of triazenes, potential in vivo alkylating agents. Ann. N.Y. Acad. Sci. 81:285-310.

35. Preussman, R., S. Ivankovic, C. Landschutz, J. Gimmy, E. Flohr, and U. Griesbach. 1974. Carcinogene Wirkung von 13 Aryldialkyltriazenen an BD-Ratten. Z. Krebsforsch. 81:285-310.

36. Preussmann, R., A. von Hodenberg, and H. Hengy. 1969. Mechanisms of carcinogenesis with 1-aryl-3,3-dialkyltriazenes. Enzymatic dealkylation by rat liver microsomal fractions in vitro. Biochem. Pharmacol. 18:1-13.

37. Malaveille, C., G.F. Kolar, and H. Bartsch. 1976. Rat and mouse tissue-mediated mutagenicity of ring-substituted 3,3-dimethyl-1-phenyltriazenes in Salmonella typhimurium. Mutat. Res. 36:1-10.

38. Giraldi, T., C. Nisi, and G. Sava. 1975. Investigation on the oxidative N-demethylation of aryl triazenes in vitro. Biochem. Pharmacol. 24:1793-1797.

39. Preussman, R., and A. von Hodenberg. 1970. Mechanism of carcinogenesis with 1-aryl-3,3-dialkyltriazenes. Biochem. Pharmacol. 19:1505-1507.

40. Ong, T.M., and F.J. deSerres. 1973. Genetic characterization of ad-3 mutants induced by chemical carcinogens 1-phenyl-3,3-dimethyltriazene and 1-phenyl-3-monomethyltriazene in Neurospora crassa. Mutat. Res. 20:17-23.

41. Margison, G.P., A.J. Likhachev, and G.F. Kolar. 1979. In vivo alkylation of fetal, maternal and normal rat tissue nucleic acids by 3-methyl-1-phenyltriazene. Chem.-Biol. Interact. 25:345-357.

42. Kleihues, P., G.F. Kolar, and G.P. Margison. 1976. Interaction of the carcinogen 3,3-dimethyl-1-phenyltriazene with nucleic acids of various rat tissues and the effect of a protein-free diet. Cancer Res. 36:2189-2193.

43. Goth, R., and M.F. Rajewsky. 1974. Molecular and cellular mechanisms associated with pulse-carcinogenesis in the rat nervous system by ethylnitrosourea: Ethylation of nucleic acids and elimination rates of ethylated bases from the DNA of different tissues. Z. Krebsforsch. 82:37-64.

44. Kleihues, P., and G.P. Margison. 1974. Carcinogenicity of N-methyl-N-nitrosourea: Possible role of excision repair of O^6-methylguanine from DNA. J. Nat. Cancer Inst. 53:1839-1841.

45. Jenssen, D., B. Beije, and C. Ramel. 1979. Mutagenicity testing on Chinese hamster V79 cells treated in the in vivo liver perfusion system. Comparative investigation of different in vitro metabolizing systems with dimethylnitrosamine and benzo[a]pyrene. Chem.-Biol. Interact. 27:27-39.

46. Khudoley, V., C. Malaveille, and H. Bartsch. 1981. Mutagenicity studies in *S. typhimurium* on some carcinogenic N-nitramines *in vitro* and in the host-mediated assay in rats. Cancer Res. 41:3205-3210.

47. Lee, I.P., and R.L. Dixon. 1978. Mutagenicity, carcinogenicity, and teratogenicity of procarbazine. Mutat. Res. 55:1-14.

48. Moriya, M., K. Kato, T. Ohta, K. Watanabe, Y. Watanabe, and Y. Shirasu. 1978. Detection of mutagenicity of the powerful colon carcinogen 1,2-dimethylhydrazine (DMH) by host-mediated assay and its inhibition by disulfiram. Mutat. Res. 54:244-245.

49. Blijleven, W.G.H., and E. Vogen. 1977. The mutational spectrum of procarbazine in *Drosophila melanogaster*. Mutat. Res. 45:47-59.

DISCUSSION

Dr. Bartsch was unable to attend the meeting and, therefore, the paper was not available for discussion.

CELL-MEDIATED MUTAGENESIS, AN APPROACH TO STUDYING ORGAN SPECIFICITY OF CHEMICAL CARCINOGENS

Robert Langenbach and Stephen Nesnow

Carcinogenesis and Metabolism Branch, Genetic Toxicology Division, Health Effects Research Laboratory, U.S. Environmental Protection Agency, Research Triangle Park, North Carolina 27711

INTRODUCTION

We have been interested in developing *in vitro* systems in which the organ and species specificity of chemical carcinogens can be studied (1-6). The phenomena of species, organ, sex, and age specificity in response to chemical carcinogens pose an intriguing problem and may be important for the extrapolation of *in vivo* and *in vitro* carcinogenesis data to humans. Many carcinogens exist in the environment in nonreactive form and must be metabolically activated to manifest their biological activity (7,8).

A number of approaches have been employed to elucidate the causes of organ and species specificity (8-15). In the earlier studies, homogenates of various tissues were used to metabolically activate the chemical (9-12); however, metabolite profiles, DNA-adduct profiles, and induced mutagenic responses of cell homogenates differ from those of intact cells (16-19). More recent studies have looked at the nature of carcinogen metabolites and DNA-adducts formed in cells or tissues or at the nature and persistence of DNA-adducts in *in vivo* tissues (15). Differences in the results from these various approaches are apparent. In addition, the nature and amount of DNA-adducts are only correlated with the biological response expected in the tissue. The ability to measure a biological response from a system as well as parameters such as chemical metabolism, DNA adducts, DNA repair, etc., would provide a useful system for elucidating some of the biological mechanisms leading to the phenomena of specificity.

In the approach described here, intact cells are obtained from adult male rat liver, lung, bladder, and kidney by enzymatic dispersion, and the cells are cocultivated with Chinese hamster V79 cells in the presence of the chemical (1-6). The mutation of the V79 cells from ouabain or 6-thioguanine (TG) sensitivity to resistance then indicates the production of mutagenic/carcinogenic metabolites of the chemical. The V79 cells alone cannot activate the chemicals being studied; therefore, the production of mutagenic intermediates reflects the specificities of activation of the different primary cell types. By using this approach, factors other than metabolism believed to be important in determining organ or species specificities (24) such as DNA repair, nature of DNA-adducts, cell uptake of the chemical, etc., can also be studied and correlated with the mutagenesis endpoint.

In the present report, carcinogens from three classes of chemicals were studied for mutagenic activity with the primary cells from the four organs: liver, lung, kidney, and bladder. The metabolism of the carcinogen benzo[*a*]pyrene (BP) was studied in detail in all cell systems by high pressure liquid chromatography (HPLC), while nitrosodimethylamine (DMN) metabolism was investigated in the liver and lung system. An attempt was made to correlate metabolism with mutagenic activities and also to correlate cell-mediated mutagenesis data with *in vivo* carcinogenesis data.

MATERIALS AND METHODS

Six- to ten-week-old male Sprague-Dawley rats were the source of the primary liver, lung, kidney, and bladder cells. Methods for preparing liver, lung, and bladder cells were reported previously (1-4). Kidney cells were dissociated enzymatically for 1.5 h at 37°C from minced kidney tissue with 0.13% trypsin and 0.01% EDTA containing 50 units/ml of collagenase. All primary cell types were more than 90% viable at the time of seeding. The medium used was Williams Medium E plus 10% heat-inactivated fetal bovine serum supplemented with 2 mM L-glutamine, penicillin (100 units/ml) and streptomycin (100 μg/ml). Cells were maintained at 37°C in humidified incubators with an atmosphere of 5% CO_2 in air.

The protocols for the mutation studies were reported previously (1-4). The background mutation frequency was 1 mutant/10^6 survivors for ouabain and $\leq$3 mutants/10^6 survivors for TG. The expression time was 2 days for ouabain resistance and 6 days for TG (2,6).

The BP and DMN metabolism studies were carried out as previously reported (2).

RESULTS

The basic protocols for carrying out the cell-mediated mutagenesis studies were reported previously (1-6). Figure 1 shows schematically how the hepatocyte or bladder cell-mediated V79 cell mutagenesis systems are performed. Due to slower attachment, the lung and kidney cells are seeded first and allowed to attach, followed by the V79 cells. In all the systems, however, the ratio of activating cells to V79 cells is about 3:1 or 4:1. Using the hepatocyte system as an example (see Figure 1), the hepatocytes attach on top of the V79 cells, forming a near monolayer. The medium is then changed to fresh medium containing the chemical, and the cocultivation is continued for 48 h. The cells are then reseeded to determine toxicity and mutation to the V79 cells. The activating cells do not reattach and grow in this procedure. In this system, the liver cell metabolizes the chemical to a reactive intermediate that is then transported, presumably via cell-to-cell junctions to the V79 cells, which are mutated. A proximity between the activating cell and the target cells may be a prerequisite for the occurrence of mutagenesis, although the more stable the intermediate or reactive form, the greater the distance it can transverse.

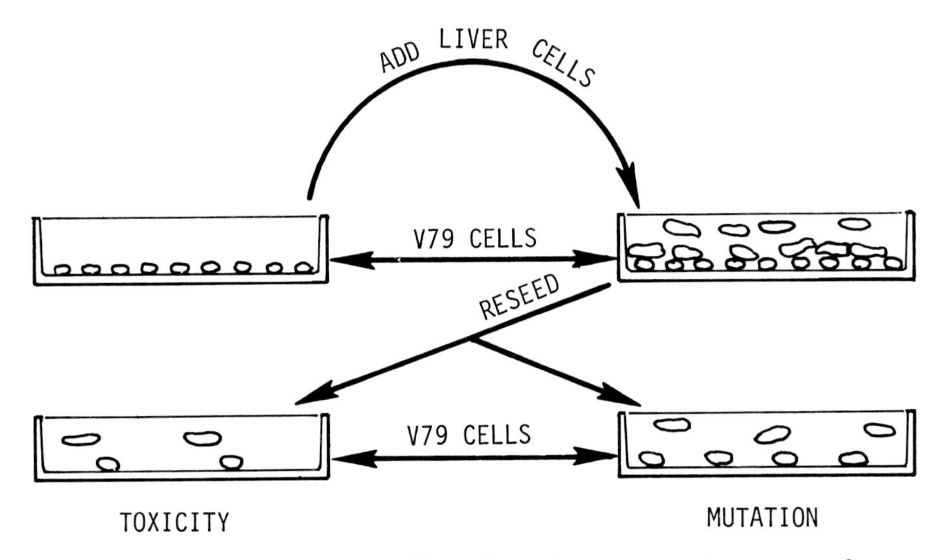

Figure 1. Diagram of cell-mediated mutagenesis protocol.

Interestingly, the hepatocyte to V79 cell arrangement shown in Figure 1 may be an _in vitro_ model for the events that occur _in vivo_ during the initiation of transformation or mutation. In other words, the differentiated cell (hepatocyte, in this instance) has the metabolic capabilities to carry out the tissues' metabolic functions, but lacks or has limited replicative capabilities. The less well differentiated cells, including stem cells (represented by the V79 cells) that possibly have less metabolic capabilities but can replicate, are arranged in proximity to the differentiated cells. Therefore, _in vivo_, the terminally differentiated cells metabolize the xenobiotic, and the activated intermediates are transported to the stem cells. The mutated or transformed stem cells on replication could give rise to the mutant colony or tumor. Such a phenomenon could also explain the long known difficulty in mutating or transforming differentiated cells from adult animal tissues _in vitro_.

The data in Table 1 summarize our initial studies to investigate the cell type specificity in the activation of chemical carcinogens. BP, a potent skin and lung carcinogen capable of also producing fibrosarcomas, and aflatoxin B_1 (AFB_1), a potent liver carcinogen, were studied for mutagenic activity in the rat embryonic fibroblast- and the adult rat hepatocyte-mediated mutagenesis system. BP was mutagenic in the embryonic fibroblast-mediated system, while in the hepatocyte-mediated system, no significant increase in mutagenic activity was observed with up to 3 μg/ml BP. In contrast, AFB_1 was not mutagenic in the fibroblast-mediated system but was mutagenic in the hepatocyte-mediated system. These studies established that a cell type specificity could be observed _in vitro_, which agreed with the _in vivo_ tumorigenic response of the two cell types.

Table 1. Mutagenic Activities of BP and AFB_1 in the Hepatocyte- and Embryonic Fibroblast-Mediated Mutagenesis System

Activating Cell	Chemical	Mutants/10^6 Survivors
None	--	1
Liver	BP	2
Liver	AFB_1	39
Fibroblasts	BP	96
Fibroblasts	AFB_1	2

We had two major concerns about this initial study. First, we were comparing mixed embryonic cells to cells from an adult animal organ. Secondly, fibroblasts were being compared to epithelial cells for activation potential, while the majority of tumors in man and animals arise in the epithelium of various organs. In an attempt to overcome the limitations of our initial approach, we began to develop a method for conducting cell-mediated mutagenesis studies with epithelial cells from various adult tissues (1,2,5,6). The data in Table 2 show the relative mutagenic activity of three potent chemical carcinogens in the liver, lung, bladder, and kidney cell-mediated mutagenesis systems. All of these studies used primary cultures of intact cells from the respective organs, and the cultures were predominantly of epithelial-like cells. As can be seen in Table 2, the noncarcinogenic hydrocarbon anthracene was not mutagenic in any of the cell-mediated systems. In the liver cell-mediated system, BP was inactive as indicated above, while 7,12-dimethylbenz[a]anthracene (DMBA) was somewhat mutagenic, and DMN was highly mutagenic in this system. By contrast in the lung cell-mediated system, the two hydrocarbons were mutagenic, while DMN was inactive. The kidney cells were able to activate the two hydrocarbons and the nitrosamine. Likewise, cells from the bladder epithelium activated all three carcinogens. The data in Table 2 are expressed as fold increase over background per 1.5×10^6 activating cells. For the liver and lung cell systems, ouabain, which gave a background of 1 mutant/10^6 surviving V79 cells (2), was used as the selective agent. However, for the kidney and bladder cell-mediated systems (6), TG was used as the selective agent, and the spontaneous frequency was 3×10^6 mutant/10^6 surviving V79 cells. We reported previously that by applying this method for certain chemicals, the relative activities can be compared even when different selective agents are used (19). However, the generality of this approach has yet to be determined.

Table 2. Relative Mutagenic Activities in the Rat Cell-Mediated Mutagenesis Systems

		Activating Cell Type			
Chemical	(μg/ml)	Liver	Lung	Kidney	Bladder
Anthracene	(3)	1	1	1	1
BP	(1)	2	56	5	6
DMBA	(1)	14	154	12	21
DMN	(100)	95	2	19	11

Having determined the mutagenic activities of the carcinogens in the various cell-mediated systems, we looked at carcinogen metabolism to determine if correlations between metabolism and mutagenesis could be discerned. The metabolism of BP was accomplished by HPLC analysis, and the metabolism of DMN was determined by CO_2 production (2).

The HPLC profiles of BP metabolism for primary cells were reported previously (1,2,6). All cell lines produce metabolites that are organically soluble or are conjugated to glucuronic acid or sulfate (2,6). The data in Table 3 show the amounts of three types of metabolites produced by the primary cells in culture. These particular metabolites were chosen for discussion here because of their potential involvement in the transformation or mutation process. The pre-9,10-diols constitute the early eluting fraction from the HPLC and presumably contain tetrols, triols, and other oxygenated metabolites, some of which probably at one stage in their metabolism were intermediates that could have reacted with cellular macromolecules. The BP-4,5-diol probably results from the BP-4,5-oxide, a species also capable of interacting with cellular constituents, although the 4,5-diol itself is inactive or weakly active as a mutagen to V79 cells (19). The BP-7,8-diol is a precursor to the BP-7,8-diol-9,10-epoxide, the presumed active metabolite of BP known (20). As can be seen in Table 3, the order of pre-9,10-diol production is lung > liver > bladder > kidney, which also is the order of total BP metabolism, including conjugates. The liver produces the greatest amount of the BP-4,5-diol. The BP-7,8-diol, thought to be a precursor to the most important biological metabolite, is formed mostly in the lung, the cell type where BP was also most mutagenic. Bladder and kidney cells, which also activate BP to mutagenic intermediates, produce significant levels of the 7,8-diol. However, liver cells, which do not activate BP to mutagenic intermediates, also produced the 7,8-diol. Therefore, the absolute amount of the BP-7,8-diol produced does not directly correlate with the mutagenic response in the cell-mediated systems.

The data in Table 4 show the metabolism of DMN by liver and lung cells. The DMN metabolism studies were carried out with cells from the two tissues immediately after their isolation, so that loss of enzyme capability due to isolation should have been minimized. DMN was metabolized to CO_2 by the liver cells (Table 4). However, lung cells, which did not metabolize DMN to mutagenic intermediates, also did not metabolize the DMN to detectable levels of CO_2. The lack of DMN metabolism by lung cells may account for its lack of mutagenicity in the lung cell-mediated system.

Table 3. BP-Diol Metabolites Formed by Liver, Lung, Bladder, and Kidney Cells

Cell Type	pmoles Formed/48 h/10 ^{6} Cells		
	Pre-9,10-diol	4,5-diol	7,8-diol
Lung	4870	90	750
Liver	2320	217	212
Bladder	2655	108	415
Kidney	765	50	115

Table 4. Metabolism of DMN to CO_2 by Liver and Lung Cells

Time (h)	DPM/10 ^{6} Cells	
	Liver	Lung
3	15,000[a]	ND[b]
6	41,000	ND

[a]DMN at 100 µg/ml, data approximately 1 and 3% metabolism at the respective times.
[b]ND, not detectable.

The data in Table 5 indicate that the cell-mediated mutagenesis approach can also be used to study species differences in the activation of chemical carcinogens. The data indicate that hamster hepatocytes are between three and four times as active at metabolizing DMN to mutagenic intermediates as are rat hepatocytes.

Table 5. Species Differences in the Activation of DMN to Mutagenic Intermediates[a]

Species	Mutants/10^6 Survivors
Control	1
Rat	95
Hamster	320

[a]DMN was used at 100 μg/ml.

DISCUSSION

The data reported herein suggest that the cell-mediated mutagenesis approach may be useful for studying some aspects of the organ and species specificity of chemical carcinogens. In Table 6 we compared the relative carcinogenic activities of the chemicals to their relative mutagenic activities in the cell-mediated system. As can be seen in Table 6, there is general agreement in the activities between the *in vivo* and *in vitro* results. The relative carcinogenic activities for liver, lung, and kidney, was assigned from literature references (21-24); rodent bladder carcinogenesis data with these chemicals are limited. DMBA has been reported to cause focal hyperplasia and papillomas in the bladder (21) and to transform bladder epithelial cells in organ culture (25). The finding that bladder epithelial cells can activate DMN is important, given its presence in urine of humans with certain types of urinary tract infections (26). While DMN has not been shown to induce bladder cancer in animals or humans, people with frequent urinary tract infections have an increased incidence of bladder cancer (27). BP also has not been shown to induce bladder cancer, although correlations between bladder cancer and smoking have been shown (28), and BP, along with other known carcinogens, is a component of cigarette smoke. The possible involvement of BP glucuronides in bladder cancer has been suggested (29). The present studies predict that these carcinogens may induce bladder cancer and demonstrate the role of the bladder epithelium in the activation of some chemical carcinogens.

Because of the differential mutagenic responses to BP and DMN in the various organs, the metabolism of these carcinogens in the primary cells was undertaken. All the cell types are capable of metabolizing BP, although quantitative differences in the total metabolism and individual metabolites existed. Glucuronidation and formation of sulfates of BP also occurred in all tissues. However, as stated above, a precise correlation between any metabolite or

Table 6. Comparison of Relative Carcinogenic and Mutagenic Activities[a]

	Target Organ or Activating Cell Type							
	Liver		Lung		Kidney		Bladder	
Chemical	Car.	Mut.	Car.	Mut.	Car.	Mut.	Car.	Mut.
BP	±	-	++	++	+	+	-	+
DMBA	+	+	++	++	++	+	±	+
DMN	++	++	±	-	++	+	?	+

[a]Mutation: -, <3 x background;
+, 4 to 25 x background;
++, >25 x background.

or pattern of metabolites and mutagenic activity could not be discerned. This finding again emphasizes that metabolism is one of many factors leading to organ and species specificity.

A major concern in developing *in vitro* systems to study various processes involved in carcinogenesis is how well the *in vitro* results simulate the *in vivo* situation. The possible similarity of the cell-mediated approach to *in vivo* cell interaction has been depicted in Figure 1. When carrying out the cell-mediated mutagenesis approach, several factors must be considered. A possible limitation of using intact cells for activation is whether the activated metabolite can transverse the distance to the DNA of the V79 cell. This transportability depends in part on the stability of the active intermediate and/or whether the proper junctions (if needed) form between the metabolizing cell and V79 cell during the short coculture time. A proximity between the activating cell and target cell has been reported to be essential (30); the extent of cell-to-cell closeness required probably will vary with the stabilities of the active intermediates. At this time, information concerning this aspect is limited, and further studies in these areas would be informative and useful. The data do indicate that several classes of carcinogens can be assayed in the cell-mediated system with various primary activating cell types. Another concern about the cell-mediated approach is the possible selection for or against certain cell types during the tissue disssociation and seeding procedures. Those cell types that are only a small proportion of the total tissue but are major sources of tumors may not be adequately represented for activation capability in the dissociated cell populations. Most of these limitations can be investigated and possibly overcome by improved cell culture methodologies and specific cell type isolation techniques. Pharmacodynamics and tissue distribution of the carcinogens are phenomena which may not be entirely simulated in the current approach. However, studies of relative cell uptake may aid in working this variable into the system.

A future worthwhile application of the cell-mediated approach would be the utilization of human cells from various tissues for metabolic activation and mutable or transformable human cells as the target cells. In this _in vitro_ all human cell system, one would be studying directly the effect of the chemical being applied to human tissues. Concommitant with this approach, the other biological parameters (i.e., DNA-adducts, etc.) could be measured. This battery of biological data then could be used to determine the target organ and potential risk of the agent to man. The accumulation of such data may provide a method for extrapolating risk to humans that would not involve extrapolation directly from _in vivo_ rodent studies. Such an approach appeals, because it does not depend on the long-term maintenance of differentiated human cells in culture, a difficult task to date. Thus, the potential utilization of the cell-mediated approach appears to have fundamental as well as applied uses in chemical carcinogenesis.

REFERENCES

1. Langenbach, R., S. Nesnow, L. Malick, R. Gingell, A. Tompa, C. Kuszynski, S. Leavitt, K. Sasseville, B. Hyatt, C. Cudak, and L. Montgomery. 1981. Organ specific activation of carcinogenic polynuclear aromatic hydrocarbons in cell culture. In: Chemical Analysis and Biological Fate: Polynuclear Aromatic Hydrocarbons. M. Cooke and A.J. Dennis, eds. Battelle Press: Columbus, OH. pp. 75-84.

2. Langenbach, R., S. Nesnow, A. Tompa, R. Gingell, and C. Kuszynski. 1981. Lung and liver cell-mediated mutagenesis systems: specificities in the activation of chemical carcinogens. Carcinogenesis 2:851-858.

3. Langenbach, R., H.J. Freed, and E. Huberman. 1978. Liver cell-mediated mutagenesis of mammalian cells by liver carcinogens. Proc. Natl. Acad. Sci. USA 75:2864-2867.

4. Langenbach, R., H.J. Freed, D. Raveh, and E. Huberman. 1978. Cell specificity in metabolic activation of aflatoxin B_1 and benzo[a]pyrene to mutagens for mammalian cells. Nature 276:277-280.

5. Tompa, A., and R. Langenbach. 1979. Culture of adult rat lung cells: Benzo[a]pyrene metabolism and mutagenesis. In Vitro 15:569-578.

6. Langenbach, R., L. Malick, and S. Nesnow. 1981. Bladder cell-mediated mutagenesis. J. Natl. Cancer Inst. 66:913-917.

7. Miller, J.A. 1970. Carcinogenesis by chemicals: an overview. Cancer Res. 30:559-576.

8. Heidelberger, C. 1975. Chemical carcinogenesis. Ann. Rev. Biochem. 44:79-121.

9. Hutton, J.J., J. Meier, and C. Hackney. 1979. Comparison of the in vitro mutagenicity and metabolism of dimethylnitrosamine and benzo[a]pyrene in tissues from inbred mice treated with phenobarbital, 3-methylcholanthrene or polychlorinated biphenyls. Mutat. Res. 66:75-94.

10. Prough, R.A., V.W. Patrizi, R.T. Okita, B.S.S. Masters, and S.W. Jakobsson. 1979. Characteristics of benzo[a]pyrene metabolism by kidney, liver, and lung microsomal fractions from rodents and humans. Cancer Res. 39:1199-1206.

11. Juchau, M.R., J. DiGiovanni, M.J. Namkung, and A.H. Jones. 1979. A comparison of the capacity of fetal and adult liver, lung, and brain to convert polycyclic aromatic hydrocarbons to mutagenic and cytotoxic metabolites in mice and rats. Toxicol. Appl. Pharmacol. 49:171-178.

12. Hundley, S.G., and R.I. Freudenthal. 1979. A comparison of benzo[a]pyrene metabolism by liver and lung microsomal enzymes from 3-methylcholanthrene-treated Rhesus monkeys and rats. Cancer Res. 37:3120-3125.

13. Bartsch, H., E. Malaveille, and R. Montesano. 1975. In vitro metabolism and microsome-mediated mutagenicity of dialkylnitrosamines in rat, hmaster, and mouse tissues. Cancer Res. 35:644-651.

14. Autrup, H., F.C. Wefald, A.M. Jeffrey, H. Tate, R.D. Schwartz, B.F. Strump, and C.C. Harris. 1980. Metabolism of benzo[a]pyrene by cultured tracheobronchial tissues from mice, rats, hamsters, bovines and humans. Int. J. Cancer 25:293-300.

15. Boroujerdi, M., H. Kung, A.G.E. Wilson, and M.W. Anderson. 1981. Metabolism and DNA binding of benzo[a]pyrene *in vivo* in the rat. Cancer Res. 41:951-957.

16. Newbold. R.F., C.B. Wigley, M.H. Thompson, and P. Brookes. 1977. Cell-mediated mutagenesis in cultured Chinese hamster cells by carcinogenic polycyclic hydrocarbons: nature and extent of the associated hydrocarbon-DNA reaction. Mutat. Res. 43:101-116.

17. Bigger, C.A.H., J.E. Thomaszewski, and A. Dipple. 1978. Differences between products of binding of 7,12-dimethylbenz[a]anthracene to DNA in mouse skin and in a rat liver microsomal system. Biochem. Biophys. Res. Commun. 80:229-235.

18. Bigger, C.A.H., J.E. Tomaszewski, A. Dipple, and R.S. Lake. 1980. Limitations of metabolic activation systems used with *in vitro* tests for carcinogens. Science 209:503-505.

19. Bradley, M.O., B. Bhuyan, M.C. Francis, R. Langenbach, A. Peterson, and E. Huberman. 1981. Mutagenesis by chemical agents in V79 Chinese hamster cells: a review and analysis of the literature. Mutat. Res. 87:81-142.

20. Yang, S.K., J. Deutsch, and H.V. Gelboin. 1978. Benzo[a]pyrene metabolism: Activation and detoxification. In: Polycyclic Hydrocarbons and Cancer. H.V. Gelboin and P.O. Ts'o, eds. Academic Press: New York. pp. 205-224.

21. Public Health Service, National Institutes of Health. 1961-1967. Survey of compounds which have been tested for carcinogenic activity. DHEW publication No. (NIH) 73-75, PHS publication No. 149. U.S. Government Printing Office: Washington, DC.

22. Marquardt, H. 1973. Carcinogenic activity of DMBA in the liver. Cancer Res. 33:1102-1109.

23. Nettesheim, P., and R.A. Griesemer. 1978. Experimental models for studies of respiratory tract carcinogensis. In: Pathogenesis and Therapy of Lung Cancer. C.C. Harris, ed. Marcel Dekker: New York. pp. 75-188.

24. Magee, P.N. 1979. Organ Specificity of Chemical Carcinogenesis. In: Carcinogenesis, Volume 1. G.P. Margison, ed. Pergamon Press: Oxford. pp. 213-221.

25. Summeshayes, I.C., and L.M. Franks. 1979. Effects of donor age on neoplastic transformation of adult mouse bladder epithelium *in vitro*. J. Natl. Cancer Inst. 62:1017-1023.

26. Radomski, J.L., D. Greenwald, W.L. Hearn, H.L. Block, and F.M. Woods. 1978. Nitrosamine formation in bladder infections and its role in the etiology of bladder cancer. J. Urol. 120:48-50.

27. Cox, C.E., A.S. Cass, and W.H. Boyce. 1969. Bladder cancer: a 26-year review. J. Urol. 101:550-565.

28. Stevens, R.G., and S.H. Moolgavkor. 1979. Estimation of relative risk from vital data: Smoking and cancers of the lung and bladder. J. Natl. Cancer Inst. 63:1351-1357.

29. Kinoshita, N., and H.V. Gelboin. 1978. β-Glucuronidase catalyzed hydrolysis of benzo[*a*]pyrene-3-glucuronide and binding to DNA. Science 199:307-309.

30. Kuroki, T., and C. Drevon. 1978. Direct or proximate contact between cells and metabolic activation systems is required for mutagenesis. Nature 271:368-370.

DISCUSSION

Q.: You told us earlier on that you had the feeling that the cooperation between the metabolizing cells and the mutable cells might be important. Then you showed us that picture of the very few bladder cells lying on top of an awful lot of these 79 cells. Have you tried any experiments to see whether the mutagenic potency will increase as you approach a monolayer or near monolayer of bladder cells on top of your V79 cells?

A.: Yes, we have. There wasn't time to point this out, but we have conducted both dose responses with all the chemicals and cell number responses with all cell types. When we carry out the mutagenesis experiments, we usually pretty nearly have a monolayer of these bladder cells on top of the V79 cells. We find that a ratio of about four activating cells per V79 cell is about optimal.

Q.: Just a couple of comments regarding your tables. One is with DMBA in the bladder system. DMBA _in vitro_ has been shown to transform bladder cells in organ culture. The other is for the kidney. The kidney is not just a kidney. It's a combination of at least seven organs, probably even more, and to just throw in a kidney cell is not going to give you the kind of answers you're looking for, particularly when you need to separate cortex and medulla.

A.: Your points are very well taken. In the organ culture studies, I don't recall which cell types were transformed. If they were fibroblast or the transformed cells gave rise to fibrosarcomas, the system is not as meaningful as if epithelial cells were transformed and carcinomas produced. In our system, we have predominantly epithelial cells for activation and I consider this significant.

Regarding the kidney, it is our goal to separate it into various cell types.

Q. I would just like to follow up on that comment. _In vivo_, one would assume that these carcinogens must pass through the endothelium (which is a major cell type in the lung), and I was wondering if you had looked at isolated endothelial cells.

A. No, we haven't as yet isolated individual lung cell types either, but in our lung population we do have endothelial cells in our lung cell preparations when we do the cell-mediated studies.

THE ACTIVATION OF CARCINOGENS BY MAMMARY CELLS: INTER-ORGAN AND INTRA-ORGAN SPECIFICITY

Michael N. Gould

Department of Human Oncology, Wisconsin Clinical Cancer Center, University of Wisconsin, Madison, Wisconsin 53792

INTRODUCTION

Evidence has been presented by epidemiologists that the etiology of the majority of human cancers has environmental factors. It is currently felt that the major environmental factor for cancers other than that of the skin is chemical (1). With the exception of alkylating and acylating agents, almost all chemical carcinogens must be metabolically activated (i.e., converted to an ultimate carcinogen) to initiate neoplasia or induce mutations (1). This activation process is important not only *in vivo*, but is crucial for *in vitro* systems that are employed to study the mechanisms of carcinogenesis and to screen for environmental chemical carcinogens. Most *in vitro* models use either various cell homogenate fractions or intact cultured cells to metabolically activate the chemical to be evaluated. For example, Ames and his collaborators (2) use an S9 fraction of liver homogenate to metabolically activate carcinogens; the metabolic derivatives are then assayed for their ability to induce bacterial mutations. Similar systems have been used that employ specific locus mutations in mammalian cells (3,4). In other models, carcinogens are activated by cultured intact mammalian cells. The activity of the metabolized carcinogen is assayed by specific locus mutation or transformation in the activating cell itself (5), or in other co-cultivated cells that have lost their ability to activate carcinogens (6). The validity of using mutagenesis as an endpoint to identify active carcinogens has been reviewed extensively (7).

While both methods are useful, whole cell activation may more closely resemble the *in vivo* situation. First, the profile of the carcinogen metabolites and the carcinogen-DNA adducts obtained with whole cell activation more nearly resembles the *in vivo* profiles than do the profiles resulting from cellular fractions (8,9,10). Also, the ability of intact cultured primary cells to activate a specific carcinogen correlates directly with the sensitivity of its organ of origin to the carcinogen (11,12). Subcellular systems lack this specificity (4). Finally, cultured primary cells can be manipulated by physiologically active agents such as hormones while activating carcinogens (Gould, unpublished data).

When intact cultured cells are used to activate carcinogens, the biological effects of the metabolized carcinogen can be assayed either in the activating cell itself, or in a co-cultured cell that itself is unable to activate carcinogens. Both systems have advantages and disadvantages when used to assay endpoints such as cytotoxicity, mutagenesis, and transformation. A cell that can be used in an *in vitro* system for both carcinogen activation and endpoint assay is difficult to obtain. These two functions, while not mutually exclusive, cannot usually be optimized in the same cell. This ability is either wholly or partially lost over a period of time as the cell is maintained in culture (13,14, and Gould, unpublished data). On the other hand, primary cells have low plating efficiency, making them difficult to use reliably in clonogenic assays of toxicity, mutagenicity or neoplastic transformation. In spite of these difficulties, several quantitative cell systems of this type have been used. These systems usually employ fibroblasts. Examples of these include those using early passage hamster embryo fibroblasts (15) and those using fibroblast-like cell lines established from mouse embryos (16).

An alternative is to use cultured primary cells to activate carcinogens and co-cultivated cells from established lines to assay the biological effects. The advantages of a co-cultivation system stems from the use of two types of cell. One cell type is used to activate the carcinogen. This can be a well-differentiated primary culture from either the stroma or parenchyma of various specific organs or tissues. A second cell type is used to assay various biological endpoints such as toxicity, mutagenicity, and transformation. It is usually taken from an established cell line chosen for this purpose.

Primary embryo fibroblasts (6,11), primary adult rat hepatocytes (11,17,18), lung cells (19), and mammary cells (12), among others, have previously been employed to activate chemicals for the induction of mutations in co-cultured cell lines. Most of these cell types have been shown to activate specific types of carcinogens and not others. For example, hepatocytes can activate carcinogens such as aflatoxin B_1 (AFB_1) that cause liver cancer when systemically administered *in vivo*. Conversely, hepatocytes will not activate polycyclic aromatic hydrocarbons such as benzo[a]pyrene (BP) (11) that do not cause liver cancer upon systemic administration. The inverse is true of embryo fibroblasts (11). While the liver cell system shows a specificity that correlates well with the in vivo situation, it is interesting to note that the liver subcellular fraction employed in certain in vitro short-term screening procedures lacks this specificity (4).

Currently, we are investigating the activation of chemical procarcinogens by mammary gland cells. A mammary cell-mediated mammalian cell mutagenesis assay is used to quantitate activation. We feel that the use of a mammary model is desirable in that it provides many unique features (e.g., hormonal manipulation, well-characterized animal models) that will aid in investigating the mechanisms of carcinogenesis, and specifically, the role of procarcinogen activation in this process. In addition, this organ-specific model provides a means to study the etiology of breast cancer, the foremost lethal cancer of American women (20).

MATERIALS AND METHODS

Most methods employed in these studies have been published in detail (12) and thus will only be summarized here.

Mammary Cell Preparation and Culture

Mammary tissue was obtained from virgin female randomly bred Sprague-Dawley (55 days old) or inbred Fischer F344 (7 to 8 weeks old) rats. The tissue was minced and exposed to collagenase for 3 h. Deoxyribonuclease (DNase) was added during the last 10 min of this incubation. The suspension was washed and then divided into a stromal-enriched and a parenchymal-enriched fraction by selective adhesion to tissue culture, plastic, and velocity centrifugation. The parenchymal-enriched fraction, consisting of mainly ductal fragments, was further dispersed by pronase treatment. Both cell populations were grown in 2-minimum essential medium (MEM) buffered with 4-(2-hydroxyethyl)-1-piperazine ethanesulfonic acid (20 mM). The media were supplemented with 10% fetal bovine serum, bovine prolactin (5 μg/ml), insulin (5 μg/ml), 17β-estradiol (0.005 μg/ml), progesterone (0.5 μg/ml), and cortisol (0.5 μg/ml).

Cultures were assessed by two methods. In the first method, they were fixed and stained, and the percentage of epithelial-like cells was estimated using conservative criteria (12). In the quantitative transplantation method, the number of cells (from Fischer rat mammary cultures) needed to produce mammary tissue at 50% of the transplant sites (alveolar dose is 50% [AD50]) was determined (21).

Carcinogen Exposure

The mammary cultures (stromal- or parenchymal-enriched) were reproductively sterilized 16 h after initial plating. After this irradiation, V79 Chinese hamster fibroblasts were co-cultivated with the mammary cells. Three h later, carcinogen was added to the cultures. The carcinogens employed, 7,12-dimethylbenz[a]anthracene (DMBA), BP, and AFB_1, were dissolved in dimethylsulfoxide (DMSO). The maximum DMSO concentration (1%) was added to cultures not treated with carcinogen. After 45 h of exposure to the carcinogen, the cultures were washed and the V79 cells removed by differential trypsinization (12).

Mutagenesis Assay

The V79 cells were assayed for carcinogen-induced cytotoxicity at the time of initial removal from the co-cultures and three days or six days after removal. Mutagenesis was estimated at the Na^+/K^+ adenosinetriphosphatase (ATPase) locus (resistance to ouabain) and at the hypoxanthine-guanine phosphoribosyl transferase locus (resistance to 6-thioguanine). A three-day expression time was allowed for mutation to ouabain resistance and a six-day expression time was allowed for mutation to 6-thioguanine resistance.

RESULTS

Mammary Cell Preparation

Photomicrographs of parenchymal- (epithelial) and stromal-enriched fractions are shown in Figure 1a and 1b. Based on conservative morphologic criteria such as epithelial cells strictly defined (12), the parenchymal-enriched fraction contained 94% epithelial-like cells, while the stromal-enriched fraction contained 4% epithelial-like cells. When these two enriched mammary populations were evaluated by quantitative transplantation into isologous recipients, we found that it took 925 (95% confidence limits, 407, 2233) cells from the parenchymal-enriched fraction and 3056 (95% confidence limits, 914, 4658) cells from the stromal-enriched fraction to produce differentiated mammary tissue at 50% of the transplant site (AD50).

Inter-Organ Specificity

DMBA, an *in vivo* mammary-specific carcinogen, was activated to mutagenic form(s) by mammary epithelial cells. The number of induced specific locus mutations in co-cultured V79 cells was related to the DMBA concentration (see Figure 2). AFB_1, a very potent _in vivo_ hepatocarcinogen that is not associated with the induction of mammary tumor was not activated by these mammary cells. In addition, DMBA, but not AFB_1, was activated to cytotoxic

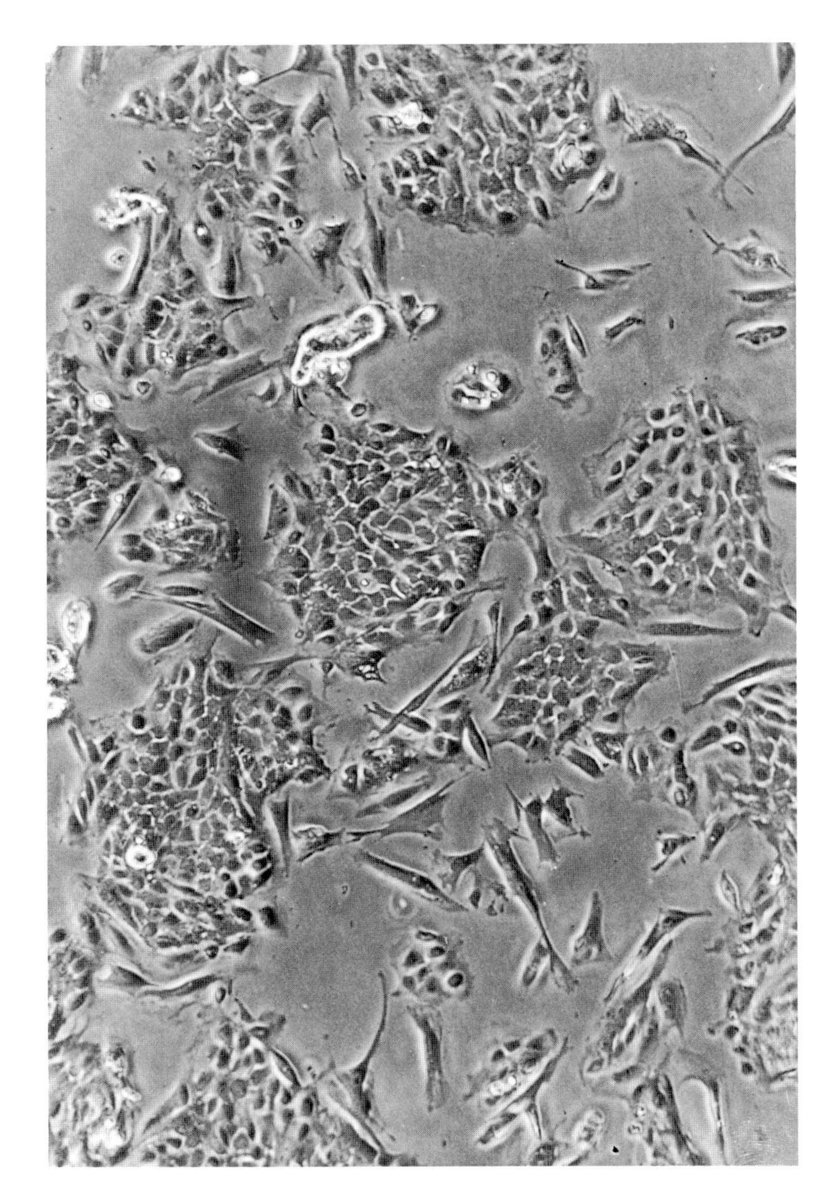

Figure 1. a) Mammary epithelial-enriched culture 72 h after plating (enlarged 170X); b) Mammary stromal-enriched culture 72 h after plating (enlarged 330X).

products by these cultures (see Figure 3.) Similar results were also found in the stromal-enriched mammary cultures (see Table 1).

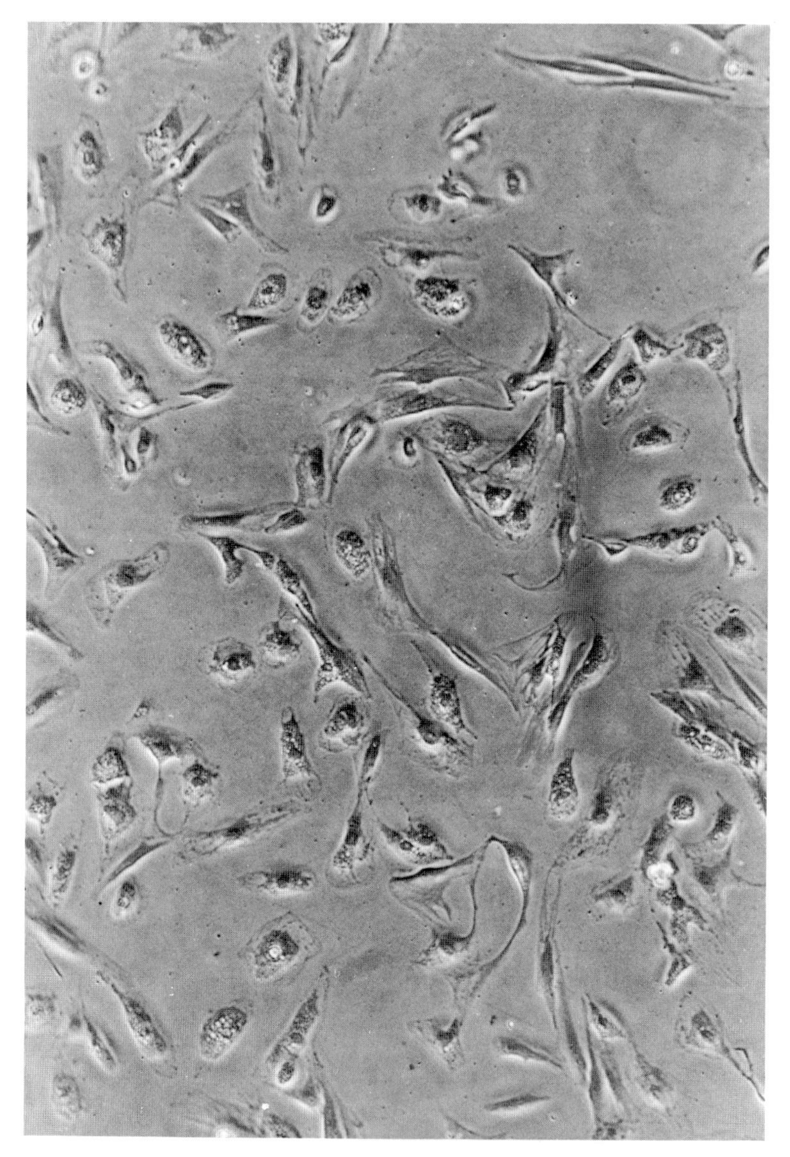

Figure 2. Dose-response curve for mutations to ouabain (A) and 6-thioguanine (B) resistance induced by DMBA or AFB_1. The V79 cells were exposed to these carcinogens in the presence of enriched mammary epithelial cells for 45 h (12).

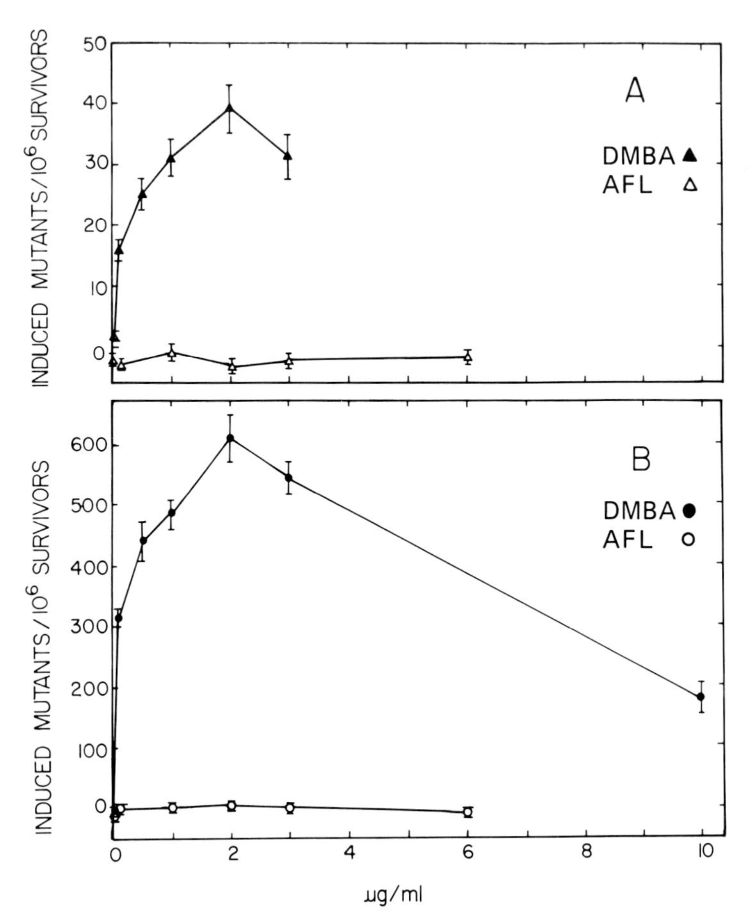

Figure 3. Dose-response curve for V79 cell cytotoxicity due to exposure of cells to DMBA or AFB_1 in the presence of enriched mammary epithelial cells (12).

Intra-Organ Specificity

As described above, both parenchymal- and stromal-enriched mammary cell populations activated the strong *in vivo* mammary carcinogen DMBA but not the non-mammary carcinogen AFB_1. However, BP, a weak *in vivo* mammary carcinogen, was activated not by the parenchymal-enriched fraction but by the mammary stromal fraction (22) (see Figure 4 and Table 1).

Table 1. *In Vivo* Relationships for Rat Mammary Gland

Ability	Procarcinogen DMBA	BP	AFB_1
To induce mammary cancer *in vivo*	+++++	+	-
Of mammary epithelial cells to activate procarcinogens	+++++	-	-
Of mammary stromal cells to activate procarcinogens	+++++	+++	-

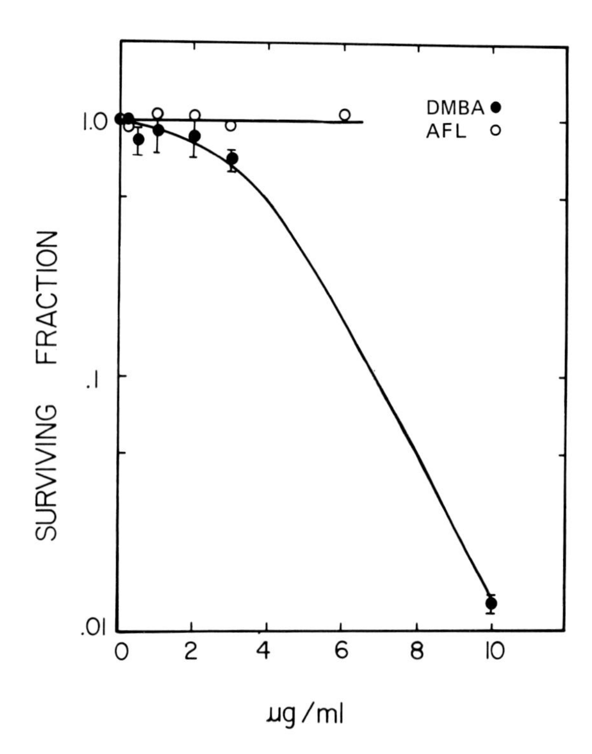

Figure 4. Dose-response curve for mutations to 6-thioguanine resistance induced by BP. The V79 cells were exposed to the carcinogen for 45 h in the presence of either enriched mammary epithelial cells or enriched mammary stromal cells (12).

DISCUSSION

The process that occurs in an organ or tissue from the time it is exposed to a chemical carcinogen to the appearance of a frank neoplasm is complex. In most cases, the compound must be activated to an ultimate carcinogen that interacts with cellular targets. The target-carcinogen complex may be eliminated through a repair process or left as an intact lesion. Either the remaining adduct or errors in the repair process may alter cell function. The occurrence of functional cellular changes may be amplified or accelerated by other environmental chemicals such as promoters, or by physiological processes such as change in hormonal balances. Finally, altered cells may progress to frank neoplasms under the influence of physiologic or xenobiotic factors. The relationship between these factors in the dynamics of neoplastic processes leading to organ and species specificity in *in vivo* oncogenesis is not fully understood.

In defining this mechanistic interrelationship, *in vitro* systems will be invaluable because of their ability to be easily manipulated and because they allow the inclusion of man in interspecies experimental comparisons. To fulfill this potential, *in vitro* models represent the *in vivo* organ and species in function as well as in name. In addition, when studying the oncogenic process for a specific organ, it is important to be able to define the role of each cell type in the interacting mixture of cells that make up the organ. Remember that the quantitative abundance, as well as the interactive relationships of these cell types, may vary among species.

Our laboratory is involved in the study of organ and species specificity in chemical and physical carcinogenesis. We are utilizing *in vivo*, *in vitro*, and *in vivo-in vitro* mammary models. In this paper, I have presented a mammary model designed to study the role of procarcinogen activation in organ specificity. The results presented give evidence that procarcinogen activation at least in part accounts for organ specificity in mammary carcinogenesis. The strong mammary carcinogen DMBA is activated by both mammary parenchymal and stromal cells, while the potent hepatocarcinogen AFB_1 is not activated by either mammary cell subpopulation. The results further suggest that it is not sufficient merely to know which organs activate which chemicals. To understand the *in vivo* situation, we must also know which cells in an organ activate the procarcinogen and which cells give rise to the neoplasm of interest. We found that the weak mammary carcinogen BP can be activated in the breast. However, BP is mainly activated by the stromal cells, while most breast tumors are carcinomas of parenchymal origin. It can therefore be postulated that BP is a weak mammary carcinogen because its ultimate carcinogenic metabolite must be transported from stromal to parenchymal cells to induce mammary carcinomas. The efficiency of this transport process is under investigation.

The above findings support the hypothesis that the activation of procarcinogens is organ specific. However, other additional processes probably contribute to organ specificity in carcinogenesis. To eliminate the complexities of chemical carcinogen distribution and activation, we are currently investigating organ specificity for the effects of ionizing radiation on parenchymal cells of various in vivo organs. Radiation organ-specific carcinogenesis is found in both rodents and man (27). As seen in Table 2, the cytotoxic action of ionizing radiation is also organ specific. This specificity occurs both in radiosensitivity (the slope of the survival curve Do) and in the ability to accumulate and repair sublethal damage (the width of the shoulder of the survival curve Dq). I believe it is important to investigate the factor(s) responsible for the cytotoxic and carcinogenic organ-specific effects of ionizing radiation.

Table 2. Organ Specificity in Radiation Cytotoxicity[a]

Organ[b]	Species (strain)	Do (rad)[c]	Dq (rad)[d]
Mammary	Rat (Fischer)	127	360
Thyroid	Rat (Fischer)	200	497
Liver	Rat (Fischer)	249	--
Bone marrow	Mouse (BDF_1)	82	0

[a]All data from in vivo irradiation with in vivo transplantation assays.
[b]See the following references for organ data: mammary (23), thyroid (24), liver (25), and bone marrow (26).
[c]Lower Do indicates more radiosensitivity.
[d]Based on experiments in which tissue was allowed to remain in situ for a post-irradiation repair period (data not available for liver).

In conclusion, I believe that inter- and intra-organ specificity in the metabolic activation of procarcinogens plays an important role in organ-specific chemical carcinogenesis. Thus, a better understanding of the role of procarcinogen activation in the context of the overall process of organ- and species-specific carcinogenesis will provide more reliable *in vitro* short-term assays for the identification of environmental carcinogens. In addition, the development of organ-specific human cell-mediated mutagenesis assays may also allow us to identify individual differences in procarcinogen activation. This in turn might allow us to identify individuals with a high risk to cancer of specific organs or tissues.

ACKNOWLEDGMENTS

I thank Ms. J.A. Robertson and Mr. D. Kolenda for skillful technical assistance. The gift of prolactin from the National Institutes of Health-NIAMDD National Pituitary Agency is gratefully acknowledged. This research is supported partly by grants R01-CA 28954, P01 CA 19298 and P30 CA 14520 from the Department of Health and Human Services, Public Health Services, National Cancer Institute, and National Institutes of Health.

REFERENCES

1. Miller, E.C. 1978. Some current perspectives on chemical carcinogenesis in humans and experimental animals: Presidential address. Cancer Res. 38:1479-1496.

2. Ames, B.N., J. McCann, and E. Yamasaki. 1975. Methods for detecting carcinogens and mutagens with the *Salmonella*/ mammalian microsome mutagenicity test. Mutat. Res. 31:347-364.

3. Kuroki, T., C. Drevon, and R. Montesano. 1977. Microsome-mediated mutagenesis of V79 Chinese hamster cells by various nitrosamines. Cancer Res. 37:1044-1050.

4. Krahn, D.F., and C. Heidelberger. 1977. Liver homogenate-mediated mutagenesis in Chinese hamster V79 cells by polycyclic aromatic hydrocarcons and aflatoxins. Mutat. Res. 46:27-44.

5. Barrett, C., and P.O.P. Ts'O. 1978. Relationship between somatic mutation and neoplastic transformation. Proc. Nat. Acad. Sci 75:3297-3301.

6. Huberman, E., and C. Sachs. 1974. Cell-mediated mutagenesis of mammalian cells with chemical carcinogen. Int. J. Cancer 13:326-333.

7. Meselson, M., and K. Russell. 1977. Comparisons of carcinogenic and mutagenic potency. In: Origins of Human Cancer, Volume C. H.H. Hiatt, J.D. Watsorund, J.A. Wingten, eds. Cold Spring Harbor Laboratory: Cold Spring Harbor, NY pp. 1473-1481.

8. Selkirk, J.K. 1977. Divergence of metabolic activation systems for short-term mutagenesis assays. Nature 270:604-607.

9. Bigger, C.A.H., J.E. Tomaszewski, and A. Dipple. 1978. Differences between products of 7,12-dimethylbenz[a]-anthracene to DNA in mouse skin and in a rat liver microsomal system. Biochem. Biophys. Res. Comm. 80:229-235.

10. Schmeltz, I., J. Tosk, and G.M. Williams. 1978. Comparisons of the metabolic profiles of benzo[a]pyrene obtained from primary cell culture and subcellular fractions derived from normal and methylcholanthrene-induced rat liver. Cancer Lett. 5:81-89.

11. Langenbach, R., H.J. Freed, D. Raveh, and E. Huberman. 1978. Cell specificity in metabolic activation of aflatoxin B_1 and benzo[a]pyrene to mutagens for mammalian cells. Nature 276:277-280.

12. Gould, M.N. 1980. Mammary gland cell-mediated mutagenesis of mammalian cells by organ-specific carcinogens. Cancer Res. 40:1836-1841.

13. Michalopoulos, G., and H.C. Pitot. 1975. Primary culture of parenchymal liver cells on collagen membranes: Morphological and biochemical observations. Exp. Cell Res. 94:70-78.

14. Michalopoulos, G., G.L. Sattier, and H.C. Pitot. 1976. Maintenance of microsomal cytochrome b_5 and P-450 in primary cultures of parenchymal liver cells on collagen membranes. Life Sci. 18:1139-1144.

15. Berwald, Y., and C. Sachs. 1965. In vitro transformation of normal cells to tumor cells by carcinogenic hydrocarbons. J. Natl. Cancer Inst. 35:641-661.

16. Reznikoff, C.A., D.N. Brankow, and C. Heidelberger. 1973. Quantitative and qualitative studies of chemical transformation of cloned C_3H mouse embryo cells sensitive to post-confluence inhibition of cell division. Cancer Res. 33:3231-3238.

17. San, R.H.C., and G.M. Williams. 1977. Rat hepatocyte primary cell culture-mediated mutagenesis of adult rat liver epithelial cells by procarcinogens. Proc. Soc. Exp. Biol. Med. 156:534-538.

18. Langenbach, R., H.J. Freed, and E. Huberman. 1978. Liver cell-mediated mutagenesis of mammalian cells by liver carcinogens. Proc. Natl. Acad. Sci. 75:2864-2867.

19. Tompa, A., and R. Langenbach. 1979. Culture of adult rat lung cells: Benzo[*a*]pyrene metabolism and mutagenesis. *In Vitro* 15:569-578.

20. American Cancer Society. 1979. Cancer facts and figures 1980. American Cancer Society: New York. 8 pp.

21. Gould, M.N., W.F. Biel, and K.H. Clifton. 1977. Morphological and quantitative studies of gland formation from inocula of monodispersed cells. Exp. Cell Res. 107:405-416.

22. Gould, M.N. (MS). Chemical carcinogen activation in the rat mammary gland; intra-organ cell specificity.

23. Gould, M.N., and K.H. Clifton. 1979. Evidence for a unique *in situ* component of the repair of radiation damage. Radiat. Res. 77:149-155.

24. Mulcahy, R.T., M.N. Gould, and K.H. Clifton. 1980. The survival of thyroid cells: *In vivo* irradiation and *in situ* repair. Radiat. Res. 84:523-528.

25. Jirtle, R.L., G. Michalopoulos, J.R. McClain, and J. Crowley. (in press). The survival of parenchymal hepatocytes exposed to ionizing radiation. Cancer Res.

26. Thomas, F., and M.N. Gould. (MS). Evidence for the repair of potentially lethal damage in irradiated bone marrow.

27. United Nations Scientific Committee on the Effects of Atomic Radiation. 1977. Sources and Effects of Ionizing Radiation. United Nations: New York.

DISCUSSION

Q.: There are some strains of rats in which the female is quite resistant to the effects of DMBA, such as the Long-Evans and the Marshall; have you tried any of those in your systems?

A.: It appears that it's not going to be the activation stage that's going to differentiate the Long-Evans and the Sprague-Dawley rat; they seem to activate at the same rate and for the experiments we've done with the epithelial cells.

We have preliminary experiments which indicate that it's also going to be the same for stromal cells. There have been some recent reports implicating that repair is going to be a difference between these two strains of rats and not activation ability.

Q.: Concerning the studies in which you transplanted in vivo irradiated cells, my question is do they produce tumors; and if so, what is the frequency of tumors relative to number of injected cells?

A.: We're just getting into these experiments and tumors are produced in a limited number of cases. The most extensive work with this type of approach has actually been done with thyroid cells, and we hope to have precise numbers soon.

STUDIES ON THE MODE OF ACTION OF CHEMICAL CARCINOGENS IN CULTURED MAMMALIAN CELLS

Carol Jones and Eliezer Huberman

Biology Division, Oak Ridge National Laboratory, P.O. Box Y, Oak Ridge, Tennessee 37830

INTRODUCTION

Researchers estimate that environmental chemicals are responsible for a portion of human cancers. These chemicals, identified as potential carcinogens by epidemiology or experimental studies, constitute a very diverse group and thus are likely to interact in the carcinogenic process at different stages and to varying degrees.

It has been shown that most carcinogens require metabolic activation to electrophilic reactants prior to exerting their toxic effects (1). Such reactive metabolites are capable of binding to cellular macromolecules, including DNA (2-6), a binding which possibly results in the production of critical mutations as the initial event in the process of tumor development (7-14). Indeed, most chemical carcinogens have been shown to act as mutagens as well. *In vitro* cell culture systems devised to investigate the mutagenic activity of chemicals may thus be valuable both in the detection of carcinogens and for elucidating their mode(s) of action. However, for an accurate assessment of the genetic risk from exposure to these chemicals, merely indicating mutagenic potential is not sufficient. One must show that a quantitative relationship exists between carcinogenicity and mutagenicity and that the same metabolites are responsible in both cases. Furthermore, one problem in cancer studies is that most carcinogens exhibit organ and species specificity, and that the exact mechanisms of the specificities are largely unknown. Therefore, in order to make a valid extrapolation from the *in vitro* systems to man, one must devise systems that also take into account the organ or species specificity of the carcinogens.

Some classes of chemicals do not appear to act via a mutational mechanism, and yet they can influence the development of tumors. These chemicals, for example the phorbol esters, are thought to act subsequent to an initiation event caused by another chemical and to amplify or promote the development of tumors (15-18). We do not know the exact mechanism by which these environmental chemicals promote tumor formation. It would, therefore, be useful to devise simple *in vitro* systems in which both the identity and mode of action of such chemicals can be investigated.

Our laboratory has been concerned with the need to develop appropriate *in vitro* systems for the study of the mechanisms of chemical carcinogenesis. In the following report, we will describe the results we have obtained from such an approach and the conclusions we have drawn from these studies.

MUTAGENICITY OF CHEMICAL CARCINOGENS

Carcinogenesis is a complex process in which tumors arise from cells that have undergone a hereditary change from the normal phenotype to malignancy. As stated earlier, it is believed that this change is initiated by the interaction of the carcinogen with the cellular DNA, resulting in the production of mutation(s) or mutation-like change(s) in the genes regulating normal cell function. *In vitro* assays have been devised for determination of the mutagenic activity of chemical agents, e.g., the *Salmonella typhimurium*-S9 assay (7,19), as a means of identifying suspect carcinogenic agents. Using such systems, a qualitative relationship between the mutagenicity and carcinogenicity of a wide variety of chemical carcinogens could be demonstrated with a high degree of correlation (19). However, quantitative correlations are now in increasing demand in order to facilitate more meaningful estimates of the genetic risks from carcinogen exposure and to assist in elucidating the critical mechanisms relating the two phenomena of carcinogenesis and mutagenesis. Recently, careful examination of the data from the *Salmonella*-S9 system has indicated some degree of correlation between mutagenicity and carcinogenicity (20,21). The difficulties in achieving a good correlation could arise from problems in the design of the *in vitro* system, i.e., in the choice of target cells and metabolic activation system. The organization and content of genetic material in bacterial systems differ markedly from those in mammalian cells (22). Membrane function and DNA repair systems may also be dissimilar. The liver-derived microsomal S9 fractions used in most of these systems differ from intact cells in their metabolic competence and can generate artifactual metabolites as evidenced by examination of the DNA adducts formed after metabolism of benzo[*a*]pyrene (BP) and 7,12-dimethylbenz[*a*]anthracene

(DMBA) (6,23,24). An approach that may hopefully circumvent some of these difficulties, described in the following parts of this paper, is the use of the mammalian cell-mediated mutagenesis assay (25-28).

Relationship Between Carcinogenicity and Mutagenicity in the Mammalian Cell-Mediated Assay

In this system, mammalian cells like Chinese hamster V79 or ovary cells (13,25,26,29) that are sensitive to various types of genetic damage are employed as the target cells. As these cells cannot activate chemical carcinogens (25), they are cocultivated with intact normal cells that can carry out the required metabolism. Mutagenic metabolites released from the activating cells are transferred to the target cells where the genetic damage is assessed in terms of the increased frequency of certain specific mutations such as resistance to ouabain, 6-thioguanine, or 8-azaguanine (26,30-32).

The relationship between the carcinogenicity and mutagenicity of a series of polycyclic aromatic hydrocarbons (PAH) was examined in such a cell-mediated assay consisting of V79 cells as the target cells and irradiated hamster embryo cells for metabolic activation (10,26). In this assay, carcinogenic PAH such as DMBA, BP, 3-methylcholanthrene, and 7-methylbenz[*a*]anthracene, induced ouabain-resistant mutants, whereas noncarcinogenic polycyclic aromatic hydrocarbons such as benzo[*e*]pyrene, benz[*a*]anthracene, phenanthrene, pyrene, and chrysene were inactive. Dibenz[*a,c*]anthracene and dibenz[*a,h*]anthracene showed a weak mutagenic effect. These results indicate that a relationship between mutagenicity and carcinogenicity could be established for PAH. To broaden the scope of the cell-mediated assay and allow the study of other classes of carcinogens, we are developing a series of assays utilizing intact cells from various adult rodent tissues such as liver, kidney, colon, and trachea as the source of activating enzymes. In the liver cell-mediated assay, the mutagenicity of liver carcinogens such as nitrosamines and aflatoxins could be determined (27,28,33). As in the case of PAH, a quantitative relationship for 26 nitrosamines could be established between their carcinogenic effectiveness in experimental animals and their mutagenic potential in this system (34) (see Figure 1).

Cell Specificity in the Activation of Chemical Carcinogens into Mutagens

The cell-mediated mutagenesis assay, which can use intact cells from various organs and tissues to metabolically activate the

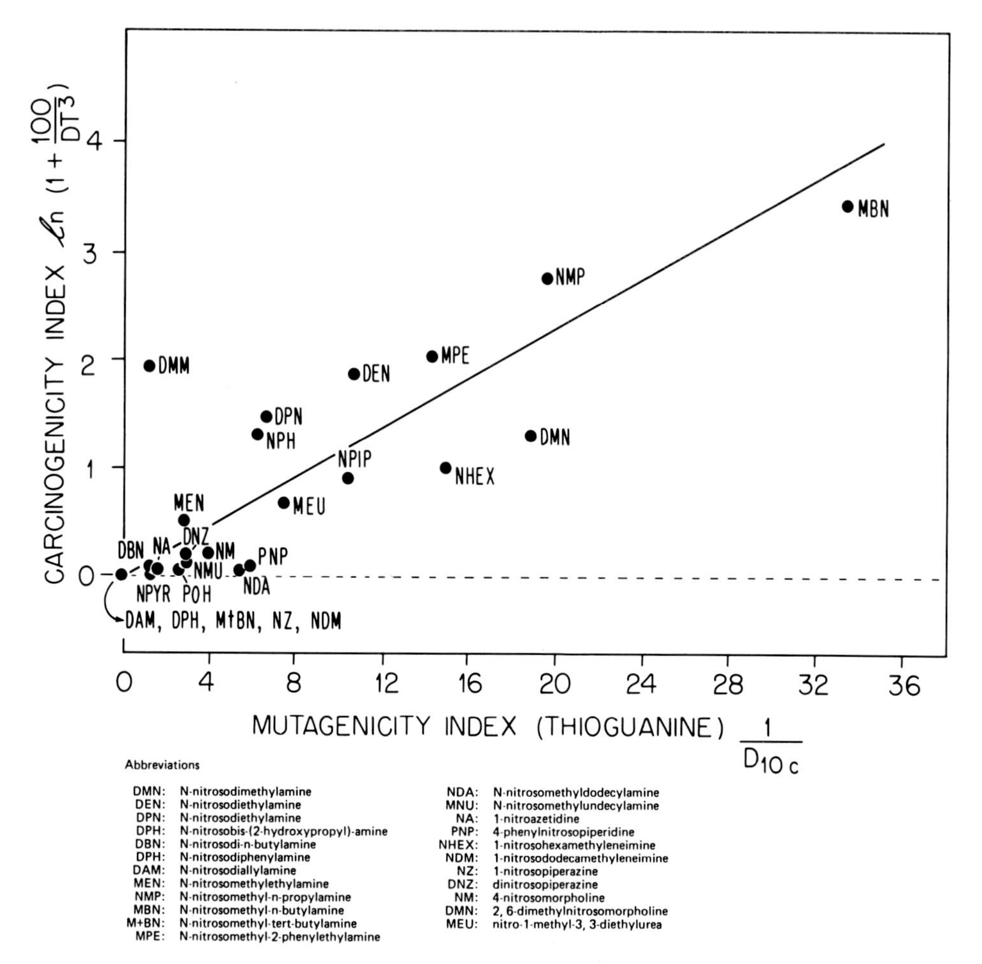

Figure 1. Relationship between carcinogenicity and mutagenicity for nitrosamines with 6-thioguanine resistance as the genetic marker. In Index of Mutagenicity, D = dose (nM) yielding a mutant frequency 10 times higher than the spontaneous mutant frequency. In Index of Carcinogenicity, D = dose (mol) at which 50% of rats die from tumors in time T (weeks).

carcinogens, might represent a useful approach for the study of organ or cell specificity in chemical carcinogenesis. To investigate such a cell specificity, we compared the abilities of rat fibroblasts (fibroblast-mediated assay) and hepatocytes (hepatocyte-mediated assay) to activate several organ-specific carcinogens. N-Nitrosodimethylamine (DMN), which can produce liver tumors but no fibrosarcomas, was activated into a potent mutagen by hepatocytes but not by fibroblasts (see Table 1). This lack of mutagenicity in the fibroblast-mediated assay may be explained by the absence in the fibroblasts of the requisite metabolizing capacity for this compound (33).

Table 1. Induction of Ouabain-Resistant Mutants in the Fibroblast- and Hepatocyte-Mediated Assay by the Carcinogens DMN, BP, and DMBA[a]

Metabolizing Cell Type	Number of Ouabain-Resistant Mutants/ 10^6 Surviving V79 Cells		
	DMN	BP	DMBA
None	1	1	1
Fibroblast	1	38	54
Hepatocyte	258	1	24

[a]Concentrations used were: 0.7 μg/ml DMN and 1 μg/ml each of BP and DMBA.

Benzo[a]pyrene, a potent lung and skin carcinogen that can induce fibrosarcomas but is not considered to be a liver carcinogen (35), was activated to a mutagen for V79 cells by fibroblasts but not by hepatocytes (see Table 1). Unlike the case of DMN, both hepatocytes and fibroblasts could extensively metabolize BP to products that bind to the cellular DNA (see Table 2) (33,36). However, in the fibroblasts the major BP adduct was derived from the reaction of diol epoxide with the deoxyguanosine nucleosides. This adduct is associated with the carcinogenic and mutagenic effects of BP (5,6,36,37). By contrast, no diol epoxide adducts of BP were detected in the hepatocytes. In these cells, the major adducts were hydrophilic nucleoside derivatives, which are presumably nonmutagenic. DMBA, which induces both liver tumors and fibrosarcomas, was mutagenic in both the hepatocyte- and fibroblast-mediated assays.

Table 2. Binding of BP to Hepatocyte and Fibroblast DNA

Concentration of BP (μg/ml)[a]	BP Residues/10^6 Nucleosides	
	Hepatocytes	Fibroblasts
0.01	0.67	0.26
0.1	10.0	1.47
1.0	31.5	3.34
12.0	147.00	ND[b]

[a]Primary liver cells (10×10^6) or fibroblasts (10×10^6) were treated with BP for 18 h. The cell monolayer was washed with phosphate-buffered saline and the cells dissociated with trypsin. After extraction of the cellular DNA, the bound adducts were separated by Sephadex LH-20 chromatography.
[b]ND = not determined.

Thus, these studies indicate that chemical carcinogens are mutagenic in the appropriate cell-mediated assay and furthermore that the carcinogenicity of the chemical can be correlated in a quantitative manner with its mutagenicity. The activation of carcinogens in the cell-mediated assays parallels more closely the activation *in vivo* and thus facilitates the study of the role of metabolism in the organ specificity exhibited by most carcinogens.

INDUCTION OF CELL DIFFERENTIATION IN HUMAN MELANOMA AND MYELOID LEUKEMIA CELLS BY TUMOR-PROMOTING PHORBOL ESTERS

The concept of carcinogenesis is one of a multistage process initiated by mutation-like processes caused by the carcinogen and followed by a stepwise development leading to the formation of tumors (15-18). Possibly, some environmental agents may act during the postinitiation period of the carcinogenic process by a nonmutational mechanism to promote the development of tumors (15-18,38,39). Since the action of these agents could be rate determining in some instances or implicated in the control of organ or species specificity in carcinogenesis, it is important to develop appropriate model systems to investigate their mode of action. One class of chemicals, the phorbol esters, has been shown to act as tumor promoters in an initiation-promotion system in mouse skin (16-18,40). Recently, phorbol esters were found to inhibit spontaneous and induced cell differentiation in certain murine and avian cell types (41-46). In other cultured cells (47-52) including the human myeloid leukemia HL-60 cells and HO melanoma cells (49,50), we and others have shown that phorbol esters induce some characteristics of terminal differentiation. These established cell lines, which have appropriate markers for cell differentiation, offer good models for study of cell growth and differentiation and the mechanisms by which environmental chemicals may interfere with these processes, in particular, for the study of those determinants that contribute to the development of tumors.

Differentiation in the HL-60 cell line can be characterized by inhibition of cell growth, attachment of cells to the surface of Petri dishes, changes in cell structure, increase in percentage of phagocytizing cells (see Figure 2), and stimulation of nonspecific esterase and lysozyme activities (48,50-52). The ability of phorbol esters to induce differentiation can be correlated with their tumor-promoting activity in mouse skin (50) (see Figure 3). Similarly, in HO melanoma cells where inhibition of cell growth, stimulation of melanin synthesis, and dendrite-like structure formation (see Figure 4) are indicative of increased differentiation, the induction of cell differentiation is correlated to the tumor-promoting activity in mouse skin (49). Phorbol esters which lack tumor-promoting ability were inactive also in producing cell differentiation. Thus, these cell systems might be useful in the identification of chemicals that may represent potential tumor promoters, and allow the study of the cellular and biochemical events that lead to the induction of differentiation by such chemicals. In the next part we shall discuss two studies so that we can understand the biochemical events involved in the induction of differentiation by tumor-promoting phorbol diesters.

Alteration in Polyamine Levels Induced by Phorbol Esters

The polyamines putrescine, spermidine, and spermine have been implicated in the control of cell growth and differentiation (53-58) and in tumor promotion (59,60). Therefore, studies were undertaken to determine the role of polyamines in the control of cell growth and differentiation in human HL-60 leukemia cells by tumor-promoting agents such as the phorbol esters.

Treatment of the HL-60 cells with either 12-O-tetradecanoyl-phorbol 13-acetate (phorbol 12-myristate-13-acetate; PMA) or phorbol 12,13-didecanoate (PDD) resulted in increased levels of putrescine (see Figure 5 and Table 3) (61). The increase in putrescine levels preceded expression of the induced PMA differentiation markers (see Figures 5 and 6). In addition to increasing putrescine levels, PMA enhanced the amount of spermidine and decreased the amount of spermine (see Figure 5). The nontumor

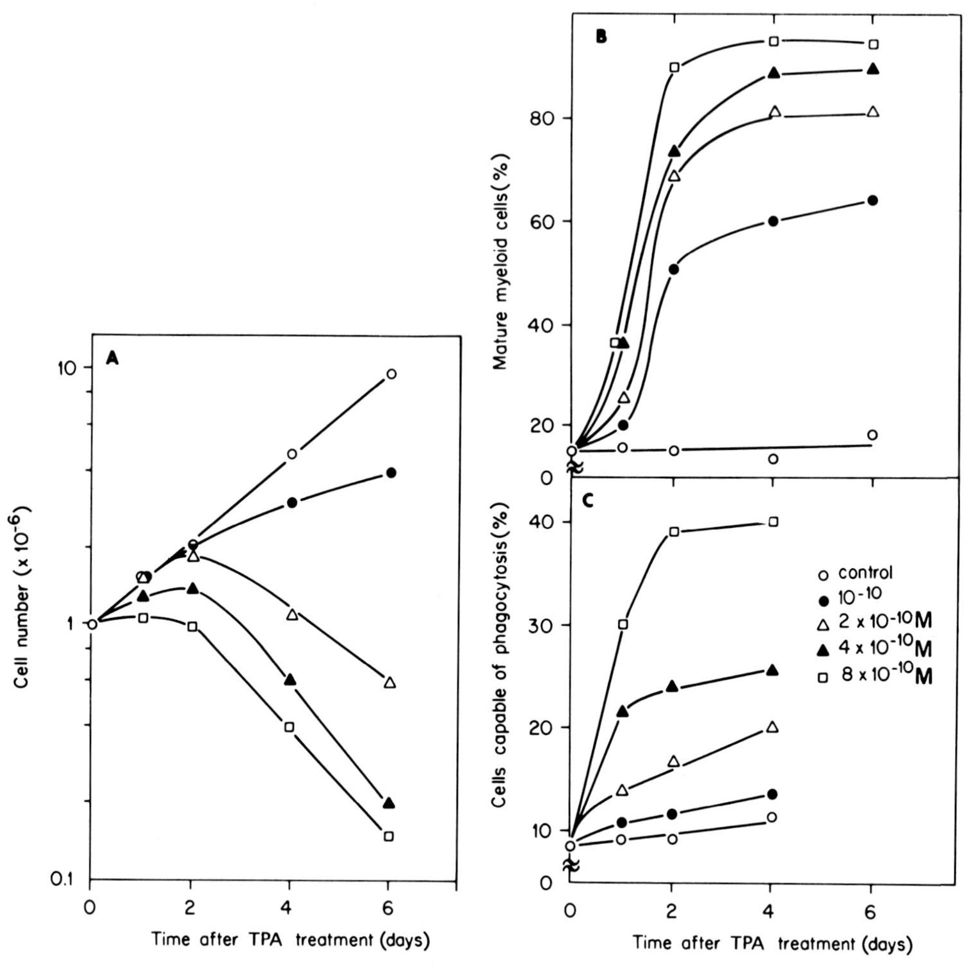

Figure 2. Cell growth (A), percentage of morphologically mature cells (B), and phagocytizing cells (C) in HL-60 cells at different times after treatment with different concentrations of PMA. The cultures were treated a day after seeding 5×10^5 cells in 5 ml growth medium in 60-mm Petri dishes. Cells were counted to determine cell growth and stained with Wright-Giemsa stain to determine the percentage of mature and phagocytizing cells. The mature cells were composed mainly of myelocytes and metamyelocytes. A small fraction of cells with banded and segmented nuclei was also observed. Phagocytosis was determined after the HL-60 cells were incubated for 30 min with 4×10^6 cells/ml diploid *Saccharomyces cerevisiae* strain XY 664 (50).

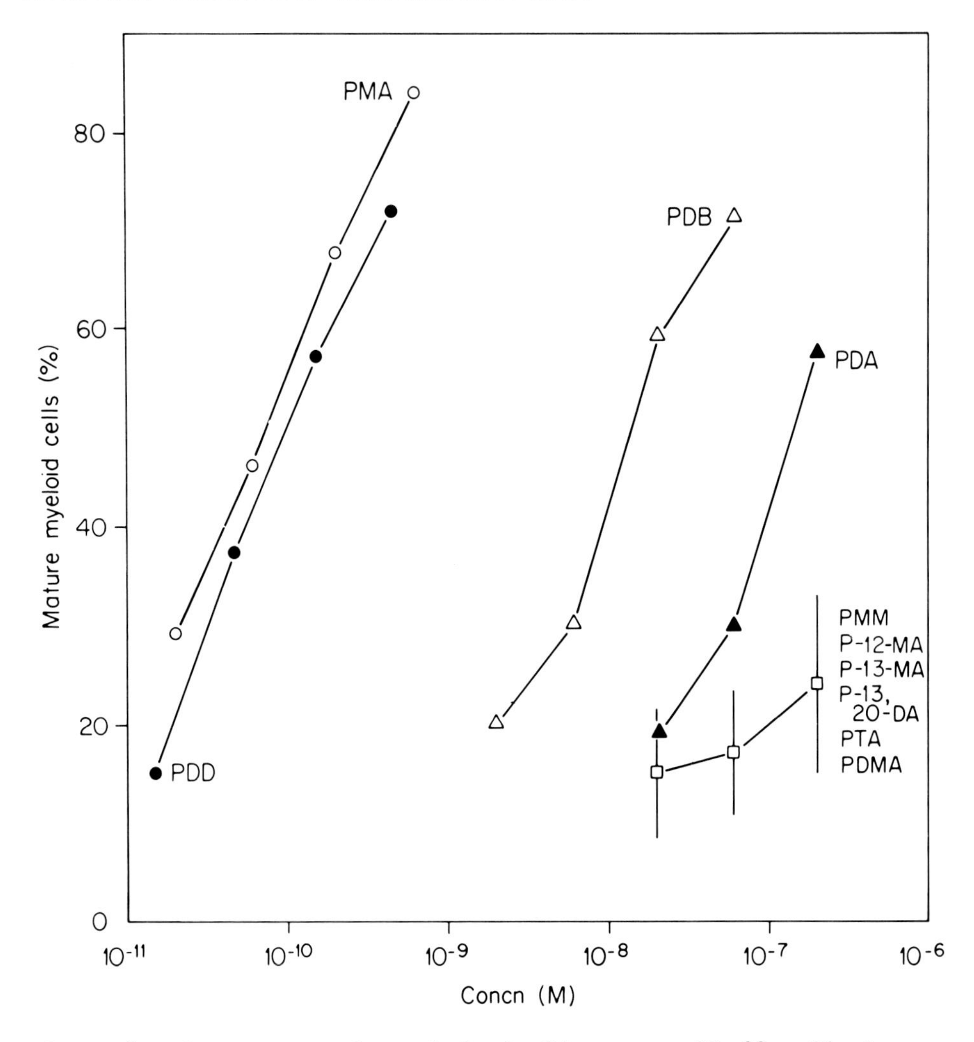

Figure 3. Percentage of morphologically mature HL-60 cells two days after treatment with different phorbol esters. The percentage of morphologically mature cells was determined after cells were stained with Wright-Giemsa. The control cultures contained about 15% mature cells (50).

promoters phorbol 12,13-diacetate (PDA) and 4-O-methyl-12-O-tetradecanoylphorbol 13-acetate (4-O-methylphorbol 12-myristate-13-acetate; 4-O-MePMA), which are not inducers of cell differentiation, did not induce changes in the polyamine levels. Neither was there a change after PMA treatment of an HL-60 variant designated R-20 which was less susceptible to PMA-induced differentiation (see Figure 6) (61).

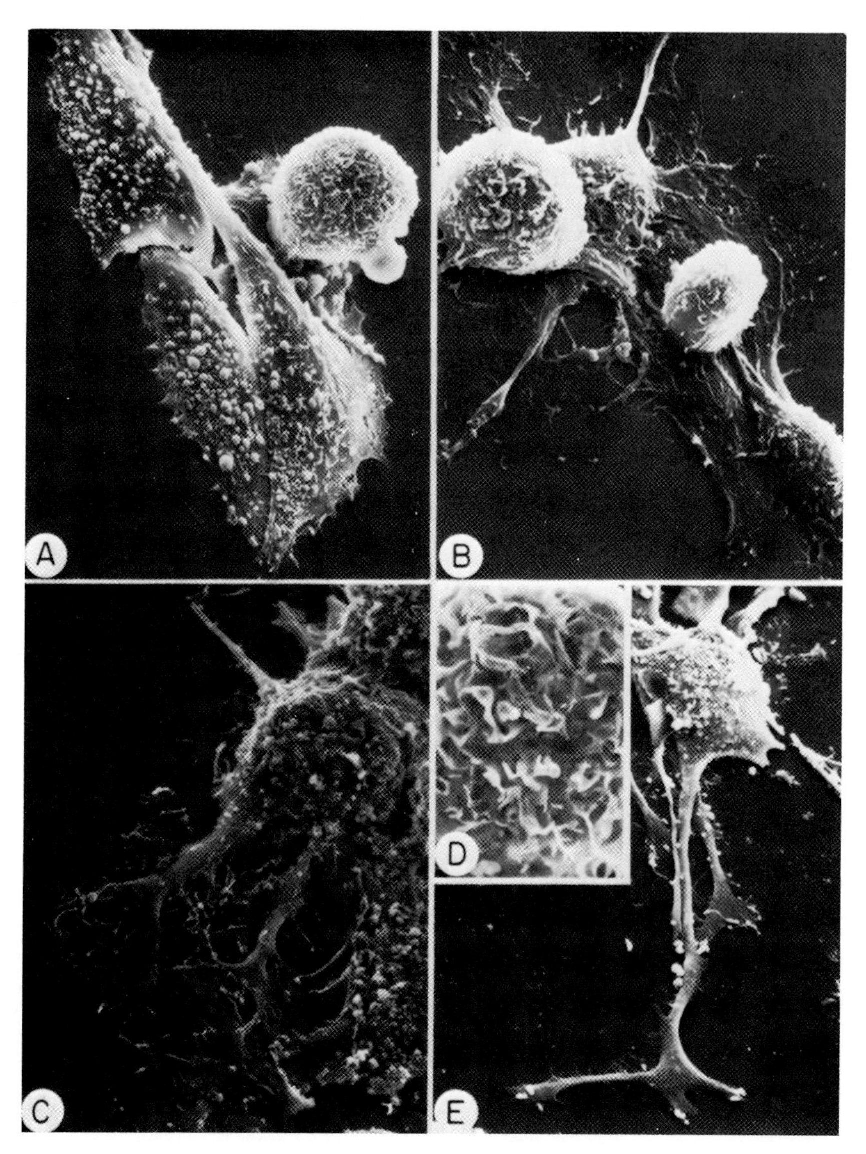

Figure 4. Scanning electron microscopic morphology of human HO melanoma cells. A is an untreated control; B, 4-h treatment with 4×10^{-8} PMA; C, 8-h treatment with PMA; D, high magnification view of ridges on the surface of an 8-h treated cell; and E, 24-h treatment with PMA. A-C are magnified 2,600 times. D is magnified 5,700 times, and E is magnified 1,800 times (49).

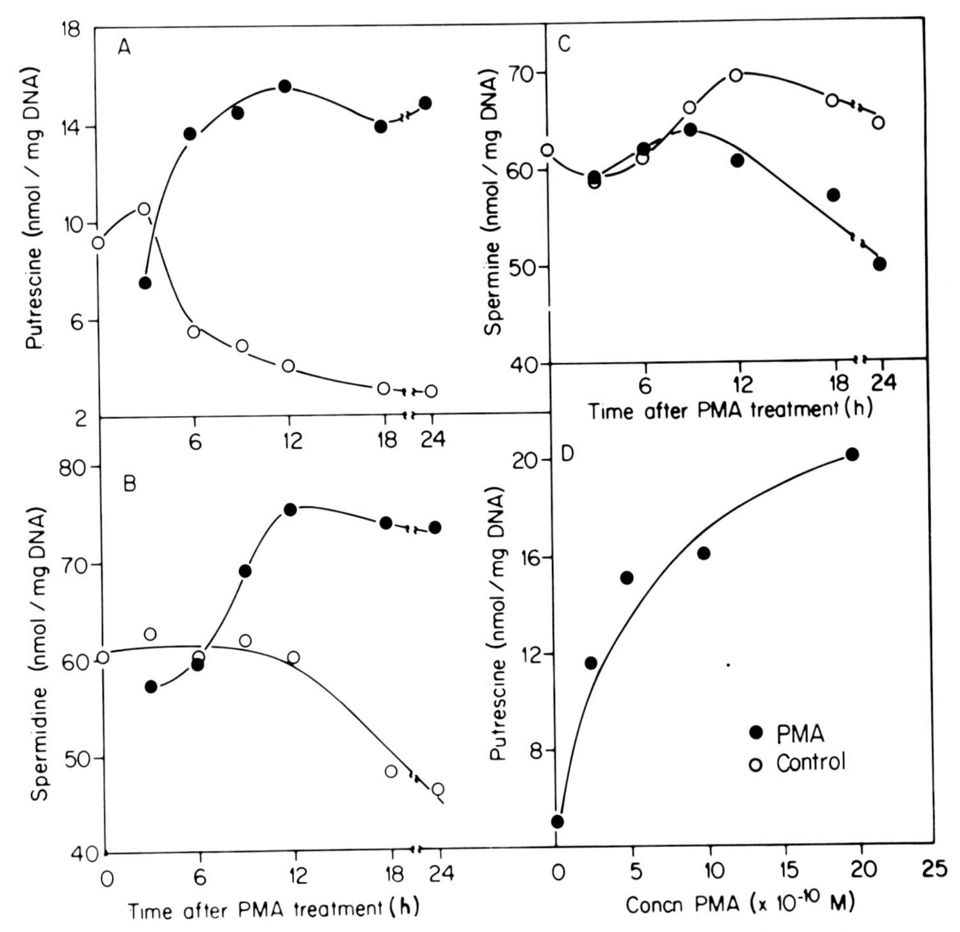

Figure 5. The level of putrescine (A), spermidine (B), and spermine (C) in HL-60 cells at different times after treatment with 5 x 10^{-10} M PMA. D is the amount of putrescine at 12 h after treatment with PMA at different concentrations (61).

The mechanisms involved in the alteration of polyamine levels are not understood. Activities of the principal enzymes of the polyamine biosynthetic pathway, namely ornithine decarboxylase and S-adenosylmethionine decarboxylase (57,58), were not changed significantly following exposure to PMA. Furthermore, inhibitors of these enzymes, α-methylornithine, α-difluoromethylornithine

Table 3. Relationship Between Percentage of Morphologically Mature HL-60 Cells and Putrescine Levels After Treatment With Phorbol Esters[a]

Treatment	Tumor-Promoting Activity	Morphologically Mature Cells (%)	Putrescine Level (nmol/mg DNA)
None	-	12	4
PDA	-	12	3
4-O-MePMA	-	15	4
PDD	+++	70	10
PMA	+++	85	13

[a]HL-60 cells were treated with 5 x 10^{-10} M of the phorbol esters. Percentage of morphologically mature cells was determined two days after incubation with the phorbol diesters. Putrescine levels were determined 12 h after treatment with the inducer (61). See text for definition of abbreviations.

(DFMO), and methylglyoxal bis-(guanylhydrazone) (62-64) did not effect differentiation in control or PMA-treated cells. Similarly, the addition of exogenous polyamines was without effect. Note that polyamines are the natural substrates for a further group of enzymes, the transglutaminases (65). These enzymes are involved in membrane and receptor functions that may constitute the initial site of action for the normal inducers of cell differentiation. Alternatively, alterations in polyamine levels may be only a consequence of induced differentiation that precedes other morphological or biochemical changes.

Specific Binding of 20-[^{3}H]phorbol 12, 13-Dibutyrate in HL-60 Cells

It was recently suggested that specific binding sites may be important in the action of the tumor-promoting phorbol esters (66). The difference in the effect of PMA on terminal differentiation and polyamine levels between normal HL-60 and the less susceptible variant R-35 (progeny of R-20) cells could thus be the result of difference in the number of binding sites for the phorbol ester 20-[^{3}H]phorbol 12,13-dibutyrate ([^{3}H]PDBu) to both cell types (67). This compound is less lipophilic than PMA and has proven valuable in the identification of specific binding sites for phorbol esters in several tissues (66). The R-35 cells were not susceptible to the induction of differentiation by either PMA or PDBu at doses u to 3 x 10^{-7} M. We found that the variance in the response of HL-60

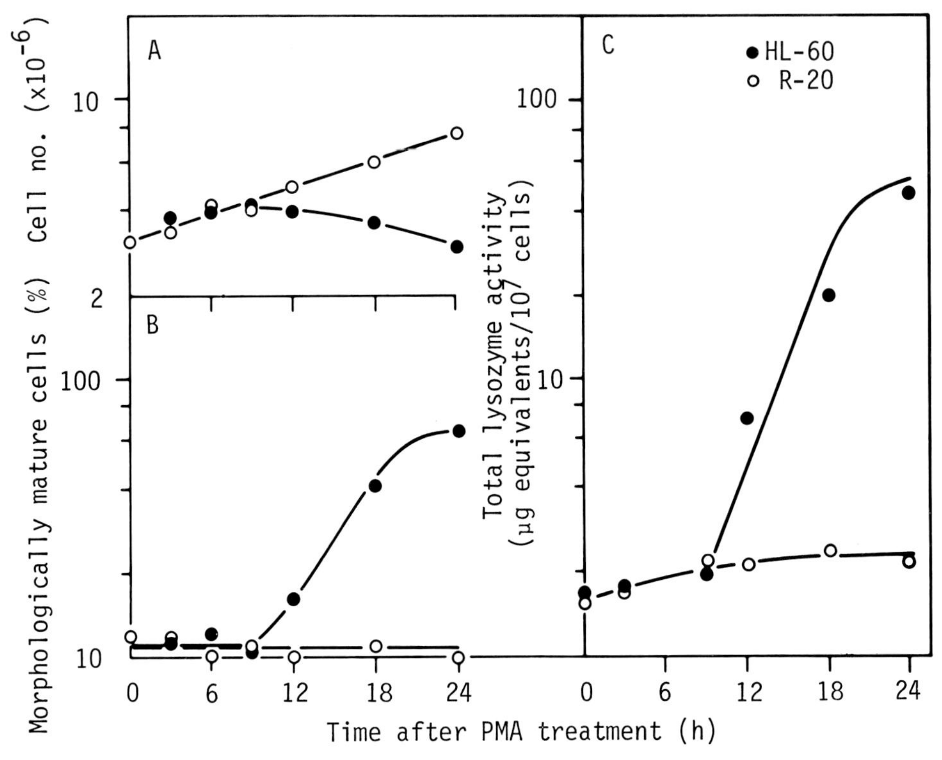

Figure 6. Cell growth (A), percentage of morphologically mature cells (B), and lysozyme activity (C) in HL-60 and R-20 cells at different times after treatment with 5×10^{-10} M PMA. Cultures were treated one day after seeding 1×10^{6} cells in 10 ml growth medium in 100-mm Petri dishes. Morphologically mature cells were composed mainly of myelocyte and metamyelocyte-like cells. A small fraction of cells with banded and segmented nuclei was observed (61).

and R-35 cells to PMA- or PDBu-induced cell differentiation was not due to either the number of binding sites or the affinity of [^{3}H]PDBu specific binding (see Figure 7), but rather to the down-regulation (i.e., loss of PDBu bound to the cells) of bound PDBu following maximum specific binding. This finding was deduced from the fact that the down-regulation of bound [^{3}H]PDBu seen in HL-60 was not observed in R-35 cells (see Figure 8 and Table 4). This down-regulation was temperature dependent, as no loss of radiolabel occurred by 1 h at 4°C, and could result from

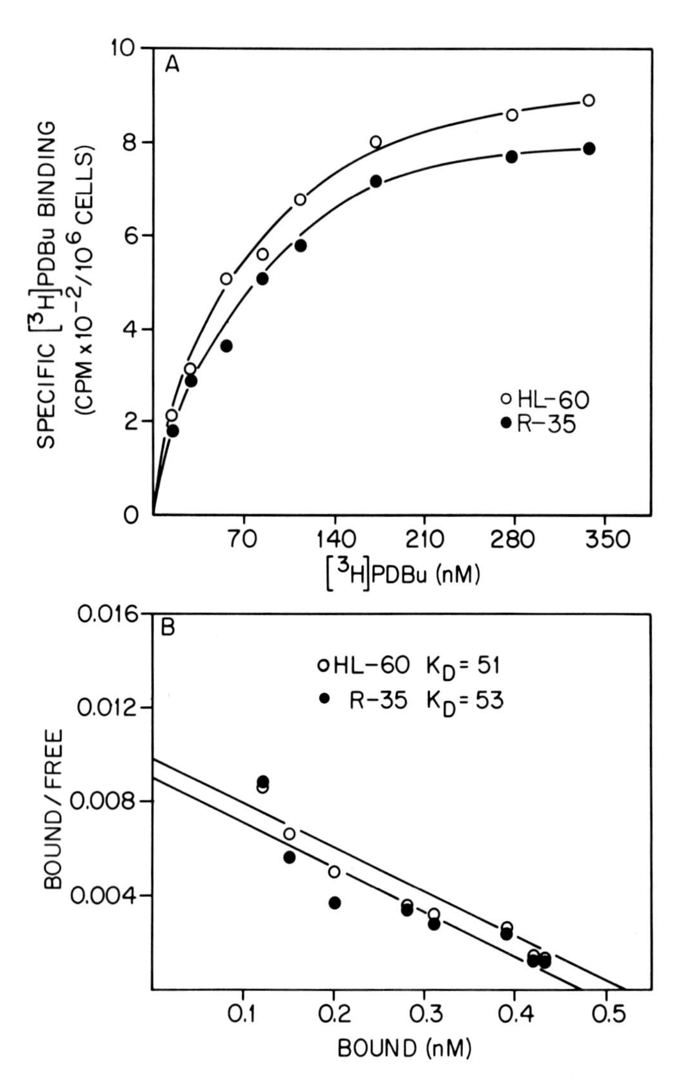

Figure 7. A is equilibrium of specific [^{3}H]PDBu binding to HL-60 and R-35 cells as a function of ligand concentration. Incubation was carried out at 4°C in the absence and presence of 30-μm unlabeled PDBu for 45 min. B is specific binding of [^{3}H]PDBu plotted by the method of Scatchard (67).

conformational changes in the PDBu-binding sites or perhaps, more likely, from internalization of the phorbol ester-binding sites and their degradation by lysosomal enzymes (68). However, it must be emphasized at this point that we do not have any data to prove either case.

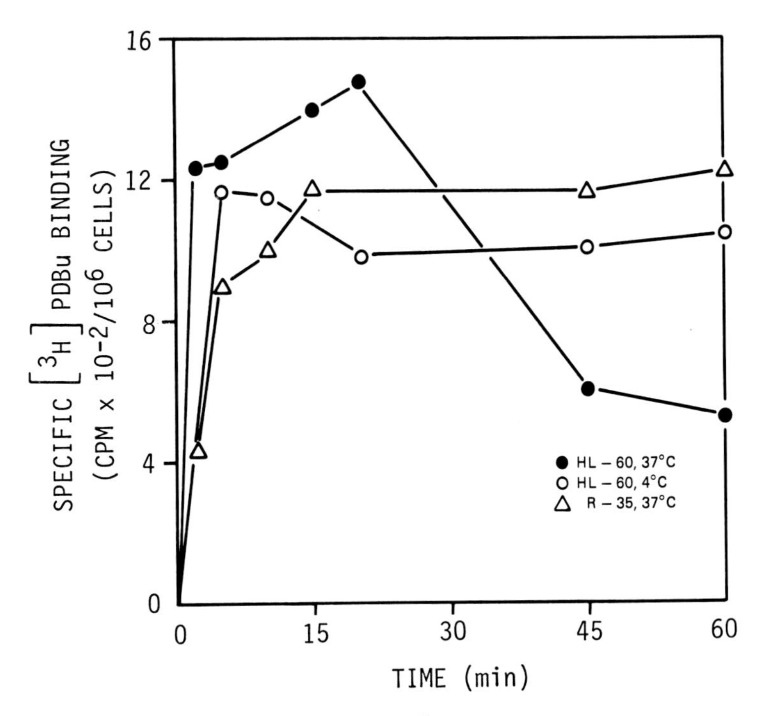

Figure 8. Time course of specific [^{3}H]PDBu binding to intact HL-60 cells at 37°C and at 4°C, and to R-35 cells at 37°C (67).

The results of these studies indicate that the down-regulation of specific [^{3}H]PDBu binding may be a crucial early event in the control of phorbol ester-induced terminal differentiation in human HL-60 cells and may also be an important mechanism in tumor promotion.

Table 4. Effect of Prior Exposure of HL-60 and R-35 Cells to PMA on Specific [^{3}H]PDBu Binding

	Specific [^{3}H]PDBu Binding (%)[a]			
	HL-60		R-35	
Pretreatment with	~27 nM	~82 nM	~27 nM	~82 nM
Saline	100	150	100	147
PMA (1 μM)	22	33	97	150

[a]Specific binding was measured at 27 nM and 82 nM labeled PDBu at 4°C, following 90-min exposure of the cells with saline or 1 μM PMA at 37°C. The amount of specific binding at 27 nM [^{3}H]PDBu without PMA pretreatment was considered as 100%. Cells were washed with 2- x 1-ml cold phosphate buffered saline (pH 7.4) before incubation at 4°C (67).

In summary, we can conclude that the human cell lines HL-60 and HO melanoma may offer a useful model for studying the mode of action of certain classes of tumor promoters and for evaluating some unknown chemicals for this activity.

CONCLUSION

In this report we have discussed cell culture systems that may be useful in evaluating the carcinogenic potential of environmental agents. The cell-mediated mutagenesis assays enable the investigation of mutagenic and hence, possibly, the tumor-initiating activity of a chemical, whereas specific chemically-induced alterations in the growth and cell differentiation of human cells, such as the HL-60 myeloid cells, may indicate a tumor-promoting potential of the chemical used.

REFERENCES

1. Miller, J.A. 1970. Carcinogenesis by chemicals: An overview - G.H.A. Clowes memorial lecture. Cancer Res. 30:559-576.

2. Brookes, P., and P.D. Lawley. 1964. Evidence for the binding of polynuclear aromatic hydrocarbons to the nucleic acids of mouse skin: Relation between carcinogenic power of hydrocarbons and their binding to deoxyribonucleic acid. Nature 202:781-784.

3. Essigmann, J.M., R.G. Croy, A.M. Hadzan, W.F. Busby, V.N. Reinhold, G. Buchi, and G.N. Wogan. 1977. Structural identification of the major DNA adduct formed by aflatoxin B_1 _in vitro_. Proc. Natl. Acad. Sci. USA 74:1870-1874.

4. Huberman, E., and L. Sachs. 1977. DNA binding and its relationship to carcinogenesis by different polycyclic hydrocarbons. Int. J. Cancer 19:122-127.

5. Jeffrey, A.M., I.B. Weinstein, K.W. Jenette, K. Grzeskowiak, K. Nakahishi, R.G. Harvey, M. Authrup, and C. Harris. 1977. Structures of benzo[_a_]pyrene-nucleic acid adducts formed in human and bovine bronchial explants. Nature 269:348-350.

6. Newbold, R.F., C.B. Wigley, M.H. Thompson, and P. Brookes. 1977. Cell-mediated mutagenesis in cultured Chinese hamster cells by carcinogenic hydrocarbons: Nature and extent of the associated hydrocarbon-DNA reaction. Mutat. Res. 43:101-116.

7. Ames, B.N. 1979. Identifying environmental chemicals causing mutations and cancer. Science 204:587-593.

8. Bouck, N., and G. DiMayorca. 1976. Somatic mutation as the basis for malignant transformation of BHK cells by chemical carcinogens. Nature (London) 264-360-361.

9. Heidelberger, C. 1970. Chemical carcinogenesis. Ann. Rev. Biochem. 44:78-121.

10. Huberman, E. 1977. Viral antigen induction and mutability of different genetic loci by metabolically activated carcinogenic polycyclic hydrocarbons in cultured mammalian cells. In: The Origins of Human Cancer, Book C. H.H. Hiatt, J.D. Watson, and J.A. Winston, eds. Cold Spring Harbor Laboratory Publications: Cold Spring Harbor, New York. pp. 1521-1535.

11. Huberman, E. 1978. Mutagens and cell transformation of mammalian cells in culture by chemical carcinogens. J. Environ. Pathol. Toxicol. 2:29-42.

12. Huberman, E., R. Mager, and L. Sachs. 1976. Mutagenesis and transformation of normal cells by chemical carcinogens. Nature 264:360-361.

13. Kao, F.T., and T.T. Puck. 1971. Genetics of somatic mammalian cells. XII: Mutagenesis by carcinogenic nitroso compounds. J. Cell. Physiol. 78:139-144.

14. Knudsen, A.G., Jr., H.W. Hetchcote, and B.W. Brown. 1975. Mutation and childhood cancer: A probabilistic model for the incidence of retinoblastoma. Proc. Natl. Acad. Sci. US 72:5116-5120.

15. Berenblum, I. 1969. A re-evaluation of the concept of cocarcinogenesis. Prog. Exp. Tumoir Res. 11:21-30.

16. Boutwell, R.K. 1974. Function and mechanism of promoters of carcinogenesis. CRC Crit. Rev. Toxicol. 2:419-447.

17. Van Duuren, B.L. 1969. Tumor-promoting agents in two stage carcinogenesis. Prog. Exp. Tumor Res. 11:31-38.

18. Diamond, L., T.G. O'Brien, and W.M. Baird. 1980. Tumor promoters and the mechanism of tumor promotion. Adv. Cancer Res. 32:1-63.

19. McCann, J.B., and B.N. Ames. 1976. Detection of carcinogens as mutagens in the *Salmonella* microsome test: Assay of 300 chemicals. Proc. Natl. Acad. Sci. USA 73:950-954.

20. Meselson, M., and K. Ruseell. 1977. Comparisons of carcinogenic and mutagenic potency. In: The Origins of Human Cancer, Book C. H.H. Hiatt, J.D. Watson, and J.A. Winston, eds. Cold Spring Harbor Laboratory Publications: Cold Spring Harbor, New York. pp. 1473-1482.

21. Scribner, N.K. B. Woodworth, G.P. Ford, and J.D. Scribner. 1980. The influence of molecular size and partition coefficients on the predictability of tumor initiation in mouse skin from mutagenicity in *Salmonella typhimurium*. Carcinogenesis 1:715-719.

22. Malling, H.V., and L.R. Valcovic. 1977. Gene mutation in mammals. In: Progress in Genetic Toxicology. D. Scott, B.A. Bridges, and F.H. Sobels, eds. Elsevier/North-Holland Biomedical Press: New York. pp. 155-164.

23. Bigger, C.A.H., J.E. Tomaszewski, and A. Dipple. 1978. Differences between products of binding of 7,12-dimethylbenz[*a*]anthracene to DNA in mouse skin and in a rat liver microsomal system. Biochem. Biophys. Res. Comm. 80:229-235.

24. Selkirk, J.K. 1977. Benzo[a]pyrene carcinogenesis - A biochemical selection mechanism. J. Toxicol. Environ. Hlth. 2:1245-1258.

25. Huberman, E., and L. Sachs. 1974. Cell-mediated mutagenesis with chemical carcinogens. Int. J. Cancer 13:326-333.

26. Huberman, E., and L. Sachs. 1976. Mutability of different genetic loci in mammalian cells by metabolically activated carcinogenic polycyclic hydrocarbons. Proc. Natl. Acad. Sci. USA 731:188-192.

27. Jones, C.A., and E. Huberman. 1980. A sensitive hepatocyte-mediated assay for the metabolism of nitrosamines to mutagens for mammalian cells. Cancer Res. 40:406-411.

28. Langenbach, R., H.J. Freed, and E. Huberman. 1978. Liver cell-mediated mutagenesis of mammalian cells with liver carcinogens. Proc. Natl. Acad. Sci. USA 75:2864-2867.

29. Chu, E.H.Y., and H.V. Malling. 1968. Mammalian cell genetics. II. Chemical induction of specific locus mutations in Chinese hamster cells *in vitro*. Proc. Natl. Acad. Sci. USA 61:1306-1312.

30. Arlett, C.F., C. Turnbull, S.A. Harcourt, A.R. Lehman, and C.M. Colletta. 1975. A comparison of the 8-azaguanine and ouabain-resistance systems for the selection of induced mutant Chinese hamster cells. Mutat. Res. 33:261-278.

31. Baker, R.M., D.M. Brunette, R. Mankovitz, L.H. Thompson, G.F. Whitmore, L. Siminovitch, and J.E. Till. 1974. Ouabain-resistant mutants of mouse and hamster cells in culture. Cell 1:9-21.

32. Van Zeeland, A.A., and J.Y.I.M. Simons. 1975. Linear dose-response relationships after prolonged expression times in V79 Chinese hamster cells. Mutat. Res. 35:129-138.

33. Langenbach, R., H.J. Freed, D. Raveh, and E. Huberman. 1978. Cell specificity in metabolic activation of aflatoxin B_1 and benzo[a]pyrene to mutagens for mammalian cells. Nature 276:277-280.

34. Jones, C.A., P.J. Marlino, W. Lijinsky, and E. Huberman. (in press). The relationship between the carcinogenicity and mutagenicity of nitrosamines in a hepatocyte-mediated mutagenicity assay. Carcinogenesis.

35. IARC Monograph Series 3. 1973. pp. 91-136.

36. Jones, C.A., R. Santella, E. Huberman, J.K. Selkirk, and D. Grunberger. MS in preparation.

37. Huberman, E., L. Sachs, S.K. Yang, and H.V. Gelboin. 1976. Identification of the mutagenic metabolites of benzo[a]pyrene in mammalian cells. Proc. Natl. Acad. Sci. USA 73:606-611.

38. Slaga, T.J., S.M. Fischer, K. Nelson, and E.L. Gleason. 1980. Studies on the mechanism of skin tumor promotion. Evidence for several stages in promotion. Proc. Natl. Acad. Sci. USA 77:3659-3663.

39. Weinstein, I.B., M. Wigler, P.B. Fisher, E. Sisskin, and C. Pietropaolo. Cell culture studies on biological effects of tumor promoters. In: Mechanisms of Tumor Promotion and Cocarcinogenesis. T.J. Slaga, A. Sivak, and R.K. Boutwell, eds. Raven Press: New York. pp. 313-333.

40. Hecker, E. 1978. Structure-activity relationships in diterpine esters irritant and cocarcinogenic to mouse skin. In: Mechanisms of Tumor Promotion and Cocarcinogenesis. T.J. Slaga, A. Sivak, and R.K. Boutwell, eds. Raven Press: New York. pp. 14-48.

41. Cohen, R., M. Pacifici, N. Rubenstein, J. Biehl, and H. Holtzer. 1977. Effect of a tumor promoter on myogenesis. Nature (London) 266-538-540.

42. Diamond, L., T.G. O'brien, and G. Rovera. 1977. Inhibition of adipose conversion of 313 fibroblasts by tumor promoters. Nature (London) 269:247-248.

43. Ishii, D., E. Fibach, H. Yamasaki, and I.B. Weinstein. 1978. Tumor promoters inhibit morphological differentiation in cultured mouse neuroblastoma cells. Science 200:556-559.

44. Lowe, M.E., M. Pacifico, and M. Holtzer. 1978. Effects of phorbol-12-myristate-13-acetate on the phenotypic program of cultured chondroblasts and fibroblasts. Cancer Res. 38:2350-2356.

45. Rovera, G., T.A. O'Brien, and L. Diamond. 1977. Tumor promoters inhibit spontaneous differentiation of Friend erythroleukemia cells in culturs. Proc. Natl. Acad. Sci. USA 74:2894-2898.

46. Yamasaki, H., E. Fibach, U. Nudel, I.B. Weinstein, R.A. Rifkind, and P.A. Marks. 1977. Tumor promoters inhibit spontaneous and induced differentiation of murine erythroleukemia cells in culture. Proc. Natl. Acad. Sci. USA 74:3451-3456.

47. Miao, R.M., A.H. Fieldsteel, and D.W. Fodge. 1978. Opposing effects of tumor promoters on erythroid differentiation. Nature 274:271-272.

48. Lotem, J., and L. Sachs. 1979. Regulation of normal differentiation in mouse and human myeloid leukemia cells by phorbol esters and the mechanism of tumor promotion. Proc. Natl. Acad. Sci. USA 76:5162.

49. Huberman, E., C. Heckman, and R. Langenbach. 1979. Stimulation of differentiated functions in human melanoma cells by tumor promoting agents and dimethylsulfoxide. Cancer Res. 39:2618-2624.

50. Huberman, E., and M. Callaham. 1979. Induction of terminal differentiation in human promyelocytic leukemia cells by tumor promoting agents. Proc. Natl. Acad. Sci. USA 76:1293-1297.

51. Rovera, G., T.G. O'Brien, and L. Diamond. 1979. Induction of differentiation in human promyelocytic leukemia cells by tumor promoters. Science 204:868-870.

52. Rovera, G., D. Santoli, and W.C. Damsk. 1979. Human promyelocytic leukemia cells in culture differentiate into macrophage-like cells when treated with a phorbol diester. Proc. Natl. Acad. Sci. USA 76:2779-2783.

53. Emanuelsson, H., and O. Heby. 1978. Inhibition of putrescine synthesis blocks development of the polychete Ophryotrocha labronica at gastrulation. Proc. Natl. Acad. Sci. USA 75:1039-1042.

54. Fozard, J.R., M-L. Part, N.J. Prakash, J. Grove, P.J. Schechter, A. Sjoerdsma, and J. Koch-Weser. 1980. L-Ornithine decarboxylase: An essential role in early mammalian embryogenesis. Science 208:505-508.

55. Gazitt, Y., and C. Friend. 1980. Polyamine biosynthesis enzymes in the induction and inhibition of differentiation in Friend erythroleukemia cells. Cancer Res. 40:1727-1732.

56. Takigawa, M., H. Ishida, T. Teruko, and F. Suzuki. 1980. Polyamine and differentiation: Induction of ornithine decarboxylase by parathyroid hormone is a good marker of differentiated chondrocytes. Proc. Natl. Acad. Sci. USA 77:1481-1485.

57. Janne, J., H. Poso, and A. Raina. 1978. Polyamines in rapid growth and cancer. Biochim. Biophys. Acta 473:241-293.

58. Tabor, C.W., and H. Tabor. 1976. 1,4-Diaminobutane (putrescine), spermidine, and spermine. Ann. Rev. Biochem. 45:285-306.

59. Weeks, C.E., and T.J. Slaga. 1979. Inhibition of phorbol ester polyamine accumulation in mouse epidermis by anti-inflammatory steroid. Biochem. Biophys. Res. Comm. 91:1488-1496.

60. Yuspa, S.H., U. Lichti, T. Ben, E. Patterson, H. Hennings, T. Slaga, N. Colburn, and W. Kelsey. 1976. Phorbol esters stimulate DNA synthesis and ornithine decarboxylase activity in mouse epidermal cell cultures. Nature 262:402-404.

61. Huberman, E., C.E. Weeks, A. Herrmann, M. Callaham, and T.J. Slaga. 1981. Alterations in polyamine levels induced by phorbol diesters and other agents that promote differentiation in human promyelocytic leukemia cells. Proc. Natl. Acad. Sci. USA 78:1062-1066.

62. Abdel-Monem, M.M., N.E. Newton, and C.E. Weeks. 1974. Inhibitors of polyamine biosynthesis. I. α-Methylornithine, an inhibitor of ornithine decarboxylase. J. Med. Chem. 17:447-451.

63. Mamont, P., M-C. Duchesne, J. Grove, and P. Bey. 1978. Antiproliferative properties of DL-α-difluoromethyl ornithine in cultured cells. A consequence of the irreversible inhibition of ornithine decarboxylase. Biochem. Biophys. Res. Comm. 81:59-66.

64. Newton, N.E., and M.M. Abdel-Monem. Inhibitors of polyamine biosynthesis. 4. Effects of α-methyl(+)-ornithine and methylglyoxal bis(guanylhydrazone) on growth and polyamine content of L1210 leukemic cells of mice. J. Med. Chem. 20:249-253.

65. Folk, J.E., M.H. Park, S.I. Chung, J. Schrode, E.P. Lester, and H.L. Cooper. 1980. Polyamines as physiological substrates for transglutaminases. J. Biol. Chem. 255:3695-3700.

66. Driedger, P.E., and P.M. Blumberg. 1980. Specific binding of phorbol ester tumor promoters. Proc. Natl. Acad. Sci. USA 77:576-581.

67. Solanki, V., T.J. Slaga, M. Callaham, and E. Huberman. 1981. The down regulation of specific binding of [20-^{3}H]phorbol 12,13-dibutyrate and phorbol ester-induced differentiation of human promyelocytic leukemia cells. Proc. Natl. Acad. Sci. USA 78:1722-1725.

68. Fox, C.F., and M. Das. 1979. Internalization and processing of the EGF receptor in the induction of DNA synthesis in cultued fibroblasts: The endocytic activation hypothesis. J. Supramol. Struct. 10:199-214.

COMPARISON OF THE SENSITIVITY OF RODENT AND HUMAN CELLS TO CHEMICAL CARCINOGENS USING VIRAL TRANSFORMATION, DNA DAMAGE, AND CYTOTOXICITY ASSAYS

Bruce C. Casto

Northrop Services, Inc., Research Triangle Park, North Carolina 27709

INTRODUCTION

The close association between the mutagenic and carcinogenic activity of chemicals and their interaction with cell DNA has focused attention on assays that directly or indirectly measure damage to cellular DNA. Three such assays -- enhancement of viral transformation, analysis of DNA breakage, and stimulation of unscheduled DNA synthesis (UDS) -- have been used extensively in hamster embryo cells to determine the potential of these assays as predictors of carcinogenic activity of various environmental chemicals.

Determining the capacity of carcinogens and mutagens to increase the frequency of hamster cell transformation by DNA viruses (1-8) has been particularly useful, since this technique responds to chemical classes (inorganic metals, hormones, hydrazines, and certain chlorinated hydrocarbons) that are not detected by conventional bacterial mutagenesis assays. In assays with more than 150 chemicals, a 95% agreement was observed between known carcinogenic activity and enhancement of viral transformation (5,9).

Direct damage to cellular DNA by chemical carcinogens can be demonstrated by sedimentation in alkaline sucrose (10-12) or by alkaline elution techniques (13), which suggests that induction of DNA breakage might be useful as a rapid assay for chemical carcinogens. These techniques can be applied to a variety of cell types *in vitro* and, in addition, lend themselves to determining DNA damage in cells isolated from tissues treated *in vivo*.

In several studies using hamster (12,14) or human (12,15) cells cultured *in vitro*, stimulation of UDS appeared to correlate well with carcinogenicity when a series of related compounds was tested. Studies that employed a variety of chemical classes (9) did not demonstrate similar correlations, although the carcinogens used in the study were positive when assayed for cell transformation. The assay for UDS in hamster cells has never yielded false-positive results with noncarcinogens; however, a large number of carcinogens, including metals and certain chlorinated hydrocarbons, fail to induce a positive response.

The extrapolation to man of the potential risk of chemical agents, based upon data from short-term *in vitro* assays in rodent cells, can be reinforced when similar effects are demonstrated in cultured human cells. This presentation compares the performance of selected chemical carcinogens in the three described assays using hamster and human embryonic fibroblasts.

MATERIALS AND METHODS

Cell Cultures

Pregnant hamsters were obtained from the Charles River Lakeview Hamstery (Boston, MA). Primary hamster embryo cell cultures were prepared by trypsinization of eviscerated and decapitated embryos after 13 to 14 days of gestation. Cells were resuspended in a modified Dulbecco's medium (MDM) (General Biochemicals, Grand Island, NY), selected for optimal growth of Syrian hamster cells (1). The medium was supplemented with 5% heat-inactivated fetal bovine serum (FBS), and 0.22% (w/w) sodium biocarbonate ($NaHCO_3$). Approximately 5 x 10^6 cells in 5 ml of medium were plated into 60-mm plastic petri dishes and incubated in a 5% carbon dioxide (CO_2) atmosphere at 36.5°C. Total cell counts after 3 days usually ranged from 3.7 to 4.5 x 10^6 cells per plate.

Continuous lines of monkey kidney cells (VERO and CV-1) were passaged weekly in 100-mm plastic petri dishes. Growth medium consisted of minimum essential medium (MEM) (General Biochemicals, Inc.) with 10% heat-inactivated FBS and 0.22% (w/w) of $NaHCO_3$.

The human male embryonic lung cells used were passaged weekly in 100-mm plastic petri dishes at a 1:4 split ratio ($\sim$ 2 x 10^6 cells/dish). Growth medium consisted of MDM with 1% bovine serum albumin (MDM-BSA), 10% FBS, and 0.30% (w/w) $NaHCO_3$.

Virus

Simian adenovirus, SA7, was inoculated into VERO cell cultures in 100-mm dishes at an input multiplicity of 2 to 3 plaque-forming units (PFU)/cell. Virus was adsorbed for 2 h and 5 ml of medium (MEM, 5% FBS) was then added to each plate. Cytopathic effects were usually complete by 72 h, after which the infected cells were harvested, frozen-thawed four times, and virus was separated from cell debris by low-speed centrifugation. Virus stocks for transformation assays were stored in 1-ml aliquots at -65°C.

Simian virus, SV40, was passaged in CV-1 cells by inoculating cells in 100-mm petri dishes at an input multiplicity of 1 to 2 PFU/cell. The virus was harvested after 4 to 5 days of incubation by four cycles of freeze-thawing, and stored at -65°C in 1-ml aliquots.

Cell Survival Assays

Primary hamster embryo cells were removed from plastic dishes by trypsinization. After centrifugation, the cells were resuspended in MDM with 10% FBS and 0.11% (w/w) $NaHCO_3$, to give 600 to 700 cells per 3 ml; 3 ml of the cell suspension was then added to 60-mm plastic petri dishes using 25 dishes for each chemical to be tested. After 24 h, 3 ml of MDM (10% FBS, 0.22% [w/w] $NaHCO_3$) containing twice the final chemical concentration was added to each of five dishes per test dilution.

The cells were treated for 2 or 24 h, rinsed once, then refed with complete medium and incubated for 8 to 9 days at 37°C. The colonies were fixed in 10% buffered formalin and stained with 0.02% crystal violet. The cloning efficiency of hamster embryo cells under these conditions was usually 7 to 10%.

Survival of human male embryonic lung cells was assayed by plating 500 cells into each 60-mm dish in 3 ml of MDM-BSA, 10% FBS, and 0.15% (w/w) $NaHCO_3$. After 24 h, the cells were treated with chemical for 2 or 24 h, rinsed once, and fed with 3 ml MDM-BSA, 10% FBS, and 0.22% (w/w) $NaHCO_3$. After 3 to 4 days, 3 ml of medium was added, and after 9 to 11 days, the colonies of cells were fixed, stained, and counted. The cloning efficiency of human male embryonic lung cells was usually 10 to 15%.

Preliminary dose-range studies were conducted using fivefold dilutions, with the highest concentration at 100 µg/ml. Final LC_{50} determinations were performed using twofold dilutions. For chemicals not lethal at 100 µg/ml, the highest concentrations employed were 1000 µg/ml; other chemicals were tested beginning with the concentration yielding 0 to 20% cell survival as determined from the preliminary screen.

Enhancement of Viral Transformation

Stock solutions of chemicals were prepared fresh each time by dissolving in acetone. Appropriate dilutions were then made in medium to give the desired final concentrations. In each experiment, two to three plates of hamster embryo cells were treated with chemical for 2 or 18 h, depending upon the nature of the agent being tested. Following incubation with the chemical, hamster embryo cells were rinsed with complete medium and inoculated with SA7. Transformation and survival assays were then performed with each treatment group as described below.

A complete description of the methodology for adenovirus transformation has been presented elsewhere (16,17). Briefly the procedure was as follows: SA7 was added to hamster embryo cells (3 to 4 x 10^7 PFU/culture) and adsorbed for 3 h; the virus-inoculated cells were removed with trypsin (0.25% in MDM with 0.1 mM calcium chloride [$CaCl_2$]), centrifuged, and resuspended to 10^6 cells/ml in MDM, 10% FBS, 0.11% (w/w) $NaHCO_3$, and 2.5 mM BES buffer. Cells were mixed vigorously and plated into 60-mm dishes using 2 or 3 x 10^5 cells per dish; 3 ml of the above medium was then added to each plate. After incubation for 2 or 3 days, the medium was changed to MDM with 0.1 mM $CaCl_2$ (18), 10% FBS, and 0.22% (w/w) $NaHCO_3$. After 6 days and 13 days, all transformation assay plates were overlaid with 5 ml of medium consisting of 0.5% Bacto-agar in MDM with 0.1 mM $CaCl_2$, 10% FBS, and 0.30% (w/w) $NaHCO_3$.

Approximately 21 days from the beginning of the experiment, 4 ml of buffered 10% formalin was added to each plate and allowed to remain for 24 h, after which the soft agar was removed and the cells stained with Giemsa. Foci were counted macroscopically against a background of fluorescent light.

For survival assays, an aliquot of cells from the suspension containing 10^6 cells/ml was diluted 1:300 to give 666 cells/0.2 ml. Onto each of five dishes, 0.2 ml was then plated, 3 ml of medium added, followed 48 to 72 h later by an additional 3 ml; the plates were fixed and stained after incubation for 8 to 9 days.

For enhancement of SV40 transformation of human male embryonic lung cells, cells were seeded into five dishes at 20,000 cells/dish in 3 ml MDM-BSA, 10% FBS, and 0.15% (w/w) $NaHCO_3$. After 24 h, SV40 was added at an input multiplicity of approximately 1000 PFU/cell. After 3 h adsorption, 3 ml of medium (MDM, 10% FBS, 0.22% (w/w) $NaHCO_3$) containing 0.5% anti-SV40 horse serum was added to each dish. Medium was changed every 3 to 4 days for 21 days, at which time all cells were fixed in buffered formalin and Giemsa-stained. SV40 foci appeared as large (5 to 10 mm in diameter), darkly stained areas composed of piled-up, fibroblastic cells against a monolayer background of lightly stained normal cells. Survival was determined from plates containing 500 cells, but treated only with chemical.

The fraction of cells surviving chemical treatment was determined from the survival assay plates which had received 500 to 700 cells per plate. The number of colonies in five plates arising from chemically-treated cells was divided by the number of colonies in five plates from control cells to give the surviving fraction of chemically-treated cells.

The number of SA7 or SV40 foci counted from five control plates, each receiving 200,000 or 20,000 cells, was taken as the total number of foci expected from untreated, virus-inoculated cells. On those plates receiving chemically-treated cells, the total number of foci per 10^6 (SA7) or 10^5 (SV40) cells was calculated by multiplying the actual number from five plates by the ratio: 1/surviving fraction of treated cells. The enhancement ratio was then determined by dividing the total number of foci per 10^6 or 10^5 treated cells by the total number of foci from the appropriate control cells.

Analysis of DNA Strand Breaks

Gradients of 5 to 35% sucrose were prepared by four cycles of freeze-thawing (19) tubes containing 20% sucrose in 0.05% EDTA, which was adjusted to pH 12.6 with 10 M sodium hydroxide (NaOH). Hamster or human fibroblast cell cultures were passaged to 60-mm plastic dishes using 4 x 10^5 cells per dish. After 24 h, the cells were pulsed with 0.5 µCi/ml of ^{3}H-labeled thymidine (^{3}H-TdR) for 24 h. After ^{3}H-TdR labeling, all cultures were changed to MDM with 0.5% FBS and 0.22% (w/w) $NaHCO_3$, and held for an additional 24 h. At this time, each dish contained approximately 10^6 cells. The test chemicals were usually prepared as 1 to 10 mg/ml stocks in acetone and added to prewarmed medium to give the desired final concentration. The cells were treated for 2 or 18 h, washed once, and removed from the dish with EDTA. Following centrifugation, the cells were resuspended in EDTA to give 10^5 cells per 0.2 ml. A 0.2-ml aliquot of the cell suspension was then added to the top of a sucrose gradient tube layered with 0.2 ml of lysing solution (1% sarcosyl in EDTA). The cells were then lysed at room temperature for 1 h, placed in an SW-50 rotor, and centrifuged for 1 h at 30,000 rpm in a Model L-2 ultracentrifuge at 20°C. Three-drop fractions were collected directly into scintillation vials following bottom puncture, neutralized with 1.0 ml of

0.2N hydrochloric acid (HCl), and prepared for counting by adding 5 ml of Bray's scintillation fluid to each vial. Counts were made in a Packard Tri-Carb scintillation spectrometer, 10 min per sample. Data were plotted as a percent of the peak count in each gradient.

Analysis of DNA Repair Synthesis

Cells were passaged to 35-mm petri dishes, each containing a 22-mm square glass coverslip, at 500,000 cells per dish. After 24 h incubation, the cultures were changed to an arginine-free medium (MDM-arg) (20) containing 1.0% FBS to inhibit scheduled DNA synthesis. After incubation in the MDM-arg for 48 to 72 h, the medium was withdrawn, and appropriate concentrations of the test chemicals in MDM-arg were added to each of four plates of cells. Depending upon the particular experiment and the chemical being tested, the exposure period was either 2 or 18 h. After treatment, the cells were rinsed once in MDM-arg, and 2.0 ml of MDM-arg with 1.0% FBS was added to each plate. To each of two plates per chemical concentration was then added ^{3}H-TdR at a concentration of 10 μCi/ml. The cultures were pulsed for 6 h (0 to 6 h), rinsed three times, fixed in Carnoy's fixative, and air-dried. The remaining two plates were labeled as above with ^{3}H-TdR, beginning 6 h after treatment and continuing through 24 h (6 to 24 h). The coverslips were fixed to slides (cell side up) with mounting medium (21), dipped in subbing solution (21), and air-dried. The coverslips were then coated with Kodak Nuclear Track emulsion (NTB2) and exposed for 14 days at 4°C. After developing, the cells were stained for 5 min in a 0.1% crystal violet-0.1 M citric acid solution. The number of grains per nucleus was counted on 100 cells per slide for each of the controls and chemical concentrations.

RESULTS

Lethal Effects of Various Organic and Inorganic Chemicals for Hamster and Human Fibroblasts

The sensitivity of hamster and human cells after 2 h treatment with chemical carcinogens did not differ substantially, with few exceptions (Table 1). Hamster cells were significantly more sensitive than human cells to the lethal effects of aflatoxin B_1 (AFB_1), 4,4-methylenebis-O-chloroaniline (MOCA), and N'N-bis-2-chloroethyl-2-naphthylamine (CE-NAP), whereas lethality induced by N-acetoxy-acetylaminofluorene (AcAAF), α-naphthylamine (α-NAP) and β-naphthylamine (β-NAP), β-propiolactone (β-PL), ethyl methanesulfonate (EMS), methyl methanesulfonate (MMS), N-methyl-N-nitro-N-nitrosoguanidine (MNNG), 4-nitrobiphenyl

(4-NBP), and 1,3-propane sultone (PS) was essentially the same. LC_{50} endpoints were not established in hamster embryo cells for α- or β-NAP and 4-NBP nor in human male embryonic lung cells for AFB_1, α- or β-NAP, or 4-NBP after only 2-h treatment. Following 18-h treatment, LC_{50} endpoints were determined for each of the above (Table 1). Hamster cells were found to be more sensitive than human cells to the cytotoxic effects of AFB_1 (4% survivors at 0.06 μg/ml in hamster embryo cells), benzo[a]pyrene (BP), 7-12-dimethylbenz[a]anthracene (DMBA), and 3-methylcholanthrene (MCA); human cells were more sensitive to cytosine arabinoside (Ara-C), 3,3'-dichlorobenzidine (DCB), and thiourea (TU). Compounds such as 1,3-diethyl-2-thiourea (DETU), ethylene thiourea (ETU), and TU are not metabolized by the hamster embryo cells used in these studies, which is apparently also true for DETU, ETU, DMBA, and MCA in the human male embryonic lung cells.

When metal salts were tested in series in hamster and human cells, cadmium, nickel, and zinc (as $ZnSO_4$) were 5- to 10-fold more toxic for hamster cells; other metal salts, including those of beryllium, chromium, mercury, manganese, titanium, and zirconium, induced essentially the same degree of cell killing in both cell types (Table 2). Certain metal salts, such as those of cadmium and zinc, produced dose-response curves in human cells that showed a 90% reduction in survivors within a single twofold dilution; mercury and zirconium produced the same type of dose response in hamster cells (data not shown).

Enhancement of Viral Transformation by Chemical Carcinogens in Hamster, Rat, and Human Cells

Hamster, rat, or human cells when pretreated with chemical carcinogens become more sensitive to transformation by DNA viruses (1-8,22-24). An example of an observed effect is shown in Table 3: Treatment of hamster and human embryonic cells with MMS resulted in an absolute increase in virally-induced transformed foci in treated cells and a dose-related increase in the frequency of viral transformation. The foci induced are typical for the virus and are not induced under these test conditions when cells are treated with chemical alone.

The lowest effective concentration that induces a significant ($p < 0.05$) enhancement response (2,25) was determined for selected carcinogens in hamster, rat, or human cells. Hamster cells were more sensitive than rat cells to the enhancing effects of AcAAF, BP, and MCA (Table 4), but were less sensitive to ETU. Both β-PL and MMS were equally effective in hamster and human cells, but hamster cells were more sensitive to the polycyclic hydrocarbons BP and MCA.

Table 1. LC_{50} of Various Chemicals for Hamster and Human Cells Treated for 2 and 18 h

	LC_{50} (μg/ml)[b]			
	2 h		18 h	
Chemical[a]	Hamster	Human	Hamster	Human
AcAAF	2.5	1.0	-	-
AFB_1	0.1	>5.0	<0.06	0.2
α-NAP	>200	>500	100	65
Ara-C	-	-	0.09	0.016
β-NAP	>200	>500	200	220
β-PL	7.0	7.0	-	-
BP	-	-	0.35	5
Caffeine	-	-	280	285
CE-NAP	0.3	2.0	-	-
DCB	-	-	250	50
DETU	-	-	>1000	>1000
DMBA	-	-	0.006	>10
EMS	>400	750	-	-
ETU	-	-	>1000	>1000
HA[c]	-	-	140	220
HU[c]	-	-	200	140
MCA	-	-	0.25	>20
MMS	50	40	-	-
MNNG	0.5	0.1	-	-
MOCA	45	270	-	-
4-NBP	>200	>200	120	100
PS	20	30	-	-
TA[c]	-	-	8	20
TU	-	-	>1000	200

[a]Hamster or human cells were plated at 500 to 700 cells per dish. Twenty-four hours after plating, the cells were treated for 2 h or 18 h with chemical, the cultures rinsed, fresh medium was added, and the cells were fixed and stained after 8 to 10 days at 37°C.
[b]Colonies were counted from five plates per chemical concentration and the percent of control was calculated for each dose. Fifty-percent endpoints were determined from line graphs representing average data from two to three experiments per chemical.

Table 2. LC_{50} of Metal Salts for Hamster and Human Cells Treated for 18 h

Metal[a]	LC_{50} (μg/ml)[b]	
	Hamster	Human
$BeSO_4$	125	100
$Cd(C_2H_3O_2)$	0.35	35
$CdCl_2$	0.80	35
$CaCrO_4$	2.0	7.5
$HgCl_2$	10	14
K_2CrO_4	3.0	5.5
$MnCl_2$	100	>50
$NiSO_4$	65	400
TiO_2	>1000	550
$ZnCl_2$	45	42
$ZnSO_4$	30	350
ZrF_4	350	240

[a,b]See legend, Table 1.

Analysis of DNA Breakage in Hamster and Human Cells Treated with Chemical Carcinogens

Hamster and human embryonic cells were treated with a series of eight chemicals. The lowest effective concentration required to induce breakage and the relative distance (ΔD) of the broken DNA peak from the peak count of control cell DNA were determined. Peaks of control cell DNA from replicate samples or DNA from cells treated with noneffective concentrations of chemical are usually clustered within one fraction from a single run (10).

All of the chemicals tested, with the exception of PS, induced breakage at lower concentrations in hamster cells (Table 5). The differences in the lowest effective concentrations required to induce breakage by AFB_1, $Cd(C_2H_3O_2)_2$, and MOCA in hamster and human cells were of the same order as the differences in the LC_{50} concentrations (see Tables 1 and 2).

Table 3. Enhancement of Viral Transformation in Hamster and Human Cells by MMS

Cell Type	MMS (μg/ml[a])	Surviving Fraction[b]	Viral Foci[c]	Enhancement Ratio[d]
Hamster	100	0.04	6	7.2
	50	0.29	30	4.9
	25	0.32	36	5.4
	12.5	0.76	45	2.8
	6.25	0.98	42	2.0[e]
	A	1.06	27	1.2
	C	1.00	21	1.0
Human	100.0	0.05	3	13.0
	50.0	0.78	20	5.2
	25.0	1.09	19	3.6
	12.5	1.04	7	1.4
	6.2	1.03	6	1.2
	A	1.04	4	0.8
	C	1.00	5	1.0

[a]Cells were treated for 2 h with MMS. After rinsing, virus was added and adsorbed for 3 h. Foci of transformed cells were counted after 21 to 25 days at 37°C. A = acetone control; C = medium control.
[b]Determined from plates receiving 500 to 700 cells. The number of surviving colonies from five treated dishes was divided by the number from five control dishes to give the surviving fraction.
[c]Total foci from 10^6 (SA7) or 10^5 (SV40) plated cells.
[d]Enhancement ratio was determined by dividing the transformation frequency (TF) of treated cells (TF = virus foci x reciprocal of the surviving fraction) by that obtained from control cells. Underlined values were significant at $p \leq 0.01$.
[e]Significant at $p \leq 0.05$.

UDS in Hamster and Human Cells Treated with Chemical Carcinogens

The typical response of human cells to chemicals capable of inducing UDS is shown in Figure 1. Most control cells (72%) and most cells treated only with solvent (77%) had no grains over the nucleus when labeled with ^{3}H-TdR for 6 h; the average counts in such preparations were 0.49 and 0.34 grains per nucleus, respectively (Figure 1). When labeled for 18 h (6 to 24 h after treatment) the average counts for medium and solvent control were 0.61 and 1.53 grains per nucleus (Figure 1). The good

Table 4. Enhancement of Viral Transformation in Hamster, Rat, and Human Embryonic Cells Treated with Chemical Carcinogens

	Cell System					
	Hamster		Rat		Human	
Chemical[a]	LEC[b]	ER[c]	LEC	ER	LEC	ER
AcAAF	1.25	2.6	10	2.2		
β-PL	10	3.4			10	3.6
BP	0.08	2.8	0.4	4.2	1.2	2.7
ETU	1000	0.9	125	1.7		
MCA	0.08	2.3	0.4	3.7	1.2	2.6
MMS	12.5	2.8	25	2.5	25	3.6

[a]Cells were treated for 2 h (AcAAF, β-PL, MMS) or 18 h with chemical. After rinsing, virus was added and adsorbed for 3 h. Foci of transformed cells were counted after 21 to 25 days at 37°C.
[b]Lowest effective concentration of chemical (μg/ml) yielding a significant response ($p < 0.05$).
[c]Enhancement ratio (ER) was obtained by dividing the transformation frequency in treated cells by the frequency in control cells.

dose-response relationship between grain counts per nucleus and treatment concentrations that is shown in this analysis allows a determination of the magnitude of the response per cell and of the percentage of the cell population undergoing UDS.

A comparison of the induction of UDS in hamster and human cells by five carcinogens is shown in Table 6. AcAAF, β-PL, and MNNG induced UDS in hamster cells at 4- to 25-fold lower concentrations than in human cells; the concentration of EMS required was approximately the same in both cell types. The sensitivity of hamster and human cells to induction of UDS with AcAAF, β-PL, and MNNG agrees well with the relative sensitivity to the same chemicals as determined by DNA breakage analysis (Table 5).

The initial UDS response to ultraviolet radiation and most chemicals on a per-cell basis is significantly higher in human cells than in hamster cells, as determined by counting the number of grains per nucleus. For example, when cells were treated with

Table 5. DNA Breakage in Hamster and Human Embryonic Cells Treated with Chemical Carcinogens

	Cell System			
	Hamster		Human	
Chemical[a]	LEC[b]	ΔD[c]	LEC	ΔD
AFB_1	1	0.30	10	0.0
AcAAF	0.4	0.12	10	0.17
β-PL	2.5	0.33	10	0.15
$Cd(C_2H_3O_2)_2$	0.25	0.33	50	0.19
MMS	25	0.35	100	0.23
MNNG	0.2	0.34	5	0.20
MOCA	30	0.61	400	0.55
PS	25	0.10	25	0.13

[a]Cells were plated at 4 x 10^5 per 60-mm dish, labeled with ^{3}H-TdR and treated with test chemical. After treatment the cells were removed with EDTA, lysed on 5 to 35% sucrose gradients (pH 12.6), and centrifuged at 30,000 rpm for 1 h at 20°C. Fractions were collected by bottom puncture, neutralized, scintillation fluid was added, and each fraction counted for 10 min in a liquid scintillation spectrometer.

[b]Lowest effective concentration of chemical (μg/ml) causing the peak of treated cell DNA to shift $>$ 6 mm ($\Delta D > 0.09$) in distance from the control cell DNA peak. (See footnote C.)

[c] ΔD = Proportionate distance from the peak count of control cell DNA when the total gradient is plotted on a scale 0 to 1.0.

the same concentrations of AcAAF, MMS, and MNNG, the median grain counts in human cells (labeled for 6 h) were three- to sevenfold higher than in hamster cells (Table 7). Similar differences were not observed in cells treated with β-PL or EMS.

DISCUSSION

Short-term *in vitro* techniques, used to determine the potential carcinogenicity of chemicals in rodent cells, can be applied to cultured human cells. Three such assays, showing a positive response in hamster cells to chemical carcinogens, were employed using cells derived from human embryonic lung.

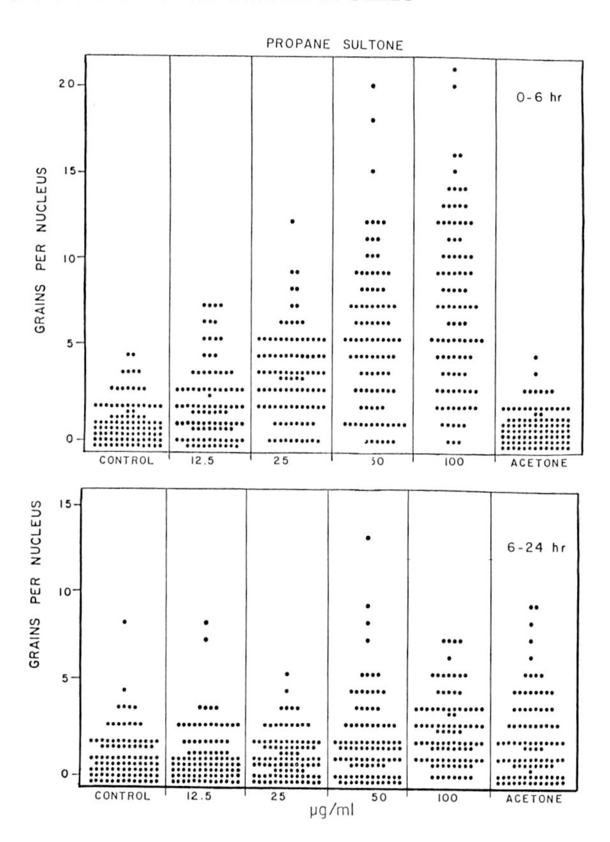

Figure 1. Autoradiographic analysis of UDS in human embryonic fibroblasts treated with PS. Cells were preincubated for 72 h in MDM-arg and treated with chemical for 2 h. One-half of the cultures were pulsed for 6 h immediately after treatment (0 to 6 h) and the remaining for 18 h beginning 6 h after chemical removal (6 to 24 h). Each point represents the number of grains per nucleus over individual cells.

Cell survival assays, conducted in human and hamster cells concurrently with the short-term carcinogenicity bioassays, revealed that the human lung embryonic cells used in these assays were equally sensitive to the lethal effects of most chemicals (64% of those tested). Three chemicals (Ara-C, DCB, and TU) were more toxic for human cells, whereas 10 others were more toxic for hamster cells when assayed for cell survival. Cell killing did not occur after treatment with certain agents, possibly because the cultured cells did not metabolize the test chemicals. For example, DETU, ETU, and TU were found negative in a variety of _in vitro_ tests in hamster embryo cells; TU has also been found to be negative in the Ames test (26). Chemicals such as α- and β-NAP,

Table 6. UDS in Hamster and Human Cells Treated with Chemical Carcinogens: Effective Dose.

Labeling Period	Chemical[a]	Hamster Cell System			Human Cell System		
		LEC[b]	Grains/ Nucleus[c]	% Cells in Repair[d]	LEC	Grains/ Nucleus	% Cells in Repair
0 to 6 h	AcAAF	0.08	7	87	1.25	28	89
	β-PL	2.5	3	21	10	4	17
	EMS	62.5	21	38	125	3	29
	MMS	1.0	7	21	<25	28	100
	MNNG	0.04	4	53	1.0	11	22
6 to 24 h	AcAAF	0.4	10	36	1.25	19	80
	β-PL	2.5	7	36	10.0	6	30
	EMS	62.5	12	53	250	8	15
	MMS	125	9	79	<25	35	97
	MNNG	0.04	6	70	0.5	19	18

[a] Cells were preincubated for 48 to 72 h in MDM-arg and treated for 2 h with chemical. After treatment, one-half of the cultures were pulsed with ^{3}H-TdR (10 μCi/ml) for 6 h (0 to 6 h); the remaining cultures were pulsed for 18 h beginning 6 h after chemical removal (6 to 24 h).

[b] Lowest effective concentration of chemical (μg/ml) causing greater than a threefold increase in the number of grains per nucleus.

[c] Median grain count per nucleus among cells in repair (>3 times above background).

[d] Percentage of cells having a grain count per nucleus threefold or greater above background. Background counts in separate experiments ranged from 0.4 to 2.0 in hamster cells and 0.2 to 4.0 in human cells.

Table 7. UDS in Hamster and Human Cells Treated with Chemical Carcinogens: Level of Response.

			Hamster Cell System			Human Cell System		
			Grains per Nucleus			Grains per Nucleus		
Labeling Period	Chemical[a]	Dose (μg/ml)	Med[b]	Avg[c]	% Cells in Repair[d]	Med	Avg	% Cells in Repair
0 to 6 h	AcAAF	1.25	9	8.9	71	28	26.2	89
	β-PL	10.0	3	3.0	29	6	4.7	30
	EMS	250	10	10.5	59	8	8.1	43
	MMS	25.0	7	7.8	38	35	38.5	100
	MNNG	0.5	6	7.4	73	19	24.8	18
6 to 24 h	AcAAF	1.25	20	15.1	70	19	20.9	80
	β-PL	10.0	10	10.8	92	4	4.7	30
	EMS	125	19	13.6	66	3	3.3	4
	MMS	25.0	6	6.8	8	28	27.4	97
	MNNG	1.0	20	21	99	21	22.5	51

[a]Cells were preincubated for 48 to 72 h in MDM-arg and treated for 2h with chemical. After treatment, one-half of the cultures were pulsed with ^{3}H-TdR (10 μCi/ml) for 6 h (0 to 6 h); the remaining cultures were pulsed for 18 h beginning 6 h after chemical removal (6 to 24 h).
[b]Median grain count per nucleus among cells in repair (>3 times above background).
[c]Average grain count per nucleus among cells in repair (>3 times above background.
[d]Percentage of cells having a grain count per nucleus threefold or greater above background. Background counts in separate experiments ranged from 0.2 to 4.0 in hamster cells and 0.2 to 4.0 in human cells.

AFB_1, and 4-NBP were not cytocidal to human cells after a 2-h exposure to concentrations that are more than 80% lethal after a 24-h exposure. Hamster cells also required a longer exposure to these agents to demonstrate maximal cell killing (with the exception of AFB_1). As would be expected when a larger number of chemicals were tested, longer exposure times (18 h versus 2 h) resulted in more cell killing at the same dose of chemical and in a lowering of the LC_{50}. Greater toxic responses were also observed if the cells were treated shortly after plating (within 5 h after cell transfer) in contrast with treatment of confluent cells, or cells plated at low density 24 h prior to treatment (data not shown).

Using the data obtained from the cytotoxicity assays, selected chemicals were tested in hamster and human cells in three short-term *in vitro* assays.

SV40 transformation of human cells was enhanced by the same chemical carcinogens that were found to enhance adenovirus transformation of hamster and rat cells, the only provision being that the human cells are able to metabolize the test chemical to an active form. With the direct-acting chemical agents, the concentration required and the degree of enhancement did not differ between hamster and human cells; however, agents such as the polycyclic hydrocarbons (BP and MCA) that require metabolic activation were more effective in hamster cells than in rat or human cells.

When assayed for breakage of cell DNA by alkaline sucrose gradients, seven of eight chemicals positive in hamster cells were also positive in human cells. (AFB_1 was negative in human cells at 10 μg/ml.) Six of those seven chemicals were more effective in producing DNA breakage in hamster cells than in human cells; the remaining chemical (PS) induced breaks at the same concentration in both hamster and human cells. With most chemicals (PS and AFB_1 being the exceptions), the dose required to induce breakage was substantially less than the LC_{50}. Moreover, several toxic chemicals did not induce breakage. The above results suggest that DNA breakage is a specific event that is exhibited independent of cell killing.

Treatment of hamster and human embryonic cells with certain chemical carcinogens stimulates UDS (10-12,14,15). Although a good correlation exists between carcinogenic potential and UDS with related carcinogens (14,15), such relationships were not observed when a series of agents from several chemical classes was assayed (9). The assay is valuable because a relatively short time is needed for demonstration, false-positives have not been observed, and the test can be applied to various target cell types that are not capable of replicating *in vitro*.

The five chemicals selected for study that induced UDS in hamster cells also induced UDS in human cells. The lowest effective concentration for three of the five chemicals was 4- to 25-fold lower in hamster cells; however, the human cells generally gave a higher response per cell (as indicated by autoradiography). Following ultraviolet or chemical treatment, the total fraction of cells demonstrating a repair response was 95 to 100% at the higher chemical concentrations, whether in hamster or human cell cultures.

The data presented show that short-term assays useful for determining the carcinogenic potential of environmental chemicals in hamster cells may be applied to human cells in culture. In comparative studies, the human cell cultures were as sensitive (with respect to the concentration necessary to induce a positive response) as hamster cells to β-PL, EMS and MMS, and PS. The human embryonic lung cells were less sensitive to AcAAF, AFB_1, BP, cadmium, MNNG, MCA, and MOCA. Certain of these short-term assays, therefore, are applicable to human cell systems in the search for the etiologic agents of human cancer.

ACKNOWLEDGMENTS

This publication is based on work performed at BioLabs, Inc., Northbrook, IL, pursuant to NIH-NCI Contract NOI-CP-45615 with the National Cancer Institute, Department of Health, Education, and Welfare. Human male embryonic lung cells were the gift of Dr. George Milo, The Ohio State University in Columbus, OH. The author wishes to thank William J. Pieczynski, Judy Meyers, Nancy Janosko, and Regina Oslapas for invaluable technical assistance during these studies.

REFERENCES

1. Casto, B.C. 1973. Enhancement of adenovirus transformation by treatment of hamster cells with UV, DNA base analogs, and dibenz[a,h]anthracene. Cancer Res. 33:402-407.

2. Casto, B.C., W.J. Pieczynski, and J.A. DiPaolo. 1973. Enhancement of adenovirus transformation by pretreatment of hamster cells with carcinogenic polycyclic hydrocarbons. Cancer Res. 33:819-824.

3. Casto, B.C., W.J. Pieczynski, and J.A. DiPaolo. 1974. Enhancement of adenovirus transformation by treatment of hamster embryo cells with diverse chemical carcinogens. Cancer Res. 34:72-78.

4. Casto, B.C., J. Meyers, and J.A. DiPaolo. 1979. Enhancement of viral transformation for evaluation of the carcinogenic or mutagenic potential of inorganic metal salts. Cancer Res. 39:193-198.

5. Casto, B.C. 1981. Detection of chemical carcinogens and mutagens in hamster cells by enhancement of adenovirus transformation. In: Advances in Modern Environmental Toxicology, Volume 1. Mammalian Cell Transformation by Chemical Carcinogens. N. Mishra, V. Dunkel, and M. Mehlman, eds. Senate Press Inc.: Princeton Junction, NJ. pp. 241-271.

6. Ledinko, N., and M. Evans. 1973. Enhancement of adenovirus transformation of hamster cells by N-methyl-N^1-nitro-N-nitrosoguanidine, caffeine, and hydroxylamine. Cancer Res. 33:2936-2938.

7. Milo, G.E., J.P. Schaller, and D.S. Yohn. 1973. Hormonal modification of adenovirus transformation of hamster cells _in vitro_. Cancer Res. 32:2338-2347.

8. Parent, R.A., and B.C. Casto. 1979. Effect of acrylonitrile on primary Syrian hamster embryo cells in culture: Transformation and DNA fragmentation. J. Natl. Cancer Inst. 62:1025-1029.

9. Casto, B.C., N. Janosko, J. Meyers, and J.A. DiPaolo. 1978. Comparison of _in vitro_ tests in Syrian hamster cells for detection of carcinogens. Proc. Am. Assoc. for Cancer Res. 19:83.

10. Casto, B.C., W.J. Pieczynski, N. Janosko, and J.A. DiPaolo. 1976. Significance of treatment interval and DNA repair in the enhancement of viral transformation by chemical carcinogens and mutagens. Chem.-Biol. Interact. 13:105-125.

11. Laishes, B.A., and H.F. Stich. 1973. Repair synthesis and sedimentation analysis of DNA of human cells exposed to dimethylnitrosamine and activated dimethylnitrosamine. Biochem. Biophys. Res. Comm. 52:827-833.

12. Stich, H.F., R.H.C. San, P.P.S. Lam, D.J. Koropatnick, L.W. Lo, and B.A. Laishes. 1976. DNA fragmentations or DNA repair as an _in vitro_ and _in vivo_ assay for chemical procarcinogens, carcinogens, and carcinogenic nitrosation products. In: Screening Tests in Chemical Carcinogenesis. R. Montesano, H. Bartsch, and L. Tomatis, eds. IARC Scientific Publications No. 12. International Agency for Research on Cancer: Lyons, France. pp. 617-636.

13. Swenberg, J.A., G.L. Petzold, and P.R. Harbach. 1976. In vitro DNA damage/alkaline elution assay for predicting carcinogenic potential. Biochem. Biophys. Res. Comm. 72:732-738.

14. Stich, H.F., R.H.C. San, and Y. Kawazoe. 1971. DNA repair synthesis in mammalian cells exposed to a series of oncogenic and nononcogenic derivations of 4-nitroquinoline-1-oxide. Nature 229:416-419.

15. San, R.H.C., and H.F. Stich. 1975. DNA repair synthesis of cultured human cells as a rapid bioassay for chemical carcinogens. Int. J. Cancer 16:284-291.

16. Casto, B.C. 1968. Adenovirus transformation of hamster embryo cells. J. Virol. 2:376-383.

17. Casto, B.C. 1973. Biologic parameters of adenovirus transformation. Prog. Exp. Tumor Res. 18. Karger: Basel/New York. pp. 166-198.

18. Freeman, A.E., P.H. Black, R. Wolford, and R.J. Huebner. 1967. Adenovirus type 12-rat embryo transformation system. J. Virol. 1:362-367.

19. Baxter-Gabbard, K.L. 1972. A simple method for the large-scale preparation of sucrose gradients. FEBS Lett. 20:117-119.

20. Freed, J.J., and S.A. Schatz. 1969. Chromosome aberrations in cultured cells deprived of a single essential amino acid. Exp. Cell Res. 55:393-409.

21. Boyd, G.A. 1955. Autoradiography in Biology and Medicine. Academic Press, Inc.: New York.

22. Hirai, K., V. Defendi, and L. Diamond. 1974. Enhancement of simian virus 40 transformation and integration by 4-nitroquinoline-1-oxide. Cancer Res. 34:3497-3500.

23. Casto, B.C. 1974. Enhancement of viral oncogenesis by chemical carcinogens. In: The Biochemistry of Disease, Volume 4. Chemical Carcinogenesis. P.O.P. Ts'o and J.A. DiPaolo, eds. Marcel Dekker, Inc.: New York. pp. 607-618.

24. Casto, B.C., and J.A. DiPaolo. 1973. Viruses, chemicals, and cancer. Prog. Med. Virol. 16:1-47.

25. Lorenz, R.J. 1962. Zur Statistik des Plaque-Testes. Arch. Gesamt. Virusforsch. 12:108-137.

26. McCann, J., E. Choi, E. Yamasaki, and B.N. Ames. 1975. Detection of carcinogens as mutagens in the *Salmonella*/microsome test: Assay of 300 chemicals. Proc. Natl. Acad. Sci. 72:5135-5139.

DISCUSSION

Q.: In the beginning of your presentation you indicated that for viral transformation hamster embryo cells derived from different organs showed very different sensitivity, which is a tantalizing piece of information. Have you followed that up with direct chemical transformation studies to relate the two processes?

A.: I agree that this is a very interesting finding, but we have not yet followed it up with further studies.

Q.: How were the humans cells obtained. Were they pools of cells or from a specific site or organ?

A.: The human cells were all obtained from human embryonic lung tissue.

TISSUE-SPECIFIC SISTER CHROMATID EXCHANGE ANALYSES IN MUTAGEN-CARCINOGEN EXPOSED ANIMALS

James W. Allen[1], Yousuf Sharief[2], Robert Langenbach[1], and Michael D. Waters[1]

[1]Genetic Toxicology Division, Health Effects Research Laboratory, U.S. Environmental Protection Agency, Research Triangle Park, North Carolina 27711, and [2]Northrop Services, Inc., Research Triangle Park, North Carolina 27709

INTRODUCTION

The phenomenon of sister chromatid exchange (SCE) has been extensively reviewed (1-5). Sister chromatid exchanges are intrachromosomal events, wherein segments of DNA are reciprocally swapped between the chromatids. They are most easily studied with 5-bromodeoxyuridine (BrdU) dye methodology (6-8), which effectively differentiates the sister chromatids so that exchanges between them are detectable as staining discontinuities. Presumably, the exchange sites are at homologous loci and no inequality in the amount of translocated material results. Sister chromatid exchange is not known to alter cell viability or function; its spontaneous frequency and biological importance are uncertain. Yet, early autoradiography studies in cultured cells revealed elevated SCE frequencies as an effect of mutagen and carcinogen exposures (9). Consequently, with the development of more expeditious BrdU methodology, a course was set for accelerated studies of SCE formation in response to mutagen- or carcinogen-DNA interactions.

A wide array of chemical mutagens and carcinogens have now been surveyed for SCE-inducing properties (4,5). Through its sensitivity and relevance as a chromosomal effect from many genotoxic agents, SCE induction has proven a meaningful index of genetic activity. Induced SCEs and gene mutations have, for some chemicals, been shown to be linearly related (10,11), although the relative efficiency of chromosomal or gene response varies with different modes of chemical-DNA interaction (10-12). Increasing evidence suggests that mechanisms of SCE induction are at least partially independent from those involved in chromosome aberrations. Most clastogenic chemicals induce significant increases in SCE at small fractions of the concentration required to cause chromosome aberrations. Yet, a few chemicals are relatively more potent for the production of chromosomal aberrations (4,5). Sister chromatid exchanges and aberrations also appear to be unrelated in their distribution (13).

Although usually accompanying other forms of induced DNA alteration, SCE is clearly a divergent expression of DNA alteration and represents a unique genetic phenomenon. It is thought to arise from a small fraction of the actual number of DNA lesions, i.e., adducts (5) or dimers (14), although the precise mechanism of SCE formation is unknown. Similarities between SCE and steps or products of various repair processes have been noted (1-5). Yet, the dependence of SCE upon DNA repair has not been demonstrated. It has recently been hypothesized that SCE may not be a direct expression of a repair process; rather, repair may be implicated only to the extent that the residual lesion is ultimately a determinant of SCE formation (15). Clearly, SCE is critically associated with DNA synthesis and requires this process for its expression (16). The replication fork has been implicated theoretically with the initiation of SCEs (3,15,17). Painter (15) has suggested that the junctions between replicon clusters may be especially susceptible to double-strand breakage with subsequent recombination between parent and daughter strands. These sites might represent a limited number of regions vulnerable to SCE formation where DNA damage remains unrepaired.

In vivo analyses account for "complete" host mediation or processing of a chemical. As such, they provide highly relevant approaches for evaluating genetic hazard. A perspective on *in vivo* tissue-specific SCE analyses in mammals is presented in the following text and the relationship of these studies to some *in vitro* approaches is discussed. As most chemical carcinogens require metabolic activation (18) and are influenced by physiological and tissue-specific variables (19,20), pertinent advantages of *in vivo* SCE systems are emphasized. Although few studies of animal tissue differences in SCE response to chemicals have been undertaken, some examples wherein such differences have been observed are noted. In these instances, further studies aimed at characterizing the influence of suspect metabolites on gene mutation and chromosomal effects *in vitro* are briefly described.

METHODOLOGY

The basic BrdU dye technique to achieve differential staining of sister chromatids depends upon sequential steps of DNA labeling, cell cycling, and chromosome staining. Cells are treated with BrdU in order to effect substitution of this base analogue for thymidine during DNA synthesis. A subsequent replication period, with or without further labeling, results in sister chromatids characterized by different amounts of BrdU substitution. When a BrdU-sensitive dye is then applied at metaphase stage, the sister chromatids become differentially stained. Options in the mode of BrdU administration, in conjunction with flexibility in the time of test agent treatment, have permitted a great deal of versatility for application within *in vitro* and *in vivo* systems (see Figure 1).

I. *In Vitro*
BrdU and test chemical treatments in culture.

II. *In Vivo*
BrdU and test chemical treatments in the intact animal.

III. Hybrid *In Vivo* - *In Vitro*
A. Test chemical treatment *in vivo*; BrdU treatment *in vitro*.

B. BrdU treatment *in vivo*; test chemical treatment *in vitro*.

Figure 1. Versatility in technical approaches for SCE analysis.

The original development (6) and predominant application of the BrdU dye technique has been as a "pure" *in vitro* method. Cells are cultured through two consecutive DNA synthesis periods in media containing BrdU and the test chemical. Thus, sister chromatids become unifilarly versus bifilarly substituted with BrdU. *In vivo* BrdU labeling methods in mammals were slower to develop because of early difficulties in achieving sufficient levels of analogue substitution for effecting chromatid dye contrast. Due to adult liver capabilities to rapidly catabolize and dehalogenate BrdU (21), techniques designed to provide continuous replenishment of analogue to the animal are necessary. Schemes developed to provide sustained BrdU exposure rely upon serial intraperitoneal injections (22,23), infusion (24,25), or internal deposition of BrdU in order to label DNA over at least one DNA synthesis period (see Figure 2). The latter "depot" methods operate on the principle of prolonged release of analogue from a subcutaneous implant of either BrdU adsorbed onto charcoal (26,27) or pure BrdU packed into a slow-dissolving tablet (28,29). The continuous infusion and BrdU tablet methods are widely used because of relative technical simplicity. Label incorporation over the first DNA replication only, or alternatively over both replications, is inconsequential to the quality of chromatid contrast achievable.

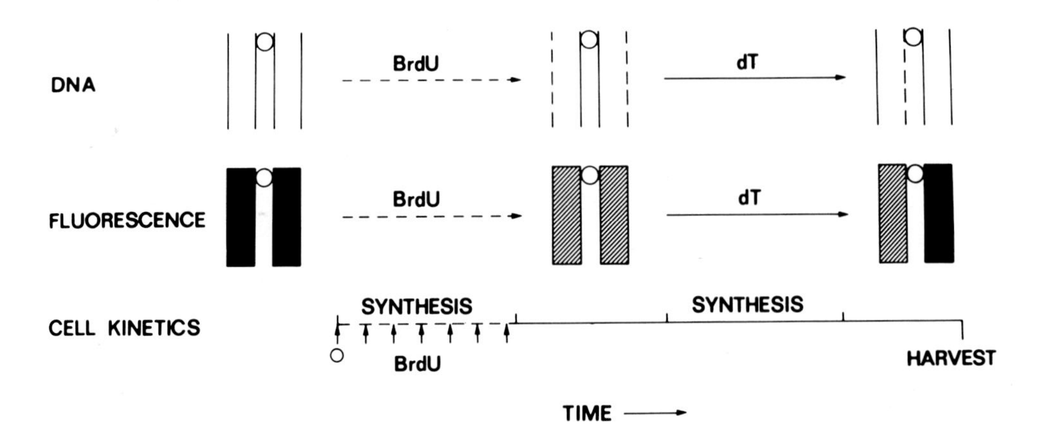

Figure 2. Diagrammatic representation of *in vivo* protocol for effecting sister chromatid differentiation. Unsubstituted DNA chains are represented by solid lines and BrdU-substituted chains by broken lines. 33258 Hoechst fluorescence is denoted as bright by black shading and dull by grey shading. Following BrdU incorporation for one DNA synthesis period, first division chromosomes are unifilarly substituted in each chromatid and exhibit dull fluorescence in chromatid arms. Subsequent replication without BrdU incorporation results in second division chromosomes with asymmetrical BrdU substitution. Bright fluorescence of unsubstituted chromatids contrasts with dull fluorescence of chromatids with single-strand substitution (26).

BrdU is thought to quench the fluorescence of 33258 Hoechst dye (see Figure 3a) by reducing the quantum yield of bound dye molecules (5). A variety of analogue and dye modifications to the basic approach have been reported. In particular, the fluorescence-plus Giemsa (FPG) dye technique (8,30) has been widely used for its advantages related to permanent staining and easy analysis. The schedule for test chemical treatment is optional, although usually the chemical is administered to the animal at a time estimated to coincide with the first or second DNA synthesis period. An advantage of the former is that chromosome insult is maximized over two replication periods; and of the latter, that heavily damaged cells which may cycle only once are not lost from analysis (see Figure 3b).

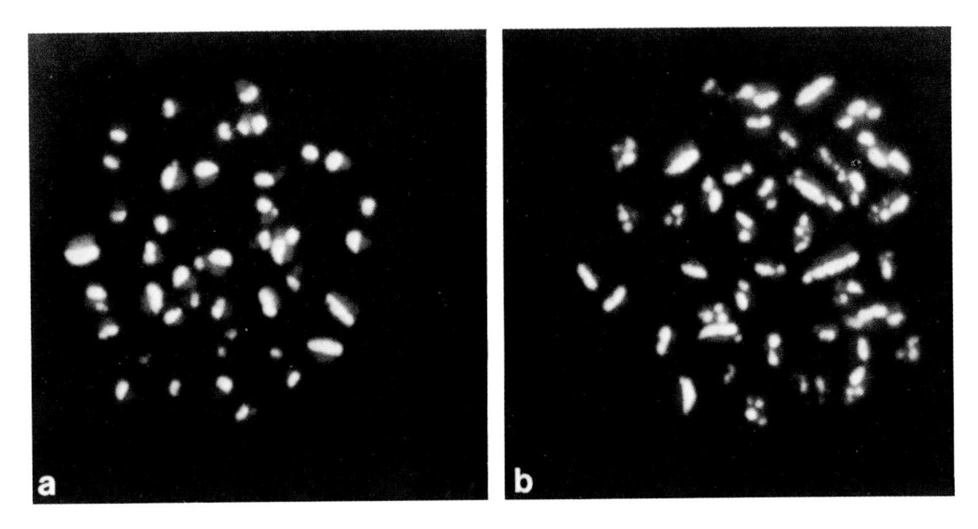

Figure 3. Sister chromatid differentiation and exchange in rat embryo liver cells after maternal treatment with a BrdU tablet and metaphase staining with 33258 Hoechst dye. Five SCEs are evident in the control cell (a). More than 40 SCEs are detectable in cell (b) after maternal intraperitoneal exposure to 10 mg/kg cyclophosphamide.

Hybrid methodology (31,32) affords expanded capabilities for analyzing in vivo SCE induction in human and animal tissues. The impropriety of administering BrdU to humans prevents direct analysis. However, following accidental or medical exposure to potentially genotoxic agents, cells may be removed for growth in vitro with BrdU and subsequent analysis of SCE formation. Although some loss in sensitivity may result from lesion repair or cell-cycling dilution of elevated SCE levels, this loss can be minimized by initiating cell culture soon after exposure. Residual elevations in lymphocyte SCE have been detectable in cancer patients at variable periods of time after chemotherapy (33-35) and in rabbits several months after drug treatment (36). Additional target tissues with characteristically low cell turnover rates can also be analyzed through in vitro stimulation of growth and BrdU substitution.

Occasional instances occur that are best served by the reverse protocol, where BrdU labeling is in vivo even though chemical testing is in vitro. For example, rodent embryos scheduled for test agent exposures under whole embryo culture conditions are most uniformly substituted in specific tissues with BrdU when labeling is via the in vivo transplacental route immediately prior to explantation (37). While the principal methodological approaches have been outlined, further variations exist. As an example, differential staining analyses of SCE have been conducted on cells cultured in diffusion chambers and implanted in animal hosts. SCE induction in both human (38) and rodent (39) cells has been analyzed in this way following in vivo BrdU and mutagen treatments of a mouse host.

IN VIVO STUDIES

Sister chromatid exchange analyses in carcinogen-exposed animals complement and extend simpler in vitro trials. Both approaches have proven adaptable for large-scale chemical surveys (31,40), although in vivo systems are often used to verify, or signal deficiencies in, results from cell culture studies. Chemicals that are direct-acting in vitro for the production of SCEs tend to be similarly effective in vivo. A few exceptions exist; for example, vitamin C causes dose-dependent SCE increases in cultured Chinese hamster ovary (CHO) cells and human lymphocytes (41,42). Yet, when this substance is administered to Chinese hamsters over a wide dose range, bone marrow cells do not reveal any increase in SCE. In this case, it is suspected that enzyme levels in the intact organism are protective (42).

On the other hand, agents such as benzo[a]pyrene (BP), 2-acetylaminofluorene, cyclophosphamide, and ethyl carbamate (urethane) are relatively ineffective SCE inducers in routinely cultured cells without an exogenous metabolic activation system (31,43,44). Under conditions of improved metabolic capabilities through addition of S9 mix (43,45,46), liver or embryo cell mediation (47,48), testing in hepatic tumor cell lines (49), or, alternatively, with in vivo exposure trials (50-53), these chemicals become competent for SCE induction. However, as illustrated in Table 1, some fundamental metabolic differences are indicated. While S9 mix effectively activates cyclophosphamide to give very positive results for the SCE end point in Chinese hamster V79 cells, the same cannot be said of ethyl carbamate. Yet, both compounds yield dramatically positive results when administered to mice (50,53). These conflicting results with ethyl carbamate are generally consistent with other studies of genotoxic effects from this chemical (44). Studies aimed at defining steps critical to the metabolic conversion of ethyl carbamate are currently in progress in our laboratory. These studies involve the evaluation of selected co-factors for S9 metabolism as well as metabolic activation provided by cocultivation with intact primary hepatocytes.

Table 1. *In Vitro* SCE Frequencies in Chinese Hamster V79 Cells Treated with Cyclophosphamide or Ethyl Carbamate[a]

Test Chemical	Dose	SCE Frequencies[b] -S9	SCE Frequencies[b] +S9
Control	--	9.9 ± 2.9	10.7 ± 2.9
Cyclophosphamide	5 μg/ml	11.6 ± 4.4	27.6 ± 7.1
	25 μg/ml	12.9 ± 5.0	60.6 ± 14.0
Ethyl carbamate	1 mg/ml	8.7 ± 3.4	10.1 ± 3.0
	10 mg/ml	9.3 ± 2.7	11.8 ± 3.5

[a]Cells were grown in Williams E media with 10% fetal calf serum. After 4 h of test chemical treatment (with or without S9 from Aroclor-1254-treated Syrian hamsters), cells were reseeded in media containing 10 μM BrdU and harvested after 22 h. Colchicine was added 2 h before cell harvest. Standard cytogenetic methodology (1) was used to prepare and stain slides.
[b]Mean ± standard deviation of the mean per sample of 25 to 40 cells.

Various physiological factors are likely to be important in determining the eventual genetic effect. Strain comparison studies have been performed in embryos and adults discrepant for the Ah locus. Mouse embryos of aryl hydrocarbon hydroxylase (AHH)-inducible strains have been shown to undergo significantly greater SCE induction than AHH-uninducible strains after culturing with media containing BP (54). However, an *in vivo* study in adult mouse strains has revealed that SCE induction by BP is not strictly dependent upon AHH inducibility. It was suggested that the inconsistent results may reflect complex developmental differences in enzymes (55).

Age and sex-hormonal influences upon SCE reactivities to mutagens have been detected in culture (49,56), although more comprehensively described *in vivo*. Mutagen-induced SCE levels reportedly increase with post-embryonic development, and then decline with advancing age (57,58). Phenobarbital-induced mice, after exposure to benzene, exhibit significant sex-related differences in marrow cell proliferation, SCE, and chromosome aberrations (59).

Whole animal assays are flexible for testing target organ carcinogens by various routes of exposure. In addition to the usual routes of chemical administration, novel combinations of pathways have permitted analyses of SCE induction from agents acting synergistically. Hamster cheek pouch epithelium, when exposed systemically to 8-methoxypsoralen or topically to near-ultraviolet light, does not reveal any increase in SCE. However, treatments together cause a tripling of the baseline SCE level (60). These findings confirm in the intact animal earlier *in vitro* observations of genetic activity stemming from these two agents administered together and further denote an element of risk to their clinical use (61,62).

Unusual SCE levels have not been consistently linked with human cancerous tissues (63). However, cultured lymphocytes and fibroblasts from patients characterized by various diseases having a predisposition to neoplasia and thought to involve defective DNA repair have revealed striking abnormalities in SCE. These abnormalities have involved enhanced or depressed levels of SCE response to mutagens or carcinogens (for recent reviews, see references 5 and 63). Unfortunately, animal models with comparable syndromes in which these observations can be pursued are not known to exist. It is interesting, however, that independent *in vivo* studies have detected significantly reduced levels of chemical-induced SCE in bone marrow cells of the leukemia-prone AKR/J strain of mice as compared with other strains (64-65).

TISSUE SPECIFICITY

The levels of chemical reactivity with DNA measured in a tissue reflect a totality of influences from pharmacokinetic, metabolic, repair, and other physiological variables. *In vivo* studies with both cyclophosphamide and ethyl carbamate have revealed tissue-specific differences in levels of SCE induction (29,37,50,66). In mice, baseline SCE frequencies in various somatic tissues, i.e., bone marrow, spleen, thymus, and regenerating liver, are typically much higher than those of spermatogonia. After exposure to cyclophosphamide or ethyl carbamate, these differences become greater due to the fact that somatic tissues undergo proportionally higher levels of SCE increase than germ cells (29,50). For example, after intraperitoneal injection of 400 mg/kg ethyl carbamate, spermatogonia incur a doubling of the control level of SCE, while marrow cells reveal increases close to six times higher (see Figure 4). Still higher levels of SCE induction from ethyl carbamate are detectable in regenerating liver (50,66) and alveolar macrophages (66). These higher levels are notable in view of liver and lung characterizations as undergoing high levels of DNA-ethyl carbamate binding, and as the tissues most susceptible to carcinogenic effects from ethyl carbamate (44,67). As discussed elsewhere (29,37,50), it is not known whether these germ and somatic cell SCE differences relate to intrinsic uniqueness at the tissue or cell level for such factors as metabolic capabilities, cell cycling, DNA vulnerability and repair, BrdU effects (see also 77) or, more simply, to pharmacokinetic differences to result in an unequal distribution of active metabolites. Perhaps replicon structure (size)/activity characteristic of relatively slowly synthesizing spermatogonial DNA is influential to the lower incidence of SCE formation.

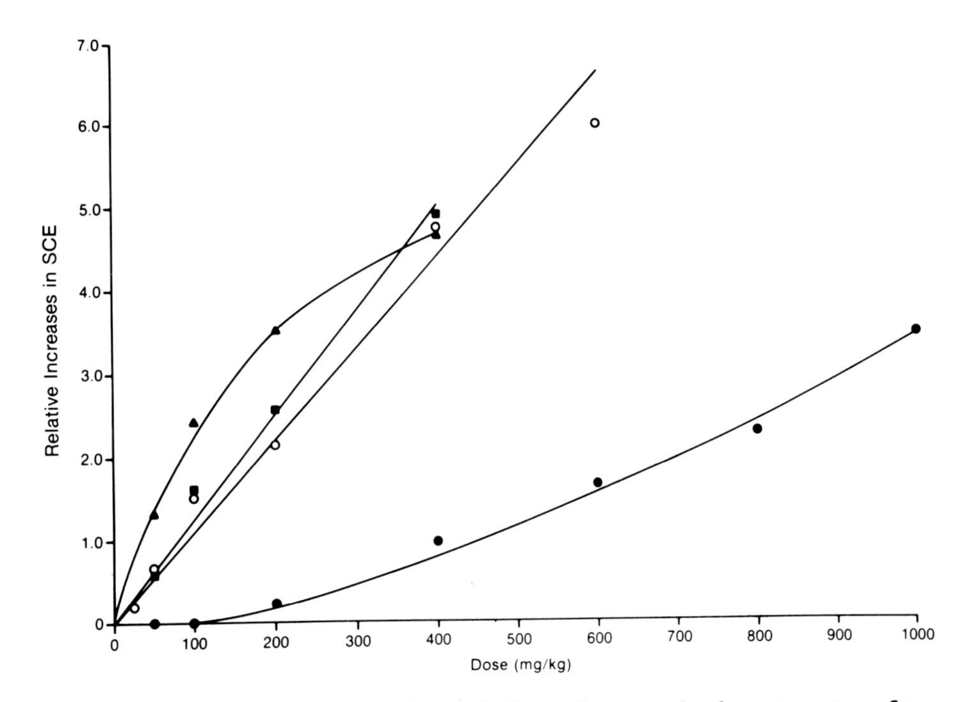

Figure 4. Induction of SCE by ethyl carbamate in hepatocytes from partially hepatectomized mice (▲), bone marrow from partially hepatectomized mice (■), bone marrow from intact mice (o), and spermatogonial cells from intact mice (●).

Cyclophosphamide has also been shown to induce different levels of SCE between maternal and fetal tissues. In intravenously-exposed pregnant mice, significantly greater increments of SCE are detectable in the mid-gestation fetus as compared with maternal bone marrow (68). With advancing gestational age, fetal SCE responses decline to levels significantly below those of maternal marrow. This observation, plus similar findings with additional chemicals, led to the suggestion that drug transport across the placenta may be reduced at later gestational ages (68). A gestational aging-related reduction in SCE has not been found in rat fetal liver transplacentally exposed to 4-nitroquinoline 1-oxide or procarbazine (69). Cyclophosphamide was not examined over a comparable time frame in the pregnant rat although this compound, after maternal intraperitoneal administration, was shown to cause significantly less SCE formation in gestation day 11 yolk sac as compared with day 14 fetal liver and maternal marrow (see Table 2). Different modes of drug transport (70) are suggested to result in inequalities in the amount of active metabolite actually reaching the target tissues. The yolk sac, nourished through endocytosis of uterine substances, may be simply the recipient of quantitatively less active metabolite than fetal liver which is nourished via both the chorioallantoic placenta and the yolk sac (37).

METABOLITES

Once a compound is identified as undergoing metabolic conversion to a product that causes SCE formation in the intact animal, known or suspect metabolites can be examined directly to determine their potential contributions to genetic activity. For example, cyclophosphamide is thought to be hydroxylated in the liver to 4-hydroxycyclophosphamide-aldophosphamide, which either before (71) or after (72) entering systemic circulation gives rise to a series of relatively noncytotoxic and cytotoxic metabolites. Among the latter is phosphoramide mustard. *In vitro* experiments with rat yolk sac tissue (see Table 3), have shown cyclophosphamide to be inactive for the induction of SCE, while phosphoramide mustard can produce SCE increases up to eight times higher than baseline. This latter activity approximates that demonstrable in yolk sac after *in vivo* exposure to cyclophosphamide (Table 2; 37). Thus, phosphoramide mustard appears to be a significant contributor to the high level of SCE induction evident in this tissue after *in vivo* exposure to cyclophosphamide. Similar results have been obtained in CHO cells (73) where, in addition, the metabolites nor-nitrogen mustard and acrolein were tested and characterized as relatively strong and weak SCE inducers, respectively.

Ethyl N-hydroxycarbamate (67) and vinyl carbamate (74,75) have been viewed as potential metabolites accounting for ethyl carbamate carcinogenicity (for review, see reference 44). We have exposed Chinese hamster V79 cells cultured with and without S9 mix to these

Table 2. SCE Frequencies in Rat Maternal and Embryonic Tissues After *In Vivo* Exposure to Cyclophosphamide.

Cyclophosphamide (mg/kg)	Maternal Bone Marrow[a]		Embryo Liver		Yolk Sac	
	SCE/Cell[b]	No. of Cells[c]	SCE/Cell	No. of Cells	SCE/Cell	No. of Cells
0	4.7 ± 0.2	125	5.1 ± 0.3	283	3.8 ± 0.1	125
5	25.2 ± 2.9	73	27.9 ± 1.5	135	8.0 ± 0.8	81
10	39.1 ± 1.5	260	33.0 ± 0.5	639	21.7 ± 1.4	174
20	44.6 ± 4.0	93	45.2 ± 2.4	212	29.2 ± 0.9	59

[a]Tissues represented include those harvested exclusively and those harvested in combinations to provide separate maternal and embryo samples from the same day 14 (liver) or day 11 (yolk sac) gestational units.

[b]Mean ± standard error of the mean.

[c]From 20 to 44 cells/tissue were harvested from a minimum of two maternal or embryo (usually two analyzed/mother) subjects at each i.p. dose (37).

Table 3. SCE Frequencies in Pregnancy Day 11 Rat Embryo Yolk Sac After *In Vivo* BrdU Substitution and *In Vitro* Exposure to Cyclophosphamide or Phosphoramide Mustard

Treatment (μg/ml)	SCE/Cell[a]	No. of Cells[b]
0 (Control)	4.7 ± 0.1	197
Cyclophosphamide		
20	4.7 ± 0.1	48
60	3.9 ± 0.4	24
100	4.3 ± 0.1	81
Phosphoramide mustard		
0.05	9.9 ± 0.5	68
0.1	9.8 ± 0.7	74
0.3	14.1 ± 1.4	25
0.5	26.2 ± 2.7	142
1.0	33.2 ± 1.7	130
2.0	37.0 ± 2.0	29

[a]Mean ± standard error of the mean.
[b]From 20 to 68 cells/tissue were assessed. Usually, two to six yolk sacs obtained from two or more separately grown pairs of embryos (from the same mother) were analyzed. Exceptions where less than 30 cells are represented reflect single yolk sac harvests (37).

agents. After reseeding for further growth, the same exposure population of cells was evaluated for SCE and gene mutagenesis for 6-thioguanine resistance. Preliminary data indicate that ethyl carbamate and ethyl N-hydroxycarbamate are either ineffective or weakly active over broad dose ranges. Vinyl carbamate, on the other hand, is a powerful dose-dependent inducer of both mutagenesis and SCE (see Figure 5) in the presence of S9. Without S9, higher doses caused comparably high levels of SCE in the absence of any significant increase in mutagenesis. Vinyl carbamate-induced SCE increases of approximately 7 times the baseline level of 10 per cell are obtainable at 0.01 mg/ml with S9 and 1.0 mg/ml without S9 exposure concentrations. Bacterial gene mutagenesis from this chemical is also reported to require exogenous activation (75). The high levels of SCE induction observable after exposure *in vivo* to ethyl carbamate (50,66) and *in vitro* to vinyl carbamate support suggestions that the latter may be a metabolite (75). From studies thus far, ethyl N-hydroxycarbamate appears to cause fewer SCEs and more chromosome aberrations *in vitro* as compared with vinyl carbamate. As induction for both of these cytogenetic end points is observed after animal exposure to ethyl carbamate (44), further studies are aimed at defining the extent to which *in vivo* SCEs and aberrations may be separately attributable to vinyl carbamate and ethyl N-hydroxycarbamate, respectively.

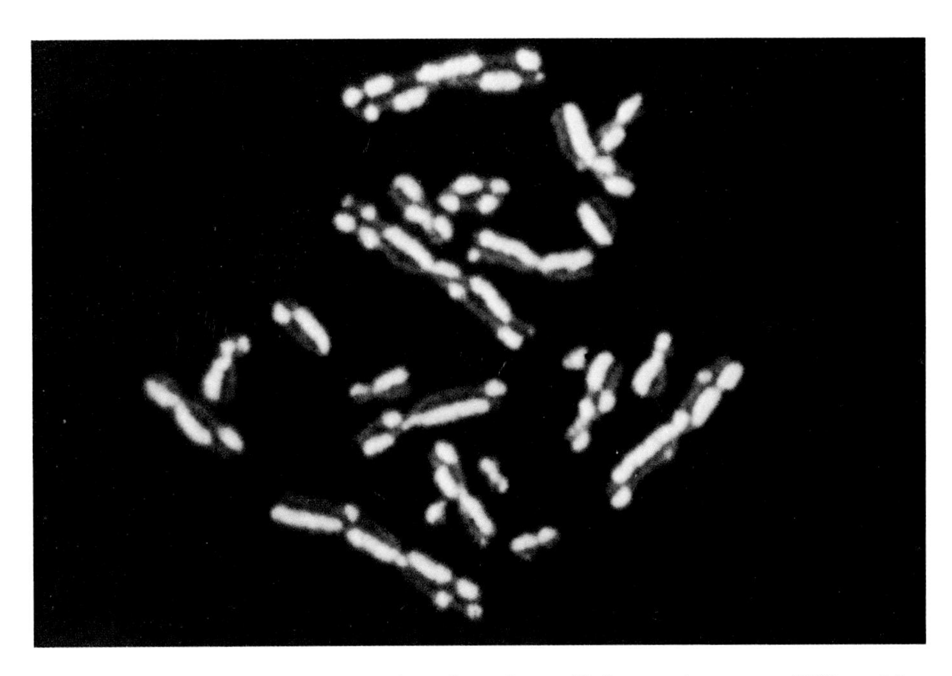

Figure 5. Extensive SCE induction in a Chinese hamster V79 cell exposed *in vitro*, in the presence of S9, to vinyl carbamate. After BrdU substitution and staining with 33258 Hoechst dye, approximately 50 SCEs are evident.

CONCLUSIONS

Sister chromatid exchange analysis variably overlaps, or interfaces, with other assays to detect genetic effects from chemical exposures. In itself, SCE represents a unique end point that offers a high level of sensitivity for studying DNA interactions with many genotoxic chemicals. A practical advantage is its versatility for studies in a wide variety of tissues under *in vitro* or *in vivo* conditions. As such, the importance of various host influences can be determined and potent metabolites for SCE induction identified. Future studies can be directed to comparisons of multiple types of genetic effects in a wide variety of tissues following *in vivo* exposure to target organ carcinogens. These determinations may afford a clearer understanding of genetic effects that are ancillary to, or correlated with, carcinogenesis. More precise investigations into the relative levels of genetic impact of teratogens, mutagens, and carcinogens upon the developing fetus and germ cells is now possible. Regarding the latter, possible relationships between SCE and meiotic crossover exchange both as fundamental processes and as genotoxic reactivity events are of interest (76). Thus, SCE analysis has broad usefulness in genotoxicity evaluations and within *in vivo* systems attains an especially high level of relevance and versatility for specific tissue considerations.

ACKNOWLEDGMENTS

Vinyl carbamate was generously provided by Dr. James Miller, McArdle Laboratory for Cancer Research, University of Wisconsin, through the courtesy of Dr. Stephen Nesnow, Health Effects Research Laboratory, U.S. Environmental Protection Agency. We thank Karen Sasseville and Sharon Leavitt for their able technical assistance in experiments with the carbamate compounds.

REFERENCES

1. Latt, S.A., J.W. Allen, W.E. Rogers, and L.A. Juergens. 1977. *In vitro* and *in vivo* analysis of sister chromatid exchange formation. In: Handbook of Mutagenicity Test Procedures. B.J. Kilbey, M. Legator, R. Nichols, and C. Ramel, eds. Elsevier-North Holland: Amsterdam. pp. 275-291.

2. Wolff, S. 1977. Sister chromatid exchange. Ann. Rev. Genet. 11:183-201.

3. Kato, H. 1977. Spontaneous and induced sister chromatid exchanges as revealed by the BrdU-labeling method. Int. Rev. Cytol. 49:55-97.

4. Perry, P.E. 1980. Chemical mutagens and sister chromatid exchange. In: Chemical Mutagens--Principles and Methods for Their Detection, Vol. 6. F.J. de Serres and A. Hollaender, eds. Plenum Press: New York. pp. 1-39.

5. Latt, S.A., R.R. Schreck, K.S. Loveday, C.P. Dougherty, and C.F. Shuler. 1980. Sister chromatid exchanges. In: Advances in Human Genetics, Vol. 10. H. Harris and K. Hirschhorn, eds. Plenum Press: New York. pp. 267-331.

6. Latt, S.A. 1973. Microfluorometric detection of DNA replication in human metaphase chromosomes. Proc. Natl. Acad. Sci. USA 70:3395-3399.

7. Latt, S.A. 1974. Sister chromatid exchanges, indices of human chromosome damage and repair: Detection by fluorescence and induction by mitomycin C. Proc. Natl. Acad. Sci. USA 71:3162-3166.

8. Perry, P., and S. Wolff. 1974. New Giemsa method for the differential staining of sister chromatids. Nature 251:256-258.

9. Kato, H. 1974. Induction of sister chromatid exchanges by chemical mutagens and its possible relevance to DNA repair. Exptl. Cell Res. 85:239-247.

10. Carrano, A.V., L.H. Thompson, P.A. Lindl, and J.L. Minkler. 1978. Sister chromatid exchange as an indicator of mutagenesis. Nature 271:551-553.

11. Turnbull, D., N.C. Popescu, J.A. DiPaolo, and B.C. Myhr. 1979. cis-Platinum (II) diamine dichloride causes mutation, transformation, and sister chromatid exchanges in cultured mammalian cells. Mutat. Res. 66:267-275.

12. Bradley, M.O., I.C. Hsu, and C.C. Harris. 1979. Relationships between sister chromatid exchange and mutagenicity, toxicity, and DNA damage. Nature 282:318-320.

13. Galloway, S.M., and S. Wolff. 1979. The relation between chemically-induced sister chromatid exchanges and chromatid breakage. Mutat. Res. 61:297-307.

14. Reynolds, R.J., A.T. Natarajan, and P.H.M. Lohman. 1979. Micrococcus luteus UV-endonuclease-sensitive sites and sister chromatid exchanges in Chinese hamster ovary cells. Mutat. Res. 64:353-356.

15. Painter, R.B. 1980. A replication model for sister chromatid exchange. Mutat. Res. 70:337-341.

16. Wolff, S., J. Bodycote, and R.B. Painter. 1974. Sister chromatid exchanges induced in Chinese hamster cells by UV irradiation of different stages of the cell cycle: The necessity for cells to pass through S. Mutat. Res. 25:73-81.

17. Ishii, Y., and M.A. Bender. 1980. Effects of inhibitors of DNA synthesis on spontaneous and ultraviolet light-induced sister chromatid exchanges in Chinese hamster cells. Mutat. Res. 79:19-32.

18. Miller, J.A., and E.C. Miller. 1979. Metabolic activation of chemicals to reactive electrophiles: An overview. In: Advances in Pharmacology and Therapeutics, Vol. 9. Y. Cohen, ed. Pergamon Press: New York. pp. 3-12.

19. Magee, P.N. 1979. Organ specificity of chemical carcinogens. In: Carcinogenesis, Vol. I. Pergamon Press: New York. pp. 213-221.

20. Langenbach, R., H.J. Freed, D. Raveh, and E. Huberman. 1978. Cell specificity in metabolic activation of aflatoxin B_1 and benzo[a]pyrene to mutagens for mammalian cells. Nature 276:277-280.

21. Kriss, J.P., Y. Maruyama, L.A. Tung, S.B. Bond, and L. Révész. 1963. The fate of 5-bromodeoxyuridine, 5-bromodeoxycytidine, and 5-iododeoxycytidine in man. Cancer Res. 23:260-268.

22. Allen, J.W., and S.A. Latt. 1976. Analysis of sister chromatid exchange formation *in vivo* in mouse spermatogonia as a new test system for environmental mutagens. Nature 260:449-451.

23. Vogel, W., and T. Bauknecht. 1976. Differential chromatid staining by *in vivo* treatment as a mutagenicity test system. Nature 260:448-449.

24. Schneider, E.L., J.F. Chaillet, and R.R. Tice. 1976. *In vivo* BrdU-labeling of mammalian chromosomes. Exp. Cell Res. 100:396-398.

25. Pera, F., and P. Mattias. 1976. Labeling of DNA and differential sister chromatid staining after BrdU treatment *in vivo*. Chromosoma 57:13-18.

26. Allen, J.W., C.F. Shuler, and S.A. Latt. 1977. Extension of BrdU dye analysis of DNA replication and sister chromatid exchange formation to in vivo systems. Stadler Symp. (U. of Missouri) 9:9-36.

27. Kanda, N., and H. Kato. 1979. A simple technique for in vivo observation of SCE in mouse ascites tumor and spermatogonial cells. Exp. Cell Res. 118:431-434.

28. Allen, J.W., C.F. Shuler, R.W. Mendes, and S.A. Latt. 1977. A simplified technique for in vivo analysis of sister chromatid exchanges using 5-bromodeoxyuridine tablets. Cytogen. Cell Genet. 18:231-237.

29. Allen, J.W., C.F. Shuler, and S.A. Latt. 1978. Bromodeoxyuridine tablet methodology for in vivo studies of DNA synthesis. Somatic Cell Genet. 4:393-405.

30. Goto, K., S. Maeda, Y. Kano, and T. Sugiyama. 1978. Factors involved in differential Giemsa-staining of sister chromatids. Chromosoma 66:351-359.

31. Perry, P., and H.J. Evans. 1975. Cytological detection of mutagen-carcinogen exposure by sister chromatid exchange. Nature 258:121-124.

32. Stetka, D.G., and S. Wolff. 1976. Sister chromatid exchange as an assay for genetic damage induced by mutagen-carcinogens. I. In vivo test for compounds requiring metabolic activation. Mutat. Res. 41:333-342.

33. Nevstad, N.P. 1978. Sister chromatid exchanges and chromosomal aberrations induced in human lymphocytes by the cytostatic drug adriamycin in vivo and in vitro. Mutat. Res. 57:253-258.

34. Raposa, T. 1978. Sister chromatid exchange studies for monitoring DNA damage and repair capacity after cytostatics in vitro and in lymphocytes of leukemic patients under cytostatic therapy. Mutat. Res. 57:241-251.

35. Lambert, B., U. Ringborg, and A. Lindblad. 1979. Prolonged increase of sister chromatid exchanges in lymphocytes of melanoma patients after CCNU treatment. Mutat. Res. 59:295-300.

36. Stetka, D.G., J. Minkler, and A.V. Carrano. 1978. Induction of long-lived chromosome damage, as manifested by sister chromatid exchange, in lymphocytes of animals exposed to mitomycin-C. Mutat. Res. 51:383-396.

37. Allen, J.W., E. El-Nahass, M.K. Sanyal, R.L. Dunn, B. Gladen, and R.L. Dixon. 1981. Sister chromatid exchange analyses in rodent maternal, embryonic, and extra-embryonic tissues. Transplacental and direct mutagen exposures. Mutat. Res. 80:297-311.

38. Huang, C.C., and M. Furukawa. 1978. Sister chromatid exchanges in human lymphoid cell lines *in vivo*: A test system for mutagenicity. Exp. Cell Res. 111:458-461.

39. Furukawa, M., and C.C. Huang. 1978. Sister chromatid exchanges induced by cyclophosphamide in V79 cells cultured in diffusion chambers in mice. Mutat. Res. 57:233-239.

40. Paika, I.J., M.T. Beauchesne, M. Randall, R.R. Schreck, and S.A. Latt. 1981. *In vivo* SCE analysis of 20 coded compounds. In: Evaluation of Short-Term Tests for Carcinogens. F. deSerres and J. Ashby, eds. Elsevier Publishers: New York. pp. 673-681.

41. Galloway, S.M., and R.B. Painter. 1979. Vitamin C is positive in the DNA synthesis inhibition and sister chromatid exchange tests. Mutat. Res. 60:321-327.

42. Speit, G., M. Wolf, and W. Vogel. 1980. The SCE-inducing capacity of vitamin C: Investigations *in vitro* and *in vivo*. Mutat. Res. 78:273-278.

43. Wolff, S., and S. Takehisa. 1977. Induction of sister chromatid exchanges in mammalian cells by low concentrations of mutagenic carcinogens that require metabolic activation as well as those that do not. In: Progress in Genetic Toxicology. D. Scott, B.A. Bridges, and F.H. Sobels, eds. Elsevier-North Holland Biomedical Press: New York. pp. 193-200.

44. Allen, J.W., Y. Sharief, and R.J. Langenbach. 1982. An overview of ethyl carbamate (urethane) and its genotoxic activity. In: The Genotoxic Effects of Airborne Agents. R. Tice, D. Costa, and K. Schaich, eds. Plenum Press: New York. pp. 443-460.

45. Takehisa, S., and S. Wolff. 1978. The induction of sister chromatid exchanges in Chinese hamster ovary cells by prolonged exposure to 2-acetylaminofluorene and S9 mix. Mutat. Res. 58:103-106.

46. Stetka, D.G., and S. Wolff. 1976. Sister chromatid exchange as an assay for genetic damage induced by mutagen-carcinogens. II. *In vitro* test for compounds requiring metabolic activation. Mutat. Res. 41:343-350.

47. Ray-Chaudhuri, R., S. Kelley, and P.T. Iype. 1980. Induction of sister chromatid exchanges by carcinogens mediated through cultured rat liver epithelial cells. Carcinogenesis 1:779-786.

48. Popescu, N.C., D. Turnbull, and J.A. DiPaolo. 1977. Sister chromatid exchange and chromosome aberration analysis with the use of several carcinogens and noncarcinogens. J. Natl. Cancer Inst. 59:289-292.

49. Dean, R., G. Bynum, D. Kram, and E.L. Schneider. 1980. Sister chromatid exchange induction by carcinogens in HTC cells. Mutat. Res. 74:477-483.

50. Roberts, G.T., and J.W. Allen. 1980. Tissue-specific induction of sister chromatid exchanges by ethyl carbamate in mice. Environ. Mutagen. 2:17-26.

51. Bayer, U., and T. Bauknecht. 1977. The dose-dependence of sister chromatid exchanges induced by 3 hydrocarbons in the *in vivo* bone marrow test with Chinese hamsters. Experientia 33:25.

52. Schreck, R.R., I.J. Paika, and S.A. Latt. 1979. *In vivo* induction of sister chromatid exchanges in liver and marrow cells by drugs requiring metabolic activation. Mutat. Res. 64:315-328.

53. Allen, J.W., and S.A. Latt. 1976. *In vivo* BrdU-33258 Hoechst analysis of DNA replication kinetics and sister chromatid exchange formation in mouse somatic and meiotic cells. Chromosoma 58:325-340.

54. Galloway, S.M., P.E. Perry, J. Meneses, D.W. Nebert, and R.A. Pedersen. 1980. Cultured mouse embryos metabolize benzo[*a*]pyrene during early gestation: Genetic differences detectable by sister chromatid exchange. Proc. Natl. Acad. Sci. USA 77:3524-3528.

55. Schreck, R.R., and S.A. Latt. 1980. Comparison of benzo[*a*]-pyrene metabolism and sister chromatid exchange induction in mice. Nature 288:407-408.

56. Schneider, E.L., and R.E. Monticone. 1978. Aging and sister chromatid exchange. II. The effect of the *in vitro* passage level of human fetal lung fibroblasts on baseline and mutagen-induced sister chromatid exchange frequencies. Exp. Cell Res. 115:269-276.

57. Nakanishi, Y., D. Kram, and E.L. Schneider. 1979. Aging and sister chromatid exchanges. IV. Reduced frequencies of mutagen-induced sister chromatid exchanges in vivo in mouse bone marrow cells with aging. Cytogenet. Cell Genet. 24:61-67.

58. Nakanishi, Y., R.A. Dein, and E.L. Schneider. 1980. Aging and sister chromatid exchange. V. The effect of post-embryonic development on mutagen-induced sister chromatid exchanges in mouse and rat bone marrow cells. Cytogenet. Cell Genet. 27:82-87.

59. Tice, R.R., D.L. Costa, and R.T. Drew. 1979. Cytogenetic effects of inhaled benzene in murine bone marrow: Induction of sister chromatid exchanges, chromosomal aberrations, and cellular proliferation inhibition in DBA/2 mice. Proc. Natl. Acad. Sci. 77:2148-2152.

60. Shuler, C.F., and S.A. Latt. 1979. Sister chromatid exchange induction resulting from systemic, topical, and systemic-topical presentations of carcinogens. Cancer Res. 39:2510-2514.

61. Carter, D.M., K. Wolff, and W. Schnedle. 1976. 8-Methoxypsoralen and UVA promote sister chromatid exchanges. J. Invest. Dermatol. 67:548-551.

62. Latt, S.A., and K.S. Loveday. 1978. Characterization of sister chromatid exchange induction by 8-methoxypsoralen plus near-UV light. Cytogenet. Cell Genet. 21:184-200.

63. Shiraishi, Y., and A.A. Sandberg. 1980. Sister chromatid exchange in human chromosomes, including observations in neoplasia. Cancer Genet. and Cytogenet. 1:363-380.

64. Kram, D., and E.L. Schneider. 1978. Reduced frequencies of mitomycin-C-induced sister chromatid exchanges in AKR mice. Human Genet. 41:45-51.

65. Biegel, J.A., S.S. Boggs, and M.K. Conner. 1980. Comparison of BCNU-induced SCE in bone marrow cells of AKR/J and BDF_1 mice. Mutat. Res. 79:87-90.

66. Cheng, M., M.K. Conner, and Y. Alarie. 1981. Multicellular in vivo sister chromatid exchanges induced by urethane. Mutat. Res. 88:223-231.

67. Mirvish. S.S. 1968. The carcinogenic action and metabolism of urethane and N-hydroxyurethane. Adv. Cancer Res. 11:1-42.

68. Kram, D., G.D. Bynum, G.C. Senula, C.K. Bickings, and E.L. Schneider. 1980. In utero analysis of sister chromatid exchange: Alterations in susceptibility to mutagenic damage as a function of fetal cell type and gestational age. Proc. Natl. Acad. Sci. 77:4784-4787.

69. Sharma, R.K., R. Dunn, and J.W. Allen. (in press). Transplacental sister chromatid exchange induction analyses in the rat. Mutat. Res. (abstract).

70. Beck, F., and J.B. Lloyd. 1977. Comparative placental transfer. In: Handbook of Teratology. J.G. Wilson and F.C. Fraser, eds. Plenum Press: New York. pp. 155-186.

71. Struck, R.K., M.C. Kirk, M.H. Witt, and W.R. Laster. 1975. Isolation and mass spectral identification of blood metabolites of cyclophosphamide: Evidence for phosphoramide mustard as the biologically active metabolite. Biomed. Mass Spectrom. 2:46-52.

72. Domeyer, B.E., and N.E. Sladek. 1980. Kinetics of cyclophosphamide biotransformation in vivo. Cancer Res. 40:174-180.

73. Au, W., O.I. Sokova, B. Kopnin, and F.E. Arrighi. 1980. Cytogenetic toxicity of cyclophosphamide and its metabolites in vitro. Cytogenet. Cell Genet. 26:108-116.

74. Dahl, G.A., E.C. Miller, and J.A. Miller. 1980. Comparative carcinogenecities and mutagenicities of vinyl carbamate, ethyl carbamate, and ethyl N-hydroxycarbamate. Cancer Res. 40:1194-1203.

75. Dahl, G.A., J.A. Miller, and E.C. Miller. 1978. Vinyl carbamate as a promutagen and a more carcinogenic analogue of ethyl carbamate. Cancer Res. 38:3793-3804.

76. Allen, J.W. 1979. BrdU-dye characterization of late replication and meiotic recombination in Armenian hamster germ cells. Chromosoma 74:189-207.

77. Davidson, R.L., E.R. Kaufman, C.P. Dougherty, A.M. Ouellette, C.M. Difolco, and S.A. Latt. 1980. Induction of sister chromatid exchanges by BrdU is largely independent of the BrdU content of DNA. Nature 284:74-76.

DISCUSSION

Q.: What kinds of chemicals appear to be required for the initiation of sister chromatid exchange?

A.: No strict pattern has emerged. SCE formation is generally quite sensitive to compounds that produce DNA adducts. Many alkylating agents have been shown to cause dramatic elevations in SCE. However, as most comprehensively noted in the Gene-Tox Committee Report on SCEs, chemicals eliciting a clearly positive response represent a wide variety of chemical classes. Radiomimetic-type chemicals that are associated with the production of double-strand DNA breakage tend to be weak inducers of SCE.

Q.: Have you looked at SCE induction by promoters-TPA?

A.: No, I haven't. As far as I'm aware, the original positive findings with TPA were not confirmed in subsequent studies carried out in the laboratories of Latt, Carrano, and others. I believe the matter is still controversial.

METABOLISM OF CHEMICAL CARCINOGENS BY TRACHEOBRONCHIAL TISSUES

Herman Autrup, Roland C. Grafstrom and Curtis C. Harris

Human Tissue Studies Section, Laboratory of Experimental Pathology, National Cancer Institute, Bethesda, Maryland 20205

INTRODUCTION

Chemical carcinogens are a large group of naturally occurring and man-made compounds of diverse molecular structures. These compounds are ubiquitous in the human environment in the food chain, the water supply, and the atmosphere and they enter the human body through the surface epithelium. The surface area of the lower respiratory tract, approximately 25 m^2, is directly exposed to some of these compounds during inhalation. In addition, chemical carcinogens and their metabolites can also reach the lung via the systemic route.

Most of the chemical carcinogens found in our environment require metabolic activation to exert their effects. The major activation pathway is by oxidative metabolism, usually catalyzed by the cytochrome P-450 dependent monooxygenase system that increases the electrophilicity and reactivity of the parent compounds. Competing with the enzymatic activation pathway(s) are several deactivation pathways; the latter generally lead to the formation of less reactive metabolites that are water soluble and rapidly excreted in the urine. The relative rates of these two pathways may be an important consideration in assessing the potential harmful effect of an environment pollutant.

The metabolism of chemical carcinogens and other xenobiotics has been extensively investigated in both subcellular and cellular preparations as well as in intact lung tissue from experimental animals and humans. The most widely studied chemical carcinogen is benzo[*a*]pyrene (BP), which is both a major component of cigarette tar and a pyrolysis product of fossil fuels. BP is emitted into the air of the United States at an estimated annual rate of 2000 tons. When BP adsorbed to particulates is instilled intratracheally, carcinomas are produced in the lungs of several animal species (1). BP has also been shown to cause in vitro malignant transformation of rat tracheal epithelial cells (2).

The oxidative metabolism of BP, often expressed as aryl hydrocarbon hydroxylase (AHH) activity, is mediated by one of the cytochrome P-450 dependent monooxygenase systems that has been resolved into at least two catalytic components, namely, a species of cytochrome P-450 and NADPH-cytochrome P-450 reductase. Cytochrome P-450 has been demonstrated in the rabbit nonciliated bronchiolar epithelium (Clara cells) by immunological and autoradiographic methods (3,4). Comparing spectral and metabolic characteristics of cytochrome P-450 shows differences between hepatic and pulmonary forms of cytochrome P-450 (5). No detectable amount of cytochrome P-450 is found in human lung microsomes, while the activity of NADPH-cytochrome P-450 reductase, estimated as NADPH-cytochrome c reductase, is similar to the activity of other tissues (6,7). Another microsomal hemoprotein, cytochrome b_5, is detected at approximately 25% of the level in human liver (6). The activity of the cytochrome P-450 system in human lung microsomes is less than 3% of the activity in liver microsomes when BP, phenacetin, or 7-ethoxycoumarin is used as substrate (8). In experimental animals, the AHH activity in the lung is about 10% of the activity found in the liver (9,10). The low level of activity found in the lung may be due in part to the difficulty associated with preparing microsomes from this organ.

Several studies indicate animal species and strain differences in the tracheobronchial capability of activating xenobiotics. Wistar rats exhibit a 10-fold higher AHH activity in microsomal preparations from the entire lung, compared to microsomes isolated from the epithelial cells of trachea (11). No differences in basal AHH activity are observed between lung microsomes isolated from either CD-1 mouse or Chinese hamster (9). When lung microsomes from CD-1 mouse are used as the activating system for BP, more mutants are observed in the Ames Salmonella test (strains TA98 and TA100) than with lung microsomes from Sprague-Dawley (SD) rats as the activating system (12). A wide inter-individual variation of the AHH activity is observed between different human lung specimens, and the activity of AHH in human lung microsomes is only 10% of that found in microsomes from BD-VI rats (13). A 20-fold variation is seen in both normal and tumorous lung tissue, and the AHH activity is generally lower in the malignant tissue. The AHH activity shows a uni-modal normal distribution. No correlation has been observed between the smoking history of the patient and the level of AHH, which is surprising, since exposure of experimental animals to cigarette smoke has been shown to increase the AHH activity in lung microsomes prepared from the exposed animals (10).

Administering a variety of substances (10) increases the AHH activity in lung tissues of experimental animals. The inducibility of AHH has been shown to be under genetic control in mice (14). Furthermore, high inducibility of AHH in the lung is correlated with the ability of 3-methylcholanthrene to induce lung tumors in inbred strains of mice (15).

Epoxide hydrolase (EH) converts BP epoxides to BP dihydrodiols. The activity of this enzyme has also been shown to vary between strains, species, and tissues. The EH activity is higher in rodent lung microsomes, compared to the liver (16). Microsomes from hamster lung exhibit higher EH activity (using BP 4,5-oxide as substrate) than microsomes from SD rats, while the lowest activity is seen in the NMRI mice (16). Epoxide hydrolase activity is also detected in microsomes prepared from human lung but shows less inter-individual variation than the cytochrome P-450 dependent activity (17). The activity of EH is inducible in the rat lung by cigarette smoke and 3-methylcholanthrene (10). The variability in content and activity of cytochrome P-450 dependent enzymes and of EH among various species and organs suggests that metabolism of BP could differ both qualitatively and quantitatively. Indeed, the patterns of BP metabolites formed by liver and lung microsomes from monkey (18) and C3H mouse (19) differ in that both animal species form relatively larger amounts of diols with lung microsomes, while phenols account for about 60% of the metabolites with liver microsomes. The BP metabolite profile formed by human lung microsomes is qualitatively similar to the profile formed by rat lung (see Table 1), but large quantitative differences in the metabolite distribution are observed with microsomal preparations isolated from different individuals.

Maintaining tracheobronchial tissues in controlled experimental conditions provides an excellent *in vitro* system to study and compare the metabolism of chemical carcinogens in experimental animals and in man. Lung tissues maintained as either isolated cells or explant cultures retain the ability to metabolically activate BP into electrophiles that bind to cellular macromolecules. This activation has been shown to occur in rat type II alveolar lung cells (21,22) and in explant cultures of human peripheral lung (23,24) and human bronchial epithelial cells (25). Several studies have demonstrated the importance of using an intact cellular system to correlate experimental data to the *in vivo* situation instead of the subcellular system. The metabolic profile of BP differs with activation systems of different levels of biological organization (28) (see Tables 2 and 3). Furthermore, this difference is also reflected in a qualitative difference of the BP-DNA adducts when microsomes or sliced tissues were used as the activating system (30). Using intact hepatocytes instead of the microsomal fraction gives an

Table 1. Species Comparisons of Benzo[a]pyrene Metabolism in Lung Microsomes[a]

Species	Dihydrodiols			Phenols		Quinones	Reference
	9,10-	4,5-	7,8-	9-OH	3-OH		
Human[b]	12.0	2.7	6.1	18.4	33.9	26.8	6
Human[c]	17.1	3.0	6.1	10.4	20.0	28.7	13
Rat (BD-IV)	4.1	2.8	3.9	15.0	19.5	54.6	13
Mouse (C3H)	7.7	7.7	23.6	7.7	38.4	23.6	19
Hamster	0.9	8.9	2.1	12.7	22.7	53.9	20
Monkey	3.9	8.3	5.2	-	26.2	48.4	18

[a]Results are expressed as percentage of total organo-soluble metabolites.
[b]Mean values of lung from 13 individuals.
[c]Mean values of lung from 6 individuals.

improved correlation of mutagenicity in a bacterial system with animal carcinogenicity for BP and several BP metabolites (31). A better approximation of the intact cell situation can be obtained by simultaneous addition of substrate and co-factors for the detoxification enzymes to the microsomes.

We have studied the metabolism of BP and its interaction with DNA in tracheobronchial tissues of several different species, using the explant culture methodology. In addition, we have investigated the capacity of human bronchial tissue to metabolize different classes of carcinogens, analyzing the resulting covalent binding to DNA.

MATERIAL AND METHODS

Tracheobronchial Tissues

Male DBA/2N (D2) and C57Bl/6N (C6) mice (6 to 8 weeks) and male CD, Buffalo and Wistar rats (4 to 5 weeks) were obtained from the Charles River Breeding Laboratories (Wilmington, MA). Male Syrian golden hamsters (6 to 8 weeks) were obtained from Lakeview Farm (Lakeview, NJ). The animals were kept under well-controlled conditions in our animal facility as previously described (32) for one week prior to the experiment. The animals were killed by asphyxiation with CO_2; the tracheas were removed aseptically and

Table 2. Benzo[a]pyrene Metabolism in Rat Lung[a]

Level of Biological Organization	Early Eluting Peak	Dihydrodiols 9,10-	4,5-	7,8-	Phenols 9-OH	3-OH	Quinones	Ref.
Microsomes (BD-IV)[b]	-	4.0	2.8	3.9	15.0	19.5	54.6	4
Perfused lung (Wistar)[c]	23.9	14.4	2.4	4.6	-	55.0	-	13, 26
Explant culture (CD)[b]	5.0	45.0	0.5	3.7	0.7	1.2	1.0	27

[a]The data are expressed as percentages (%) of total organo-extractable metabolites.
[b]Analyzed by HPLC.
[c]Analyzed by TLC.

Table 3. Benzo[a]pyrene Metabolism in Human Lung Tissues and Cells[a]

Level of Biological Organization	Early Eluting Peak	Dihydrodiols 9,10-	4,5-	7,8-	Phenols 9-OH	3-OH	Quinones	Ref.
Microsomes								
Lung	-	12.0	2.7	6.1	18.4	33.9	26.8	6
Bronchial	-	8.8	2.1	9.6	12.1	16.7	31.9	-
Cells								
Epithelial	21.4	44.9	0.4	5.1	1.5	1.9	-	25
Fibroblast	32.4	50.6	0.1	4.8	1.1	-	-	25
Explants								
Peripheral	51.8	4.4	-	11.4	-	3.2	4.0	23
Bronchus	36.8	21.2	3.9	4.4	4.1	2.4	11.5	29
Trachea	21.4	28.4	3.9	4.9	4.1	2.4	26.4	29

[a]The data are expressed as percentages (%).

immediately immersed in L-15 medium for 1 to 2 h at 4°C until culture. Human bronchi were obtained at the time of autopsy (33) and were immersed in L-15 medium at 4°C for 4 to 8 h until culture (see [34] for donor information). Human bronchi were cut into 1-cm^2 pieces and cultured in a chemically-defined medium as previously described (35). Animal tracheas were cultured unopened as tubes. The medium was changed every other day. The human explants were cultured for 6 to 7 days prior to BP exposure, and the animal explants were cultured for 1 to 2 days prior to BP exposure, to minimize the effect of exogenous factors before culture.

Treatment with Carcinogen

[^{3}H]BP (1.5 μM) dissolved in dimethyl sulfoxide (final concentration: 0.5%) was added to the medium, and the explants were incubated for another 24 h (26); approximately 50% of the BP was metabolized. After incubation with [^{3}H]BP, the mucosal layer was removed from the connective tissues with a surgical blade and forceps. Histological examination revealed that more than 90% of the epithelial cells were removed. Ten explants each from mice, rats, and hamsters, and four to five explants from each human bronchus were pooled for a single determination. The mucosa from 10 to 20 explants were pooled to identify BP-DNA adducts. The analytical procedures for isolating DNA and determining the level of binding to DNA, water- and organo-soluble BP metabolites and BP-DNA adducts have been published previously (36-38).

RESULTS AND DISCUSSION

Metabolism of Benzo[a]pyrene

Tracheobronchial tissues from all the experimental animals and humans metabolized BP into both organo-soluble and water-soluble metabolites (see Table 4). The metabolism of BP was highest in tissues from human, hamster, and C6 mice; BP has been shown to induce lung cancer in the latter two species. A higher ratio of organo-soluble to water-soluble metabolites was also seen in trachea from hamster and C6 mice, indicating that these species were less efficient in converting potentially procarcinogenic metabolites to less toxic water-soluble metabolites. These findings could in part explain the higher susceptibility of these species to lung cancer caused by carcinogenic polynuclear aromatic hydrocarbons (PAHs). Human bronchus varied widely in both the total metabolism of BP and the ability to form water-soluble metabolites that accounted for 30 to 80% of the total metabolism. The ratio of organo-soluble to water-soluble metabolites of BP was higher in nontumorous lung tissue from donors with lung cancer (29,34) than from donors without cancer. It is at present unknown whether these results are due to the presence of the tumor or characteristics of the patients who develop lung cancer. More cases will have to be investigated.

Table 4. Metabolism of Benzo[a]pyrene by Cultured Tracheobronchial Tissues[a]

Species	BP[b] (pmoles)	BP[c] (nmoles)	Ratio Organo-/Water-Soluble Metab.
Human	32	64.5	0.4
Rat			
CD	13	6.5	0.2
Buffalo	15	6.2	0.2
Wistar	22	6.2	0.2
Mouse			
C57BL/6N	11	10.0	1.4
DBA/2N	9	4.0	0.5
Hamster	26	13.4	1.2

[a]The results from experimental animals represent the mean of 3 individual experiments. The results from humans represent 15 tissues obtained from immediate autopsy of donors without cancer.
[b]Bound/10 mg DNA.
[c]Metabolized/10 mg DNA.

Separating the water-soluble metabolites into three major fractions, sulfate esters, glucuronides, and glutathione conjugates, indicated that the formation of sulfate esters is the major conjugation pathway under our experimental conditions. However, additional chromatography on a Lipadex-DEAP column with a methanol-water gradient resolved the sulfate ester fraction into several more components. Enzymatic treatment of these fractions with arylsulfatase did not convert all the fractions into organo-soluble metabolites, indicating the presence of other unidentified types of BP conjugates. These undigested compounds must have a pK_a value similar to that of sulfate esters, as the initial separation by liquid chromatography is based upon the acidity of the conjugates. Using a different approach, Cohen et al. (39) have shown that sulfate esters are the major detoxification products in normal human bronchus, while glucuronidation seems to be the most prominent pathway in tumorous tissue (40).

Binding of a carcinogen to DNA is one measure of the generation of reactive, electrophilic metabolites. All the tissues could activate BP into metabolites that bound to DNA. The highest mean binding value was seen in human bronchus and Syrian golden hamster, the level of modification being approximately 1 BP molecule/10^6 nucleotides. Similar amounts of BP-DNA adducts were observed in the various anatomical segments of the bronchus from the same individual (27). On the other hand, the binding value in human bronchi from donors without cancer (15 cases) showed a wide inter-individual variation (15-fold), although the variation was less than that seen in bronchi from a larger group of donors, some of whom had lung cancer (41,42). Similar variations in the activation of BP were observed in other human tissues (29).

The variation in our studies is similar in magnitude to the variation in studies on drug metabolism in mono- and dizygotic twins; the latter studies suggest that genetic factors are important in controlling metabolism of xenobiotics. An interesting observation is that the mean binding value in C6 and D2 mice was similar, although these two strains of mice have different susceptibility to peripheral lung tumorigenesis caused by PAHs (15). Since no correlation seems to exist between the binding level and the total metabolism, the determination of the total metabolism is not a measure of the production of potential harmful lesions in the DNA that it is related to a more specific BP metabolite. Both the epithelial surface cells and the stroma cells of human bronchus activated BP into metabolites that bind to macromolecules. By using autoradiographic methods, we found that bronchial epithelial cells bound approximately fourfold more BP than did the stromal fibroblasts (43). Using fibroblast and primary bronchial cell cultures initiated from the same individual, a threefold higher binding level of BP metabolite to DNA was seen in the bronchial epithelial cells (25).

The importance of carcinogen-DNA interaction in the carcinogenic process remains unclear. Both the extent of binding of PAHs and their metabolites to cellular DNA and their mutagenicity in mammalian cells are correlated with their carcinogenicity (44,45). Furthermore, it is known that binding of BP to DNA modifies the proper functioning of DNA in both cell-free and cellular systems (46-48). It is important both to quantitate and qualitate BP-DNA interactions before any correlation to biological effects can be made. In the case of alkylating carcinogens, the predominant alkylation product is 7-alkylguanine, a modification product that has been shown to be without any known significant mutagenic effect. The major reaction product of BP product of BP with DNA is formed between the C-10 position of BP diolepoxide and the exocyclic 2-amino group of guanine. At a high level of modification, this lesion inhibits the cellular replication, whereas no effect is observed at a lower amount of modification (46). The reaction between BP 7,8-dihydro-7,8-dihydroxy-9,10-oxide (BPDE) and DNA does not show intergenic preference when DNA molecules, SV40 DNA, or BHK-DNA, are incubated _in vitro_ with BPDE (49,50). However, when BHK cells are treated with BP, a comparatively higher level of modification is seen in the highly repetitive sequences (50). These observations point to the potential difficulties in correlating the "total binding data" with pathological responses. Thus, these data are only indicative of the cells' ability to convert chemical carcinogens into electropositive intermediates.

BP-DNA Adducts

Formation of the major BP-DNA adducts in intact tissues proceeds through the proximate carcinogenic metabolite (-)-BP 7,8-diol, which was further metabolized into both BPDE I and II, the former being the predominant metabolite in most cellular systems and also the most potent carcinogenic and mutagenic form of BP. Although both metabolites reacted with DNA, isolation of the BP-DNA adducts by high pressure liquid chromatography (HPLC) indicated that the major adduct was formed between BPDE-I and the 2-amino group of deoxyguanosine. The BPDE I-deoxyguanosine adducts accounted for more than 70% of the BP-DNA adducts in cultured tracheobronchial tissues (see Table 5). Both stereoisomeric forms of BPDE I reacted with deoxyguanosine. Although the 7_R_-form is usually more predominant than the 7_S_-form, the relative distribution appeared to vary between species (26,52). Minor amounts of unidentified BP-DNA adducts with retention-time similar to that of the BP-deoxycytosine adducts were also observed. The adducts formed by tracheobronchial tissues did not differ qualitatively from the adducts formed in other tissues and cell types (29,53,54).

We previously reported the presence of substantial amounts of BPDE I/II deoxyadenosine in both rat trachea and colon from CD rats, although these adducts were not detectable in tracheobronchial tissues from other animal species (26). In a more detailed study of the BP-DNA adducts in rat strains CD, Wistar, and Buffalo, we found that more than 15% of the adducts cochromatographed with BPDE I/II deoxyadenosine reference compounds. This was accompanied by a decrease in the amount of 7_R_-BPDE deoxyguanosine (see Table 5) (52). The presence of BP-deoxyadenine adduct in rat tissues but not in tracheobronchial

Table 5. Adducts Formed Between DNA and Benzo[a]pyrene in Cultured Tracheobronchial Tissues[a]

Species	Unknown I	Unknown II	7S-BPDE I Gua	7R-BPDE I Gua	BPDE II Gua	BPDE I/II Ade
Human	9	8	21	56	7	-
Rat						
CD	2	10	7	41	21	19
Buffalo	3	11	12	45	13	16
Wistar	5	13	10	36	16	20
Mouse						
C57BL/6N	-	3	4	83	10	-
DBA/2N	-	8	20	63	9	-
Hamster	-	6	7	71	16	0

[a]The results are expressed as percentage of total amounts of identified adducts. About 30 explants from each group were incubated with [^{3}H]BP (1.5 μM) for 24 h. The DNA was isolated from the mucosal scrapings, hydrolyzed enzymatically (27) and the BP-nucleosides were anlyzed by HPLC using a μBondapak C-18 column and a concave water-methanol gradient (38).

tissues from other animal species under the same experimental conditions could be due to a differential rate of removal of the various BPDE-DNA adducts. Such repair processes are observed in both a lung tumor cell line (53) and in hamster embryo cells (54), where the BP-adenine adducts are removed at a faster rate than the other adducts. The biological significance of the BP-adenine adduct is as yet unknown.

Using a direct-reacting PAH, Dipple and co-workers have shown that an increased ratio of arylation of the N-6 position in adenine and the 2-position in guanine is associated with increased carcinogenic potency (55). A positive correlation has also been found between the order of binding of PAHs to poly(A) after their activation with mouse epidermal microsomes and their skin carcinogenicity (56). In our cellular system, no adducts were formed between the 7-position of guanine and BPDE, although this reaction product has been detected after reaction of BPDE with DNA in a cell-free system (57,58). A large proportion of the radioactivity associated with rat tracheal DNA elutes in the early fractions (52). The identity of these reaction products is unknown, but recent experiments using mouse skin indicate that tritium incorporation into deoxynucleotides accounts for a substantial proportion of the total radioactivity associated with DNA (59).

Organo-Soluble Metabolites

Organo-soluble metabolites were extracted from the culture media with ethylacetate/acetone and were separated by HPLC (see Table 6). The metabolic profiles from all experimental animals and humans were qualitatively similar in tracheobronchial tissue. BP tetrols and BP 9,10-diol were the predominant metabolites formed by cultured human tissues and hamster trachea, while relatively minor amounts of phenols were seen, compared with studies using microsomes (see Table 3). The low level of phenols is probably associated with the presence of sulfotransferase and glucuronsoyl transferase in intact cells, which may convert the toxic phenolic metabolites into less toxic water-soluble metabolites. Some of the sulfate esters may be extracted by organic solvents under our conditions, and these metabolites may elute prior to BP tetrols by the HPLC separation. This initial peak in the HPLC separation accounts for 5 to 20% of the radioactivity for most of the species except for the rats, where it accounted for about 40%. The phenols could also serve as substrate for oxidation by the monooxygenase system to form BP triols and BP polyphenols.

BP tetrols can be formed either enzymatically or by non-enzymatic hydrolysis of the ultimate carcinogenic form of BP. The amount of these metabolites is another indication of the cells' ability to form the ultimate carcinogen. However, no correlation is observed between the amount of BP tetrols and the level of BP binding to cellular DNA in human tissues (34), which could indicate that the ultimate carcinogen is substrate for other cellular reactions such as glutathione transferase and other macromolecules.

The metabolic precursor of BPDE, BP 7,8-diol, accounted for less than 10% of the organo-soluble metabolites. More BP 7,8-diol was formed by trachea from C6 mice than from D2 mice, which is similar to the results with lung microsomes from the same mice strains (62). A relatively high level of BP quinones was detected in the media from D2 mouse trachea. BP quinones were previously considered to be end products in the metabolism of BP. However, recent investigation has shown that hamster trachea explant cultures metabolize quinones to metabolites that are conjugated with glucuronic acid (61). The ratio between the amounts of tetrols and diols is higher in rats, D2 mice, and hamster trachea than in the other tissues. This could indicate that the enzymes

Table 6. Organo-Soluble Metabolites Formed by Cultured Tracheobronchial Tissues[a]

Species	Tetrols	Diols			Phenols		Quinones
		9,10-	4,5-	7,8-	3-	9-	
Human	27[b]	33	1	9	11	0.5	3
Rat							
CD	5	45	1	4	1	1	1
Buffalo	3	35	1	14	1	2	n.d.
Wistar	6	30	5	13	3	7	1
Mouse							
C57BL/6N	12	9	1	16	3	6	6
DBA/2N	29	12	4	4	6	3	28
Hamster	38	22	1	6	3	3	3

[a]After incubation of the explants with [^{3}H]BP (1.5 μM) for 24 h, the media were extracted with ethylacetate/acetone (2/1), and the extracted metabolites were analyzed by HPLC using a Zorbax ODS column and a linear water-methanol gradient. The results are expressed as the mean of at least 3 different experiments (the human results were from 15 cases).
[b]Percent formed.

responsible for the further oxidation of the diols to tetrols are either less efficient or of a different type in these three species. Different forms of cytochrome P-450 have been shown to be involved in the conversion of BP to BP epoxides and BP diols to BP diolepoxides (62). The concentration of BP in the incubation mixture has also been shown to affect the relative level of BP diols to BP phenols, with BP diols being highest at the BP concentration similar to our incubation conditions (63). No significant differences are observed in the metabolite distribution formed by the different anatomical segments of the human respiratory tract -- trachea, main-stem bronchus, and secondary or tertiary bronchus (26). The metabolic profile of BP is similar in explants and primary epithelial cell cultures derived from the same patient (25).

Metabolism of Other Carcinogens

The metabolism of other classes of chemical carcinogens has only been studied in cultured human bronchus. In addition to BP, several other PAHs, 7,12-dimethylbenz[a]anthracene (DMBA), 3-methylcholanthrene, BP 7,8-diol, have been metabolized into reactive species that bind to cellular DNA (see Table 7) (64-66). The highest mean binding level is seen with DMBA. The major DMBA-DNA adduct in human bronchus is formed by the reaction of DMBA-3,4-dihydro-3,4-dihydroxy-1,2-oxide and the exocyclic 2-amino group of guanine (A.M. Jeffrey, to be published), similar to the adducts formed in other intact cells. The binding level of the proximate carcinogenic form of BP, BP 7,8-diol, is several-fold higher than that of the parent compound, while BP phenols and BP 9,10-diol bind to a lesser extent (66). The extent of binding of the PAHs to human bronchus gives a fairly good correlation with the carcinogenic potency of the PAHs in experimental animals.

Table 7. Metabolism of Chemical Carcinogens by Cultured Human Tissues

Compound	Carcinogen[a] pmoles	No. of Cases
Polycyclic aromatic hydrocarbons[b]		
Benzo[a]pyrene 7,8-diol	471	3
7,12-Dimethylbenz[a]anthracene	118	28
3-Methylcholanthrene	34	2
Benzo[a]pyrene	32	15
Dibenz[a,h]anthracene	28	4
Mycotoxin[b]		
Aflatoxin B_1	14	17
N-Nitrosamines[c]		
Nitrosodimethylamine	906	15
Nitrosodiethylamine	264	4
Nitrosopyrrolidine	183	4

[a]Bound/10 mg DNA.
[b]1.5 μM.
[c]100 μM.

N-Nitrosamines are another group of environmental carcinogens that may be involved in the etiology of human lung cancer, as this class of compounds is also found in cigarette smoke. N-Nitrosamines show a remarkable organ and species specificity in their carcinogenic effects. It is generally believed that the metabolism of the N-nitrosamines by the target cells may be partly responsible for this organ susceptibility. Human bronchus metabolizes both cyclic and acyclic N-nitrosamines (N-nitrosodimethylamine [DMN], N-nitrosodiethylamine, N-nitrosopyrrolidine), as measured by carbon dioxide (CO_2) formation and by radioactivity associated with DNA (67-68). The highest number of DNA modifications are seen with DMN. The major alkylation products formed by this reaction are O^6- and N^7-methylguanine. Although both DMN and BP are activated by the cytochrome P-450 system, no correlation between the binding level to DNA is seen (34). This may be due to the involvement of different forms of cytochrome P-450, since kinetic studies of DMN metabolism in liver microsomes indicate that at least two enzymes with different substrate specificity are involved in the conversion of DMN to CO_2 (69). Lung slices from humans and experimental animals could also metabolize DMN into CO_2. The activity decreased in the following order: hamster, mouse, human, and rat (70).

Aflatoxin B_1 (AFB_1), a mycotoxin that induces liver cancer in experimental animals, is also activated by human bronchus. The major AFB_1-DNA adduct is formed between the 3-position of AFB_1 and the 7-position of guanine, although minor adducts have been formed with other bases (71). This major adduct is similar to the adduct formed in the rat liver.

CONCLUSION

Understanding the metabolic activation of environmental contaminants by human tissues is important in evaluating the human risk factor of a certain compound. By using an explant culture system, we have shown that human bronchus can activate several classes of environmental carcinogens into metabolites that damage DNA. In addition, extensive studies using BP indicate that metabolism of BP in the explant culture system is qualitatively similar to that in experimental animals in which BP is carcinogenic. The results emphasize the advantage of an intact cellular system instead of a subcellular system for the study of carcinogen metabolism, since the cellular system possesses intact activation and deactivation enzymes and, therefore, resembles the *in vivo* situation.

ACKNOWLEDGMENTS

This project is the result of a collaboration between our laboratory, Dr. A.M. Jeffrey, Institute of Cancer Research, Columbia University, Dr. J.M. Essigmann, Department of Nutrition and Food Science, Massachusetts Institute of Technology, and Dr. B.F. Trump, Department of Pathology, University of Maryland. The technical assistance of R. Schwartz, M. Brugh, H. Tate, and F. Wefald is greatly appreciated.

REFERENCES

1. Nettesheim, P., and R.A. Griesemer. 1978. Experimental models for studies of respiratory tract carcinogenesis. In: Pathogenesis and Therapy of Lung Cancer. C.C. Harris, ed. Marcel Dekker, Inc.: New York. pp. 75-188.

2. Steele, V.E., A.C. Marchok, and G.M. Cohen. 1980. Transformation of rat tracheal epithelial cells by benzo[a]pyrene and its metabolites. Cancer Lett. 8:291-298.

3. Serabjit-Singh, C.J., C.R. Wolf, R.M. Philpot, and C.G. Plopper. 1980. Cytochrome P-450: Localization in rabbit lung. Science 207:1469-70.

4. Boyd, M.R. 1977. Evidence for the Clara cell as a site of cytochrome P-450 dependent mixed-function oxidase activity in lung. Nature 269:713-715.

5. Vadi, H., B. Jernstrom, and S. Orrenius. 1976. Recent studies on benzo[a]pyrene metabolism in rat liver and lung. In: Carcinogenesis - A Comprehensive Survey. R. Freudenthal, and P.W. Jones, eds. Raven Press: New York. pp. 45-61.

6. Sipal, Z., T. Ahlenius, A. Bergstrand, L. Rodriquez, and S.W. Jakobsson. 1979. Oxidative biotransformation of benzo[a]pyrene by human lung microsomal fractions prepared from surgical specimens. Xenobiotica 9:633-645.

7. Prough, R.A., Z. Sipal, and S.W. Jakobsson. 1977. Metabolism of benzo[a]pyrene by human lung microsomal fractions. Life Sci. 21:1629-1636.

8. McManus, M.E., A.R. Boobis, G.M. Pacifici, R.Y. Frempong, M.J. Brodie, G.C. Kahn, C. Whyte, and D.S. Davies. 1979. Xenobiotic metabolism in the human lung. Life Sci. 26:481-487.

9. Mitchell, C.E. 1980. Induction of aryl hydrocarbon hydroxylase in Chinese hamsters and mice following intratracheal instillation of benzo[a]pyrene. Res. Comm. Chem. Pathol. Pharmacol. 28:65-78.

10. Dansette, P.M., K. Alexandrov, R. Azerad, and C.H. Frayssinet. 1979. The effect of some mixed-function oxidase inducers on aryl hydrocarbon hydroxylase and epoxide hydrase in nuclei and microsomes from rat liver and lung: The effect of cigarette smoke. Eur. J. Cancer 18:915-922.

11. Simberg, N., and P. Uotila. 1978. Stimulatory effect of cigarette smoke on the metabolism and covalent binding of benzo[a]pyrene in the trachea of the rat. Int. J. Cancer 22:28-31.

12. Juchau, M.R., T. DiGiovanni, M.J. Namkung, and A.H. Jones. 1979. A comparison of the capacity of fetal and adult liver, lung, and brain to convert polycyclic aromatic hydrocarbons to mutagenic and cytotoxic metabolites in mice and rats. Toxicol. Appl. Pharmacol. 49:171-178.

13. Sabadie, N., H.B. Richter-Reichhelm, R. Saracci, U. Mohr, and H. Bartsch. 1981. Studies on inter-individual differences in oxidative benzo[a]pyrene metabolism by normal and tumorous surgical lung specimens from 105 lung cancer patients. Int. J. Cancer 24:417-426.

14. Kouri, R.E., T. Rude, P.E. Thomas, and C.E. Whitmire. 1976. Studies on pulmonary aryl hydrocarbon hydroxylase activity in inbred strains of mice. Chem.-Biol. Interact. 13:317-331.

15. Kouri, R.E., H.L. Billups, T.H. Rude, C.E. Whitmire, B. Sass, and C.J. Henry. 1980. Correlations of inducibility of aryl hydrocarbon hydroxylase with susceptibility to 3-methylcholanthrene-induced lung cancer. Cancer Lett. 9:277-284.

16. Oesch, F., and H. Schmassmann. 1979. Species and organ specificity of the trans-stilbene oxide-induced effects on epoxide hydratase and benzo[a]pyrene monooxygenase activity in rodents. Biochem. Pharmacol. 28:171-176.

17. Oesch, F., H. Schmassmann, E. Ohnhaus, U. Althaus, and T. Lorenz. 1980. Monooxygenase, epoxide hydrolase, and glutathione-S-transferase activities in human lung. Variation between groups of bronchogenic carcinoma and noncancer patients and inter-individual differences. Carcinogenesis 1:827-835.

18. Hundley, S.G., and R.I. Freudenthal. 1977. Comparison of benzo[a]pyrene metabolism by liver and lung microsomal enzymes from 3-methylcholanthrene-treated rhesus monkeys and rats. Cancer Res. 37:244-249.

19. Gehly, E.B., W.E. Fahl, C.R. Jefcoate and C. Heidelberger. 1979. The metabolism of benzo[a]pyrene by cytochrome P-450 in transformable and non-transformable C3H mouse fibroblast. J. Biol. Chem. 254:5041-5048.

20. Bornstein, W.A., M.D. Lamden, A.H.L. Chuang, R.L. Gross, P.M. Newberne, and E. Bresnick. 1978. Inability of vitamin A deficiency to alter benzo[a]pyrene metabolism in Syrian hamsters. Cancer Res. 38:1497-1501.

21. Teel, R.W., and W.H.T. Douglas. 1980. Aryl hydrocarbon hydroxylase activity in type II alveolar lung cells. Experientia 36:107.

22. Teel, R.W. 1979. Induction of aryl hydrocarbon in primary cultures of type II alveolar lung cells and binding of metabolically activated benzo[a]pyrene to nuclear macromolecules. Cancer Lett. 7:349-355.

23. Stoner, G.D., C.C. Harris, A. Autrup, B.F. Trump, E.W. Kingsbury, and G.A. Myers. 1978. Explant culture of human peripheral lung tissues. I. Metabolism of benzo[a]pyrene. Lab. Invest. 38:685-692.

24. Mehta, R., M. Meredith-Brown, and G.M. Cohen. 1979. Metabolism and covalent binding of benzo[a]pyrene in human peripheral lung. Chem.-Biol. Interact. 28:345-358.

25. Lechner, J.F., A. Haugen, H. Autrup, I.A. McClendon, B.F. Trump, and C.C. Harris. 1981. Clonal growth of epithelial cells from normal adult human bronchus. Cancer Res. 41:2294-2304.

26. Cohen, G.M., P. Uotila, J. Hartiala, L.-M. Suolinna, N. Simberg, and O. Pelkonen. 1979. Metabolism and covalent binding of [^{3}H]benzo[a]pyrene by isolated perfused lung and short-term tracheal organ culture of cigarette-exposed rats. Cancer Res. 37:2147-2155.

27. Autrup, H., F.C. Wefald, A.M. Jeffrey, H. Tate, R.D. Schwartz, B.F. Trump, and C.C. Harris. 1980. Metabolism of benzo[a]pyrene by cultured tracheobronchial tissues from mice, rats, hamsters, bovine, and humans. Int. J. Cancer 25:293-300.

28. Selkirk, J.K. 1977. Divergence of metabolic activation systems for short-term mutagenesis assays. Nature 270:604-607.

29. Autrup, H., A.M. Jeffrey, and C.C. Harris. 1980. Metabolism of benzo[a]pyrene by cultured human tissues. In: Polynuclear aromatic hydrocarbons: Chemistry and biological effects. A. Bjorseth and A.J. Dennis, eds. Battelle Press: Columbus. pp. 89-106.

30. Kahl, G.F., E. Klaus, C. Legraverend, D.W. Nebert, and O. Pelkonen. 1979. Formation of benzo[a]pyrene metabolite-nucleoside adducts in isolated perfused rat and mouse liver and in mouse lung slices. Biochem. Pharmacol. 28:1051-1056.

31. Glatt, H.R., R. Billings, K.L. Platt, and F. Oesch. 1981. Improvement of the correlation of the bacterial mutagenicity with carcinogenicity of benzo[a]pyrene and four of its major metabolites by activation with intact liver cells instead of cell homogenate. Cancer Res. 41:270-277.

32. Autrup, H., G.D. Stoner, F. Jackson, C.C. Harris, A.K.M. Shamsuddin, L.A. Barrett, and B.F. Trump. 1978. Explant culture of rat colon: A model system for studying metabolism of chemical carcinogens. In Vitro 14:868-877.

33. Trump, B., E. McDowell, L. Barrett, A. Frank, and C.C. Harris. 1974. Studies of ultrastructure, cytochemistry, and organ culture of human bronchial epithelium. In: Experimental Lung Cancer. E. Karbe, and J.J. Park, eds. Springer-Verlag: New York. pp. 548-588.

34. Autrup, H., R.C. Graftstrom, M. Brugh, J. Lechner, A. Haugen, B.F. Trump, and C.C. Harris. (in press). Comparison of benzo[a]pyrene metabolism in bronchus, colon, esophagus, and duodenum from the same individual. Cancer Res.

35. Harris, C.C., A.L. Frank, C. van Haaften, D.G. Kaufman, R. Connor, F.E. Jackson, L.A. Barrett, E.M. McDowell, and B.F. Trump. 1976. Binding of [^{3}H]benzo[a]pyrene to DNA in cultured human bronchus. Cancer Res. 36:1011-1018.

36. Autrup, H. 1979. Separation of water-soluble metabolites from cultured human colon. Biochem. Pharmacol. 28:1727-1730.

37. Yang, S.K., P.P. Roller, and H.V. Gelboin. 1977. Enzymatic mechanism of benzo[a]pyrene conversion to phenols and diols and an improved high pressure liquid chromatographic separation of benzo[a]pyrene derivatives. Biochemistry 16:3680-3686.

38. Jeffrey, A.M., I.B. Weinstein, K.W. Jennette, K. Grezeskowiak, K. Nakanishi, R.G. Harvey, H. Autrup, and C.C. Harris. 1977. Structures of benzo[a]pyrene-nucleic acid adducts formed in human and bovine bronchial explants. Nature 269:348-350.

39. Cohen, G.M., S.M. Haws, B.P. Moore, and J.W. Bridges. 1976. Benzo[a]pyrene-3-yl hydrogen sulphate, a major ethyl acetate-extractable metabolite in human, hamster, and rat lung cultures. Biochem. Pharmacol. 25:2561-2570.

40. Mehta, R., and G.M. Cohen. 1979. Major differences in the extent of conjugation with glucuronic acid and sulphate in human peripheral lung. Biochem. Pharmacol. 28:2479-2484.

41. Harris, C.C., H. Autrup, R. Connor, L.A. Barrett, E.M. McDowell, and B.F. Trump. 1976. Inter-individual variation in binding of benzo[a]pyrene to DNA in cultured human bronchi. Science 194:1067-1069.

42. Cohen, G.M., R. Mehta, and M. Meredith-Brown. 1979. Large inter-individual variations in metabolism of benzo[a]pyrene by peripheral lung tissues from lung cancer patients. Int. J. Cancer 24:129-133.

43. Harris, C.C., H. Autrup, G. Stoner, and B.F. Trump. 1978. Model systems using human lung for carcinogenesis studies. In: Pathogenesis and Therapy of Lung Cancer. C. Harris, ed. M. Dekker: New York. pp. 559-597.

44. Wigley, C.B., R.F. Newbold, J. Amos, and P. Brookes. 1979. Cell-mediated mutagenesis in cultured Chinese hamster cells by polycyclic hydrocarbons: Mutagenicity and DNA reaction related to carcinogenicity in a series of compounds. Int. J. Cancer 23: 691-696.

45. Newbold, R.F., P. Brookes, and R.G. Harvey. 1979. A quantitative comparison of the mutagenicity of carcinogenic polycyclic hydrocarbon derivatives in cultured mammalian cells. Int. J. Cancer 24:203-209.

46. Moore, P., and B.S. Strauss. 1979. Sites of inhibition of *in vitro* DNA synthesis in carcinogen- and UV-treated ϕ x 174 DNA. Nature 278:664-666.

47. Sagher, D., R.G. Harvey, W.-T. Hsu, and S.B. Weiss. 1979. Effect of benzo[a]pyrenediolepoxide on infectivity and in vitro translation of phage MS2 RNA. Proc. Natl. Acad. Sci. USA 76:620-624.

48. Yamaura, I., H. Marquardt, and L.F. Cavelieri. 1978. Effects of benzo[a]pyrene adducts on DNA synthesis in vitro. Chem.-Biol. Interact. 23:399-407.

49. Jack, P., and P. Brookes. 1980. The binding of benzo[a]pyrene to DNA components of differing sequence complexity. Int. J. Cancer 25:789-795.

50. Pulkrabek, P., S. Leffler, D. Grunberger, and I.B. Weinstein. 1979. Modification of deoxyribonucleic acid by a diol epoxide of BP. Relation to deoxyribonucleic acid structure and confirmation and effects on transfectional activity. Biochemistry 18:5128-5134.

51. Autrup, H., R.D. Schwartz, J.M. Essigmann, L. Smith, B.F. Trump, and C.C. Harris. 1980. Metabolism of aflatoxin B_1, benzo[a]pyrene and 1,2-dimethylhydrazine by cultured rat and human colon. Teratogen. Carcinogen. and Mutagen. 1:3-13.

52. Grafstrom, R.G., H. Autrup, and C.C. Harris. (MS). Metabolism of benzo[a]pyrene by explant cultures of tracheobronchial, esophageal, and colonic tissues from three different rat strains.

53. Cerutti, P., K. Shinohara, M.-L. Ide, and J. Remsen. 1978. Formation and repair of benzo[a]pyrene-induced DNA damage in mammalian cells. In: Polycyclic Hydrocarbons and Cancer, Volume 2. H.V. Gelboin, and P.O.P. T'so, eds. Academic Press: New York. pp. 203-212.

54. Ivanovic, V., N.E. Geacintor, H. Yamasaki, and I.B. Weinstein. 1978. DNA and RNA adducts formed in hamster embryo cell cultures exposed to benzo[a]pyrene. Biochemistry 17:1597-1603.

55. Dipple, A. 1976. Polynuclear aromatic hydrocarbons. American Chemical Society monograph 173:245-314.

56. DiGiovanni, J., J.R. Romson, D. Linville, and M.R. Juchau. 1979. Covalent binding of polynuclear aromatic hydrocarbons to adenine correlates with tumorigenesis in mouse skin. Cancer Lett. 7:39-43.

57. King, H.W.S., M.R. Osborne, and P. Brookes. 1979. The in vitro and in vivo reactions at the N^7-position of guanine of the ultimate carcinogen derived from benzo[a]pyrene. Chem.-Biol. Interact. 24:345-353.

58. Haseltine, W.A., K.M. Lo, and A.D. D'Andrea. 1980. Preferred sites of strand-scission in DNA modified by anti-diol epoxide of benzo[a]pyrene. Science 209:929-931.

59. Phillips, D.H., P.L. Grover, and P. Sims. 1978. A quantitative determination of the covalent binding of a series of polycyclic hydrocarbons to DNA in mouse skin. Int. J. Cancer 23:201-208.

60. Seifried, H.E., D.J. Birkett, W. Levin, A.Y.H. Lu, A.H. Conney, and D.M. Jerina. 1977. Metabolism of benzo[a]pyrene: Effect of 3-methylcholanthrene pretreatment on metabolism by microsomes from lungs of genetically "responsive" and "non-responsive" mice. Arch. Biochem. Biophys. 178:256-263.

61. Mass, M.J., and D.G. Kaufman. 1979. Benzo[a]pyrene quinone metabolism in tracheal organ cultures. Biochem. Biophys. Res. Comm. 89:885-892.

62. Deutsch, J., R.P. Vatsis, M.J. Coon, J.C. Leutz, and H.V. Gelboin. 1979. Catalytic activity and stereoselectivity of purified form of rabbit liver microsomal cytochrome P-450 in the oxygenation of the (-)- and (+)-enantioners of trans 7,8-diohydroxy-7,8 dihydro-benzo[a]pyrene. Molec. Pharmacol. 16:1011-1018.

63. Namkung, M.J., and M.R. Juchau. 1980. On the capacity of human placental enzymes to catalyze the formation of diols by benzo[a]pyrene. Toxicol. Appl. Pharmacol. 55:253-259.

64. Harris, C., V. Genta, A. Frank, D. Kaufman, L. Barrett, E.M. McDowell, and B.F. Trump. 1974. Carcinogenic polynuclear hydrocarbons bind to macromolecules in cultured human bronchi. Nature 252:68-69.

65. Harris, C.C., H. Autrup, G. Stoner, S.K. Yang, J.C. Leutz, H.V. Gelboin, J.K. Selkirk, R.J. Connor, L.A. Barrett, R.T. Jones, E.M. McDowell, and B.F. Trump. 1977. Metabolism of benzo[a]pyrene and 7,12-dimethylbenz[a]anthracene in cultured human tissues: Bronchus and pancreatic duct. Cancer Res. 37:3349-3355.

66. Yang, S.K., H.V. Gelboin, B.F. Trump, H. Autrup, and C.C. Harris. 1977. Metabolic activation and DNA binding of benzo[a]pyrene in cultured human bronchus. Cancer Res. 37:1207-1212.

67. Harris, C.C., H. Autrup, G.D. Stoner, E.M. McDowell, B.F. Trump, and P. Schafer. 1977. Metabolism of dimethylnitrosamine and 1,2-dimethylhydrazine in cultured human bronchi. Cancer Res. 37:2309-2311.

68. Harris, C.C., H. Autrup, G.D. Stoner, E.M. McDowell, B.F. Trump, and P. Schafer. 1977. Metabolisms of acyclic and cyclic N-nitrosamines in cultured human bronchus. J. Natl. Cancer Inst. 59:1401-1406.

69. Kroeger-Koepke, M.B., and C.J. Michejda. 1979. Evidence for several dimethylase enzymes in the oxidation of dimethylnitrosamine and phenylmethylnitrosamine by rat liver fractions. Cancer Res. 39:1587-1591.

70. Den Engelse, L., M. Gebbink, and P. Emmelot. 1975. Studies on lung tumors. III. Oxidative metabolism of dimethylnitrosamine by rodent and human lung tissue. Chem.-Biol. Interact. 11:535-544.

71. Autrup, H., J.M. Essigmann, R.G. Croy, B.F. Trump, G.N. Wogan, and C.C. Harris. 1979. Metabolism of aflatoxin B_1 and identification of the major aflatoxin B_1-DNA adducts formed in cultured human bronchus and colon. Cancer Res. 39:694-698.

DISCUSSION

Q.: You showed that the A, B blood types were correlated with this greater risk; did you have enough samples of people with other blood types to make it significant, because A and B types are the most common.

A.: No. Those are the only types we have looked at and at the present time we have only 100 cases in our data bank. Within the next few years we hope to be able to answer your question.

Q.: Two questions: first, how do binding levels compare with the different levels of tissue organization, and second, can you compare adducts from organ to organ to predict a response?

A.: The first point with respect to an *in vivo* situation compares with an *in vitro* system. I think it is clear that we have to be very careful to compare one level of biological organization to the next one. For example, if you use microsomes to activate the benzo[*a*]pyrene, then you get a completely different adduct pattern than you would in the intact tissues. This is something I think Dr. Bigger is going to talk about tomorrow.

Furthermore, there is a difference between tissues. I've reported some studies with human bladder cells and I don't see any of the BP-DNA adducts observed in tracheobronchial tissues. But I see some adducts that I suspect are formed between phenol epoxides. So even correlation from one type cell to another one is very difficult.

INTRODUCTION: DNA DAMAGE AND REPAIR

P. N. Magee

Fels Research Institute and Department of Pathology, Temple University School of Medicine, Philadelphia, Pennsylvania 19140

INTRODUCTION

The concept that cancer may be induced by the interaction of a carcinogen with DNA is widely accepted, although it is becoming increasingly clear that some carcinogens do not interact with DNA to a detectable extent. The carcinogens have been classified into two broad categories, genotoxic and non-genotoxic or epigenetic. Genotoxic carcinogens damage DNA, whereas epigenetic or non-genotoxic carcinogens appear to operate by other mechanisms, such as chronic tissue injury, immunosuppression, solid-state effects, hormonal imbalance, cocarcinogenicity, and promotion (1). This presentation will be concerned only with agents that cause DNA damage and repair.

Many of the known genotoxic carcinogens require metabolic activation by tissue enzymes to form their carcinogenically active products, or ultimate carcinogens, namely electrophiles that react with nucleophilic sites in the cell (2). The nature of the crucial cellular target for malignant transformation is not known with complete certainty, but is generally thought to be macromolecular, including proteins, RNA, and DNA. DNA, in particular, is being considered the crucial target.

THE INVOLVEMENT OF DNA IN CARCINOGENESIS

The viral genome of the DNA oncogenic viruses is known to be incorporated, to a greater or lesser extent, in the DNA of transformed or tumor cells (3). This process is thought to be crucially related to the causal mechanism of tumor induction. The same mechanism appears to be involved in oncogenesis by RNA tumor viruses, after the complimentary DNA has been synthesized by the RNA-dependent DNA polymerase (reverse transcriptase) of the virus (4,5). New genetic material is being added that apparently carries the message for oncogenesis into the genome of the cells, which subsequently become transformed.

Weinberg (6) and Cooper (7) have recently obtained similar evidence, namely that the altered phenotype of virally- or chemically-transformed cells can be transmitted to untransformed cells by transfection of purified DNA. Shih and his colleagues (6) prepared DNA from 15 different mouse or rat cell lines transformed by chemical carcinogens *in vitro* or *in vivo* and transfected them to NIH3T3 mouse fibroblast cultures using the calcium phosphate transfection technique. Five of the donor DNAs induced foci of transformed cells in the recipients; the other donor DNAs and DNAs from untransformed control cells produced no foci. These findings indicated that the chemically-induced transformed phenotype was encoded in DNA and support the idea that DNA is the crucial target for chemical carcinogenesis. Similarly, Cooper and his colleagues (7) found that DNA fragments of chemically-transformed and normal avian and murine cells could induce transformation of NlH3T3 mouse cells with low frequencies. Secondary transfection assays with high-molecular-weight DNA prepared from these transformed cells resulted in transformation with high frequencies. The authors concluded that endogenous transforming genes of untreated cells could be activated and transmitted by transfection and that their results supported the hypothesis that normal cells contain genes able to induce transformation if they are expressed at abnormal levels.

Barrett and his colleagues (8) have provided further evidence. These investigators have clearly demonstrated that neoplastic transformation can be induced by a direct perturbation of DNA resulting from treatment of cells in culture with 5-bromodeoxyuridine (BrdU) and near-ultraviolet light. The specificity of these experiments depends on the fact that BrdU is incorporated into cellular DNA exclusively in place of thymidine and that such substituted DNA has an ultraviolet absorption spectrum that is shifted to longer wavelengths. For this reason, irradiation with light of wavelengths greater than 300 nm produces photochemical lesions in the DNA that result in chromosome damage, cytotoxicity, and somatic mutation. Barrett and his colleagues showed that combined treatment of Syrian hamster embryo cells in cultures with BrdU and near-ultraviolet light resulted in neoplastic transformation, whereas treatment with either agent alone did not. This finding strongly supports the role of DNA damage in neoplastic transformation.

Perhaps the most widely quoted evidence in support of DNA as the target for carcinogens is Cleaver's finding that human fibroblasts from individuals suffering from the disease *Xeroderma pigmentosum* have a defective capacity to repair ultraviolet light-induced lesions in their DNA (9). *Xeroderma pigmentosum* is an autosomal recessive hereditary condition characterized by a greatly increased incidence of cancer of the skin in areas exposed to sunlight (10,11). An interesting extension of this argument has been developed by Hart, Setlow, and Woodhead (12) in their studies using the gynogenetic fish *Poecilia formosa* (Amazon Molly). Because this species grows in clones, cells and tissues can be transplanted from one fish to another without rejection. Irradiation of cells from the thyroid and adjacent tissues with ultraviolet light, followed by injection into the abdominal cavities of recipients, led to extensive growth of the transplanted tissue, which was diagnosed as tumor. If the ultraviolet irradiation was followed by photoreactivation by exposure to visible light, the yield of thyroid growths in the recipient fish was greatly reduced. Since photoreactivation is known to convert the pyrimidine dimers induced by ultraviolet light to monomers, these interesting findings indicate that pyrimidine dimers in DNA can give rise to tumors. The work on *Xeroderma* and on *Poecilia formosa* also emphasize the probable importance of DNA repair in carcinogenesis.

In addition to the direct evidence for DNA involvement in carcinogenesis described above, there is a substantial body of indirect evidence. The idea that cancer may arise from a mutation in a somatic cell dates back to the work of Boveri (13), in 1914. Subsequent studies on mechanisms of chemical carcinogenesis have shown that many chemical carcinogens, after appropriate metabolic activation, yield products that are mutagenic. Much of this work has been reported by Bruce Ames and his colleagues in a series of papers, one entitled simply "Carcinogens are mutagens" (14). Many carcinogens seem to act by non-genetic mechanisms; nevertheless, the number of chemicals known to be both mutagenic and carcinogenic after appropriate metabolic activation is constantly increasing (15,16). Since mutagenesis, by definition, requires a change in the base sequence of DNA, the close parallels between mutagens and carcinogens strongly support the role of DNA as a target for carcinogenesis as well as mutagenesis.

Further indirect evidence comes from studies of the binding of chemical carcinogens to DNA *in vivo* and *in vitro*. Many organic chemicals, after being administered to animals, yield metabolic products that bind covalently to DNA of liver and other organs. The extensive literature on this subject has been comprehensively reviewed by Lutz (17), who concluded that a good correlation exists between the hepatocarcinogenic potency of a chemical and its extent of covalent binding to liver DNA after administration to the intact animal. This correlation is expressed as the Covalent Binding Index, which takes into account the measured extent of binding of the carcinogen to DNA in relation to the size of the dose. More detailed studies of the organ specificities and persistence of certain DNA adducts in animals treated with various alkylating carcinogens are also consistent with DNA as the target for these agents (18,19). This area will be discussed later by Drs. Kleihues, Montesano, and Pegg.

DNA REPAIR

Genetic continuity was formerly thought to be dependent on the stability of the DNA molecule, but it is now known that certain cellular mechanisms involving various enzyme systems repair damage to DNA in microbial and mammalian cells (20,21). If cancer can result from damage to DNA, it follows that efficient DNA repair processes might be able to prevent its occurrence by removal of the potentially carcinogenic lesion before cellular replication has perpetuated it, resulting in neoplasia.

Three types of repairable DNA damage are recognized: 1) missing, incorrect, or altered bases; 2) interstrand cross links; and 3) strand breaks. The nature of the DNA lesions that result in malignancy is not clear, but current thinking links the formation of covalently bound adducts of the activated forms of precarcinogens with DNA as the most likely initial step. DNA repair in mammalian cells can occur by at least two different processes, excision and post-replication repair. A third form, photoreactivation repair by visible light, which is exemplified by the reversal of pyrimidine dimerization in bacterial, may also occur.

Excision repair is the mechanism that has been most extensively studied in relation to carcinogenesis. It involves either the removal of a modified base by a glycosylase, leaving an apurinic or an apyrimidinic site (AP site) that can be recognized by an endonuclease, or recognition of a structural defect, such as a pyrimidine dimer or carcinogen adduct, by damage-specific endonucleases. Excision of the AP site or the carcinogen-DNA adduct then occurs by the action of an exonuclease; the gap is filled by a DNA polymerase, using the undamaged strand as a template, and the newly formed base sequence is joined by the enzyme DNA ligase. DNA glycosylases and AP endonucleases have been comprehensively reviewed by Lindahl (22). A third enzymic mechanism for repair of damage to DNA has recently been discovered in studies with carcinogenic methylating agents, such as nitrosodimethylamine and nitrosomethylurea. In a series of investigations on the cytotoxic and mutagenic effects of *N*-methyl-*N*'-nitro-*N*-nitrosoguanidine (MNNG), Cairns and his colleagues discovered an adaptive enzyme that apparently removes the methyl group from the O^6-position of guanines in DNA by a process of simple demethylation, without base or nucleotide excision (23). Olsson and Lindahl (24) have recently shown that the enzyme transfers the methyl group from the guanine of the DNA to a sulphydryl group of the enzyme protein itself. This enzyme has been found in mammalian cells and will be discussed later in this Symposium by Dr. A.E. Pegg. Removal of carcinogen-DNA adducts by enzymes is summarized in Table 1 (22). Not included in this review are the recently discovered glycosylases that remove 7-methylguanine (25-27).

Table 1. Removal of Carcinogen-DNA Adducts by Enzymes

Product	Enzyme	Adduct
Oligonucleotide Nucleotide	Endonuclease/exonuclease	Thymine dimer Probably aromatic amine, polycyclic hydrocarbon, etc.
Base	DNA glycosylase/exonuclease	3-Methyladenine 7-Methylguanine Uracil Hypoxanthine
Adduct itself (O^6-methylguanine)	Adaptive enzyme Methyl transferase	Methyl group

INDUCTION OF DNA REPAIR ENZYMES IN REGENERATING RAT LIVER

In 1979, Michael Sirover (28) investigated the induction of the DNA repair enzyme uracil-DNA glycosylase in human lymphocytes stimulated to proliferate by phytohemagglutinin. He showed that its activity was increased 10-fold and that the stimulation was coordinate with the asynchronous activation of DNA synthesis and of DNA polymerase activity. This stimulation required transcription and translation. In later work, Gupta and Sirover (29) extended these studies to another human cell, the WI-38 diploid human fibroblast. They examined two parameters of the base-excision repair pathway: the induction of the DNA repair enzyme, uracil DNA glycosylase, which functions in an initial step in base-excision repair; and also cell-mediated base-excision repair, as measured by unscheduled DNA synthesis after exposure to sodium bisulfite or to methyl methanesulfonate.

Uracil may occur in DNA under several circumstances. It may be incorporated as deoxyuridine-5'-monophosphate biosynthetically by certain microbial enzymes during DNA replication, and it can be formed in situ by treating DNA with heat or other agents that cause deamination of cystosine. Sodium bisulfite deaminates cytosine specifically in DNA to leave uracil. Methyl methanesulfonate, of course, alkylates DNA to give a variety of methylated bases, including 7-methylguanine and 3-methyladenine but very little O^6-methylguanine. Gupta and Sirover (29) found that uracil DNA glycosylase activity was stimulated during cell proliferation and made the very interesting observation that the repair enzyme was stimulated about 4 h earlier than were DNA replication and the induction of DNA polymerase. Their findings led them to suggest that some form of DNA-repair complex might be formed prior to DNA replication that could prescreen the DNA and thus prevent the transfer of erroneous genetic information to the daughter cells. However, the question was raised as to whether this inducibility of DNA repair enzymes is universal or constitutive in other species and cell types. Clearly, the mammalian liver regenerating after partial hepatectomy is an appropriate model for such an investigation, and the rat is highly suitable because a great deal is known about hepatic regeneration and carcinogenesis in this species. Uracil DNA glycosylase and 3-methyladenine DNA glycosylase were measured, therefore, at increasing time intervals after partial hepatectomy in the rat; the induction of DNA replication and the stimulation of DNA polymerase were also measured (30). Table 2 shows that both DNA synthesis and DNA polymerase reach maximal levels 20 to 24 h after partial hepatectomy and then decline. This growth and decline occurred particularly rapidly in the case of the polymerase, which reached basal levels at 48 h. Figure 1 shows the activation of the two DNA repair enzymes at increasing time intervals after hepatectomy. In both cases, the enzyme activities reach their maximal levels at 20 to 24 h and then decline rapidly. These results clearly show that the rat hepatocyte, like the human lymphocyte and fibroblast, modulates the activities of its DNA repair enzymes during cell proliferation. No increase in enzyme activities was found in sham-operated controls.

These results may seem difficult to reconcile with reports by Valda Craddock and others that regenerating liver is more susceptible to the induction of cancer than resting liver (31). This effect applies particularly to single doses of nitrosodimethylamine which rarely induce liver tumors in the rat unless the animal has undergone partial hepatectomy. However, the dose of nitrosodimethylamine used in these experiments was relatively large and may well have overwhelmed the repair

Table 2. Induction of DNA Replication and DNA Polymerase After Partial Hepatectomy[a]

Time After Hepatectomy (h)	DNA Synthesis [^{3}H]Thymidine Inc (cpm) DNA / (μg)	DNA Polymerase (units/mg protein)	-Fold Increase (Polymerase)
0	0.5 ± 0.2	104 ± 40	1.0
16	4.2 ± 2.1	271 ± 40	2.6
20	49.6 ± 16.7	287 ± 48	2.7
24	47.8 ± 35.0	242 ± 134	2.3
48	18.5 ± 9.8	124 ± 26	1.2

[a]One unit of enzyme activity equals that amount of DNA polymerase which incorporates 1 pmol of [α^{32}P]dTMP into acid-insoluble material in 60 min at 37°C (30). All experiments were performed in duplicate and standard deviations were determined.

mechanisms. According to Kleihues and Margison (32), the capacity for removal of O^6-methylguanine from DNA in rat liver may be exhausted under some circumstances. Whereas O^6-methylguanine may be the base in carcinogenesis crucially altered by methylating nitroso compounds, some apparently conflicting evidence suggests that its repair enzyme may be modulated during cell proliferation. Rabes and his colleagues (33) found that disappearance of the labeled methyl group was enhanced during S-phase in regenerating liver synchronized *in vivo* by hydroxyurea while Smith, Kaufman, and Grisham (34) reported decreased excision of O^6-methylguanine and 7-methylguanine during the S-phase of 10T1/2 cells *in vitro*.

ACKNOWLEDGMENTS

The author is indebted to the editor of *Carcinogenesis* for permission to reproduce Table 2 and Figure 1 from Reference 30. He would also like to acknowledge support from grants CA12227 and CA23451 from the National Cancer Institute and from the Samuel S. Fels Fund of Philadelphia.

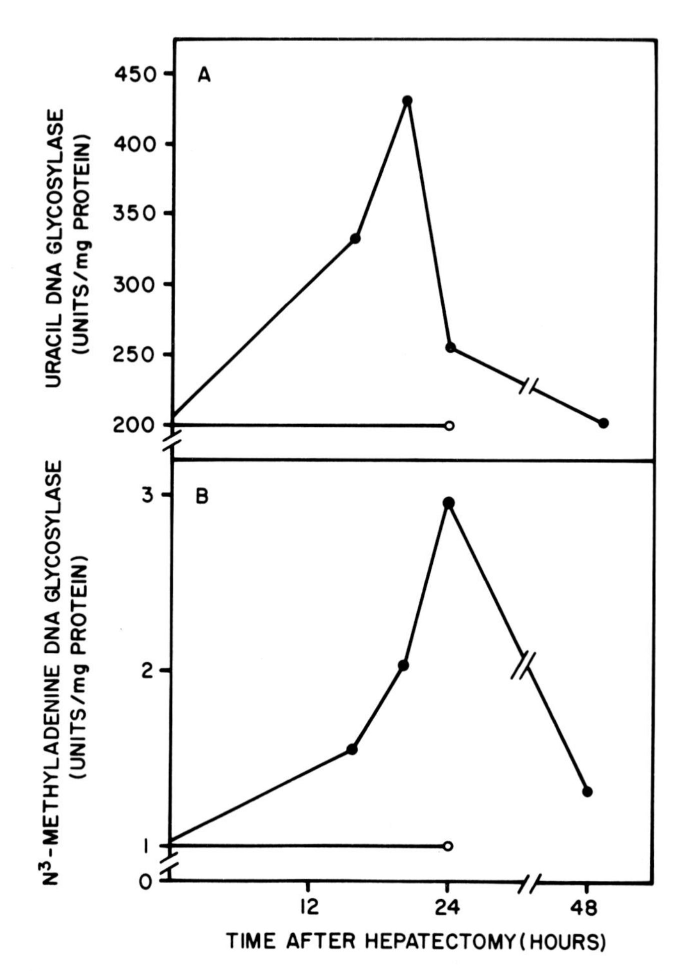

Figure 1. Induction of the DNA repair enzymes uracil DNA glycosylase and N^3-methyladenine DNA glycosylase in regenerating rat liver (30). A. Uracil DNA glycosylase. B. 3-MeA DNA glycosylase. (● = specific activity in regenerating liver; o = specific activity in livers from sham-operated control rats.)

REFERENCES

1. Williams, G.M. 1980. Classification of genotoxic and epigenetic hepatocarcinogens using liver culture assays. Ann. N.Y. Acad. Sci. 349:273-282.

2. Miller, E.C., and J.A. Miller. 1966. Mechanisms of chemical carcinogenesis: Nature of proximate carcinogens and interactions with macromolecules. Pharmacol. Rev. 18:805-838.

3. Westphal, H., and R. Dulbecco. 1968. Viral DNA in polyoma- and SV40-transformed cell lines. Proc. Natl. Acad. Sci. USA 59:1158-1165.

4. Temin, H., and S. Mizutani. 1970. RNA-dependent DNA polymerase in virions of Rous sarcoma virus. Nature 226:1211-1213.

5. Baltimore, D. 1970. RNA-dependent DNA polymerase in virions of RNA tumor viruses. Nature 226:1209-1211.

6. Shih, C., B.Z. Shilo, M.P. Goldfarb, A. Dannenberg, and R.A. Weinberg. 1979. Passage of phenotypes of chemically transformed cells via transfection of DNA and chromatin. Proc. Natl. Acad. Sci. USA 76:5714-5718.

7. Cooper, G.M., S. Okenquist, and S. Silverman. 1980. Transforming activity of DNA of chemically transformed and normal cells. Nature 284:418-421.

8. Barrett, J.C., T. Tsutsui, and P.O.P. Ts'o. 1978. Neoplastic transformation induced by a direct perturbation of DNA. Nature 274:229-232.

9. Cleaver, J.E. 1968. Defective repair replication of DNA in Xeroderma pigmentosum. Nature 218:652-656.

10. Robbins, J.H., K.H. Kraemer, M.A. Lutzner, B.W. Festoff, and H.G. Coon. 1974. Xeroderma pigmentosum: An inherited disease with sun sensitivity, multiple cutaneous neoplasms, and abnormal DNA repair. Ann. Intern. Med. 80:221-248.

11. Cleaver, J.E., and D. Bootsma. 1975. Xeroderma pigmentosum: Biochemical and genetic characteristics. Ann. Rev. Genet. 9:19-38.

12. Hart, R.W., R.B. Setlow, and A.D. Woodhead. 1977. Evidence that pyrimidine dimers in DNA can give rise to tumors. Proc. Natl. Acad. Sci. USA 74:5574-5578.

13. Boveri, T.H. 1914. Zur Frage der Entstehung maligner Tumoren. Gustav Fischer: Yena. 64 pp.

14. Ames, B.N., W. Durston, E. Yamasaki, and F. Lee. 1973. Carcinogens are mutagens: A simple test system combining liver homogenates for activation and bacteria for detection. Proc. Natl. Acad. Sci. USA 70:2281-2285.

15. McCann, J., E. Choi., E. Yamasaki, and B.N. Ames. 1975. Detection of carcinogens as mutagens in the *Salmonella*/ microsome test: Assay of 300 chemicals. Proc. Natl. Acad. Sci. USA 72:5135-5139.

16. Sugimura, T., S. Sato, M. Nagao, T. Yahagi, T. Matsushima, Y. Seino, M. Takeuchi, and T. Kawachi. 1976. Overlapping of carcinogens and mutagens. In: Fundamentals in Cancer Prevention. P.N. Magee, S. Takayama, T. Sugimura, and T. Matshushima, eds. Univ. Tokyo Press: Tokyo/Univ.; Park Press: Baltimore, MD. pp. 191-215.

17. Lutz, W.K. 1979. *In vivo* covalent binding of organic chemicals to DNA as a quantitative indicator in the process of chemical carcinogenesis. Mutat. Res. 65:289-356.

18. Goth, R., and M.F. Rajewsky. 1974. Persistence of O^6-ethylguanine in rat-brain DNA: Correlation with nervous system-specific carcinogenesis by ethylnitrosourea. Proc. Natl. Acad. Sci. USA 71:639-643.

19. Margison, G.P., and P. Kleihues. 1975. Chemical carcinogenesis in the nervous system. Preferential accumulation of O^6-methylguanine in rat brain deoxyribonucleic acid during repetitive administration of *N*-methyl-*N*-nitrosourea. Biochem. J. 148:521-525.

20. Cleaver, J.E. 1975. Methods for studying repair of DNA damaged by physical and chemical carcinogens. Meth. Cancer Res. 11:123-165.

21. Hanawalt, P.C., P.K. Cooper, A.K. Ganesan, and C.A. Smith. 1979. DNA repair in bacteria and mammalian cells. Ann. Rev. Biochem. 48:783-836.

22. Lindahl, T. 1979. DNA glycosylases, endonucleases for apurinic/apyrimidinic sites, and base excision-repair. Prog. Nucl. Acid Res. Molec. Biol. 22:25-192.

23. Cairns, J. 1980. Bacteria as proper subjects for cancer research. Proc. R. Soc. Lond. B. 208:121-133.

24. Olsson, M., and T. Lindahl. 1980. Repair of alkylated DNA in *Escherichia coli*. Methyl group transfer from O^6-methylguanine to a protein cysteine residue. J. Biol. Chem. 255:10569-10571.

25. Laval, J., J. Pierre., and F. Laval. 1981. Release of 7-methylguanine residues from alkylated DNA by extracts of *Micrococcus luteus* and *Escherichia coli*. Proc. Natl. Acad. Sci. USA 78:852-855.

26. Singer, B., and T.P. Brent. 1981. Human lymphoblasts contain DNA glycosylase activity excising N-3 and N-7 methyl and ethyl purines but not O^6-alkylguanines or 1-alkyladenines. Proc. Natl. Acad. Sci. USA 78:856-860.

27. Margison, G.P., and A.E. Pegg. 1981. Enzymatic release of 7-methylguanine from methylated DNA by rodent liver extracts. Proc. Natl. Acad. Sci. USA 78:861-865.

28. Sirover, M.A. 1979. Induction of the DNA repair enzyme uracil-DNA glycosylase in stimulated human lymphocytes. Cancer Res. 39:2090-2095.

29. Gupta, P.K., and M.A. Sirover. 1980. Sequential stimulation of DNA repair and DNA replication in normal human cells. Mutat. Res. 72:273-284.

30. Gombar, C.T., E.J. Katz, P.N. Magee, and M.A. Sirover. 1981. Induction of the DNA repair enzymes uracil DNA glycosylase and 3-methyladenine DNA glycosylase in regenerating rat liver. Carcinogenesis 2:595-599.

31. Craddock, V.M. 1976. Cell proliferation and experimental liver cancer. In: Liver Cell Cancer, Vol. 8. H.M. Cameron, D.A. Linsell, and G.P. Warwick, eds. Elsevier Publishing Company: Amsterdam, New York, and Oxford. pp. 153-201.

32. Kleihues, P., and G.P. Margison. 1976. Exhaustion and recovery of repair excision of O^6-methylguanine from rat liver DNA. Nature 259:153-155.

33. Rabes, H.M., R. Kerler, R. Wilhelm, G. Rode, and H. Riess. 1979. Alkylation of DNA and RNA by [^{14}C]dimethylnitrosamine in hydroxyurea-synchronized regenerating rat liver. Cancer Res. 39:4228-4236.

34. Smith, G.J., D.G. Kaufman, and J.W. Grisham. 1980. Decreased excision of O^6-methylguanine and N^7-methylguanine during the S phase in 10T1/2 cells. Biochem. Biophys. Res. Commun. 92:787-794.

DNA MODIFICATION AND REPAIR *IN VIVO*: TOWARDS A BIOCHEMICAL BASIS OF ORGAN-SPECIFIC CARCINOGENESIS BY METHYLATING AGENTS

Paul Kleihues[1], Ruth M. Hodgson[1], Christof Veit[1], Fritz Schweinsberg[2], and Manfred Wiessler[3]

[1]Abteilung Neuropathologie, Pathologisches Institut, Universitat Freiburg, Freiburg, Federal Republic of Germany, [2]Hygiene Institut, Universitat Tubingen, Tubingen, Federal Republic of Germany, and [3]Deutsches Krebsforschungszentrum, Heidelberg, Federal Republic of Germany

INTRODUCTION

The elucidation of the biological basis of organ-specific tumor induction by chemicals is a major objective of cancer research. For many carcinogens, the principal site of tumor induction has been shown to vary with species, dose, route of administration, and age or developmental stage. Some species also exhibit marked differences in their overall susceptibility to certain classes of chemical carcinogens. Accordingly, to accurately predict the adverse effects of genotoxic agents in humans, the basic mechanisms underlying organ and species specificity must first be understood.

This report summarizes data on the reaction of methylating carcinogens with DNA in the intact animal. The experiments were carried out under conditions similar to those used in chronic carcinogenicity studies and designed to detect possible correlations between the initial or cumulative extent of DNA modification and the preferential site of tumor induction. To facilitate comparative evaluation, we concentrated on carcinogens that after chronic administration selectively induce tumors in different rat tissues (see Table 1). All of these carcinogens methylate DNA and other cellular macromolecules *in vivo*, and there is evidence that this methylation is mediated through a common ultimate carcinogen, methyl diazonium ion (1). They apparently produce an identical pattern of reaction products with cellular DNA, characterized by a high proportion of O-alkylated bases (O^6-methylguanine, O^4-methylthymine, O^2-methylthymine, and O^2-methylcytosine). Under physiological conditions *in vitro*, these carcinogens cause the formation of O^6-methylguanine and

Table 1. Organ-Specific Tumor Induction by Methylation Agents in Rats.

Carcinogen			
Structure	Name	Route	Target Organ
$O{=}N{-}N(CH_3){-}CH_2{-}O{-}CO{-}CH_3$	**Nitrosomethyl(acetoxymethyl)amine** (DMN-OAc)	i.v. i.p.	Lung Intestine
$O{=}N{-}N(CH_3){-}CH_2{-}C_6H_5$	N-Nitrosomethylbenzylamine (MBN)	oral,s.c.	Esophagus
$CH_3{-}NH{-}NH{-}CH_3$	1,2-Dimethylhydrazine (SDMH)	s.c.	Colon
$O{=}N{-}N(CH_3){-}CO{-}NH_2$	**N-Nitroso-N-methylurea** (MNU)	i.v.	Brain

7-methylguanine at a ratio of 0.11 (2-4). It is further assumed that the initial pattern of DNA modification produced by these agents depends entirely on the chemical reactivity of their common ultimate intermediate and is, therefore, identical in target and nontarget tissues (5).

ORGAN SPECIFICITY DUE TO INSUFFICIENT SYSTEMIC DISTRIBUTION OF THE PARENT CARCINOGEN (FIRST-PASS EFFECT)

For many carcinogens, the predominant site of tumor induction is identical to the site of administration. This correlation is most frequent after skin painting, topical instillations (e.g., intratracheal, intravesicular, intrarectal, intragastric), and subcutaneous or oral administration, if the parent carcinogen is very unstable or locally metabolized before any significant resorption into the systemic circulation can occur. However, an apparent organ specificity may also result from insufficient distribution after uptake of the carcinogen into the systemic circulation.

Tumor Induction in Lung and Intestines by Nitrosomethyl(acetoxymethyl)amine (DMN-OAc)

Nitrosomethyl(acetoxymethyl)amine (DMN-OAc) is a stable derivative of the α-hydroxy intermediate of the hepatocarcinogen nitrosodimethylamine. Under physiological conditions *in vitro* (pH 7.2; 37°C), it decomposes with a half-life of 26 h. In the presence of esterases, the heterolytic decomposition of DMN-OAc is greatly enhanced due to enzymic cleavage of the acetoxy moiety. Using DMN-OAc as substrate, esterase activity was present in supernatant fractions from all rat tissues investigated, with the highest levels in kidney and liver (3). Pretreatment of tissue extracts with the esterase inhibitor diisopropyl fluorophosphate (10^{-4} M) was found to reduce both the decomposition of DMN-OAc and DNA alkylation *in vitro* by more than 90% (3).

The location of tumors induced by DMN-OAc depends primarily on the route of application. A single i.p. injection of 0.1 mmol/kg body weight induces intestinal tumors in up to 86% of experimental animals (6), with most neoplasms originating from epithelial cells of the small intestine (7). Intravenous injections, on the other hand, led to the formation of lung tumors in more than 70% of the animals (8,9). In addition, some tumors were observed in kidney, brain, ear duct, and heart, with the latter originating from endocardial nerves (8,9). Following i.v. injection of [^{14}C]DMN-OAc *in vivo* (3), by far the highest levels of DNA alkylation were found in the lung, the principal target organ for this route of application. Concentrations of methylated bases somewhat lower than those in lung were present in kidney and brain DNA, which again correlates with the results of chronic carcinogenicity studies (8,9). In DNA of lung, kidney, and brain, the extent of O^6-alkylation of guanine was 9, 8, and 36 times higher after i.v. injection than after a single i.p. dose. In contrast, i.p. injection of [^{14}C]DMN-OAc resulted in a preferential alkylation of organs bordering the abdominal cavity, with the highest levels of alkylation in the target organs for this route of application, i.e., colon and ileum (see Figure 1). These data indicate that a substantial proportion of DMN-OAc administered i.p. is directly absorbed through the peritoneum and activated by organs bordering the abdominal cavity. After i.v. injection, esterase activity in the lung is sufficiently high to metabolize a substantial amount of the carcinogen during its first pass through the pulmonary circulation, thus reducing its systemic distribution to other tissues. This is in agreement with the work of Frank et al. (38) who determined a half-life of 16 sec for the hydrolysis of DMN-OAc *in vivo*. These studies also show that many rat tissues are basically susceptible to the carcinogenicity of DMN-OAc and related methylating agents. However, a high extent of initial DNA alkylation appears to be required to cause a significant tumor incidence.

Several N-nitrosamides have also been shown to induce lung tumors after i.v. administration in rats, including N-methyl-N'-nitro-N'-nitrosoguanidine (10), N-nitroso-N-methylurethane (11), and N-nitroso-N-methylpropionamide (12). These carcinogens do not require enzymic activation but rapidly decompose after reaction with thiol compounds (e.g., cysteine). Again, the apparent organ specificity results from preferential DNA alkylation in the target tissue due to the breakdown of a substantial proportion of the parent carcinogen during its first pass through the pulmonary circulation. The selective induction of liver tumors following oral administration of low doses of nitrosodimethylamine has also been interpreted to result from a first-pass effect (13,14). After uptake into portal veins, very small oral doses are metabolized to a great extent during their first pass through the hepatic circulation. In contrast to i.v. injections or high oral doses ($>$ 1 mg/kg), this method has been shown to result in almost exclusive alkylation of liver DNA.

PREFERENTIAL BIOACTIVATION IN THE TARGET ORGAN

Since most carcinogens require enzymic activation *in vivo*, it would be reasonable to expect that tumors usually originate in the tissues that contain the highest activity of microsomal enzymes involved in the breakdown of the parent compound. However, this is often not the case. Although the vast majority of environmental carcinogens, including nitrosamines, are predominantly metabolized

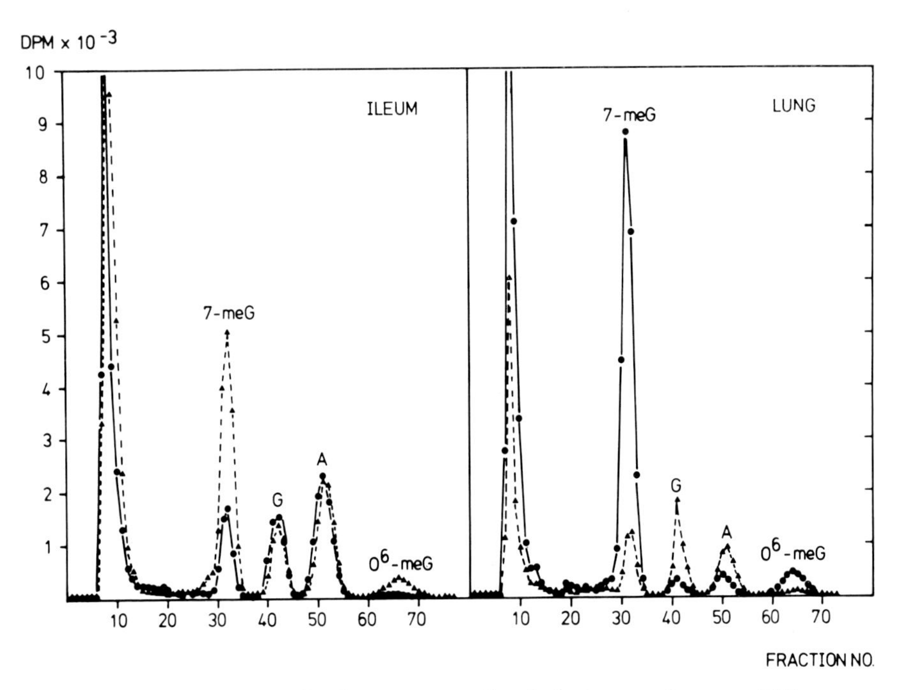

Figure 1. Influence of the route of administration on DNA methylation in ileum and lung by a single dose of DMN-OAc (3). Male CD rats received an i.v. (●) or i.p. (▲) injection of [^{14}C]DMN-OAc (12 mg/kg) and were killed 12 h later. Radioactivity profiles from two chromatographic separations of acid DNA hydrolysates on Sephadex G-10 columns were superimposed and adjusted to similar amounts of DNA.

in the liver, only a few induce a high incidence of liver tumors. In fact, high doses of most carcinogens fail to produce hepatic tumors in rats. Among nonhepatic tissues, however, the principal target organ often exhibits the highest levels of metabolism and the greatest initial extent of DNA modification.

Induction of Esophagus and Forestomach Tumors by N-Nitrosomethylbenzylamine (MBN)

Structure-activity studies by Druckrey et al. (11) have shown that in rats symmetrical N-dialkylnitrosamines produce predominantly liver tumors, whereas most asymmetrical nitrosamines, including N-nitrosomethylbenzylamine (MBN), selectively induce esophageal carcinomas. This organ specificity is largely independent of the route of application. MBN induces esophageal tumors after both oral (11) and s.c. (15) administration. Studies on the metabolism of MBN in rats were carried out with the parent carcinogen [^{14}C]-labeled in either the methyl group or in the methylene bridge of the benzyl moiety (see Figure 2). Within 10 min after a single i.v. dose of [^{14}C-methyl]MBN (2.5 mg/kg), labeled metabolites (methanol, formic acid) accounted for 50% of the total radioactivity present in the esophagus, for approximately 25% in liver and forestomach, and for less than 20% in all other organs investigated (16). Four hours after the injection, methylation of purine bases in DNA was most extensive in the esophagus, followed by liver, lung, and forestomach (see Figure 3). In the remaining tissues, DNA methylation was either considerably less (kidney, glandular stomach, spleen) or not detectable (ileum, colon, brain). At this time the concentration of the promutagenic base O^6-methylguanine in esophageal DNA was six times higher than in lung DNA and nine times higher than in hepatic DNA (see Table 2). These data suggest that in the rat the selective induction of esophageal tumors by MBN and related asymmetrical nitrosamines is mediated by a preferential bioactivation of the carcinogen in the target organ.

Table 2. DNA Alkylation in Wistar Rats and NMRI Mice by MBN[1]

Organ	7-meG[b]		O^6-meG[b]	
	Rat	Mouse	Rat	Mouse
Liver	120	163	4.9	11.8
Esophagus	344	18	46.1	1.5
Forestomach	10	23	n.d.[c]	1.7
Lung	65	46	7.7	4.8

[a]Animals received a single s.c. (rats) or i.p. (mice) injection of [^{14}C-methyl]MBN (2.5 mg/kg) and were killed 4 (rats) or 6 (mice) h later (16,18).
[b]Expressed as fraction of guanine x 10^6.
[c]n.d. = not detectable.

After injection of a similar dose of [^{14}C-methylene]MBN, no benzylation of DNA was detectable (17), suggesting that enzymic hydroxylation of MBN occurs predominantly, if not exclusively, in the methylene bridge. This response is in accordance with *in vitro* studies using microsomes from rat liver and esophagus (19). Incubation with MBN and an NADPH-generating system yielded benzaldehyde but no formaldehyde.

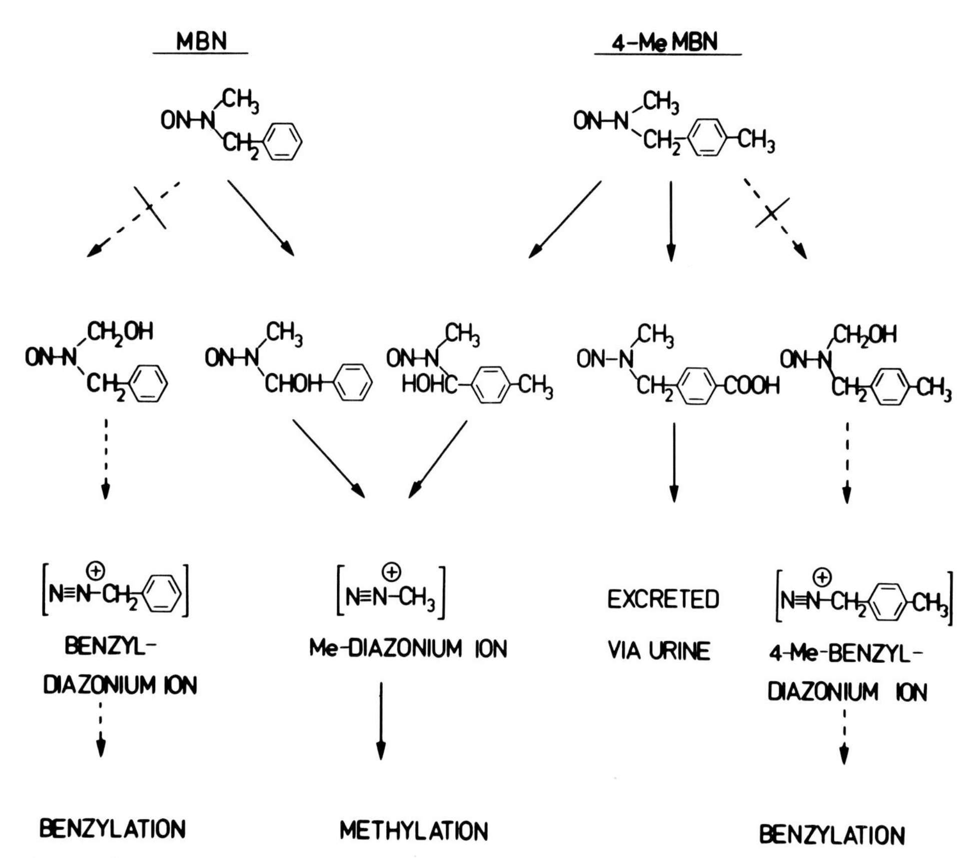

Figure 2. Metabolic pathways potentially involved in the bioactivation of MBN and its ring-methylated analogue, nitrosomethyl-(4-methylbenzyl)amine (4-MeMBN) (17). Metabolic routes, indicated by broken arrows, were found to be largely inoperative *in vivo*.

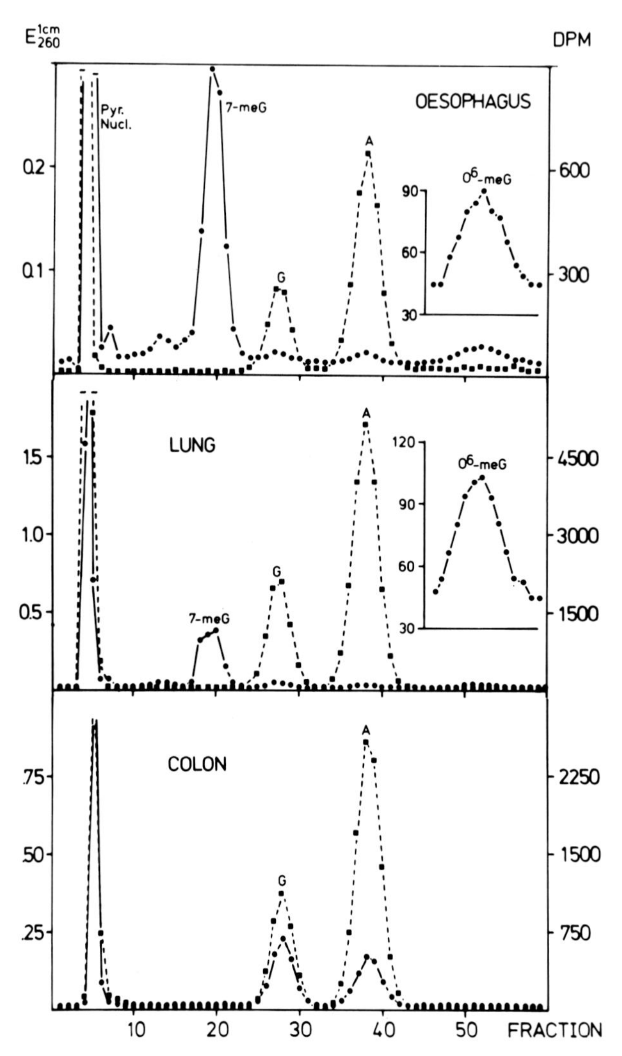

Figure 3. DNA methylation by MBN in vivo (16). Adult rats received a single i.v. injection of [^{14}C-Methyl]MBN (2.5 mg/kg) and were killed 4 h later. Acid DNA hydrolysates from esophagus, lung, and colon were separated on Sephasorb HP columns, eluted with 10 mM phosphate buffer (pH 5.5) at a flow rate of 1.6 ml/min (fraction vol. 3.8 ml) (■----■ E_{260}^{1cm}; ●----● dpm).

Schweinsberg et al. (20) have shown that methyl substitution in the para position of the phenyl moiety of MBN greatly reduces the toxicity of MBN, increasing the LD_{50} from 18 to 400 mg/kg. After chronic administration in the drinking water, N-nitrosomethyl(4-methylbenzyl)amine (4-MeMBN) produced a high incidence of esophageal tumors, whereas after multiple s.c. injections no tumors have been observed thus far (experiments are in progress). Biochemical studies (17,21) revealed that after systemic administration of 4-MeMBN more than 60% of the carcinogen is excreted via the urine as benzoic acid derivative (see Figure 2). Due to this detoxification pathway, the extent of DNA methylation by 4-MeMBN was considerably lower than that produced by the non-modified carcinogen. However, at approximately equitoxic doses (18 and 393 mg/kg, corresponding to 0.12 and 2.4 mmol/kg) both agents produced similar amounts of 7-methylguanine in nucleic acids of the esophagus (see Figure 4). In contrast to MBN, DNA alkylation by 4-MeMBN was more extensive in the liver than in the esophagus, indicating that even minor modifications of these carcinogens markedly alter their substrate specificity for hydroxylation by microsomal P-450 enzymes. These data indicate that after systemic administration of equimolar doses, 4-MeMBN should be considerably less carcinogenic than MBN. The high incidence of esophageal tumors observed after chronic oral administration of 4-MeMBN is probably due to direct uptake from the drinking water into the esophageal mucosa, thus avoiding the hepatic detoxification pathway.

In mice, multiple i.p. doses of MBN (2.5 mg/kg/week) induce a high incidence of forestomach carcinomas and lung adenomas but no esophageal tumors (22). Analysis of methylation by [^{14}C-methyl]MBN in various mouse tissues showed highest concentrations of 7-methylguanine and O^6-methylguanine in liver, followed by the principal target tissues, lung, and forestomach (see Table 2). DNA methylation in the esophagus was only 21% less than in the forestomach, suggesting tht despite their anatomical similarities the level of initial DNA modification required for malignant transformation differs considerably in these tissues. Oral administration of MBN is likely to lead to more extensive DNA methylation in the esophagus due to direct uptake from the drinking water and has indeed been shown to result in a 100% tumor incidence in both esophagus and forestomach (22).

Induction of Colon Tumors by 1,2-Dimethylhydrazine (SDMH)

Weekly s.c. injections of 1,2-dimethylhydrazine (SDMH) in rats and mice cause a selective induction of colon carcinomas. Following a single s.c. dose of [^{14}C]SDMH in adult rats, maximum alkylation of nucleic acids is reached within 12 h, with the highest level found in liver, followed by colon, kidney, and

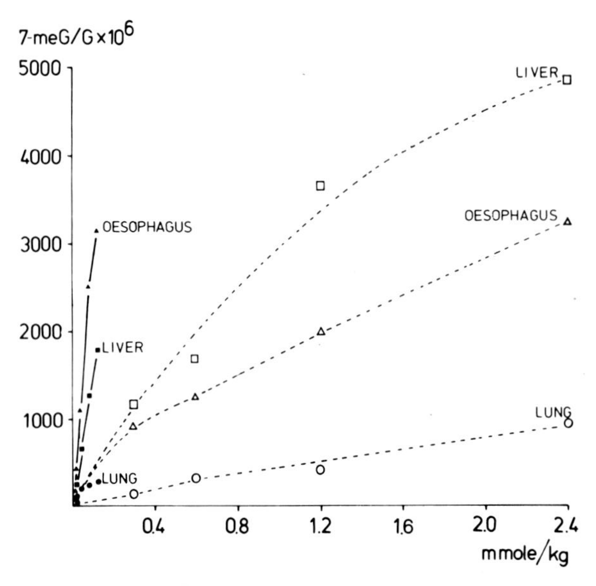

Figure 4. Formation of 7-methylguanine in nucleic acids (DNA and RNA) of esophagus, liver, and lung from rats that received a single s.c. injection of [^{14}C-methyl]MBN (continuous line) or 4-Me[^{14}C-methyl]MBN (broken line) at doses ranging from 0.0067 to 2.4 mmol/kg (12 h survival time) (17).

ileum (23,24). No detectable levels of alkylation were found in stomach and brain. Although the initial level of DNA methylation was several times higher in liver than in the principal target tissue (colon), evidence was found that the extent of colonic DNA modifcation is very critical with respect to the incidence and latency period of colon carcinomas. In mice with genetically low susceptibility to SDMH-induced colon carcinogenesis (C57Bl/Ha), concentrations of 7-methylguanine and O^6-methylguanine in DNA of colon, ileum, and kidney (but not liver), were 40 to 60% less than in mice with a high incidence of colonic tumors (ICR/Ha). The repair of O^6-methylguanine was similar in both strains (see Figure 5). In conclusion, SDMH is one of the many carcinogens that cause the most extensive DNA modification in the liver followed by the principal target tissue. Only chronic oral administration of small doses of SDMH induces liver tumors, possibly due to a first-pass effect after uptake into the portal circulation (25).

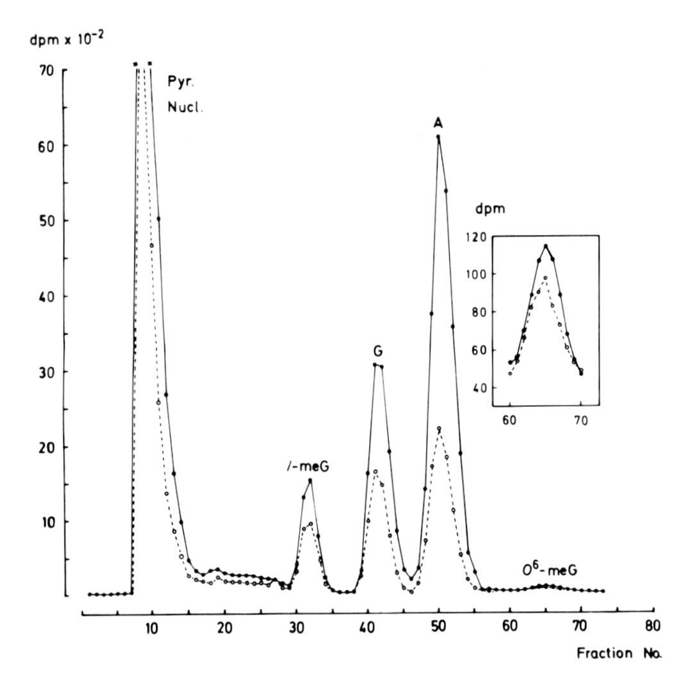

Figure 5. Methylation of colon DNA in mice with high (ICR/Ha; continuous line) and low susceptibility (C57Bl/Ha; broken line) to SDMH-induced colon carcinogenesis (26). Animals received a single s.c. injection of [^{14}C]SDMH (15 mg/kg) and were killed 12 h later. Radioactivity profiles from two chromatographic runs (Sephadex G-10) were superimposed and adjusted to similar amounts of DNA on each column.

DEFICIENT REPAIR OF O^6-METHYLGUANINE IN THE TARGET TISSUE

Increasing evidence indicates that O^6-alkylation of guanine in DNA is a promutagenic lesion likely to be involved in the initiation of malignant transformation (2,4). O^6-Methylguanine can be enzymically removed by a repair enzyme recently identified as a transmethylase (27,28). Since this type of repair is error-free, enzymic removal of O^6-methylguanine could play an important role in the prevention of stable mutations and of malignant transformation after exposure to methylating carcinogens. Several *in vivo* experiments show a deficient repair of O^6-alkylguanine in the target tissue.

Induction of Nervous System Tumors by Methylnitrosourea (MNU) and Related Carcinogens

Evidence for a differential excision repair capacity of various organs was first demonstrated for the neuro-oncogenic alkylnitrosoureas. O^6-Ethylguanine produced by a single injection of ^{14}C-nitrosoethylurea (75 mg/kg) in 10-day-old rats was found to be removed at a much slower rate from DNA of the brain, the principal target organ, than from that of liver, a nontarget organ in this animal model (29). Similarly, O^6-methylguanine produced by a single dose of N-nitroso-N-[^3H]methylurea ([^3H]MNU) to adult (30) or 10-day-old rats (see Figures 6 and 7) persisted considerably longer in brain DNA than in DNA of other rat organs, whereas for 7-alkylguanine no such differences exist. The initial loss from brain DNA was found to proceed at a similar rate for both O^6-ethylguanine and O^6-methylguanine, the apparent half-lives being in the range of 9 to 11 days. Studies in adult BD-IX rats have shown that after 2 weeks the rate of removal of O^6-methylguanine from cerebral DNA decreases greatly (see Figure 6). Six months after the injection of a single dose of 10 mg/kg of [^3H]MNU, approximately 25% of the initial (4 h) concentration was still present in brain DNA (31). Extrapolation of these data suggests that complete removal would require approximately 1 year. It is possible that the different slopes of the excision curve (see Figure 6) for removal of O^6-methylguanine from brain DNA represent different cell populations, e.g., neuronal and glial cells.

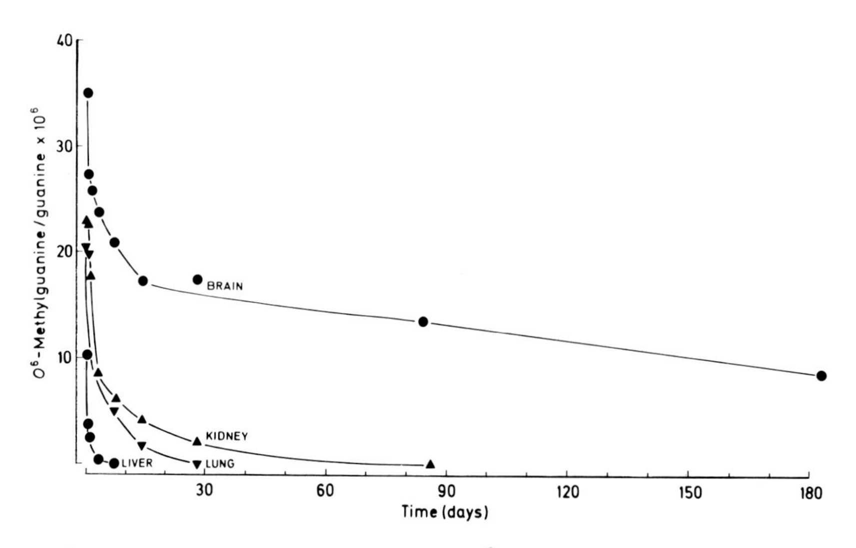

Figure 6. Long-term persistence of O^6-methylguanine in rat brain DNA (31). Adult BD-IX rats received a single i.v. injection of [^3H]MNU (10 mg/kg) and were killed at time intervals ranging from 4 h to 184 days.

In adult rats, the selective induction of nervous system tumors is possible only by repeated administration of small doses of neuro-oncogenic compounds. When [^{3}H]MNU was given as weekly doses of 10 mg/kg over a period of 5 weeks, the amount of O^6-methylguanine accumulated in brain DNA greatly exceeded that in kidney, spleen, and intestine (32). Similarly, an accumulation of O^6-methylguanine was found in cerebral DNA of rats after multiple doses of the neuro-oncogenic agent 3,3-dimethyl-1-phenyltriazene. These and other experiments (for review see reference 4) support the hypothesis that the preferential induction of tumors in certain tissues may be due to deficient repair in the target organ. However, experiments in other species have shown that the location of tumors does not solely depend on the formation and persistence of O^6-alkylguanine in DNA. In mice, alkylnitrosoureas and related carcinogens induce predominantly lung and lymphoid tumors, whereas neural tumors are generally rare (usually less than 10% of experimental animals). The repair of O^6-methylguanine in cerebral DNA was, as in rats (see Figure 7), considerably slower than in DNA of liver, spleen, and intestine. Furthermore, the rate of excision from cerebral DNA was similar in A/J and C3HeB/FeJ mice, although these strains differ significantly in their response to the neuro-oncogenic effect of alkylnitrosoureas.

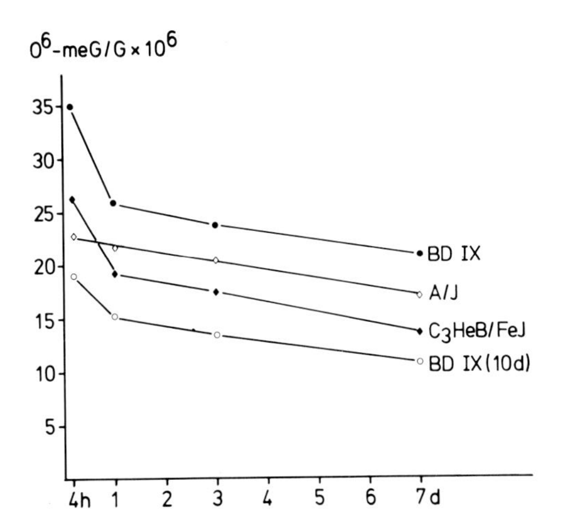

Figure 7. Loss of O^6-methylguanine from cerebral DNA of rats and mice (34). Female BD-IX rats (adult and 10-day-old), and adult female mice (A/J and C3HeB/FeJ) received a single dose of [^{3}H]MNU and were killed at various time intervals ranging from 4 h to 7 days. The carcinogen was administered i.v., with the exception of 10-day-old BD-IX rats, which received an i.p. injection.

Attempts to induce nervous system tumors by MNU and nitrosoethylurea in the Mongolian gerbil (Meriones unguiculatus) have completely failed. In this species, enzymatic removal of the promutagenic base O^6-methylguanine, as in rats, is most effective in the liver, followed by kidney, lung, and brain (35). In cerebral DNA, 40% of the initial concentration was still present after 6 months (see Figure 8). Since the gerbil brain is apparently not susceptible to the oncogenic effect of methylnitrosourea and related carcinogens, these data indicate that the formation and persistence of O^6-alkylguanine may consistitute a necessary although not sufficient event for the initiation of organ-specific carcinogenesis by monofunctional alkylating agents.

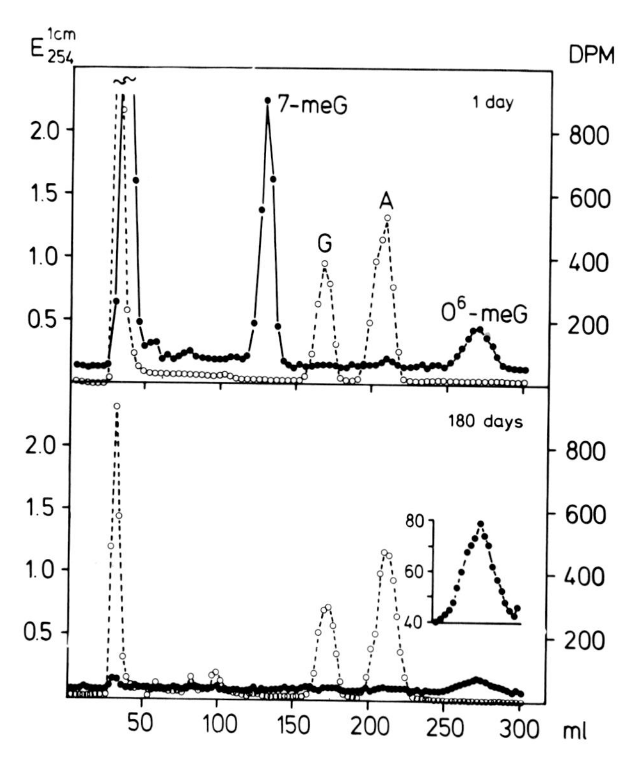

Figure 8. Long-term persistence of O^6-methylguanine in cerebral DNA of gerbils (Meriones unguiculatus) (35). Animals received a single i.v. injection of [^{14}C]MNU (10 mg/kg) and were allowed to survive for 1 day (upper) or 180 days (lower). Sephadex G-10 columns were eluted with 0.05 M ammonium formate (pH 6.2). The fraction volume was 3.8 (upper) and 2.8 ml (lower) (o ----o E^{1cm}_{260}; ● ---- ● dpm.).

CONCLUSIONS

The biological basis of organ and species specificity is complex. Even if we restrict ourselves to simple methylating agents, which all share a common ultimate carcinogen, the available experimental data are insufficient to compose a unifying theory that would enable us to reliably predict the principle target tissues and species susceptibility for compounds not yet tested in chronic carcinogenicity studies. In this review, we concentrated on the initial extent of DNA alkylation and the persistence of the promutagenic base O^6-methylguanine. With the analytical methods previously available, it was not possible to determine minor methylated bases of potential biological importance, e.g., O^4-methylthymine. In addition, the rate of DNA synthesis was not determined under the various experimental conditions. A further limitation of these studies is that the data refer to whole tissue preparations. In organs like brain, kidney, and liver, malignant transformation is often restricted to only one cell population. Lewis and Swenberg (36) have recently shown that DNA alkylation and repair differ markedly in hepatocytes and nonparenchymal liver cells. Despite these limitations, the experiments reported from our and other laboratories (4) allow four general conclusions (4):

1. In many rat tissues basically susceptible to malignant transformation by methylating agents, the incidence and location of tumors is closely correlated with the initial extent of DNA methylation. As shown in other studies (4,34,37), this correlation is particularly true for the potentially mutagenic base O^6-methylguanine. For several nonhepatic rat tissues (e.g., the different segments of the gastrointestinal tract) it would be possible to experimentally determine the level of O^6-alkylation of guanine in DNA required to produce a tumor incidence higher than 50% within a certain latency period.

2. For several agents and experimental conditions, organ specificity can be explained by insufficient systemic distribution of the parent carcinogen (first-pass effect). The location of tumors induced by these carcinogens changes with dose and/or route of application.

3. Microsomal enzyme systems mediating the metabolism of carcinogens exhibit a marked variation between different organs. Formation of the ultimate electrophile intermediate may be restricted to or preferentially occur in the target tissue (e.g., induction of esophageal tumors by MBN in rats). However, in most cases the initial extent of DNA modification is highest in liver, followed by the principal target tissue(s). The reasons for the resistance of liver cells to single or multiple high doses of methylating carcinogens remain unclear.

4. O^6-Alkylguanine can be enzymically removed from DNA, and in several rat tissues tumor induction has been shown to correlate with a relative repair deficiency in the target organ. However, species and strain differences in the response to methylating carcinogens are not paralleled by differences in the repair capacity for O^6-methylguanine.

ACKNOWLEDGMENTS

This work is supported by grants from the Deutsche Forschungsgemeinschaft, Bundesministerium Forschung und Technologie, and the Ubelmesser-Passera Stiftung.

REFERENCES

1. Hathway, D.E., and G.F. Kolar. 1980. Mechanisms of reaction between ultimate chemical carcinogens and nucleic acid. Chem. Society Rev. 9:241-264.

2. Pegg, A.E. 1977. Formation and metabolism of alkylated nucleosides: Possible role in carcinogenesis by nitroso compounds and alkylating agents. Adv. Cancer Res. 25:195-269.

3. Kleihues, P., G. Doerjer, L.K. Keefer, J.M. Rice, P.P. Roller, and R.M. Hodgson. 1979. Correlation of DNA methylation by methyl(acetoxymethyl)nitrosamine with organ-specific carcinogenicity in rats. Cancer Res. 39:5136-5140.

4. O'Connor, P.J. 1981. Interaction of chemical carcinogens with macromolecules. J. Cancer Res. Clinic. Oncol. 99:167-186.

5. Singer, B., W.J. Bodell, J.E. Cleaver, G.H. Thomas, M.F. Rajewsky, and W. Thon. 1978. Oxygens in DNA are main targets for ethylnitrosourea in normal and xeroderma pigmentosum fibroblasts and fetal rat brain cells. Nature 276:85-88.

6. Joshi, S.R., J.M. Rice, M.L. Wenk, P.P. Roller, and L.K. Keefer. 1977. Selective induction of intestinal tumors in rats by methyl(acetoxymethyl)nitrosamine, an ester of the presumed reactive metabolite of dimethylnitrosamine. J. Natl. Cancer Inst. 58:1531-1535.

7. Ward, J.M., J.M. Rice, P.P. Roller, and M.L. Wenk. 1977. Natural history of intestinal neoplasms induced in rats by a single injection of methyl(acetoxymethyl)nitrosamine. Cancer Res. 37:3046-3052.

8. Berman, J.J., J.M. Rice, M.L. Wenk, and P.P. Roller. 1979. Dependence on route of administration of tumor spectrum in Sprague-Dawley rats resulting from single or multiple injections of methyl(acetoxymethyl)nitrosamine. J. Natl. Cancer Inst. 63:93-100.

9. Habs, M., D. Schmähl, and M. Wiessler. 1978. Carcinogenicity of acetoxymethyl-methyl-nitrosamine after subcutaneous, intravenous, and intrarectal application in rats. Z. Krebsforsch. 91:217-221.

10. Stekar, J., and J. Gimmy. 1980. Induction of lung tumours in rats by i.v. injection of N-methyl-N'-nitro-N-nitrosoguanidine. Eur. J. Cancer 16:395-400.

11. Druckrey, H., R. Preussman, S. Ivankovic, and D. Schmähl. 1967. Organotrope carcinogene Wirkungen bei 65 verschiedenen N-Nitroso-Verbindungen an BD-Ratten. Z. Krebsforsch. 69:103-201.

12. Stekar, J. 1977. Pulmotropic carcinogenic activity of N-methyl-N-nitrosopropionamide. Eur. J. Cancer 13:1183-1189.

13. Diaz Gomez, M.I., P.F. Swann, and P.N. Magee. 1977. The absorption and metabolism in rats of small oral doses of dimethylnitrosamine. Biochem. J. 164:497-500.

14. Pegg, A.E. 1980. Formation and subsequent repair of alkylation lesions in tissues of rodents treated with nitrosamines. Arch. Toxicol. Suppl. 3:55-68.

15. Stinson, S.F., R.A. Squire, and M.B. Sporn. 1978. Pathology of esophageal neoplasms and associated proliferative lesions induced in rats by N-methyl-N-benzylnitrosamine. J. Natl. Cancer Inst. 61:1471-1475.

16. Hodgson, R.M., M. Wiessler, and P. Kleihues. 1980. Preferential methylation of target organ DNA by the oesophageal carcinogen N-nitrosomethylbenzylamine. Carcinogenesis 1:861-865.

17. Hodgson, R.M., F. Schweinsberg, M. Wiessler, and P. Kleihues. 1982. Mechanism of esophageal tumor induction by N-nitrosomethylbenzylamine and its ring-methylated analog N-nitrosomethyl(4-methylbenzyl)amine. Submitted for publication.

18. Kleihues, P., Ch. Veit, M. Wiessler, and R.M. Hodgson. 1981. DNA alkylation by N-Nitrosomethylbenzylamine in target and non-target tissues of NMRI mice. Carcinogenesis 2:897-899.

19. Schweinsberg, F., and M. Kouros. 1979. Reactions of N-methyl-N-nitrosobenzylamine and related substrates with enzyme-containing cell fractions isolated from various organs of rats and mice. Cancer Lett. 7:115-120.

20. Schweinsberg, F., P. Schott-Kollat, and G. Bürkle. 1977. Veränderung der Toxizität und Carcinogenität von N-Methyl-N-Nitrosobenzylamin durch Methylsubstitution am Phenylrest bei Ratten. Z. Krebsforsch. 88:231-236.

21. Schweinsberg, F., G. Döring, and M. Kouros. 1979. Metabolism of isomeric N-methyl-N-nitroso-(methylphenyl)-methylamines. Cancer Lett. 8:125-132.

22. Sander, J., and F. Schweinsberg. 1973. Tumorinduktion bei Mäusen durch N-Methylbenzyl-nitrosamin in niedriger Dosierung. Z. Krebsforsch. 79:157-161.

23. Rogers, K.J., and A.E. Pegg. 1977. Formation of O^6-methylguanine by alkylation of rat liver, colon, and kidney DNA following administration of 1,2-dimethylhydrazine. Cancer Res. 37:4082-4088.

24. Swenberg, J.A., H.K. Cooper, J. Bücheler, and P. Kleihues. 1979. 1,2-Dimethylhydrazine-induced methylation of DNA bases in various rat organs and the effect of pretreatment with disulfiram. Cancer Res. 39:465-467.

25. Swenburg, J.A., M.A. Bendell, K.C. Billings, and J.G. Lewis. 1982. Cell specificity in DNA Damage and Repair. In: Organ and Species Specificity in Chemical Carcinogenesis. R. Langenbach, S. Nesnow, and J. Rice, eds. Plenum Press: New York. pp. 605-617.

26. Cooper, H.K., J. Bücheler, and P. Kleihues. 1978. DNA alkylation in mice with genetically different susceptibility to 1,2-dimethylhydrazine-induced colon carcinogenesis. Cancer Res. 38:3063-3065.

27. Olsson, M., and T. Lindahl. 1980. Repair of alkylated DNA in *Escherichia coli*. Methyl group transfer from O^6-methylguanine to a protein cysteine residue. J. Biol. Chem. 22:10569-10571.

28. Foote, R.S., S. Mitra, and B.C. Pal. 1980. Demethylation of O^6-methylguanine in a synthetic DNA polymer by an inducible activity in *Escherichia coli*. Biochem. Biophys. Res. Comm. 2:654-659.

29. Goth, R., and M.F. Rajewsky. 1974. Persistence of O^6-ethylguanine in rat-brain DNA: Correlation with nervous system-specific carcinogenesis by ethylnitrosourea. Proc. Natl. Acad. Sci. USA 71:639-643.

30. Kleihues, P., and G.P. Margison. 1974. Carcinogenicity of N-methyl-N-nitrosourea: Possible role of repair excision of O^6-methylguanine from DNA. J. Natl. Cancer Inst. 53:1839-1842.

31. Kleihues, P., and J. Bücheler. 1977. Long-term persistence of O^6-methylguanine in rat brain DNA. Nature 269:625-626.

32. Margison, G.P., and P. Kleihues. 1975. Chemical carcinogenesis in the nervous system. Preferential accumulation of O^6-methylguanine in rat brain deoxyribonucleic acid during repetitive administration of N-methyl-N-nitrosourea. Biochem. J. 148:521-525.

33. Kleihues, P., H.K. Cooper, J. Bucheler, and G.F. Kolar. 1979. Investigations on the mechanism of perinatal tumor induction by neuro-oncogenic alkylnitrosoureas and dialkyl-aryltriazenes. Natl. Cancer Inst. Monogr. 51:227-231.

34. Kleihues, P. G. Doerjer, J.A. Swenberg, E. Hauenstein, J. Bucheler, and H.K. Cooper. 1979. DNA repair as a regulatory factor in the organotropy of alkylating carcinogens. Arch. Toxicol. Suppl. 2:253-261.

35. Kleihues, P., St. Bamborschke, and G. Doerjer. 1980. Persistence of alkylated DNA bases in the Mongolian gerbil (*Meriones unguiculatus*) following a single dose of methylnitrosourea. Carcinogenesis 1:111-113.

36. Lewis, J.G., and J.A. Swenberg. 1980. Differential repair of O^6-methylguanine in DNA of rat hepatocytes and nonparenchymal cells. Nature 288:185-187.

37. Frei, J.V., D.H. Swenson, W. Warren, and P.D. Lawley. 1978. Alkylation of deoxyribonucleic acid *in vivo* in various organs of C57BL mice by the carcinogens N-methyl-N-nitrosourea, N-ethyl-N-nitrosourea and ethyl methanesulphonate in relation to induction of thymic lymphoma. Biochem. J. 174:1031-1044.

38. Frank, N., C. Janzowski, and M. Wiessler. 1980. Stability of Nitrosoacetoxymethylmethylamine in *in vitro* systems and *in vivo* and its excretion by the rat organism. Biochem. Pharmacol. 29:383-387.

DISCUSSION

Q.: I must compliment you on your elegant work on nitrosomethylbenzylamine, but it poses a dilemma for me. Some years ago, we did an experiment with nitrosomethylcyclohexylamine which is also an esophageal carcinogen, and we found extremely high alkylation of guanine at the 7-position in the liver, but none whatsoever in the esophagus. And I think we had enough sensitivity. The reason I tested that compound was to compare it with nitrosomethylphenylamine (nitrosomethylaniline), because nitrosomethylphenylamine cannot form a methylating agent and yet it's still an esophageal carcinogen. I'd like to know what your comments are on that.

A.: Well, I must say that the latter is indeed an extremely interesting compound and since I know you are working with it, I'll stay away and work with the other ones. Nitrosomethylphenylamine cannot be hydroxylated in the phenyl moiety. So it cannot be converted into a methylating species, and indeed we have in earlier years tried this and it does not. So another ultimate carcinogen is necessary in this case.

I do not say that all these asymmetrical nitroso compounds, which induce esophageal tumors, are preferentially metabolized in the target organ. I don't think that's necessary. But I would predict that most of them produce the highest level of alkylation in rat liver, followed by the esophagus as the principal target tissue. Rat liver is indeed a special case. And why rat liver rarely develops tumors after high doses of various methylating carcinogens is, I think, one of the most interesting problems we are dealing with.

Q.: A question about your study on colon carcinogenesis. As you probably have seen, when you kill the animal, you only find tumor in the lower part of the colon; when you do your alkylation experiment you have probably taken the whole colon. Is that the right way of predicting susceptibility?

A.: Well, the most detailed study on the location of tumors in the colon of BD IX rats is that by Dr. Maskens (Cancer Res. 36:1585-1592, 1976). He found that about 50% of tumors originate in the midsection of the colon. So I think there are segments of the colon where there are more tumors than in other parts, but I don't think you can say that they are only in the lower part.

MODIFICATION OF DNA REPAIR PROCESSES INDUCED BY NITROSAMINES

R. Montesano[1], H. Bresil[1], G. Planche-Martel[1], A. E. Pegg[2], and G. Margison[3]

[1]International Agency for Research on Cancer, Lyons, France, [2]Milton Hershey Medical Center, Pennsylvania State University, Hershey, Pennsylvania 17033, and [3]Paterson Laboratories, Christie Hospital and Holt Radium Institute, Manchester, Great Britain

INTRODUCTION

The repair of DNA damage induced by various chemical and physical carcinogenic agents appears to be a critical determinant of mutagenesis and of the initiation of the carcinogenic process (1-3). The alkylating agents, especially the N-nitroso compounds, show a high degree of species, tissue, and cell specificity in their carcinogenic effects, which appear to be governed by the following major factors: systemic distribution of the carcinogens, the metabolic capacity of the target tissue or cell, the specificity and extent of DNA damage, the capacity to repair the damage, the accuracy of DNA polymerases, and cell turnover rate. The mutagenic and carcinogenic effects of the nitroso compounds have been associated with the formation in the DNA of O^6-alkylguanine (4-8), which is one of 12 DNA modifications induced by these alkylating agents (9,10). This chemically stable product is removed from DNA by the transfer of the alkyl group from the O^6 position of guanine to a receptor protein (11). Other DNA adducts, like 3-alkyladenine and 7-alkylguanine, are removed by specific N-glycosylases (12).

A series of experiments has been carried out in our laboratories to determine the capacity of the liver of Syrian golden hamsters and rats to repair DNA damages after a single or multiple treatment with nitrosodimethylamine (DMN). The results are discussed in relation to the carcinogenic response.

RESULTS

Liver DNA Alkylation After a Single Dose of DMN to Hamsters or Rats

Nitrosodimethylamine is metabolized equally well by the livers of the Syrian golden hamster and of the rat, although Syrian golden hamsters are sensitive to the induction of liver tumors by single doses of DMN, while rats are not (13). A single dose of DMN produces a 30% incidence of liver tumors in hamsters (14). Table 1 shows the amounts (micromole per mole of guanine) of *N*-7-methylguanine and O^6-methylguanine found in hamster-liver DNA 5 and 24 h after administration of various doses of DMN (0.01 to 25 mg/kg bw). The amounts of *N*-7-methylguanine formed were directly proportional to the dose of DMN. In the case of O^6-methylguanine, proportionality with the dose of DMN was observed for 0.5 to 25 mg/kg bw, when a ratio of about 0.185 O^6-methylguanine:*N*-7-methylguanine was seen as an average. For 0.25 mg/kg bw and less, the ratios at 24 h were 0.027 (0.25 mg/kg bw), 0.018 (0.1 mg/kg bw), and 0.005 (0.01 mg/kg bw). Since there is no reason to believe that the initial ratio of alkylated bases produced in DNA would be different for different doses of DMN, these results indicate that removal of O^6-methylguanine from hamster-liver DNA takes place after exposure to low doses of DMN. However, when higher doses (0.5 mg/kg bw or more) are given, the system responsible for the removal is much less effective. In fact, little or no O^6-methylguanine was removed from hamster-liver DNA after alkylation produced by doses of 0.5 mg/kg of DMN or more (15,16).

Different results were seen in rat liver after administration of similar doses of DMN (17). Removal of O^6-methylguanine from DNA was much more efficient after exposure to low doses of DMN, but still occurred after exposure to higher doses. Figure 1 shows the ratios of O^6-methylguanine:*N*-7-methylguanine in rat- and hamster-liver DNA after administering DMN over a similar dose range. Two major differences were observed: (a) in rat liver, O^6-methylguanine was lost much more rapidly than was *N*-7-methylguanine, resulting in ratios of less than 0.1, although for doses up to and including 2.5 mg/kg, an order of magnitude greater than the doses needed to produce an equivalent ratio in hamster liver resulted; and (b) even for doses of 20 mg/kg in the rat, O^6-methylguanine was lost at least as rapidly as N^7-methylguanine, so that the ratio of O^6-methylguanine:*N*-7-methylguanine did not rise above 0.12.

The limited ability of hamster liver to remove this promutagenic base could be responsible for its much greater sensitivity to tumor induction by a single dose of DMN. Similar considerations also apply to Chinese hamster liver, which is susceptible to the induction of tumors after a single dose of

Table 1. Methylated Guanine Derivatives Present in Hamster Liver After Injection of Various Doses of DMN (16)

Dose of DMN (mg/kg)	Time[a] (h)	Methylated Guanine Content of DNA (μmol/mol of guanine): N-7-Methyl-guanine	O^6-Methyl-guanine	O^6-Methylguanine: N-7-Methylguanine Ratio
0.01	5	2	0.02	0.010
0.10	5	16	0.33	0.021
0.25	5	42	1.3	0.031
0.50	5	94	12	0.128
0.75	5	146	19	0.130
1.00	5	245	21	0.086
2.50	5	594	77	0.130
2.50	7	638	70	0.110
5.0	5	835	104	0.125
10.0	5	2130	258	0.121
20.0	5	3995	471	0.118
25.0	7	4210	546	0.130
0.01	24	1.8	0.01	0.005
0.10	24	10	0.18	0.018
0.25	24	26	0.7	0.027
0.50	24	58	10	0.172
0.75	24	83	19	0.229
1.0	24	141	19	0.135
2.5	24	366	60	0.164
5.0	24	632	114	0.180
10.0	24	1567	267	0.170
15.0	24	2315	493	0.213
20.0	24	2308	464	0.201
25.0	24	2902	620	0.214

[a]The hamsters were killed at the times shown after i.p. injection of labeled DMN, and the content of methylated guanine derivatives in the hepatic DNA was measured.

DMN (18). A significant incidence of liver tumors can be induced in rats when the single dose of DMN is given 24 h after partial hepatectomy, i.e., at the time of maximal DNA synthesis (19), or during continuous treatment with DMN.

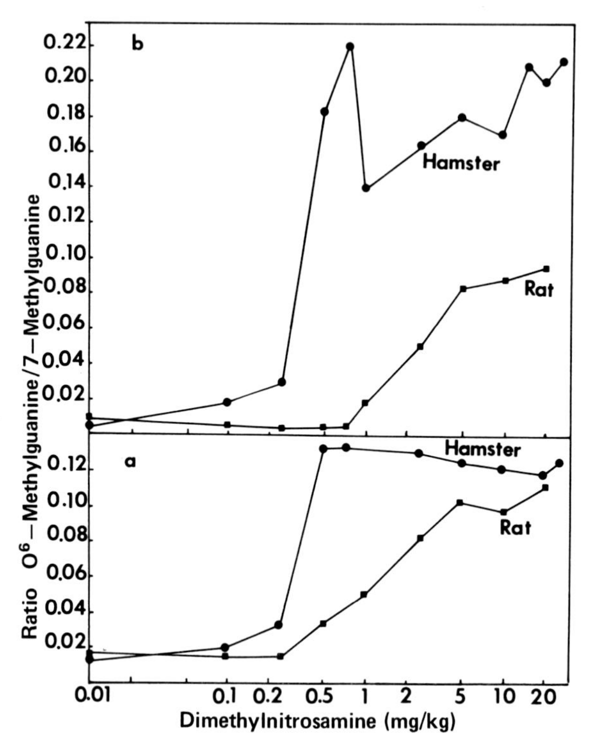

Figure 1. Ratio of O^6-methylguanine:N-7methylguanine in hamster (●) and rat (■) liver 4 or 5 h (a) and 24 h (b) after administration of DMN. Values for rat liver were calculated from data of Pegg and Hui (17) on alkylation 4 and 24 h after administration of DMN. Values for hamster liver were calculated from results in Table 1 on alkylation 5 and 24 h after DMN treatment (16).

Rat Liver DNA Alkylation After Multiple DMN Treatments

A greater rate of removal of O^6-methylguanine from liver DNA results from repeated administration of low doses of DMN to rats than from rats treated with a single dose (20). This effect appears to be specific for O^6-methylguanine, since it was not observed for other DNA adducts, such as *N*-7-methylguanine or 3-methyladenine. The effect is mediated by an induced enzymic process, as liver extracts from pretreated rats specifically remove O^6-methylguanine from DNA alkylated *in vitro*, unlike extracts from control rats (21). This increased removal of O^6-methylguanine occurred within 2 weeks of daily pretreatment with 2 mg/kg bw of DMN (see Table 2) and depended on the dose at which the animals were pretreated (21).

Under these experimental conditions, it was also found (22,23) that the increased removal can be detected within 10 min after administration of a challenging dose (2 mg/kg bw) of ^{14}C-DMN. After that time, the liver again has a "normal" capacity to remove O^6-methylguanine. These findings were confirmed when rats were given five daily doses (2 mg/kg) of labeled ^{14}C-DMN, and DNA alkylation was determined 5, 12, and 24 h after the last treatment. The O^6-methylguanine:*N*-7-methylguanine ratios at 5 and 12 h were half those observed in the liver DNA of rats treated with a single dose (2 mg/kg) of ^{14}C-DMN (see Figure 2). A lower ratio was also observed at 24 h (24).

Following the initial rapid removal of O^6-methylguanine, the subsequent rate of loss of this DNA adduct did not appear to be significantly different in pretreated and control rats, perhaps indicating the existence of two processes for the removal of O^6-methylguanine. Similar results have been obtained in another strain of rats by Swann and Mace (25).

These results are in marked contrast to the finding that inhibition of O^6-methylguanine removal is produced by large single doses of alkylating agents (18,26-28). In these experiments, relatively short pretreatment intervals were examined and recent reports show that after longer periods, repair of O^6-methylguanine is increased. Recently, partial hepatectomy has been shown to enhance O^6-methylguanine repair in the rat (29); these effects may be related to cell proliferation due to the hepatotoxicity of the pretreatment. However, the effect is also produced by very low doses of nitrosamines, which are not considered to be hepatotoxic (30).

Long-term carcinogenicity studies (31) for a wide range of DMN doses indicate that, with doses of DMN above a certain level, the risk of liver cancer in rats increases rapidly, resulting in a more

Table 2. Alkylated Purines in Liver DNA of BD IV Rats Six Hours After Administration of ^{14}C-DMN (21) (μmol/mol of parent base).

Length of Pretreatment (Week)	N-7-Methylguanine		3-Methyladenine		O^6-Methylguanine	
	Pretreated[a]	Control[b]	Pretreated[a]	Control[b]	Pretreated[a]	Control[b]
1	428	441	13	13	27	43
2	370		11		10	
3	450		14		10	
4	523		13		9.2	
6	502	504	16	15	9.2	47

[a]Alkylated purines were measured in liver DNA of BD IV rats pretreated for different periods with unlabeled DMN (2 mg/kg); measurements were also taken 6 h after administration of ^{14}C-DMN (2 mg/kg; 16.25 mCi/mmol).
[b]Controls received ^{14}C-DMN only.

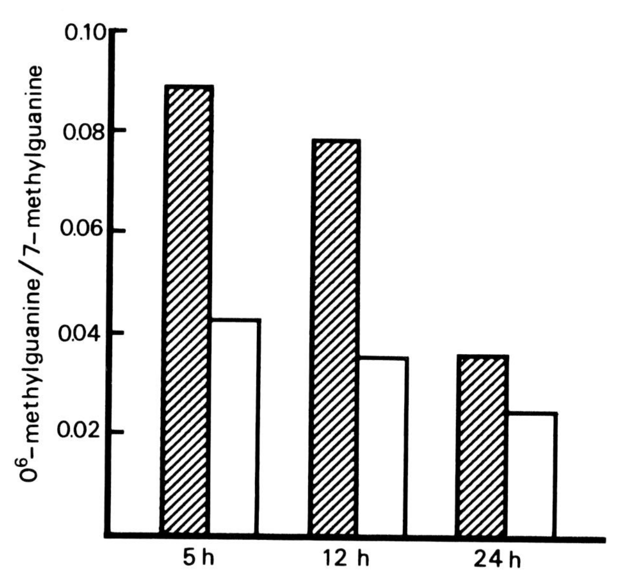

Figure 2. O^6-Methylguanine:N-7-methylguanine ratios in liver DNA of BD IV rats at various times after 5 daily doses of ^{14}C-DMN (2 mg/kg) (□), or after a single dose of ^{14}C-DMN (2 mg/kg) (▨).

than 1000-fold increase in tumor incidence with a 10-fold increase in daily dose rate. This type of response is consistent with the kinetics of repair of O^6-methylguanine in liver DNA during continuous treatment with various doses of DMN. Thus, these repair processes may be further activated by exposure to low levels of alkylating agents; however, high doses of such agents may overtax the capacity of the constitutive and even of the induced DNA repair process(es), substantially increasing the risk of cancer in animals which receive large doses. Further studies are required to substantiate such a conclusion.

Table 3 lists the various animal systems that have been examined for the effect of pretreatment with various carcinogens on the removal from liver DNA of O^6-methyl- or O^6-ethylguanine. The possible mechanism(s) underlying these findings and their similarity to the phenomenon of "adaptation" in *Escherichia coli* treated with N-methyl-N'-nitro-N-nitrosoguanidine (originally discovered by Samson and Cairns [32]), are discussed in a separate publication (see Reference 8).

DISCUSSION

The results obtained in hamster and rat liver indicate that some DNA alkylation adducts, like O^6-methylguanine, are critical in the initiation of the carcinogenic process induced by DMN, while others, like *N*-7-methylguanine and 3-methyladenine, are not. Some minor alkylation adducts (e.g., O^4-methylthymine), which are known to be promutagenic (33), have not been analyzed. However, the persistence of these promutagenic lesions in the DNA, which are attributed to the efficiency of DNA repair processes, and the rate of cell proliferation should be considered when determining the probability of initiation of carcinogenesis in a target organ.

Substantial evidence, from both *in vivo* and *in vitro* systems and with various types of carcinogenic agents, indicates the probability of an organ developing a tumor, a mutagenic effect, or neoplastic transformation of cells in culture, resulting from the complex interplay among formation and persistence of specific DNA adducts, the repair of such adducts, and DNA synthesis. Experimental studies have shown that a single dose of a carcinogen usually induces liver cancer only when it is administered at the time of active cell proliferation, e.g., after partial hepatectomy or during the perinatal period (19,34). Ying et al. (35) have demonstrated that acute liver necrosis and the compensatory liver-cell proliferation play a critical role in the induction of the early phases of liver carcinogenesis by nitrosamines. *In vitro* studies have shown that the frequency of mutation or transformation induced by chemical or physical agents decreases if the time between the introduction of the DNA lesions and the start of DNA synthesis is increased, thus permitting the excision repair processes to remove promutagenic bases (3,36,37).

In experimental situations where a carcinogenic effect in a target organ is the result of a single administration of a carcinogen, it is easier to distinguish the role played by these various determinants. However, chronic treatment results in a modulation of the various determinants and in more complicated situations. Also, during the process of neoplastic transformation of cultured cells or of carcinogenesis *in vivo* (37-41), additional

Table 3. Effect of Chronic Administration of Various Carcinogens[a] on the Removal of O-6-Alkylguanine from Rat Liver DNA (8)

Pretreatment	Challenge	Species: Rat	Species: Hamster	Effect[b]
DMN	DMN	BD IV		+
		Sprague-Dawley		+
		Wistar		+
1,2-DMH	DMN	Sprague-Dawley		+
		Wistar		+
DEN	DMN	Wistar		+
		Sprague-Dawley		+
AAF	DMN	Wistar		+
MNU	DMN	Wistar		-
MMS	DMN	Wistar		-
DMN	MNU	BD IV		-
MNU	MNU	Wistar		-
MMS	MNU	Wistar		-
DMN	DMN		Chinese	-
DMN	DMN		Syrian golden	-
DEN	DEN		Syrian golden	-
DEN	DEN	Wistar		+
DMPT	DMPT	BD IX		+

[a]DMN, nitrosodimethylamine; 1,2-DMH, 1,2-dimethylhydrazine; DEN, nitrosodiethylamine; AAF, N-acetylaminofluorene; MNU, nitrosomethylurea; MMS, methylmethanesulfonate; DMPT, 3,3-dimethyl-1-phenyltriazene.

[b](+) indicates that increased removal from DNA of O^6-alkylguanine, but not of 7-alkylguanine or 3-alkyladenine, was observed as compared with control rats.

events are required to bring about the clonal growth of initiated cells and their development into overt neoplasia.

REFERENCES

1. Setlow, R.B. 1978. Repair deficient human disorders and cancer. Nature 271:713-717.

2. Cleaver, J.E., and E.C. Friedberg. 1977. Xeroderma pigmentosum: Cellular and enzymatic defects in repair of radiation- and carcinogen-induced damage to DNA. Excerpta Medica International Congress Series No. 411, Human Genetics. Excerpta Medica: Amsterdam. pp. 347-354.

3. Maher, V.M., L.L. Yang, and J.J. McCormick. 1980. The role of DNA repair in preventing the cytotoxic and mutagenic effects of carcinogens in human cells. In: Carcinogenesis: Fundamental Mechanisms and Environmental Effects. B. Pullman, P.O.P. Ts'o, and H. Gelboin, eds. D. Reidel Pub. Co.: Dordrecht, Holland. pp. 479-490.

4. Lawley, P.D. 1974. Some chemical aspects of dose-response relationships in alkylation mutagenesis. Mutat. Res. 23:283-295.

5. Goth, R., and M.F. Rajewsky. 1974. Persistence of O^6-ethylguanine in rat brain DNA: Correlation with nervous system-specific carcinogenesis by ethyl-nitrosourea. Proc. Natl. Acad. Sci. USA 71:639-643.

6. Pegg, A.E. 1977. Formation and metabolism of alkylated nucleosides: Possible role in carcinogenesis by nitroso compounds and alkylating agents. Adv. Cancer Res. 25:195-269.

7. Margison, G.P., and P.J. O'Connor. 1979. Nucleic acid modification by N-nitroso compounds. In: Chemical Carcinogens and DNA. P.L. Grover, ed. CRC Press: Baltimore. pp. 111-159.

8. Montesano, R. 1981. Alkylation of DNA and tissue specificities in nitrosamine carcinognesis. J. Supramol. Struct. Cell. Biochem. 17:259-273.

9. Singer, B. 1979. N-Nitroso alkylating agents: Formation and persistence of alkyl derivatives in mammalian nucleic acids as contributing factors in carcinogenesis. J. Natl. Cancer Inst. 62:1329-1339.

10. Singer, B. (In press). Mutagenesis from a chemical perspective: Nucleic acid reactions, repair, translation and transcription. In: Molecular and Cellular Mechanisms of Mutagenesis. J.F. Lemontt and R.M. Generoso, eds. Plenum Press: New York.

11. Olsson, M., and T. Lindhal. 1980. Repair of alkylated DNA in E. coli: Methyl group transfer from O^6-methylguanine to a protein cysteine residue. J. Biol. Chem. 255:10569-10572.

12. Pegg, A.E. 1982. Repair of alkylated DNA by cell extracts from various organs and species. In: Organ and Species Specificity in Chemical Carcinogenesis. R. Langenbach, S. Nesnow, and J. Rice, eds. Plenum Press: New York. pp. 545-563.

13. IARC. 1978. Monographs on the Evaluation of the Carcinogenic Risk of Chemicals to Humans, Vol. 17: Some N-nitroso compounds. International Agency for Research on Cancer: Lyons, France.

14. Tomatis, L., and F. Cefis. 1967. The effects of multiple and single administration of dimethylnitrosamine to hamsters. Tumori 53:447-452.

15. Margison, G.P., J.M. Margison, and R. Montesano. 1976. Methylated purines in the deoxyribonucleic acid of various Syrian golden hamster tissues after administration of a hepatocarcinogenic dose of dimethylnitrosamine. Biochem. J. 157:627-634.

16. Stumpf, R., G.P. Margison, R. Montesano, and A.E. Pegg. 1979. Formation and loss of alkylated purines from DNA of hamster liver after administration of dimethylnitrosamine. Cancer Res. 39:50-54.

17. Pegg, A.E., and G. Hui. 1978. Formation and subsequent removal of O^6-methylguanine from deoxyribonucleic acid in rat liver and kidney after small doses of dimethylnitrosamine. Biochem. J. 173:739-748.

18. Margison, G.P., J.A. Swindell, C.H. Ockey, and A.W. Craig. 1980. The effects of a single dose of dimethylnitrosamine in the Chinese hamster and the persistence of DNA alkylation products in selected tissues. Carcinogenesis 1:91-95.

19. Craddock. V.M. 1978. Cell proliferation and induction of liver cancer. In: Primary Liver Tumors. H. Remmer, H.M. Bolt, P. Bannash, and H. Popper, eds. MTP Press Ltd. pp. 377-385.

20. Montesano, R., H. Bresil, and G.P. Margison. 1979. Increased excision of O^6-methylguanine from rat liver DNA after chronic administration of dimethylnitrosamine. Cancer Res. 39:1798-1802.

21. Montesano, R., H. Bresil, G. Planche-Martel, G.P. Margison, and A.E. Pegg. 1980. Effect of chronic treatment of rats with dimethylnitrosamine on the removal of O-^{6}methylguanine from DNA. Cancer Res. 40:452-458.

22. Montesano, R., H. Bresil, G. Planche-Martel, and G.P. Margison. 1980. Modulation of removal of O^6-methylguanine from liver DNA of rats treated chronically with dimethylnitrosamine. Proc. AACR/ASCO 21:2.

23. Montesano, R., and G.P. Margison. 1980. Modulation of repair of DNA damages induced by nitrosamines. In: Carcinogenesis: Fundamental Mechanisms and Environmental Effects. B. Pullman, P.O.P. Ts'o, and H. Gelboin, eds. D. Reidel Pub. Co.: Dordrecht, Holland. pp. 445-451.

24. Montesano, R. (Unpublished data).

25. Swann, P.F., and R. Macé. 1980. Changes in O^6-methylguanine disappearance from rat liver DNA during chronic dimethylnitrosamine administration. A possible similarity between the system removing O^6-methylguanine from DNA in rat liver and in Escherichia coli adapted to N-methyl-N'-nitro-N-nitrosoguanidine. Chem. Biol. Interactions 31:239-245.

26. Kleihues, P., and G.P. Margison. 1976. Exhaustion and recovery of repair excision of O^6-methylguanine from rat liver DNA. Nature 259:153-155.

27. Pegg, A.E. 1977. Alkylation of rat liver DNA by dimethylnitrosamine: Effect of dosage on O^6-methylguanine levels. J. Natl. Cancer Inst. 58:281-287.

28. Pegg, A.E. 1978. Effect of pretreatment with other dialkylnitrosamines on excision from hepatic DNA of O^6-methylguanine produced by dimethylnitrosamine. Chem. Biol. Interact. 22:109-116.

29. Pegg, A.E., W. Perry, and R.A. Bennett. 1981. Effect of partial hepatectomy on removal of O^6-methylguanine from alkylated DNA by rat liver extracts. Biochem. J. 197:195-201.

30. Margison, G.P. 1982. Chronic or acute administration of various dialkylnitrosamines enhances the removal of O^6-methylguanine from rat liver DNA *in vivo*. Chem. Biol. Interact. 38:189-201.

31. Peto, R. (Personal communication).

32. Samson, L., and J. Cairns. 1977. A new pathway for DNA repair in *E. coli*. Nature 267:281-283.

33. Singer, B., S. Spengler, and W.J. Bodell. 1981. Tissue-dependent enzyme-mediated repair of removal of *O*-ethyl pyrimidines and ethyl purines in carcinogen-treated rats. Carcinogenesis 2:1069-1073.

34. Columbano, A., S. Rajalakshmi, and D.S.R. Sarma. 1981. Requirement of cell proliferation for the initiation of liver carcinogenesis as assayed by three different procedures. Cancer Res. 41:2079-2083.

35. Ying, T.S., D.S.R. Sarma, and E. Farber. 1981. Role of acute hepatic necrosis in the induction of early steps in liver carcinogenesis by diethylnitrosamine. Cancer Res. 41:2096-2102.

36. Borek, C., and L. Sachs. 1968. The number of cell generations required to fix the transformed state in X-ray-induced transformation. Proc. Natl. Acad. Sci. USA 59:83-85.

37. Kakunaga, T., K.Y. Lo, J. Leavitt, and M. Ikenaga. 1981. Relationship between transformation and mutation in mammalian cells. In: Carcinogenesis: Fundamental Mechanisms and Environmental Effects. B. Pullman, P.O.P. Ts'o, and H. Gelboin, eds. D. Reidel Pub. Co.: Dordrecht, Holland. pp. 527-439.

38. Barrett, J.C., and P.O.P. Ts'o. 1978. Relationship between somatic mutation and neoplastic transformation. Proc. Natl. Acad. Sci. USA 75:3297-3301.

39. Barrett, J.C., and P.O.P. Ts'o. 1978. Evidence for the progressive nature of neoplastic transformation *in vitro*. Proc. Natl. Acad. Sci. USA 75:3761-3765.

40. Farber, E. 1980. The sequential analysis of liver cancer induction. Biochim. Biophys. Acta 605:149-166.

41. Foulds, L. 1965. Multiple etiologic factors in neoplastic development. Cancer Res. 25:1339-1347.

REPAIR OF ALKYLATED DNA BY CELL EXTRACTS FROM VARIOUS ORGANS AND SPECIES

Anthony E. Pegg

Department of Physiology and Specialized Cancer Research Center, Pennsylvania State University, School of Medicine, Hershey, Pennsylvania 17033

INTRODUCTION

Simple alkylating agents form an interesting class of chemical carcinogens whose interaction with DNA is relatively well understood (1-7). These carcinogens include agents such as alkyl alkanesulfonates, alkylnitrosamides, alkylnitrosoguanidines, and monoalkyltriazines that are direct acting and the chemically-stable nitrosamines, dialkylhydrazines, and dialkyltriazines that require enzymatic activation to generate the alkylating species. The major adducts formed by these agents on reaction with DNA in target and nontarget tissues have been quantitated and their persistence with time measured (1,2,5,6). These studies have suggested that certain adducts are more likely to be responsible for the initiation of tumors than others; particular emphasis has been placed on the potential role of O^6-alkylguanine. O^6-Alkylguanine is known to miscode in nucleic acid synthesis and to lead to mutations. Furthermore, its rate of removal from DNA differs from tissue to tissue, and the persistence correlates with sensitivity to tumor initiation (1,2,5). These results underline the significant role that DNA repair may play in preventing a carcinogenesis by alkylating agents. Other alkylated bases may also have the potential to initiate tumors, but the rapid removal would minimize their effect.

Knowledge of the repair processes to which alkylated DNA is subject has been obtained in three ways: by following the levels of radioactive alkylated bases in DNA as a function of time after giving labeled carcinogens; by studying the physical structure of DNA in cells after treatment with carcinogens; and by measuring the activities of DNA repair enzymes in cell extracts *in vitro*. The persistence of alkylation products in vivo is discussed extensively in several recent reviews (1-6) and in other chapters of this volume. Although much work has been applied to measurements of changes in the physical structure of DNA after exposure to carcinogens (e.g., the appearance and disappearance of single strand breaks), these studies cannot distinguish between the responses to widely varying alkylation products. Only recently by using in vitro assays could specific removal of individual alkylated bases from DNA be demonstrated. These studies are summarized in this paper.

MATERIALS AND METHODS

Four different enzymes catalyzing reactions involved in the repair of alkylated DNA have been characterized in extracts from mammalian cells. They are 3-methyladenine DNA glycosylase, 7-methylguanine DNA glycosylase, ring-opened-7-methylguanine DNA glycosylase (rom^{7}G) and O^6-methylguanine DNA transmethylase. Full details of the experimental methodology are given in several recent publications (7-11).

Assay of 3-Methyladenine DNA Glycosylase

For the assay of 3-methyladenine DNA glycosylase, extracts were prepared by homogenization in two volumes of ice-cold 1 mM 2-mercaptoethanol, 1 mM EDTA, 0.05 M Tris-hydrochloric acid (pH 8.0) using a Polytron homogenizer (Brinkman Instruments, NY). The extract was centrifuged at 3,000 g for 10 min and the supernatant saved. The pellet was rehomogenized in 2 volumes of the extraction buffer, and the mixture combined with the original supernatant and centrifuged at 105,000 g for 60 min. The supernatant was removed and used for the assays. The activity was assayed by following the release of [^{3}H]-3-methyladenine from [^{3}H-methylated] DNA. The substrate for this reaction was prepared by reacting 32 mg of calf thymus DNA with 5 mCi of [^{3}H-methyl]dimethylsulfate (2.4 Ci/mmol, New England Nuclear [NEN], Boston, MA) in 40 ml of 0.2 M sodium cacodylate (pH 7.2) for 1.5 h at 37°C. The DNA was precipitated by the addition of 2 volumes of cold ethanol and washed with 80% ethanol. Then the DNA was dissolved in 6 ml of 10 mM NaCl and dialyzed overnight against 100 volumes of this solution. Finally, aliquots of the DNA solution were used for the enzyme assays. The assays were carried out by incubating a total volume of 0.35 ml containing: 0.3 ml of the tissue extract prepared as described above and diluted with the extraction buffer so that up to 5 mg of protein was added, 35 μmol of KCl, 25 μmol of HEPES-KOH (pH 7.8), 0.35 μmol EDTA, 0.35 μmol dithiothreitol, and 15 μg of [^{3}H-methyl]methylated DNA (55 nCi containing about 4.6 pmol of 3-methyladenine). After incubation at

37°C for 1 h, the reaction was halted by the addition of 0.035 ml of 2 M NaCl and 1.05 ml ethanol at 2°C. The tubes were left in ice for 10 min, and the precipitate removed by centrifugation at maximum speed in an Eppendorf 3400 microcentrifuge at 4°C. Aliquots of the supernatant were removed, evaported to dryness, dissolved in 0.5 ml of 0.1N HCl, and analyzed by high pressure liquid chromatography (HPLC) (7,8) after addition of unlabeled markers of 7-methylguanine and 3-methyladenine. Results were expressed as fmol of 3-methyladenine released per hour per mg protein. The 3-methyladenine released into the supernatant fraction by spontaneous hydrolysis was determined in parallel incubations containing bovine serum albumin instead of the tissue protein and was subtracted from the 3-methyladenine released in the enzyme assays.

Assay of 7-Methylguanine DNA Glycosylase

In most experiments, this activity was measured as described above for 3-methyladenine DNA glycosylase, since the labeled DNA substrate contained about 23 pmol of 7-methylguanine. In some experiments, the [^{3}H-methylated] DNA was incubated with 3-methyladenine DNA glycosylase from *Escherichia coli* to remove all 3-methyladenine (7). The assays were then carried out by incubation of 1 μg of the treated [^{3}H-methyl]methylated DNA (containing about 1.7 pmol of 7-methylguanine), 35 μmol of KCl, 25 μmol of HEPES-KOH (pH 7.8), 0.35 μmol EDTA, 0.35 μmol dithiothreitol, and 0.3 ml of the diluted tissue extract containing up to 4 mg of protein. After incubation at 37°C for 1 h, the reaction was stopped and the radioactivity released into the alcohol supernatant fraction was determined as for the assay of 3-methyladenine DNA glycosylase. High pressure liquid chromatography analysis of this radioactivity revealed that more than 95% corresponded to 7-methylguanine. The results were corrected by subtraction of the 7-methylguanine released into the supernatant by spontaneous hydrolysis measured by parallel incubations in the presence of bovine serum albumin. In some cases, this amount was 30 to 45% of that observed in the enzymatic reaction.

Assay of Ring-Opened-7-Methylguanine DNA Glycosylase

The substrate was prepared by taking 5 mg (about 1 ml) of the [^{3}H-methyl]methylated DNA prepared as described above and dialyzing against 100 ml of 0.05 M Na_2HPO_4 adjusted to pH 11.4 with NaOH for 36 h at 4°C. The solution was then incubated at room temperature for 24 h and dialyzed into 0.02 M Tris-HCL, 1 mM EDTA pH 7.5 and stored at -20°C. This treatment (12) converted about 50% of the 7-methylguanine present into the imidazole-ring-opened forms (8).

Activity was measured using extracts and the assay conditions described above for 3-methyladenine glycosylase. The products were separated either by HPLC or by chromatography on Sephadex G10 columns as described by Margison and Pegg (8). The ring-opened form of rom^{7}G runs as a double peak in both systems, but it is easily separated from 7-methylguanine and from 3-methyladenine when chromatographed on Sephadex G10 after application of the sample at pH 5 (8).

Assay of O^6-Methylguanine Removal

[^{3}H-Methyl]methylated DNA was prepared by reacting 84 mg of calf thymus DNA (Sigma Chemical Co., St. Louis, MO) with 1 mCi of N-nitroso-N-[^{3}H]methylurea (1.01 Ci/mmol, NEN) in 16 ml of 0.08 M Na_2HPO_4 (pH 8) for 30 min at 37°C. The DNA was then precipitated by the addition of two volumes of ethoxyethanol, washed four times with ethanol and once with ether, dissolved in assay buffer, and dialyzed overnight before use. The assays contained 0.8 mg of [^{3}H-methyl]methylated DNA (containing 2.6 pmol of O^6-methylguanine), 200 µmol of Tris-HCl (final pH 8.3), 4 µmol of dithiothreitol, 1 µmol of EDTA, and 0.5 to 12 mg of protein in a total volume of 3 ml. After incubation at 37°C for 30 min (in some experiments linearity of reaction for up to 90 min was tested), the reaction was stopped by the addition of 1.0 ml of cold 1N perchloric acid. The precipitate was collected by centrifugation (all centrifugations were at 10,000 g for 10 min) at 2°C, and the pellet was washed twice at 2°C with cold 0.25 N perchloric acid. The precipitated DNA was then hydrolyzed by suspension in 0.75 ml of 0.1 N HCl and heated at 70°C for 30 min. The mixture was centrifuged and the supernatant removed. The pellet was suspended again in 0.75 ml of 0.1 N HCl and heated at 70°C for 30 min. After centrifugation the supernatant was combined with the earlier supernatant, and an aliquot was subjected to HPLC for separation of the methylated bases. The 0.75 ml was applied with appropriate marker bases to a column (0.46 cm x 25 cm) packed with Partisil 10SCX cation exchange medium (Whatman, Inc., Clifton, NJ). The column was eluted at 50°C with 0.02 M ammonium formate (pH 4) at a flow rate of 2 ml/min (7), and fractions corresponding to adenine, guanine, 7-methylguanine, and O^6-methylguanine were collected. The recovery of adenine and guanine was determined by measuring absorbance and the amounts of the methylated purines, determined by adding two volumes of Formula 947 liquid scintillation cocktail (NEN) and counting in a Beckman liquid scintillation spectrometer at an efficiency of 28%. The results of incubation with the protein extracts were compared to the content of methylated bases in DNA from tubes in which the reaction was stopped at zero time or incubated without protein. Only O^6-methylguanine was lost from DNA under these incubation conditions. Less than 5% of the 7-methylguanine or purine bases was removed from the acid-precipitable DNA during a 1-h incubation, showing that the reaction observed was specific for O^6-methylguanine.

Tissue extracts for the assay of O^6-methylguanine removal activity were prepared by homogenization in three volumes of ice-cold buffer solution containing 1 mM dithiothreitol, 50 mM Tris-HCl (pH 7.5), and 0.2 mM EDTA using a Polytron homogenizer. The homogenate was centrifuged at 12,000 g for 5 min; the supernatant was removed and saved. A second volume of the buffer solution equal to the original weight of the tissue was added to the precipitate; after homogenization the homogenate was sonicated for three periods of 30 sec each as described (13). Next the sonicated extract was combined with the original supernatant fraction and centrifuged at 22,000 g for 30 min. The supernatant was removed, and ammonium sulfate added to 80% saturation. The resulting precipitate was collected by centrifugation at 22,000 g for 10 min, dissolved in 50 mM Tris-HCl (pH 7.5), 1 mM dithiothreitol, and 0.1 mM EDTA, and dialyzed overnight against 100 volumes of this solution. The dialyzed sample was centrifuged at 22,000 g for 15 min, and the supernatant was used for the assays. Approximately 55% of the total activity was present in the original supernatant solution; the remaining 45% was released from the crude nuclear pellet by the sonication treatment. The two fractions were combined to assess the total activity.

Other Methods

Protein was determined using reagents from Bio-Rad Laboratories and bovine serum albumin as standard (14). Methylated purine bases, nitrosodimethylamine, and other reagents were obtained or synthesized as described previously (7,13,15).

RESULTS AND DISCUSSION

Importance of Liver in Activation of Alkylating Agents

A number of tissues are able to convert dialkylhydrazines, dialkylnitrosamines, alkylacylnitrosamines, and dialkyltriazines to chemically-reactive alkylating agents, but this activity is by far the greatest in the liver (15,16). Yet most of these agents produce tumors more readily at extrahepatic sites, particularly when given as large single doses, and only produce liver tumors on chronic administration at lower levels in the diet. One possible explanation for this effect is that DNA repair processes are much more efficient in the liver, particularly in the hepatocytes (1,2,5). However, this reason still does not explain the change in tumor site with dose. One possible explanation is provided by the results in Table 1 in which the alkylation of liver and kidney DNA was measured as a function of dose of nitrosodimethylamine given either orally or via intravenous injection. Irrespective of the amount of the carcinogen given, the amount of interaction with the liver DNA was invariably about nine times that with the kidney, which fits well with work showing that the capacity to metabolize nitrosodimethylamine in the liver is about 6 to 10 times greater than in the kidney (17-19). However, when the nitrosodimethylamine was given by oral administration, this ratio was seen only when doses of more than 1 mg/kg were given. At lower doses, the ratio was much greater owing to a greater proportion of the dose being metabolized in the liver (20). Similar results were obtained by Diaz Gomez et al. (21). These findings can be explained best by the rapid metabolic clearance of nitrosodimethylamine from the portal blood by the liver, so that the compound absorbed from the gastrointestinal tract is metabolized in the liver and does not become available for metabolism by extrahepatic tissues such as the kidney or the lung. Consequently, exposure via chronic treatment in the diet may lead to significant interaction only with the liver, which would be the only organ in which tumors could be produced. Therefore, the ability of liver cells to carry out DNA repair reactions reducing the chances of tumor initiation is of particular importance, and the physiological factors influencing these reactions are of particular interest.

Table 1. Ratio of Production of 7-Methylguanine in Liver and Kidney DNA after Administration of Nitrosodimethylamine by Oral and Intravenous Injection

Dose of Nitrosodimethylamine (μg/kg body wt.)	Ratio of 7-Methylguanine in Liver DNA as Compared to Kidney DNA	
	Following Oral Administration	Following i.v. Administration
5	125	11
10	83	9
50	57	8
100	36	9
1,000	18	9
5,000	10	10
10,000	9	9

Removal of 3-Methyladenine from DNA

3-Methyladenine is removed from DNA in bacteria (22,23) and in human cells (24) by the action of a glycosylase, which liberates the free base and leaves behind an apurinic site. A similar enzyme is present in rodent liver (8,25) and in extracts from all other rodent tissues that we have examined. As shown in Table 2, there was an excellent correlation between the amount of 3-methyladenine lost from DNA and that found as the free base in the ethanol supernatant, indicating that depurination appeared to be the only signficant pathway for loss of this product. 3-Methyladenine is unstable in DNA even at neutral pH and is lost with a half-life of about 30 h (1-3), but the rate of loss is increased five- to sevenfold by the liver enzyme (see Table 1).

Table 2. Removal of 3-Methyladenine from Methylated DNA on Incubation with Liver Extracts

Extract Added	Incubation Time (h)	3-Methyladenine (pmol) Present in	
		DNA	Free Base
None	0	4.99	0
10 mg Rat liver protein	2	3.46	1.52
10 mg Hamster liver protein	2	3.01	1.94
10 mg Bovine serum albumin	2	4.62	0.29

Removal of 7-Methylguanine from DNA

7-Methylguanine is a major product of the reaction of alkylating agents with DNA and is lost from DNA *in vivo* more slowly than 3-methyladenine (1-4). Since it is also unstable in DNA, being lost by spontaneous hydrolysis, some doubt exists as to whether it was enzymatically removed. However, recently three separate groups have reported finding a glycosylase that acts on this base in bacteria (26), cultured human cells (27), and in rodent liver (8,25). As shown in Table 3, the presence of rat or hamster liver extracts significantly increased the production of 7-methylguanine on incubation of alkylated DNA above that found when DNA was alkylated alone. This activity was considerably more active in the hamster extracts, which is consistent with the more rapid loss of 7-methylguanine from the hamster DNA _in vivo_ (1,2). In fact, the rat may be unusual in its relatively low capacity to remove 7-methylguanine from DNA, since human, mouse, and hamster cells all seem to be able to reduce the content of 7-methylguanine in DNA more rapidly than rat cells (27-29).

Table 3. Removal of 7-Methylguanine from Methylated DNA on Incubation with Liver Extracts

Extract Added	Incubation Time (h)	7-Methylguanine (pmol) Present in	
		DNA	Free Base
None	0	19.8	0
20 mg Rat liver protein	2	18.1	1.38
20 mg Hamster liver protein	2	17.2	2.59
20 mg Bovine serum albumin	2	19.2	0.45

When polynucleotides containing 7-methylguanine are exposed to alkaline pH, the imidazole ring of the 7-methylguanine is cleaved (30). Such DNA is a substrate for the action of a glycosylase present in _E. coli_ (12) and in rodent liver (8). This enzyme is considerably more active than that removing 7-methylguanine itself (Table 4), but its function _in vivo_ is at present quite unclear. The rate of ring opening of 7-methylguanine at physiological pH would be expected to be extremely slow, and rom^{7}G has never been reported to have been found in the DNA of animals treated with alkylating agents. However, it may be formed in small amounts and very rapidly removed by the rom^{7}G DNA glycosylase. This possibility could be an important protective mechanism, because rom^{7}G is likely to miscode. Alternately, the enzyme may have another substrate and be able to remove a more probable adduct from DNA, since it seems rather unlikely that an enzyme would be present to remove specifically a base such as rom^{7}G, which would be unlikely to occur under normal circumstances.

Table 4. Removal of 7-Methylguanine and Ring-Opened 7-Methylguanine from Methylated DNA

Extract Added	7-Methylguanine Released (pmol/2 h)	rom^{7}G Released (pmol/2 h)
10 mg Rat liver protein	0.64	3.62
10 mg Hamster liver protein	0.98	3.54
10 mg Bovine serum albumin	0.25	0.01

Removal of O^6-Methylguanine from DNA

An enzyme catalyzing the loss of O^6-methylguanine has been obtained from rodent and human liver and from some other tissues (7,9-10,13,20). The activity of this enzyme was much greater in the rat liver (100%) than in kidney (37%) and very much more than in lung (5%), colon (8%), small intestine (9%), and brain (3%), which corresponds with the rates of removal *in vivo* (1,2,9). The activity of the enzyme was lost from rat kidney when rats were pretreated with large doses (25 mg/kg) of nitrosodimethylamine (11), which also correlates with the inhibition of this activity *in vivo* after such doses of the carcinogen (1,2). The enzyme was able to remove O^6-ethylguanine from ethylated DNA at rates comparable to the loss of O^6-methylguanine (10).

This enzyme is not a glycosylase (9,10) and does not lead to the appearance of free O^6-alkylguanine in the supernatant after reaction with alkylated DNA. With crude extracts from rat liver and methylated DNA as a substrate, the radioactivity released from the DNA appeared as methanol, suggesting that the enzyme may be a transmethylase or a demethylase (9). With more purified extracts or with ethylated DNA as a substrate, the radioactivity released from DNA was found to be bound to protein (10,20) (see Table 5). In this respect, the rat liver enzyme appears to resemble closely the enzyme recently isolated by Lindahl and colleagues from *E. coli* (31). In an earlier paper, this group claimed that the *E. coli* enzyme resulted in the degradation of O^6-methylguanine in

DNA in a way that left the methyl group attached to the DNA from which it could be released by DNase (32). This claim is not consistent with our results with rat liver extracts, although Reynard and Verley (33) claimed that a chromatin factor from liver did lead to a similar reaction. Since the more recent work on _E. coli_ (31) contradicts the previous findings (32), it appears that the bacterial enzyme and the rat liver enzyme studied in my laboratory carry out a similar reaction, namely, the transfer of the methyl group to an acceptor protein. Whether the acceptor site in rat liver is a cysteine residue, as shown for the _E. coli_ enzyme (31), is not yet clear. The relationship to the activity described by Reynard and Verley (33) is also unclear. (An early abstract from this group [34] claimed that a glycosylase for O^6-ethylguanine removal had been isolated from rat liver, but this claim has not been confirmed and is not consistent with their later paper [33].)

Table 5. Loss of O^6-Methylguanine from Methylated DNA on Incubation with Rat Liver Enzyme for 30 minutes

Extract Added	O^6-Methylguanine Remaining in DNA (pmol)	O^6-Methylguanine in Supernatant (pmol)	$[C^3H_3]$Bound to Protein (pmol)
None	2.5	> 0.1	> 0.1
0.5 mg Rat liver protein	1.1	> 0.1	1.5
0.25 mg Rat liver protein	1.7	> 0.1	0.7

One of the most interesting properties of the hepatic system removing O^6-methylguanine from DNA is that it appears to be inducible in response to chronic treatment with nitrosodimethylamine (20,35). Such a response has been seen both _in vivo_ and _in vitro_ (see Table 6). As Table 6 shows, treatment with nitrosodimethylamine (2 mg/kg/day) for 44 days increased the activity of the O^6-methylguanine removal system about threefold, but had no effect on the activity of 3-methyladenine DNA glycosylase or 7-methylguanine DNA glycosylase. This treatment gives a maximal response of the O^6-methylguanine system; further administration did not continue to increase the activity (35). A considerably larger increase is produced by partial hepatectomy (7) (see Table 6). The activity of O^6-methylguanine removal, but not the glycosylases, is increased sixfold 72 h after two-thirds of the liver is removed. The increase, which is not seen in sham-operated rats, is about threefold after 24 h, maximal at sixfold at 48 to 72 h, and then declines. It corresponds quite well to the increased period of DNA synthesis brought about by partial hepatectomy. According to one published report, O^6-methylguanine removal may be enhanced *in vivo* by partial hepatectomy, at times corresponding to the increase seen here (36). The recent report describing treatment of rats with acetylaminofluorene enhancing the removal of O^6-methylguanine (37) is probably explained by the increased cellular proliferation produced by the extensive treatment with the aromatic amine. However, whether the induction by nitrosodimethylamine can be explained in this way is not yet clear. Although such chronic treatment with nitrosodimethylamine would certainly produce sufficient cell damage to induce replication, the degree to which this effect would be realized within 2 to 4 weeks is much less than after partial hepatectomy, whereas the rise in O^6-methylguanine removal is half of that produced by the surgery. Also, the increase due to nitrosodimethylamine is complete within a few weeks, whereas the degree of cell proliferation might be expected to increase more progressively. Nevertheless, it may be premature to claim that the increased O^6-methylguanine removal activity caused by 3,3-dimethyl-1-phenyltriazine (38), nitrosodimethylamine (20,35), nitrosodiethylamine (39), and 1,2-dimethylhydrazine (A.E. Pegg, unpublished observations) is a specific induction in response to the presence of alkylated bases in the tissue considered. Further study is needed to test this possibility. Although obvious parallels exist between these results and the so-called "adaptive response" in *E. coli* (40,41), the change in O^6-methylguanine removal activity in this bacterium resulting from exposure to methylating agents amounts to more than a 100-fold increase within a few minutes; however, the change with liver requires several weeks and is at most threefold.

CONCLUSIONS

The results described in this paper show clearly the presence of at least four distinct enzymes handling methylated purines in alkylated DNA. Each enzyme is separate, specific for its own product, and regulated differently, as shown by the specific response of the O^6-methylguanine removal system to partial hepatectomy. Other methylated purines, specifically 3-methylguanine, 1-methyladenine, and 7-methyladenine, are known to be produced by alkylating agents acting on DNA and it is probable that enzymes also exist in mammalian cells for these products (although 7-methyladenine is so readily lost by spontaneous

Table 6. Effect of Chronic Treatment with Nitrosodimethylamine of Partial Hepatectomy on Ability of Liver Extracts to Catalyze Removal of Alkylated Bases from DNA

Treatment of Rats	% Control Activity for Removal of		
	O^6-Methylguanine	3-Methyladenine	7-Methylguanine
Control	100 ± 10	100 ± 9	100 ± 16
Treated nitrosodimethylamine (2 mg/kg/day for 44 days)	294 ± 30	90 ± 19	89 ± 16
72 h after partial hepactectomy	603 ± 92	75 ± 15	98 ± 6

hydrolysis an enzyme may not be necessary). It is also quite possible that other enzymatic pathways for the loss of the methylated bases discussed in this paper are also present. However, the parallel between the persistence of the alkylation product *in vivo* and the activity of the enzymes *in vitro* when different species are compared (for example, in the loss of 7-methylguanine) or when different organs are compared (for example, the loss of O^6-methylguanine in the brain and liver) argues strongly for the physiological significance of the enzymes described here. The availability of isolated enzyme systems in which these enzymes can be assayed is a great advantage in studying the regulation of such DNA repair and its cellular distribution. It appears very likely that in addition to varying from one organ to another the removal of O^6-methylguanine may differ from one cell to another. Indeed, recent results suggest that this is the case in the liver where after administration of 1,2-dimethylhydrazine, O^6-methylguanine is lost more rapidly from hepatocytes than from non-hepatocytes (42). Studies of the isolated enzymes present in these cells would be of considerable interest and is readily possible with the assays described here.

The finding that the removal of O^6-methylguanine is enhanced in the liver following chronic treatment with nitrosodimethylamine and related agents has obvious potential importance whether or not the effect is caused by cell proliferation in response to damage by the carcinogen. It should be noted that the finding that this activity increases during liver regeneration is not inconsistent with its having a protective action against tumor initiation, even though it is known that partial hepatectomy increases the carcinogenic potential of nitrosodimethylamine (43). The degree of increase in cell replication brought about by partial hepatectomy is substantially greater than the degree of enhancement of O^6-methylguanine removal so the probability that cell replication will take place on a template containing O^6-methylguanine is still increased. These results raise the possibility that it may be possible to find an agent that will bring about a specific increase in O^6-methylguanine removal activity without itself being carcinogenic or producing a great deal of cell replication. Such a compound could be used to test the hypothesis that the persistence of O^6-methylguanine in DNA is related to the initiation of tumors by alkylating agents.

ACKNOWLEDGMENTS

This research was supported by Grant CA 18137 from the National Cancer Institute. I also wish to thank Mrs. Bonnie Merlino for help in the preparation of this manuscript.

REFERENCES

1. Pegg, A.E. 1977. Formation and metabolism of alkylated purines: Possible role in carcinogenesis by N-nitroso compounds and alkylating agents. Adv. Cancer Res. 25:195-269.

2. Margison, G.P., and P.J. O'Connor. 1979. Nucleic acid modification by N-nitroso compounds. In: Chemical Carcinogens and DNA. P.L. Grover, ed. CRC Press: FL. pp. 111-159.

3. Singer, B. 1979. N-Nitroso alkylating agents: Formation and persistence of alkyl derivatives in mammalian nucleic acids as contributing factors in carcinogenesis. J. Natl. Cancer Inst. 62:1329-1339.

4. Lawley, P.D. 1976. Carcinogenesis by alkylating agents. In: Chemical Carcinogens. C.E. Searle, ed. ACS Monograph Series no. 173. American Chemical Society: Washington, DC. pp. 83-244.

5. Rajewsky, M.F., R. Goth, O.D. Laerum, H. Biessmann, and D.F. Hulser. 1976. Molecular and cellular mechanisms in nervous system-specific carcinogenesis by N-ethyl-N-nitrosourea. In: Fundamentals in Cancer Prevention. Proc. 6th Int. Res. Symp. of the Princess Takamatsu Cancer Research Fund, Tokyo. P.N. Magee, S. Takayama, T. Sugimura, and T. Matsushima, eds. University Park Press: Baltimore. pp. 313-334.

6. Lawley, P.D. 1980. DNA as a target of alkylating carcinogens. Brit. Med. Bull. 36:19-24.

7. Pegg, A.E., W. Perry, and R.A. Bennett. 1981. Effect of partial hepatectomy on removal of O^6-methylguanine from alkylated DNA by rat liver extracts. Biochem. J. 197:195-201.

8. Margison, G.P., and A.E. Pegg. 1981. Enzymatic release of 7-methylguanine from methylated DNA by rodent liver extracts. Proc. Natl. Acad. Sci. 78:861-865.

9. Pegg, A.E. 1978. Enzymatic removal of O^6-methylguanine from DNA by mammalian cell extracts. Biochem. Biophys. Res. Comm. 84:166-173.

10. Pegg, A.E., and B. Balog. 1979. Formation and subsequent excision of O^6-ethylguanine from DNA of rat liver following administration of diethylnitrosamine. Cancer Res. 39:5003-5009.

11. Pegg, A.E. 1978. Dimethylnitrosamine inhibits enzymatic removal of O^6-methylguanine from DNA. Nature 274:182-184.

12. Chetsanga, C.J., and T. Lindahl. 1979. Release of 7-methylguanine residues whose imidazole rings have been opened from damaged DNA by a DNA glycosylase from _Escherichia coli_. Nucl. Acid Res. 6:3673-3684.

13. Pegg, A.E., and G. Hui. 1978. Formation and subsequent removal of O^6-methylguanine from DNA in rat liver and kidney after small doses of dimethylnitrosamine. Biochem. J. 173:739-748.

14. Bradford, M.M. 1976. A rapid and sensitive method for quantitation of microgram quantities of protein utilizing the principle of protein-dye binding. Anal. Biochem. 72:248-254.

15. Druckrey, H., R. Preussman, S. Ivankovic, and D. Schmähl. 1967. Organotrope carcinogene Wirkungen bei 65 verschiedenen N. Nitroso-Verbindungen an BD-Ratten. Z. Krebsforsch. 69:103-201.

16. Magee, P.N., R. Montesano, and R. Preussman. 1976. N-Nitroso compounds and related carcinogens. In: Chemical Carcinogens. C.E. Searle, ed. ACS Monograph Series no. 173. American Chemical Society: Washington, DC. pp. 491-625.

17. Swann, P.F., and A.E.M. McLean. 1971. Cellular injury and carcinogenesis. The effect of a protein-free, high carbohydrate diet on the metabolism of dimethylnitrosamine in the rat. Biochem. J. 124:283-228.

18. Montesano, R., and P.N. Magee. 1974. Comparative metabolism _in vitro_ of nitrosamines in various animal species including man. In: Chemical Carcinogenesis Essays. R. Montesano and L. Tomatis, eds. IARC Scientific publication no. 10. International Agency for Cancer Research: Lyons, France. pp. 39-56.

19. Pegg, A.E. 1980. Metabolism of N-nitrosodimethylamine. In: Molecular and Cellular Aspects of Carcinogen Screening Tests. R. Montesano, H. Bartsch, and L. Tomatis, eds. IARC Scientific publication no. 27. International Agency for Cancer Research: Lyons, France. pp. 3-22.

20. Pegg, A.E. 1980. Formation and subsequent repair of alkylation lesions in tissues of rodents treated with nitrosamines. Arch. Toxicol., Suppl. 3:55-58.

21. Diaz Gomez, M.I., P.F. Swann, and P.N. Magee. 1977. The absorption and metabolism in rats of small oral doses of dimethylnitrosamine. Biochem. J. 164:417-500.

22. Lindahl, T. 1976. New class of enzymes acting on damaged DNA. Nature 259:64-66.

23. Riazuddin, S., and T. Lindahl. 1978. Properties of 3-methyladenine DNA glycosylase from _Escherichia coli_. Biochemistry 17:2110-2118.

24. Brent, T.P. 1979. Partial purification and characterization of human 3-methyladenine DNA glycosylase. Biochemistry 18:911-916.

25. Cathcart, R., and D.A. Goldthwait. 1981. Enzymatic excision of 3-methyladenine and 7-methylguanine by a rat liver nuclear fraction. Biochemistry 20:273-280.

26. Laval, J., J. Pierre, and F. Laval. 1981. Release of free 7-methylguanine residues by cell extracts of _Micrococcus luteus_ and _Escherichia coli_ from alkylated DNA. Proc. Natl. Acad. Sci. 78:852-855.

27. Singer, B., and T.P. Brent. 1981. Human lymphoblasts contain DNA glycosylase activity excising N-3 and N-7 methyl and ethyl purines, but not O^6-alkylguanine or 1-alkyladenine. Proc. Natl. Acad. Sci. 78:856-860.

28. Nemoto, N., and S. Takayama. 1974. Rapid loss of 7-methylguanine from liver nucleic acids in mice during the initial stage of liver carcinogenesis induced by DMN. Biochem. Biophys. Res. Comm. 58:242-249.

29. Stumpf, R., G.P. Margison, R. Montesano, and A.E. Pegg. 1979. Formation and loss of alkylated purines from DNA of hamster liver after administration of dimethylnitrosamine. Cancer Res. 39:50-54.

30. Lawley, P.D., and S.A. Shah. 1972. Methylation of ribonucleic acid by the carcinogens dimethyl sulphate, N-methyl-N-nitrosourea and N-methyl-N'-nitro-N-nitrosoguanidine: Comparisons of chemical analyses at the nucleoside and base levels. Biochem. J. 128:117-132.

31. Olsson, M., and T. Lindahl. 1980. Repair of alkylated DNA in _Escherichia coli_. J. Biol. Chem. 255:10569-10571.

32. Karren, P., T. Lindahl, and B. Griffin. 1979. Adaptive response to alkylating agents involves alteration _in situ_ of O^6-methylguanine residues in DNA. Nature 280:76-77.

33. Renard, A., and W.G. Verly. 1980. A chromatin factor in rat liver which destroys O^6-ethylguanine in DNA. FEBS Lett. 114:98-102.

34. Renard, A., L. Thibodeau, and W.G. Verly. 1978. O^6-Ethylguanine excision from DNA of liver nuclei treated with ethylnitrosourea. Fed. Proc. 37:1412.

35. Motesano, R., H. Brésil, G. Planche-Martel, G.P. Margison, and A.E. Pegg. 1980. Effect of chronic treatment of rats with dimethylnitrosamine on the removal of O^6-methylguanine from DNA. Cancer Res. 40:452-458.

36. Rabes, H.M., R. Kerler, R. Wilhelm, G. Rode, and H. Riess. 1979. Alkylation of DNA and RNA by [^{14}C]dimethylnitrosamine in hydroxyurea-synchronized regenerating rat liver. Cancer Res. 39:4228-4236.

37. Buckley, J.D., P.J. O'Connor, and A.W. Craig. 1979. Pretreatment with acetylaminofluorene enhances the repair of O^6-methylguanine in DNA. Nature 281:403-404.

38. Cooper, H.K., E. Hauenstein, G.F. Kolar, and P. Kleihues. 1978. DNA alkylation and neuro-oncogenesis by 3,3-dimethyl-1-phenyltriazine. Acta Neuropathol. (Berl.) 43:105-109.

39. Margison, G.P., N.J. Curtin, K. Snell, and A.W. Craig. 1979. Effect of chronic N,N-diethylnitrosamine on the excision of O^6-ethylguanine from rat liver DNA. Brit. J. Cancer 40:809-813.

40. Samson, L., and J. Cairns. 1977. A new pathway for DNA repair in *Escherichia coli*. Nature 267:281-282.

41. Schendel, P.F., M. Defais, P. Jeggo, L. Samson, and J. Cairns. 1978. Pathways of mutagenesis and repair in *Escherichia coli* exposed to low levels of simple alkylating agents. J. Bacteriol. 135:466-475.

42. Lewis, J.G., and J.A. Swenberg. 1980. Differential repair of O^6-methylguanine in DNA of rat hepatocytes and nonparenchymal cells. Nature 288:185-187.

43. Craddock, V.M. 1971. Liver carcinomas induced in rats by single administration of dimethylnitrosamine after partial hepatectomy. J. Natl. Cancer Inst. 47:899-907.

DISCUSSION

Q.: Most of the studies you have described are with purified DNA which was methylated with high doses of the methylating agents. Such DNA may behave very differently from that in an intact cell. Have you conducted any studies that may approximate what is happening in a target tissue?

A.: Let me mention some recent studies that I did not have time to present. We have been doing some studies with isolated hepatocytes at low doses of DMN and looking at methylation of cellular as well as exogenously added DNA. We found that the hepatocytes effectively metabolized the DMN and both the endogenous and exogenous DNA was methylated, which indicates that an activated species is stable enough to diffuse or in some way pass out of the hepatocyte. Furthermore, only within the hepatocyte did the O^6 to N-7 ratio decrease with time.

Q.: One more question with respect to removal of the O^6-methyl. Can you be certain it is enzymatic removal? For example, to what extent is removal specific enough so that if you added more protein to your system, you would see a greater removal?

A.: Well, that is a concern since the activities are so low. However, partial hepatectomy enhances activity six-fold where you've got the same amount of protein, and it's very reasonable evidence that there is some enzymatic component. Also when different tissues are used, like brain, you don't see any removal.

Q.: I just wanted you to speculate about the stability of the 7-methylguanine. If you look at three different carcinogens there seem to be different stabilities. The benzo[*a*]pyrene reaction product with guanine is so unstable that it has only been shown by an indirect method. With the aflatoxin-guanine adduct, you've got a half-life about 7.5 h, while the 7-methylguanine is stable and does not ring open or is released from the DNA. Can you speculate why there are different stabilities?

A.: It could be the bulkiness of the adduct but there are probably additional factors as well.

Q.: You've observed the effect of partial hepatectomy on removal of the O^6-methylguanine and I'm wondering if you've looked at the proliferating cells of fetal and neo-natal liver or any other tissues.

A.: We are in the process of doing that and I can't say much at this time except that it is not higher in the neo-natal liver.

Q.: I'd like to make a comment to that. A single dose of DNA given to a newborn rat does produce an uncommon incidence of liver tumors.

A.: I'm glad you said that, because that enables me to make a comment I'd forgotten. If you simplistically think of initiation being a race between DNA repair and cell division, then even with the six-fold induction with partial hepatectomy, you are still losing, because the increase of cell division is more than six-fold. So, the results I am showing are not inconsistent with the ideal of the O^6 removal being a protective mechanism against carcinogenesis -- even though Craddock has shown that you get more liver tumors after partial hepatectomy. As Dr. Magee said, you get liver tumors in very young animals, where the liver is also dividing.

Q.: You mentioned that the O^6-methylguanine was transferred to protein. Is that protein the glycosylase, and if it is, does the methylation affect the enzyme's activity?

A.: Whether the methyl group is transferred to the enzyme, I really don't know. There are quite striking differences between this reaction and the reaction which has been seen in *E. coli*. With crude extracts from liver the reaction is linear, whereas with the crude extracts with *E. coli* you get a very rapid reaction, which then inactivates the enzyme. So, there are two possibilities: one is that it's still going to the enzyme itself and this is being regenerated in some way; or that it goes to some other receptor. We've purified this enzyme about 500-fold and we're just about in a position to answer that question.

TIME-DEPENDENT DIFFERENCES IN THE BENZO[a]PYRENE-DNA ADDUCTS PRESENT IN CELL CULTURES FROM DIFFERENT SPECIES

William M. Baird[1], Ranjana U. Dumaswala[2], and Leila Diamond[2]

[1]Department of Medicinal Chemistry and Pharmacognosy, School of Pharmacy and Pharmacal Sciences, Purdue University, West Lafayette, Indiana 47907, and [2]The Wistar Institute of Anatomy and Biology, 36th Street at Spruce, Philadelphia, Pennsylvania 19104

INTRODUCTION

Carcinogenic polycyclic aromatic hydrocarbons are metabolized in cells in which they induce biological effects (1,2). A small portion of the metabolites formed are reactive derivatives that bind covalently to cellular macromolecules; this binding process can lead to the induction of biological effects (1). Several lines of evidence (reviewed in 1-4) suggest that the interaction of hydrocarbon metabolites with DNA is involved in the initiation of carcinogenesis *in vivo* and the induction of mutagenesis in cells in culture. The major DNA-binding metabolites formed from several hydrocarbons in cells in culture and tissues *in vivo* are dihydrodiol-epoxides, usually at the "bay-region" of the molecule (5-9). Diol epoxides are formed on other regions of some hydrocarbons and are involved in the DNA-binding of these hydrocarbons (10,11).

The best characterized hydrocarbon-DNA interactions are those of benzo[a]pyrene (BP), a widespread environmental contaminant (1). The major DNA-binding metabolite formed from BP in cells in culture and tissues *in vivo* is the "bay-region" diol epoxide, BP-7,8-diol 9,10-oxide (BPDE) (12). Recent evidence suggests that a small portion of the BP applied to mouse skin can bind to DNA through 9-hydroxy-BP-4,5-oxide, a phenolic derivative of a BP "K-region" epoxide (13).

There are two isomeric forms of BPDE: the (±)-7β,8α-dihydroxy-9α,10α-epoxy-7,8,9,10-tetrahydrobenzo[a]pyrene (anti-BPDE) with the epoxide and 7-hydroxyl on opposite sides of the ring, and (±)-7β,8α-dihydroxy-9β,10β-epoxy-7,8,9,10-tetrahydrobenzo[a]pyrene (syn-BPDE) with the epoxide and 7-hydroxyl on the same side of the ring (14). In addition, two optical enantiometers of each isomer exist, and a stereochemical specificity in the reaction of these enantiomers with DNA (15) has been shown. Most studies on the structure of BP-DNA adducts have used anti-BPDE as a model compound. It has been shown to bind to DNA on the 2-NH_2 of guanine (16-19), the 6-NH_2 of adenine (20), and on cytidine (21) (probably on the 4-NH_2); it can also react to form phosphotriesters (22) and with the N-7 of guanine of DNA in aqueous solution (23,24).

The anti-isomer is the major DNA-binding metabolite of BP in several types of cell and explant cultures (e.g., 25-27); however, both syn- and anti-isomers are involved in the binding of BP to DNA in most cell types such as mouse embryo, hamster embryo and BHK/21, and human lung cells (28-31). Shinohara and Cerutti (28) studied the removal of the major syn- and anti-BPDE DNA adducts from BP-treated hamster, mouse, and human cells and found that the syn and anti lesions were removed at a similar rate, although the overall rate of adduct removal depended on the cell type. Autrup et al. (26) found that the relative proportions of specific BP-DNA adducts in hamster trachea cultures were similar after 12 or 24 h of exposure to BP and after incubation for 24 h following removal of the BP. Baird and Diamond (30) found that the BP-DNA adducts in hamster embryo cell cultures differed after short exposures (4 to 6 h) and long exposures (24 to 72 h) to BP. At short times there were similar proportions of the syn -and anti-adducts; at late times there was a greater proportion of anti-adducts. Ivanovic et al (32) used high pressure liquid chromatography (HPLC) to analyze the individual base adducts present in the DNA of hamster embryo cells after 18 h of exposure to BP and after 21 h of exposure to BP followed by a 24-h incubation in the absence of BP. They concluded that the different adduct peaks undergo differential rates of excision. In hamster embryo cells after 5, 24, and 72 h of exposure to a low dose of BP, Baird and Dumaswala (33) found differences in the BP-DNA adducts present and in the proportions of the two diol epoxide isomers responsible for the binding. The BP-deoxyadenosine adducts were rapidly removed, a result similar to that reported for 7-bromomethylbenz[a]anthracene-deoxyadenosine adducts in several cell lines (34,35). Kakefuda and Yamamoto (36,37) reported that anti-BPDE-deoxyadenosine adducts caused local denaturations of the DNA that were sensitive to S_1 nuclease. However, Pulkrabek et al. (38,39) found that no adducts were selectively removed by S_1 treatment of plasmid DNA reacted with anti-BPDE.

In the present study, the species specificity of BP-DNA adducts was examined by comparing the BP-DNA adducts present after various durations of exposure to BP in embryo cell preparations from hamsters and from two strains of rats and in a human liver-derived cell line, Hep G2.

MATERIALS AND METHODS

Preparation of [^{3}H]BP-DNA

Embryo cell cultures were prepared from 17- to 19-day-old rat embryos (Wistar-Lewis, M.A. Bioproducts, Walkersville, MD, or Sprague-Dawley, Charles River Breeding Laboratories, Wilmington, MA) or 12- to 13-day-old hamster embryos (Lakeview Hamster Colony, Newfield, NJ) as described previously (40,41). Secondary monolayer cultures were prepared in 150 cm^2 (Corning Glass Works, Corning, NY) or 175 cm^2 (Falcon, Oxnard, CA) culture flasks with 50.0 ml Eagle's minimum essential medium containing 10% fetal bovine serum. Hep G2 cells were grown as described previously (42). [G-^{3}H]BP (Amersham, Arlington Heights, IL) was diluted with unlabeled BP (Gold Label, Aldrich Chemical Co., Milwaukee, WI) to the desired specific activity and added to cultures for the times specified. DNA was isolated from the cell pellet by a phenol extraction procedure (40) or by chromatography on a hydroxylapatite column by a modification of the method of Beland et al. (43). DNA was degraded to deoxyribonucleosides with deoxyribonuclease from bovine pancreas, phosphodiesterase from *Crotalus atrox* venom and alkaline phosphatase from *Escherichia coli* (40).

Preparation of BPDE-DNA Adducts

[^{14}C]Anti-BPDE (sp. activity 29.3 mCi/mmol) and [^{3}H]syn-BPDE (sp. activity 214 mCi/mmol) were provided by the research program of the National Cancer Institute, Division of Cancer Cause and Prevention, Bethesda, MD. Markers of BPDE-DNA adducts were prepared by reacting BPDE with DNA, polydeoxyguanylic-polydeoxycytidylic acid, polydeoxyadenylic-thymidylic acid, and polydeoxycytidylic-deoxyinosinic acid; the BP-deoxyribonucleoside adducts were isolated as described previously (33).

Chromatography on Sephadex LH20 Columns

BP-DNA samples were analyzed by a modification (33) of the borate-methanol elution procedure (44). After application of the DNA digest, a column (25 x 1.5 cm) packed with Sephadex LH20 (Pharmacia, Piscataway, NJ) was eluted with 60 ml methanol:0.05 M sodium borate, pH 8.7 (1:1), and then with a linear gradient of 100 ml methanol:0.05 M sodium borate (1:1) and 100 ml methanol:0.05 M sodium borate (8:2). One hundred and ten 2.0 ml fractions were collected, and 0.5-ml samples were counted by liquid scintillation counting. Absorbance at 260 nm of deoxyribonucleosides was measured for the first 30 fractions. A marker of p-nitrobenzylpyridine was added to each column, and its elution position was detected by UV absorption.

High Pressure Liquid Chromatography

Enzyme-digested samples of DNA were applied to prepacked Sephadex LH20 columns (Sep Pak Columns, Isolabs, Akron, OH) and washed with 25.0 ml of glass distilled water to remove deoxyribonucleosides (33). The modified nucleosides were eluted with 100% methanol. Eight fractions of 2.0 ml each were collected. The fractions containing radioactivity were pooled and evaporated with N_2 to a low volume. Samples (50 µl) were chromatographed on an Altex 25 cm x 4.6 mm Ultrasphere Octyl C_8 reverse-phase column at room temperature on an Altex Model 312 HPLC instrument (Altex Scientific, Berkeley, CA). A precolumn of CO:PELL ODS (Whatman, Clifton, NJ) was used for all samples. The samples were eluted for 35 min with methanol:water (55:45), then for 10 min with a linear gradient of methanol:water (55:45 to 65:35), followed by 5 min at 65:35 methanol:water at a flow rate of 1.0 ml/min (33). One hundred and sixty fractions of 0.3 min each were collected in scintillation vials and counted by liquid scintillation counting.

RESULTS

LH20 Chromatography of HE and WLRE Cell BP-DNA

DNA was isolated from confluent cultures of Wistar-Lewis rat embryo (WLRE) cells and Syrian hamster embryo (HE) cells after 5- or 24-h exposure to [^{3}H]BP. The DNA samples were enzymatically degraded and chromatographed on Sephadex LH20 columns eluted with borate buffer containing methanol:water gradients (see Figure 1). The anti-BPDE-DNA adduct markers eluted in peak (A); the syn-BPDE-DNA adduct markers eluted in peak (B). The anti-BPDE-DNA adduct peak (A) contained only 60% as much radioactivity as the syn-BPDE-DNA adduct peak (B) in the 5-h DNA sample from WLRE cells; both peaks contained similar amounts of material in the 5-h DNA sample from HE cells (see Figure 1). After 24 h of exposure to BP, the WLRE cell DNA contained almost identical amounts of material in peaks (A) and (B); the HE cell DNA contained 20% more material in the anti-BPDE-DNA adduct peak (A) than in the syn-BPDE-DNA adduct peak (B).

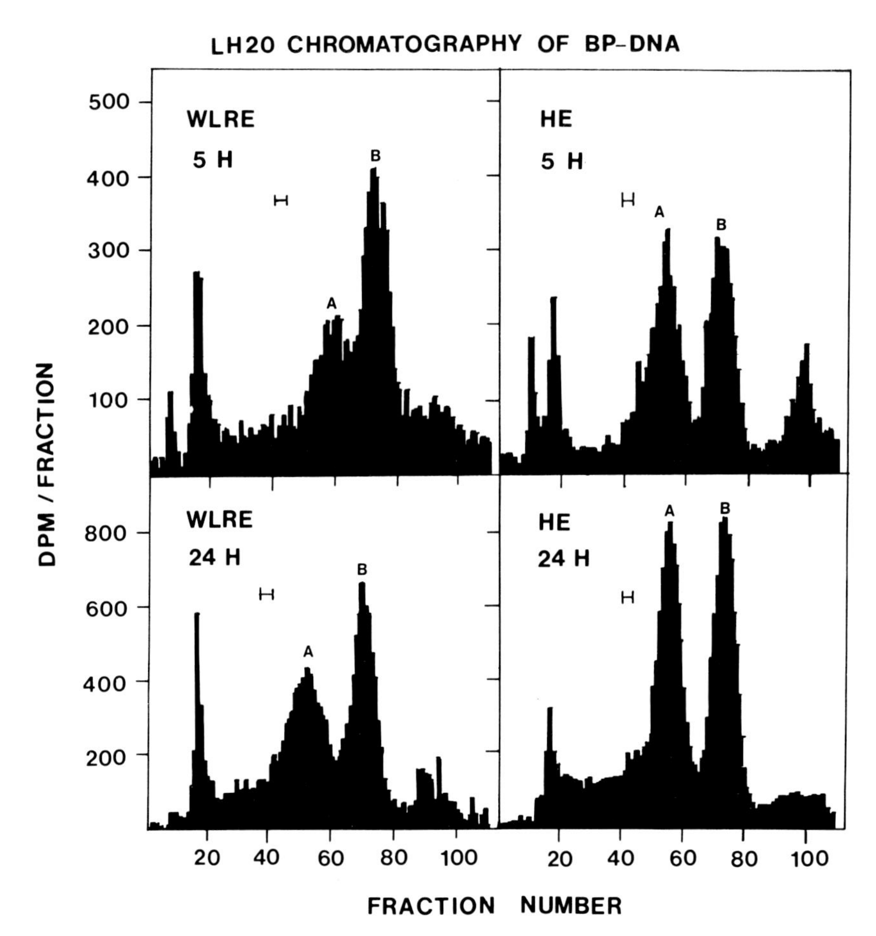

Figure 1. Sephadex LH20 column elution profiles of enzymatically degraded samples of DNA from HE and WLRE cells exposed to [^{3}H]BP. Confluent cultures of secondary HE or WLRE cells were exposed to 0.5 nmol [^{3}H]BP/ml medium (sp. activity 5 Ci/mmol) for 5 or 24 h. The elution position of a p-nitrobenzylpyridine marker is shown by H. DNA-adduct markers prepared by reaction of anti-BPDE with DNA eluted in the same position as peak (A); syn-BPDE-DNA markers eluted in the same position as peak (B).

HPLC of HE, WLRE, and SDRE Cell BP-DNA

The individual BP-DNA adducts present in BP-treated embryo cell cultures from rats and hamsters were analyzed by HPLC on a C_8 reverse-phase column eluted with a methanol:water gradient. The elution positions of adducts formed by the reaction of anti- and syn-BPDE with DNA (top) and with polydeoxyribonucleotides (bottom) are shown in Figure 2. Based upon these results and the structural elucidation studies of others (16-21), peak 1 was tentatively identified as [^{14}C]anti-BPDE-deoxycytidine (dC), peak 2 as [^{14}C]anti-7S-BPDE-deoxyguanosine (dG), peak 3 as a mixture of [^{3}H]syn-BPDE-dC and [^{3}H]syn-BPDE-dG, peak 4 as [^{14}C]anti-7R-BPDE-dG, and peak 5 as [^{3}H]syn-BPDE-dG. Peak 6 represents an unidentified [^{3}H]syn-BPDE derivative that may result from the breakdown of an unstable adduct to release a tetrol; this peak was not observed in BP-treated cells. The anti- and syn-BPDE-deoxyadenosine (dA) adducts eluted between fractions 110 and 140 (not shown on Figure 2) and were designated peak 7.

The BP-DNA adducts formed in WLRE, Sprague-Dawley (SDRE), and HE cells were analyzed after 5, 24, and 72 h of exposure to BP. After 5 h of exposure, the anti-7R-BPDE-dG (peak 4) adduct peak was the largest peak in the HE cells (see Figure 3, top), but there were large amounts of syn-BPDE-dG (peak 5) and a mixture of syn-BPDE-dG and syn-BPDE-dC (peak 3). In contrast, peak 4 was absent from the WLRE-DNA (see Figure 3, middle) and the major adducts were syn-BPDE-dG and syn-BPDE-dC (peaks 3 and 5) and anti-BPDE-dC (peak 1). The SDRE-DNA contained some anti-BPDE-dG (peak 4), but the anti-BPDE-dC (peak 1) and syn-BPDE-dG and syn-BPDE-dC (peaks 3 and 5) were the major adducts. All three cell types had a peak of dA adducts (peak 7) that probably resulted from reactions by both BPDE isomers.

After 24 h of BP exposure (see Figure 4), the predominant adduct in the HE cells (see Figure 3, top) was the anti-BPDE-dG (peak 4), although the anti-BPDE-dC (peak 1) and syn-BPDE-dG (peak 5) peaks still represented major adducts. In the WLRE cells, the major adduct peaks were the syn-BPDE-dG and syn-BPDE-dC (peaks 3 and 5) and anti-BPDE-dC (peak 1) peaks. However, there was a substantial amount of material in peak 4 (anti-BPDE-dG) at 24 h. The SDRE cells had an adduct profile similar to the HE cells, although more material was present in anti-BPDE-dC (peak 1).

After 72 h (see Figure 5), the two major peaks in HE cell DNA were anti-BPDE-dG (peak 4) and syn-BPDE-dG (peak 5). The WLRE cell DNA contained major peaks of anti-BPDE-dC and anti-BPDE-dG (peaks 1 and 4) and syn-BPDE-dG and syn-BPDE-dC (peaks 3 and 5). The SDRE cell BP-DNA adduct profile was similar to that of HE cell DNA.

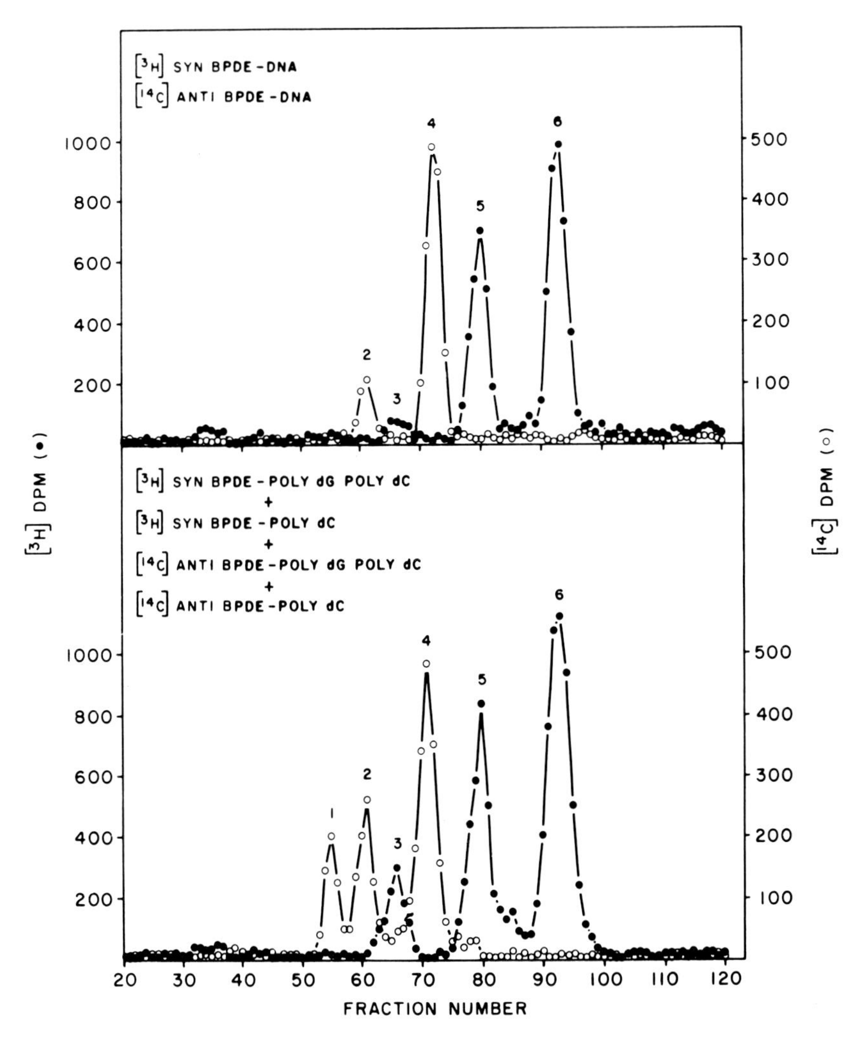

Figure 2. HPLC profiles of syn- and anti-BPDE deoxyribonucleoside markers. The fractions (0.3 ml) were collected, and radioactivity was measured by liquid scintillation counting. ● gives the $[^3H]$dpm/fraction; ○ the $[^{14}C]$dpm/fraction. The identities of the peaks are discussed in Results.

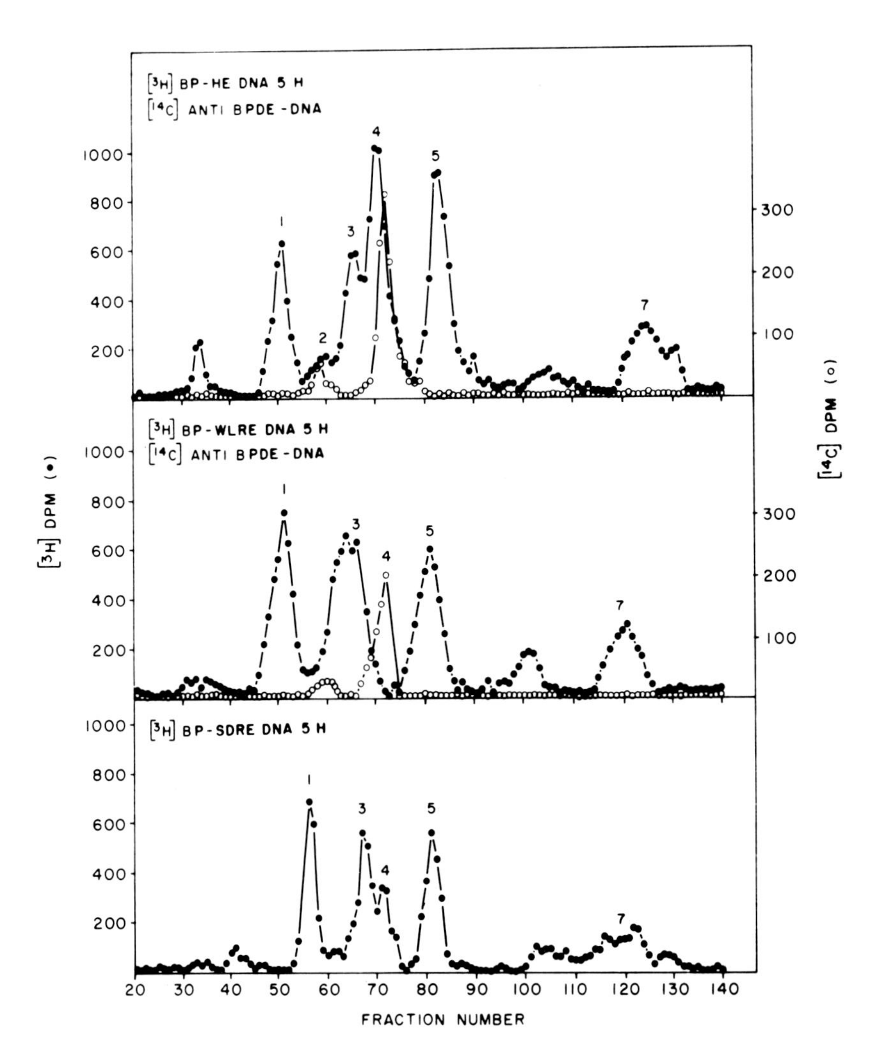

Figure 3. HPLC profiles of DNA from cells exposed to [^{3}H]BP for 5 h. Confluent secondary cultures of HE, WLRE, and SDRE cells were exposed to 0.5 nmol (0.13 μg) [^{3}H]BP/ml medium (sp. activity 5 Ci/mmol) for 5 h. The pmole BP bound/mg DNA were: HE, 4.0; WLRE, 5.6; SDRE, 1.6. ● gives the dpm/0.3 ml fraction.

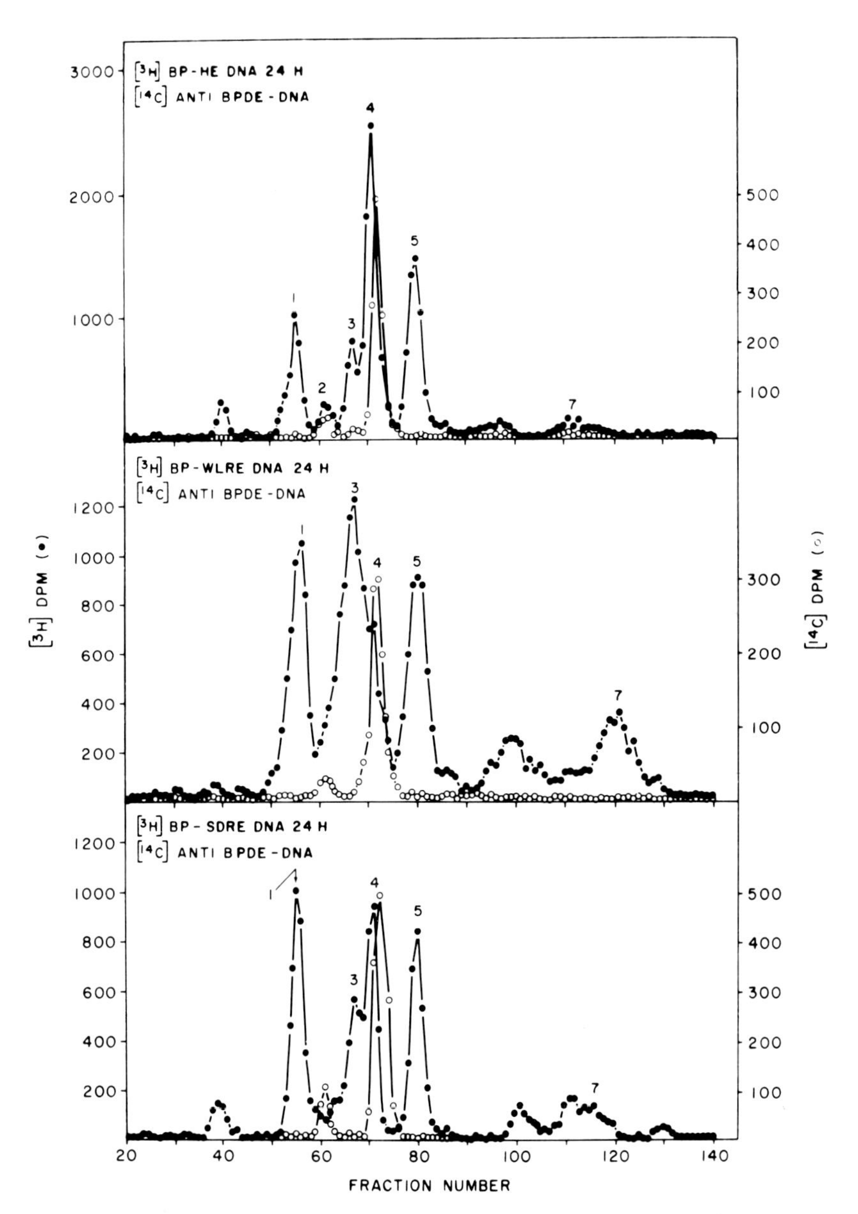

Figure 4. HPLC profiles of DNA from cells exposed to [^{3}H]BP for 24 h. The values for pmole BP bound/mg DNA were: HE, 6.0; WLRE, 14.2; SDRE, 4.0. ● gives the dpm/0.3 ml fraction.

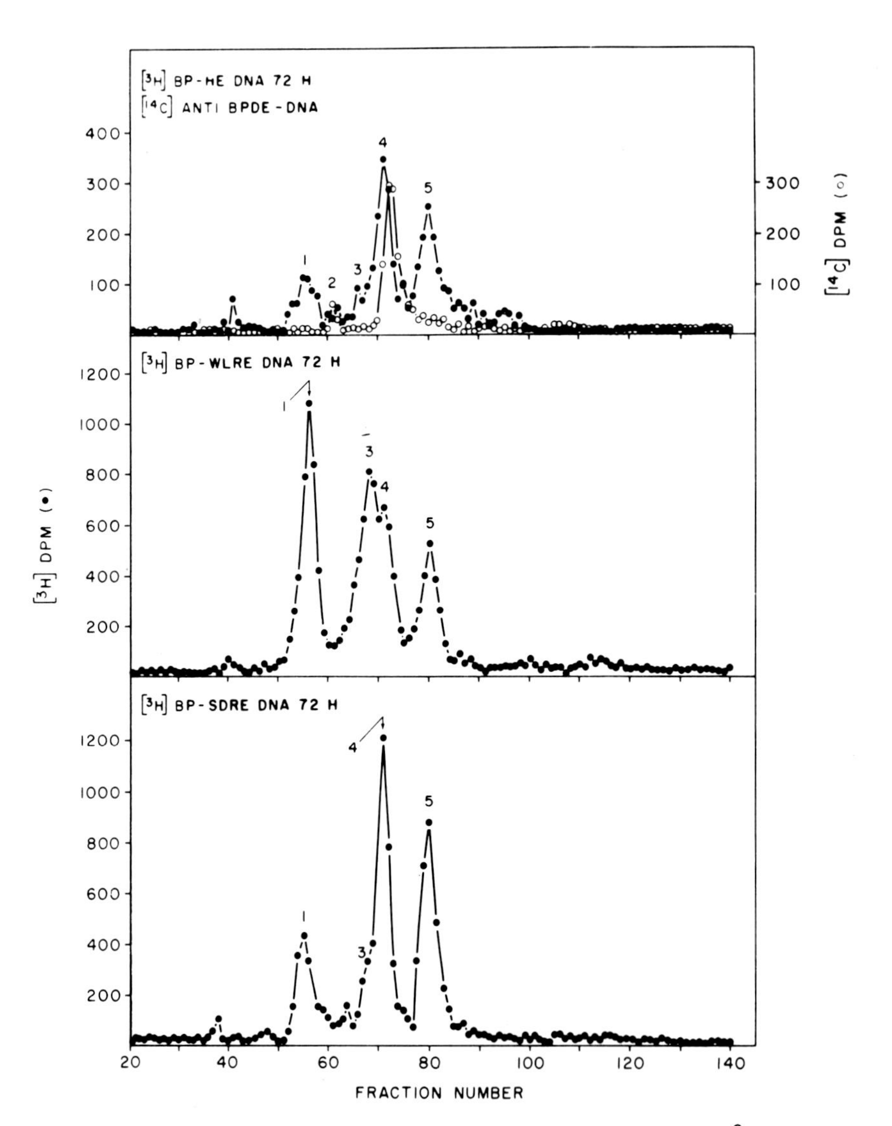

Figure 5. HPLC profiles of DNA from cells exposed to $[^{3}H]$BP for 72 h. The values for pmole BP bound/mg DNA were: HE, 3.2; WLRE, 8.5; SDRE, 2.8. ● gives the dpm/0.3 ml fraction.

The actual amount of each BP-DNA adduct present (pmoles/mg DNA) at 5, 24, and 72 h is shown in Figure 6. Comparison of the patterns of adducts present shows that there are similarities between the HE and SDRE cells and that the adduct pattern in the WLRE cells differs substantially from that of the other cells. In all three cells, the proportion of syn-BPDE adducts decreased with increased duration of exposure to BP, with alteration in the proportions of adducts being greatest between 5 and 24 h. In all cells, there was a selective loss of dA adducts (peak 7); these adducts were essentially absent in all cells by 72 h. The proportion of dA adducts decreased between 5 and 24 h. In all cases, there was a decrease in the proportion of material in the syn-BPDE-DNA-adduct peak 3 (syn-BPDE-dG and/or syn-BPDE-dC) between 24 and 72 h.

HPLC of Hep G2 Cell BP-DNA

The BP-DNA adducts formed in the liver-derived human cell line Hep G2 were analyzed after 6- and 48-h exposure to BP. At both times, the major adduct was peak 4 (anti-BPDE-dG), although smaller amounts of peak 1 (anti-BPDE-dC) and peak 5 (syn-BPDE-dG) were present. The actual amounts of BP-DNA adduct present in each peak at 6 and 48 h were similar. The values in pmole BP-DNA adduct/mg DNA were: 6 h peak 1 -- 0.7, peak 4 -- 11.4, peak 5 -- 2.7; 48 h peak 1 -- 1.2, peak 4 -- 11.4, peak 5 -- 3.7. No BP-dA adducts (peak 7) were observed at either 6 or 48 h.

DISCUSSION

Differences in the hydrocarbon-DNA adducts formed in various organs and species could provide a method for predicting the species and site specificity of carcinogenesis by hydrocarbons. The formation and persistence of specific alkylated DNA bases such as O^6-methylguanine correlate with the organ specificity and relative carcinogenic potency of several alkylating agents (reviewed in 45, 46, and other chapters of this book). Similar studies could provide valuable information about the biological importance of the hydrocarbon-DNA adducts formed in various species and organs, but first it is essential to establish that specific hydrocarbon-DNA adducts are important for such effects. The differences between the BP-DNA adduct profiles of DNA from BP-treated cells (Figure 3) and DNA reacted with BPDE in aqueous solution (Figure 2) complicate determination of the specific hydrocarbon adducts responsible for the induction of various biological effects.

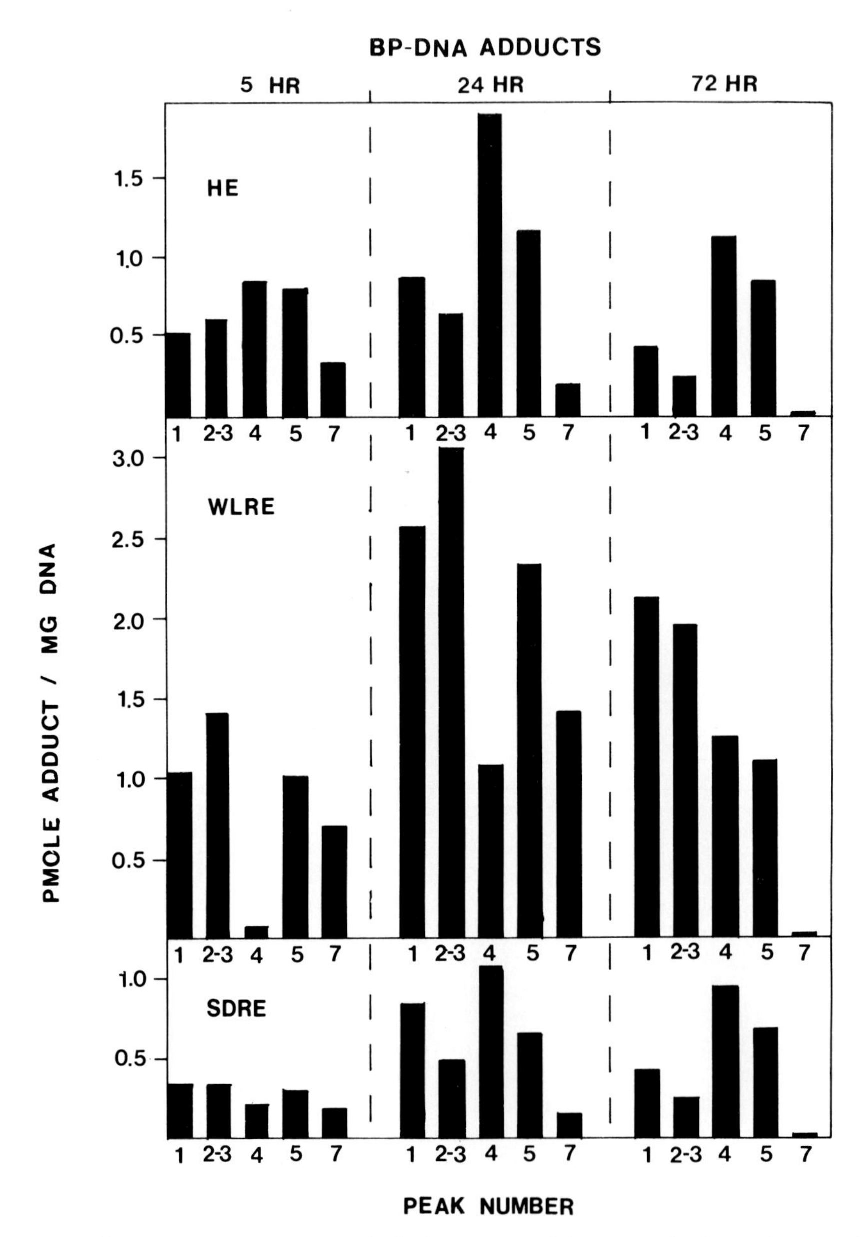

Figure 6. Amount of material in each adduct peak for the HPLC analyses shown in Figures 3, 4, and 5.

To determine how the formation and removal of specific hydrocarbon adducts are related to the induction of biological effects, it was first necessary to determine whether the BP-DNA adduct profiles in various cells are independent of the length of time of exposure to BP. The BP-DNA adducts present differed in the three types of rodent embryo cell cultures that were examined, with the largest differences in the BP-DNA adduct profiles being observed after the 5-h period of incubation with BP (Figure 3). The largest adduct peak in HE cell DNA, peak 4 (anti-BPDE-dG), was absent in WLRE cell DNA and was a minor peak in SDRE cell DNA (Figure 6). After 24 h of BP exposure (Figure 4), the adduct profiles of the three DNAs differed, but after 72-h exposure, the relative proportions of the adduct peaks in the HE and SDRE cell DNAs were similar (Figures 5 and 6). The WLRE cell BP-DNA adduct profile after 72 h of BP treatment differed from that of the SDRE and HE cells.

The BP-DNA adducts present in the HE, WLRE, and SDRE cells changed with the length of time of exposure to BP, but the adducts in the Hep G2 cells were independent of exposure time. Both the LH20 column chromatography (Figure 1) and HPLC results (Figures 3, 4, 5) demonstrate that in the rodent cells the ratio of anti- to syn-BPDE adducts increased with increased length of time of exposure to BP. The relative proportions of HE and SDRE BP-DNA adducts in peaks 4 and 5 (anti-BPDE-dG and syn-BPDE-dG, respectively) increased, between 5 and 24 h as total binding increased, and between 24 and 72 h as total binding decreased. In the WLRE cells, the relative proportions of peaks 1, 2-3, 5, and 7 were similar at 5 and 24 h; the proportion of peak 4 increased between 5 and 24 h. By 72 h, the relative proportions of peaks 2-3 (syn-BPDE-dG, syn-BPDE-dC), peak 5 (syn-BPDE-dG), and 7 (BPDE-dA adducts) decreased. Some of the BP-DNA adduct profile changes, such as the decrease in peak 7 (BPDE-dA adducts) observed in all three cells (Figure 6), probably result from selective excision. The dA adducts of 7-bromomethylbenz[a]anthracene are also selectively removed by some cells (34,35). Other changes in the adduct profile, such as the increase in peak 4 in the WLRE cells between 5 and 24 h, suggest that these were also time-dependent changes in BP-DNA adduct formation.

The BP-DNA adduct profiles obtained from Hep G2 cells after 6 and 48 h of BP treatment were almost identical (see Figure 7). No adducts were observed at either time. Thus, if such adducts were formed, they must have been excised relatively rapidly. The absence of dA adducts and time-dependent changes could also have resulted from more stable rates of adduct formation and removal in these cells than in the rodent cells.

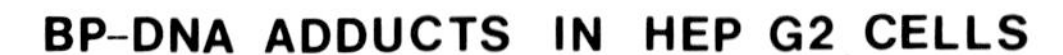

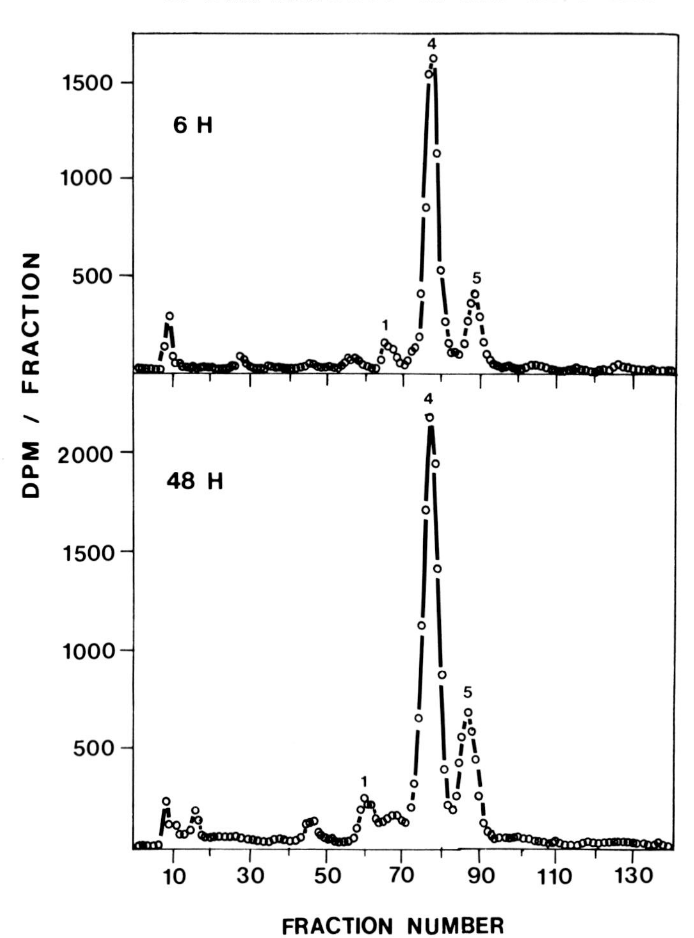

Figure 7. HPLC profiles of DNA from Hep G2 cells exposed to [^{3}H]BP for 6 and 48 h. Confluent cultures of Hep G2 cells were exposed to 4.0 nmol (1.0 μg) [^{3}H]BP/ml medium (sp. activity 0.63 Ci/mmol) for 6 or 48 h. The values for pmole BP bound/mg DNA were: 6 h, 21.6; 48 h, 28.2. o gives the dpm/0.3 ml fraction.

Biological effects induced by BP were shown to differ when the hydrocarbon was activated by HE and WLRE cells (42). Under the conditions of a clonal transformation assay, BP was much more toxic with a WLRE cell feeder layer than with an HE cell feeder layer, whereas, under conditions of a cell-mediated mutation assay, BP-induced toxicity was comparable (42).

Comparison of the BP-DNA adducts present in cells from various strains and species with the biological effects induced when BP is activated by the same cells will help to establish the role of specific BP-DNA adducts and combinations of specific adducts in the induction of biological effects. An understanding of the time-dependent variations in the BP-DNA adducts present in each cell type will be essential for the interpretation of such comparisons.

ACKNOWLEDGMENTS

We thank Francis Kruszewski, Kathryn Jones, Andrew Nebzydoski, and Janet Nargang for excellent technical assistance. The Hep G2 cells were provided by Drs. Barbara Knowles and David Aden of the Wistar Institute. This work was supported by grants CA28825, CA21778, and CA23168 from the Department of Health and Human Services, an institutional grant to Purdue University from the American Cancer Society, and a grant from the Showalter Trust Fund, Indianapolis, IN.

REFERENCES

1. Gelboin, H.V., and P.O.P. Ts'o, eds. 1978. Polycyclic Hydrocarbons and Cancer, Volumes 1 and 2. Academic Press: NY.

2. Bjørseth, A., and A.J. Dennis, eds. 1980. Polynuclear Aromatic Hydrocarbons: Chemistry and Biological Effects. Battelle Press: Columbus, OH.

3. Grover, P.L., ed. 1979. Chemical Carcinogens and DNA, Volumes 1 and 2. CRC Press, Inc.: Boca Raton, FL.

4. Newbold, R.F., P. Brookes, and R.G. Harvey. 1979. A quantitative comparison of the mutagenicity of carcinogenic polycyclic hydrocarbon derivatives in cultured mammalian cells. Int. J. Cancer 24:203-209.

5. Jerina, D.M., and J.W. Daly. 1976. Oxidation at carbon. In: Drug Metabolism - From Microbe to Man. D.V. Parke and R.L. Smith, eds. Taylor and Francis, Ltd.: London. pp. 13-32.

6. Phillips, D.H., and P. Sims. 1979. Polycyclic aromatic hydrocarbon metabolites: Their reactions with nucleic acids. In: Chemical Carcinogens and DNA, Volume 2. P.L. Grover, ed. CRC Press, Inc.: Boca Raton, FL. pp. 29-57.

7. Baird, W.M. 1979. The use of radioactive carcinogens to detect DNA modifications. In: Chemical Carcinogens and DNA, Volume 1. P.L. Grover, ed. CRC Press, Inc.: Boca Raton, FL. pp. 59-83.

8. Hecht, S.S., E. LaVoie, R. Mazzarese, S. Amin, V. Bedenko, and D. Hoffman. 1978. 1,2-Dihydro-1,2-dihydroxy-5-methylchrysene, a major activated metabolite of the environmental carcinogen 5-methylchrysene. Cancer Res. 38:2191-2194.

9. Dipple, A., and J.A. Nebzydoski. 1978. Evidence for the involvement of a diol-epoxide in the binding of 7,12-dimethylbenz[a]anthracene to DNA in cells in culture. Chem.-Biol. Interact. 20:17-26.

10. Cary, P.D., C.H. Turner, C.S. Cooper, O. Ribeiro, P.L. Grover, and P. Sims. 1980. Metabolic activation of benz[a]anthracene in hamster embryo cells: The structure of a guanosine-anti-BA-8,9-diol 10,11-oxide adduct. Carcinogenesis 1:505-512.

11. Cooper, C.S., O. Ribeiro, A. Hewer, C. Walsh, K. Pal, P.L. Grover, and P. Sims. 1980. The involvement of a "bay-region" and a non-"bay-region" diol-epoxide in the metabolic activation of benz[a]anthracene in mouse skin and in hamster embryo cells. Carcinogenesis 1:233-243.

12. Sims, P., P.L. Grover, A. Swaisland, K. Pal, and A. Hewer. 1974. Metabolic activation of benzo[a]pyrene proceeds by a diol-epoxide. Nature 252:326-328.

13. Vigny, P., Y.M. Ginot, M. Kindts, C.S. Cooper, P.L. Grover, and P. Sims. 1980. Fluorescence spectral evidence that benzo[a]pyrene is activated by metabolism in mouse skin to a diol-epoxide and a phenol-epoxide. Carcinogenesis 1:945-950.

14. Hulbert, P.B. 1975. Carbonium ion as ultimate carcinogen of polycyclic aromatic hydrocarbons. Nature 256:146-148.

15. Meehan, T., and K. Straub. 1979. Double-stranded DNA stereoselectively binds benzo[a]pyrene diol epoxides. Nature 277:410-412.

16. Weinstein, I.B., A.M. Jeffrey, K.W. Jennette, S.H. Blobstein, R.G. Harvey, C. Harris, H. Autrup, H. Kasai, and K. Nakanishi. 1976. Benzo[a]pyrene diol epoxides as intermediates in nucleic acid binding *in vitro* and *in vivo*. Science 193:592-595.

17. Meehan, T., K. Straub, and M. Calvin. 1977. Benzo[a]pyrene diol epoxide covalently binds to deoxyguanosine and deoxyadenosine in DNA. Nature 269:725-727.

18. Koreeda, M., P.D. Moore, P.G. Wislocki, W. Levin, A.H. Conney, H. Yagi, and D.M. Jerina. 1978. Binding of benzo[a]pyrene 7,8-diol-9,10-epoxides to DNA, RNA, and protein of mouse skin occurs with high stereoselectivity. Science 199:778-781.

19. Osborne, M.R., F.A. Beland, R.G. Harvey, and P. Brookes. 1976. The reaction of (±)-7α,8β-dihydroxy-9β,10β-epoxy-7,8,9,10-tetrahydrobenzo[a]pyrene with DNA. Int. J. Cancer 18:362-366.

20. Jeffrey, A.M., K. Grzeskowiak, I.B. Weinstein, K. Nakanishi, P. Roller, and R.G. Harvey. 1979. Benzo[a]pyrene-7,8-dihydrodiol 9,10-oxide adenosine and deoxyadenosine adducts: Structure and stereochemistry. Science 206:1309-1311.

21. Jennette, K.W., A.M. Jeffrey, S.H. Blobstein, F.A. Beland, R.G. Harvey, and I.B. Weinstein. 1977. Nucleoside adducts from the *in vitro* reaction of benzo[a]pyrene-7,8-dihydrodiol 9,10-oxide or benzo[a]pyrene 4,5-oxide with nucleic acids. Biochemistry 16:932-938.

22. Gamper, H.B., A.S.-C. Tung, K. Straub, J.C. Bartholomew, and M. Calvin. 1977. DNA strand scission by benzo[a]pyrene diol epoxides. Science 197-671-674.

23. King, H.W.S., M.R. Osborne, and P. Brookes. 1979. The *in vitro* and *in vivo* reaction at the N^7-position of guanine of the ultimate carcinogen derived from benzo[a]pyrene. Chem.-Biol. Interact. 24:345-353.

24. Osborne, M.R., R.G. Harvey, and P. Brookes. 1978. The reaction of trans-7,8-dihydroxy-anti-9,10-epoxy-7,8,9,10-tetrahydrobenzo[a]pyrene with DNA involves attack at the N^7-position of guanine moieties. Chem.-Biol. Interact. 20:123-130.

25. Jeffrey, A.M., I.B. Weinstein, K.W. Jennette, K. Grzeskowiak, K. Nakanishi, R.G. Harvey, H. Autrup, and C. Harris. 1977. Structures of benzo[a]pyrene-nucleic acid adducts formed in human and bovine bronchial explants. Nature 269:348-350.

26. Autrup, H., F.C. Wefald, A.M. Jeffrey, H. Tate, R.D. Schwartz, B.F. Trump, and C.C. Harris. 1980. Metabolism of benzo[a]pyrene by cultured tracheobronchial tissues from mice, rats. hamsters, bovines, and humans. Int. J. Cancer 25:293-300.

27. Harris, C.C., H. Autrup, G.D. Stoner, B.F. Trump, E. Hillman, P.W. Schafer, I.B. Weinstein, and A.M. Jeffrey. 1979. Metabolism of benzo[a]pyrene and identification of the major carcinogen-DNA adducts formed in cultured human esophagus. Cancer Res. 39:4401-4406.

28. Shinohara, K., and P.A. Cerutti. 1977. Excision repair of benzo[a]pyrene-deoxyguanosine adducts in baby hamster kidney 21/C13 cells and in secondary mouse embryo fibroblasts C57BL/6J. Proc. Natl. Acad. Sci. USA 74:979-983.

29. Baird, W.M., and L. Diamond. 1978. Metabolism and DNA binding of polycyclic aromatic hydrocarbons by human diploid fibroblasts. Int. J. Cancer 22:189-195.

30. Baird, W.M., and L. Diamond. 1977. The nature of benzo[a]pyrene-DNA adducts formed in hamster embryo cells depends on the length of time of exposure to benzo[a]pyrene. Biochem. Biophys. Res. Comm. 77:162-167.

31. Feldman, G., J. Remsen, K. Shinohara, and P. Cerutti. 1978. Excisability and persistence of benzo[a]pyrene DNA adducts in epithelioid human lung cells. Nature 274:796-798.

32. Ivanovic, V., N.E. Geacintov, H. Yamasaki, and I.B. Weinstein. 1978. DNA and RNA adducts formed in hamster embryo cell cultures exposed to benzo[a]pyrene. Biochemistry 17:1597-1603.

33. Baird, W.M., and R.U. Dumaswala. 1980. Benzo[a]pyrene-DNA adduct formation in cells: Time-dependent differences in the benzo[a]pyrene-DNA adducts present. In: Polynuclear Aromatic Hydrocarbons: Chemistry and Biological Effects. A. Bjorseth and A. Dennis, eds. Battelle Press: Columbus, OH. pp. 471-488.

34. Dipple, A., and J.J. Roberts. 1977. Excision of 7-bromomethylbenz[a]anthracene-DNA adducts in replicating mammalian cells. Biochemistry 16:1499-1503.

35. McCaw, B.A., A. Dipple, S. Young, and J.J. Roberts. 1978. Excision of hydrocarbon-DNA adducts and consequent cell survival in normal and repair defective human cells. Chem.-Biol. Interact. 22:139-151.

36. Kakefuda, T., and H. Yamamoto. 1978. Modification of DNA by the benzo[a]pyrene metabolite diol-epoxide r-7, t-8-dihydroxy-t-9,10-oxy-7,8,9,10-tetrahydrobenzo[a]pyrene. Proc. Natl. Acad. Sci. USA 75:415-419.

37. Kakefuda, T., and H. Yamamoto. 1978. Modification of DNA by benzo[a]pyrene diol epoxide I. In: Polycyclic Hydrocarbons and Cancer, Volume 2. H.V. Gelboin and P.O.P. Ts'o, eds. Academic Press: New York. pp. 63-74.

38. Pulkrabek, P., S. Leffler, I.B. Weinstein, and D. Grunberger. 1977. Conformation of DNA modified with a dihydrodiol epoxide derivative of benzo[a]pyrene. Biochemistry 16:3127-3132.

39. Pulkrabek, P., S. Leffler, D. Grunberger, and I.B. Weinstein. 1979. Modification of deoxyribonucleic acid by a diol epoxide of benzo[a]pyrene. Relation to deoxyribonucleic acid structure and conformation and effects on transfectional activity. Biochemistry 18:5128-5134.

40. Baird, W.M., and L. Diamond. 1976. Effect of 7,8-benzoflavone on the formation of benzo[a]pyrene-DNA-bound products in hamster embryo cells. Chem.-Biol. Interact. 13:67-75.

41. Baird, W.M., T.G. O'Brien, and L. Diamond. 1981. Comparison of the metabolism of benzo[a]pyrene and its activation to biologically active metabolites by low-passage hamster and rat embryo cells. Carcinogenesis 2:81-88.

42. Diamond, L., F. Kruszewski, D.P. Aden, B. Knowles, and W.M. Baird. 1980. Metabolic activation of benzo[a]pyrene by a human hepatoma cell line. Carcinogenesis 1:871-874.

43. Beland, F.A., K.L. Dooley, and D.A. Casciano. 1979. Rapid isolation of carcinogen-bound DNA and RNA by hydroxyapatite chromatography. J. Chromatog. 174:177-186.

44. King, H.W.S., M.R. Osborne, F.A. Beland, R.G. Harvey, and P. Brookes. 1976. (±)-7α,8β-Dihydroxy-9β,10β-epoxy-7,8,9,10-tetrahydrobenzo[a]pyrene is an intermediate in the metabolism and binding to DNA of benzo[a]pyrene. Proc. Natl. Acad. Sci. USA 73:2679-2681.

45. Lawley, P.D. 1979. Approaches to chemical dosimetry in mutagenesis and carcinogenesis: The relevance of reactions of chemical mutagens and carcinogens with DNA. In: Chemical Carcinogens and DNA, Volume 1. P.L. Grover, ed. CRC Press, Inc.: Boca Raton, FL. pp. 1-36.

46. Margison, G.P., and P.J. O'Connor. 1979. Nucleic acid modification by N-nitroso compounds. In: Chemical Carcinogens and DNA, Volume 1. P.L. Grover, ed. CRC Press, Inc.: Boca Raton, FL. pp. 111-159.

DISCUSSION

Q.: We've seen a variety of patterns for benzo[a]pyrene adduct formation. We've also seen that the state of the cells, whether they're dividing or not, has some influence on the kinds of adducts one sees. Have you any information or ideas as to whether cell division is playing a role in the data you have presented?

A.: We have treated all of these cells in very confluent cultures which we refed at least 48 h before BP addition to prevent any serum stimulation of division. So we have specifically tried to avoid the issue of the effects of cell division. We would like to determine the effect of cell division on adduct type and persistence, but we have not done it yet.

Q.: Several comments. We've carried out *in vivo* studies with benzo[a]pyrene in several species, Sprague-Dawley rats and several mice strains, and basically our patterns look very much like your HEP-G-6 cells in that the major adduct in the mouse strains was the guanine adduct.

We also have what you're calling peak 1. We're not sure, but it could be a recycled BP-phenol adduct. However, in our system it chromatographs in the same region as the deoxycytidine adduct. We see this adduct in the Sprague-Dawley rat but only a little of it in the AJ and C57 mouse. In these mice we see mostly the BP-diolepoxide adducts.

As for repair of the different adducts in the AJ mouse lung, we could not find differences. They disappeared with a half-life of about 15 days and we were not sure whether that was repair or cell turnover.

A.: Let me try to answer those in sequence. First, as to peak 1, we do know it is not the same as you would get from BP-9-hydroxy-4,5-oxide. We have prepared that through microsomal incubation and it would run about five fractions earlier on this gradient. If there is a minor adduct coming from a BP phenolepoxide, which is possible in this case, we might not have detected it if it were less than 5%, as our recoveries are 95% and up.

I know Vigney et al. have a paper in Carcinogenesis (ref. 13) suggesting that adducts can be formed in this way. We have not looked specifically for them.

We have done one experiment of prelabeling the cells with tritiated cytidine. In that case, using unlabeled benzo[a]pyrene, we found a peak that elutes in the region you described, but we have not been able to do an absolute structural characterization of the peak.

As to the causes of changes in the adduct, I would say that probably what we're seeing between 24 and 72 h we could attribute mainly to repair.

The changes between 5 and 24 h I think could very well be due more to changes in the metabolic pattern of the BP. The point I wanted to make is if you just pick a single time point to look for adducts, you can get different impressions of what is being formed. In the case of the adenine adducts which we're seeing early, if we had looked at later times, we would have concluded that they were absent.

Q.: We have seen this morning that methylating and alkylating carcinogens producing different adducts have obviously different biological consequences. Brookes and others have recently pointed out that perhaps the type of adduct, whether it's attached to guanine or adenine, may not be that important. Would you like to speculate on whether the same is true for the different BP-DNA adducts which you find here?

A.: That is difficult to answer because obviously we don't have the data. It is what we would like to find out. I think that if you have a big molecule like hydrocarbon-DNA, the odds are you're going to have some sort of an effect. But the biological effect may depend both on the nature of the adduct and its persistence in the DNA.

One point I failed to make is, when you react the diolepoxides specifically with DNA in large excess of DNA, you do get much more selective reaction with the guanine than we see in the case of the cells treated with the benzo[a]pyrene. We really don't know quite why this occurs, whether it is the structure of the chromatin, or some other factor. But I think there are significant differences between treating with the parent hydrocarbons or diolepoxide alone.

DNA BINDING AS A PROBE FOR METABOLIC ACTIVATION IN VARIOUS SYSTEMS

C. Anita H. Bigger and Anthony Dipple

Chemical Carcinogenesis Program, Frederick Cancer Research Center, Frederick, Maryland 21701

INTRODUCTION

The metabolic activation of chemical carcinogens has been studied intensively over the last 20 years. Classically, the pathway of activation was recognized by identifying a metabolite that exhibited greater carcinogenic potency than the parent carcinogen (1). For the polycyclic hydrocarbon carcinogens, this approach met with little success. However, theoretical chemists emphasized the K-regions as likely sites for interactions of these hydrocarbons with cellular components (2), and this theorization found a basis in the potent activity of hydrocarbon K-region oxides in various *in vitro* systems (3). As a result, there was a growing acceptance of these K-region oxides as the active forms of the hydrocarbon carcinogens, despite their very limited carcinogenic activities in *in vivo* animal test systems (4). The limited carcinogenic activity of these compounds was rationalized by the theory that their chemical reactivity led to their destruction before they reached the appropriate target cells or macromolecules.

However, in 1973 Baird et al. (5) demonstrated that the 7-methylbenz[*a*]anthracene metabolite that bound to DNA in mouse embryo cell cultures was not the K-region oxide. Also in 1973, Borgen et al. (6) demonstrated that the 7,8-dihydrodiol metabolite of benzo[*a*]pyrene was bound to DNA in the presence of microsomes far more extensively than was benzo[*a*]pyrene itself. These two studies led Sims and his colleages (7) to formulate the vicinal diol-epoxide mechanism of metabolic activation of hydrocarbons. This mechanism is now widely accepted and substantiated by the carcinogenic activities of the appropriate metabolites (8).

In addition to the understanding of hydrocarbon activation that these studies generated, they stressed that biological activity in *in vitro* systems does not always reflect the more complex situation *in vivo*, and they indicated that DNA binding was a reliable probe for metabolic activation. DNA binding clearly monitors the generation of chemically reactive metabolites and, as long as there is no highly selective repair of the adducts generated by one particular reactive metabolite, it monitors the cumulative production of such metabolites over any time interval. In contrast, direct measurement of metabolites is confused by the large number of different structures formed, and the further metabolism of primary metabolites means that metabolite profiles reflect the fate of the carcinogen only at the time of observation.

For these reasons, we have investigated various systems using DNA binding as a primary probe for metabolic activation. These investigations have concentrated on one particular carcinogen, 7,12-dimethylbenz[*a*]anthracene (DMBA). This carcinogen was chosen for study because it is the most potent hydrocarbon carcinogen, and because collaborative studies (9-14) with Baird (Purdue University) and with Moschel and Tomaszewski (now of Tracor-Jitco) at Frederick Cancer Research Center had provided evidence that this carcinogen, despite the presence of a methyl group in the "bay region" (Figure 1) is activated for DNA binding in mouse embryo cells through a "bay region" diol-epoxide, i.e., a 3,4-diol-1,2-epoxide.

To compare the products of DMBA binding to DNA in various systems, tritium-labeled DMBA was used for binding, and DNA was isolated and then enzymically hydrolyzed to deoxyribonucleosides using deoxyribonuclease, snake venom phosphodiesterase, and bacterial alkaline phosphatase. The deoxyribonucleoside digest so obtained, along with various marker compounds, was then subjected to chromatography on the Sephadex LH-20-methanol/water gradient system of Baird and Brookes (15). The most frequently used markers were: 4-(p-nitrobenzyl)pyridine, added to facilitate comparison of one chromatogram with another; the UV-absorbing products of reaction of the K-region epoxide of DMBA with DNA (digested to deoxyribonucleosides); and carbon-14-labeled adducts from DMBA binding to DNA in mouse embryo cells, these adducts representing the diol-epoxide DNA adducts.

RESULTS AND DISCUSSION

DMBA-DNA Binding Catalyzed by Aroclor-Induced Rat Liver Microsomes

Our initial studies (11) showed that while the diol-epoxide DNA adducts formed in mouse embryo cells were clearly distinguishable from the K-region epoxide adducts (Figure 2a), the DMBA-DNA adducts formed in the presence of rat liver microsomes

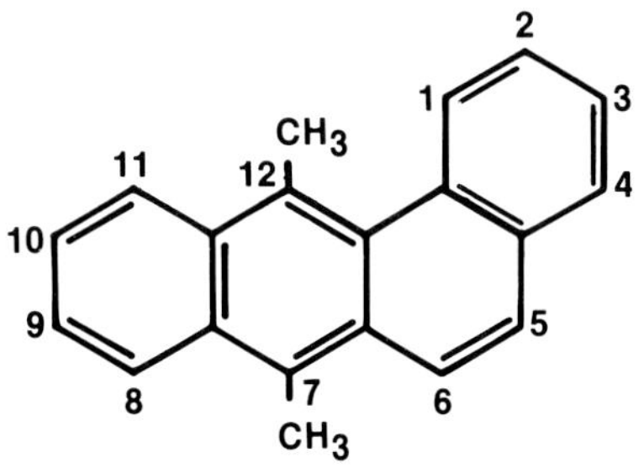

7,12-dimethylbenz(a)anthracene
(DMBA)

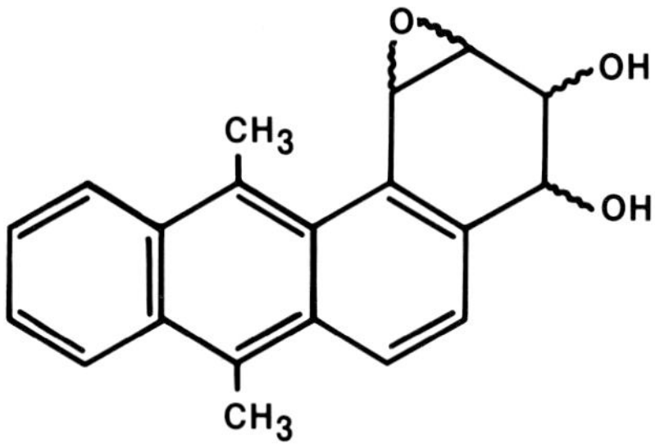

***trans*-3,4-dihydro-3,4-dihydroxy-**
7,12-dimethylbenz(a)anthracene-1,2-oxide
(3,4-DIOL-1,2-EPOXIDE)

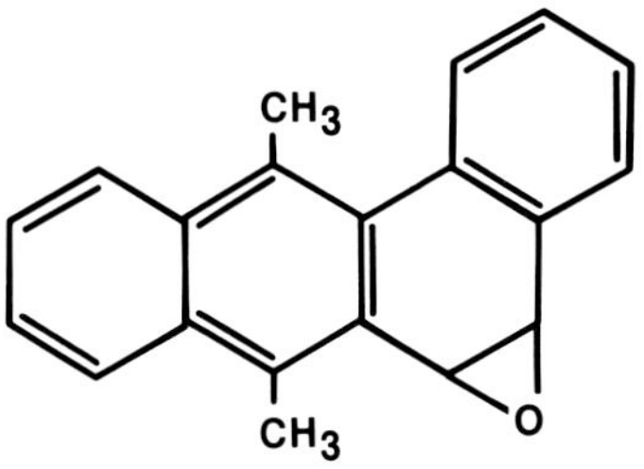

7,12-dimethylbenz(a)anthracene-5,6-oxide
(K-Region Epoxide)

Figure 1. Structures of 7,12-dimethylbenz[a]anthracene and derivatives.

were clearly due to the reaction of the K-region epoxide of DMBA with DNA (Figure 2b). Thus, microsomal systems do not necessarily provide a good model for the metabolic activation occurring in cellular systems. Since results from different laboratories were apparently in conflict concerning the activation of benzo[a]pyrene in microsomal systems (16,17), a more thorough investigation of the microsomal system was necessary, particularly with regard to the effect of magnesium ion on the system. For example, Meehan et al. (16) reported that benzo[a]pyrene bound to DNA in the presence of rat liver microsomes exclusively through the bay region diol-epoxide route, while King et al. (17) found that binding occurred primarily through other routes. Meehan et al. (16) suggested that this difference was due to the inclusion of magnesium ions in the reaction mixture used by King et al. However, since these differing results were obtained using different concentrations of benzo[a]pyrene, we examined different DMBA/microsomal protein ratios in this study (Figure 3).

As reported elsewhere (18), these experiments indicated that, at a given ratio of DMBA to microsomal protein, the presence or absence of magnesium ion had little effect on the type of DMBA-DNA adducts formed (compare Figure 3a to 3c and Figure 3b to 3d). However, at different substrate-to-microsomal-protein ratios, substantial changes in binding products were obtained. Thus, while at the high ratio (320 nmol DMBA per mg microsomal protein) the major products are again eluted with the K-region epoxide-deoxyribonucleoside markers (Figure 3a and 3c), this is not the case for the low substrate concentration experiment (24 nmol DMBA per mg microsomal protein, Figure 3b and 3d). In order to determine whether DMBA diol-epoxide-DNA adducts were generated at the low substrate concentration, these tritium-labeled adducts were chromatographed with carbon-14-labeled diol-epoxide adducts from mouse embryo cells (Figure 4). The results shown suggest that diol-epoxide adducts are formed at low substrate concentrations in the microsomal system but that, unlike the mouse embryo cell situation, other types of adduct are also generated.

DMBA-DNA Binding Catalyzed by Aroclor-Induced Rat Liver 9000 g Supernatant (S9 Fraction)

In view of the variations with substrate concentration found using microsomal systems, a similar study using an S9 fraction normally used in bacterial mutation assays (19) was undertaken (20). Again, major variations in the DMBA-DNA adducts formed were found when different substrate concentrations were used (Figure 5). More detailed analyses (20) indicated that, at the high substrate-to-S9-protein ratio (Figure 5a), the major products resulted from reaction between DMBA K-region epoxide and the added calf thymus DNA (peaks D and E). These peaks constitute a smaller

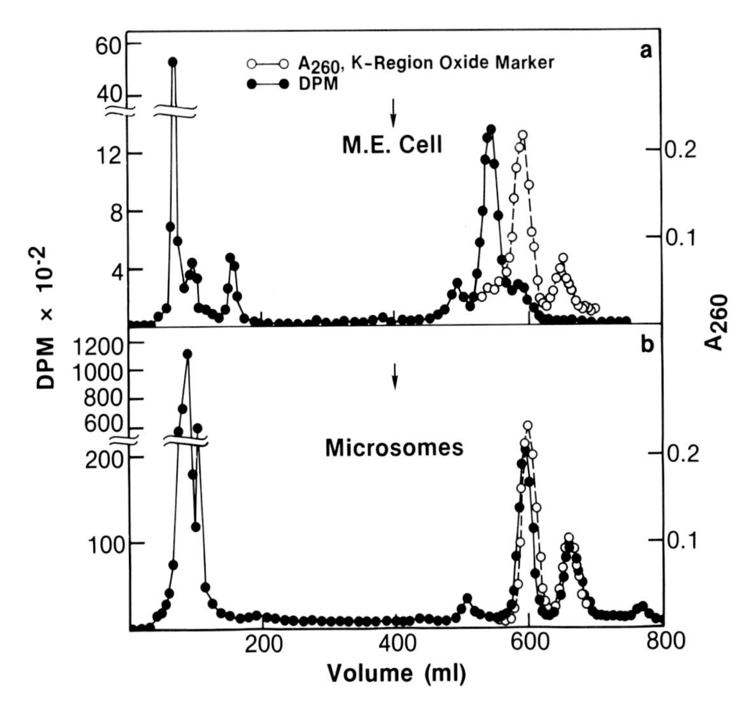

Figure 2. Comparison of Sephadex LH-20 column chromatography of DMBA 5,6-oxide-nucleoside products (o---o) formed by enzymatic digestion of calf thymus DNA which had been reacted with DMBA 5,6-oxide _in vitro_ with enzymatically digested DMBA-DNA products from (a) mouse embryo cell cultures treated 24 h with [^{3}H]DMBA and (b) calf thymus DNA treated with [^{3}H]DMBA for 2 h in the presence of Aroclor-stimulated rat microsomes. The single-headed arrow denotes the position of elution of added 4-(p-nitrobenzyl)-pyridine, a UV-absorbing marker; ●---●, dpm; o---o, absorbance at 260 nm.

fraction of the total adducts at lower substrate concentrations (Figure 5b, c). In contrast, peak C, which elutes with a carbon-14-labeled marker for diol-epoxide adducts after recovery and further analysis by high pressure liquid chromatography (HPLC) (20), tends to increase as a fraction of total adducts at lower substrate concentrations (Figure 5). Cochromatography of the adducts formed in the presence of S9 fraction and of the adducts from mouse embryo cells illustrates this point more clearly for two different substrate concentrations (Figure 6). Again however, the

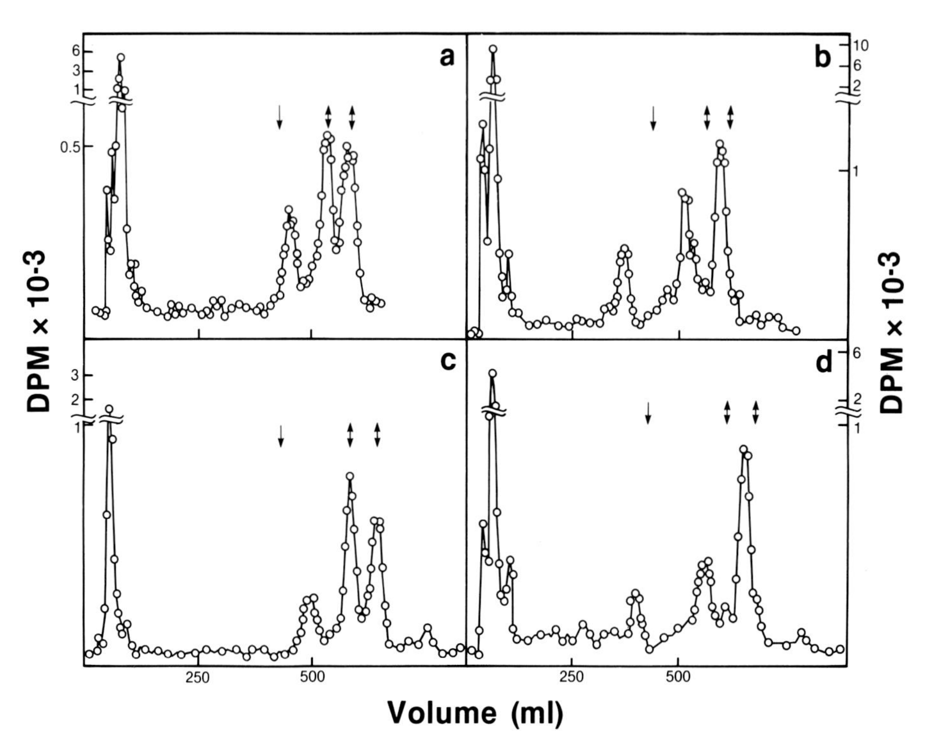

Figure 3. Sephadex LH-20 column chromatography of DMBA-deoxyribonucleoside adducts formed by enzymatic digestion of calf thymus DNA that had been treated for 2 h in the presence of Aroclor-induced rat liver microsomes with (a and c) 320 nmol or (b and d) 24 nmol [^{3}H]DMBA per mg microsomal protein in the presence of (a and b) or absence (c and d) of an $MgCL_2$-containing NADPH-generating system. The single-headed arrow denotes the position of elution of an added UV-absorbing marker 4-(p-nitrobenzyl)-pyridine. The double arrow denotes the position of elution of added DMBA 5,6-oxide-deoxyribonucleoside UV-absorbing markers.

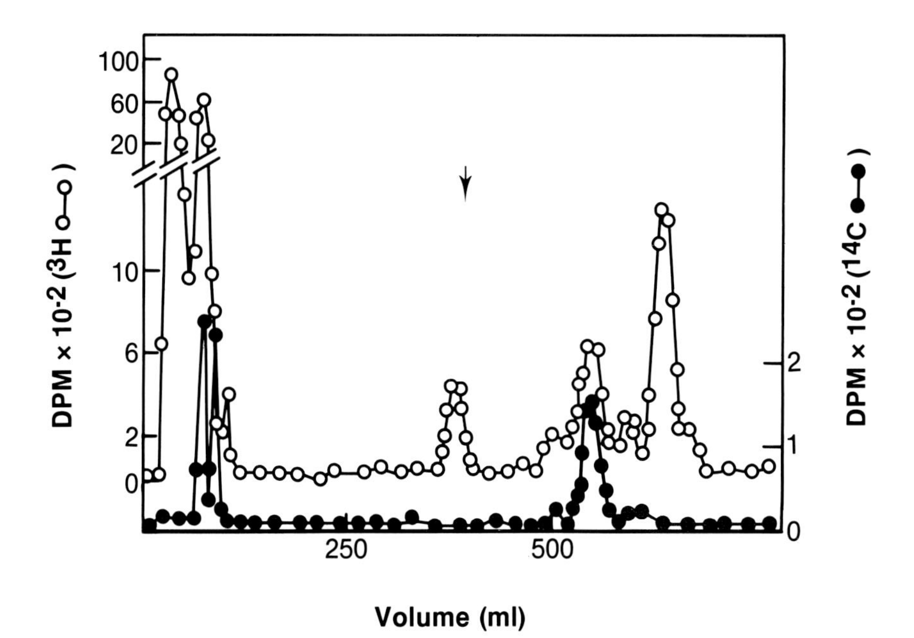

Figure 4. Sephadex LH-20 column chromatography of DMBA-deoxyribonucleoside adducts formed by enzymatic digestion of DNA from mouse embryo cells exposed to [^{14}C]DMBA for 24 h (●---●) and of calf thymus DNA incubated with microsomes and 24 nmol [^{3}H]DMBA per mg microsomal protein (o---o). The arrow is as defined in Figure 2.

diol-epoxide adducts are not a major fraction of total adducts, even at the low substrate concentration; so that, like the microsomal system, the S9 system is not an ideal model for cellular systems.

Adducts Formed at Different DMBA Doses in Mouse Skin and Mouse Embryo Cells

In contrast to the concentration-dependent qualitative changes in adducts formed in the microsomal and S9 systems, such changes were not observed in mouse embryo cell cultures nor in mouse skin (Figure 7). While quantitative increases in binding with dose were noted, the adducts behaved chromatographically like the diol-epoxide adducts in all cases. While it is difficult to equate

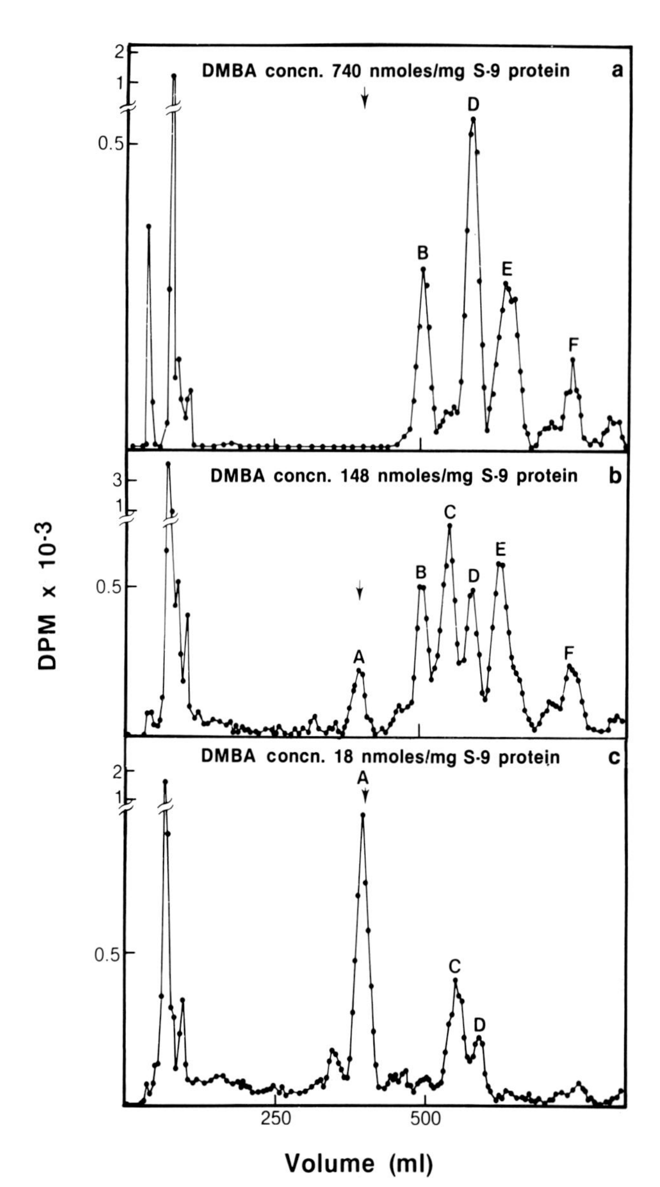

Figure 5. Comparison of Sephadex LH-20 column chromatography of DMBA-deoxyribonucleoside adducts formed by enzymatic digestion of calf thymus DNA that had been treated for 2 h in the presence of Aroclor-induced rat liver S9 fraction with (a) 740, (b) 148, or (c) 18 nmol [^{3}H]DMBA per mg S9 fraction protein. Peaks eluting with the same volume eluant in different experiments are labeled A-F for convenient reference. The arrow is as defined in Figure 2.

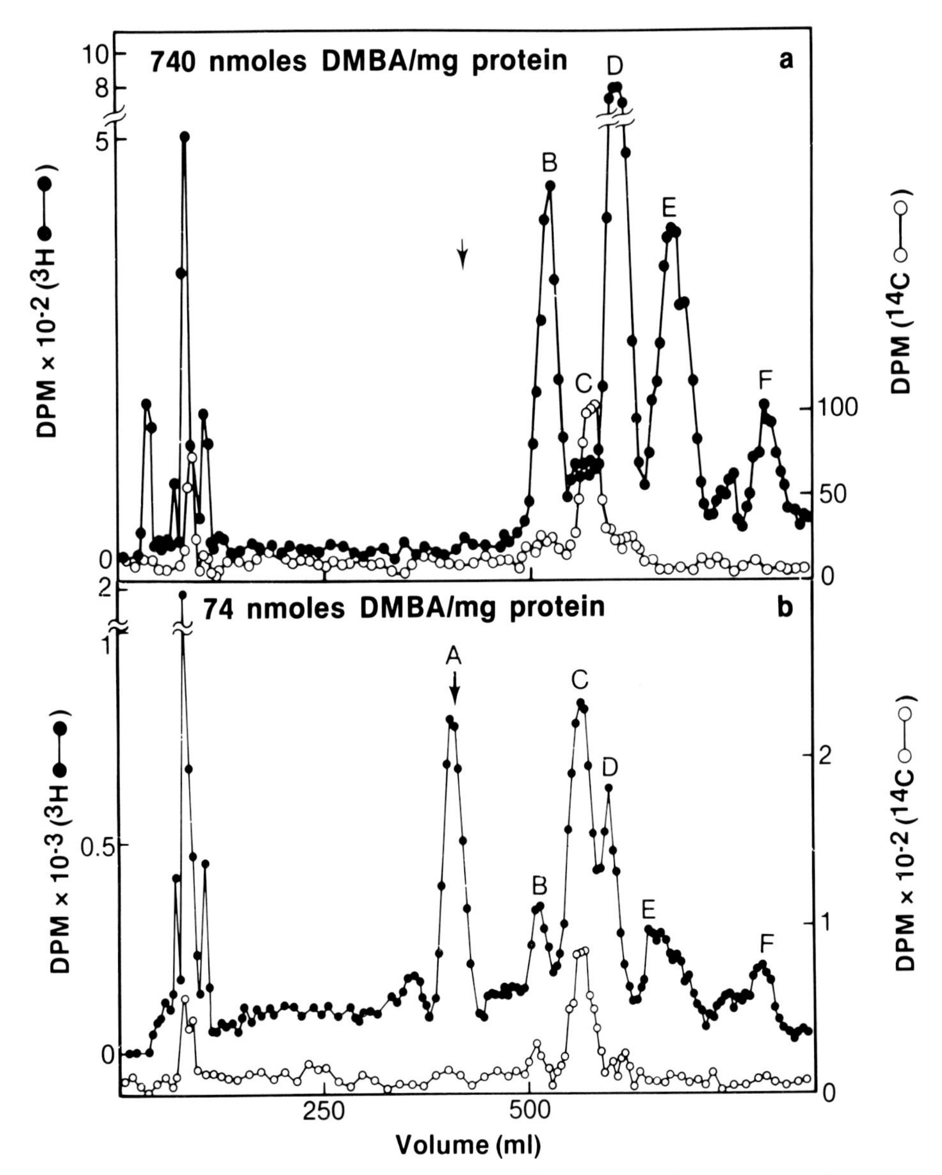

Figure 6. Comparison of Sephadex LH-20 column chromatography of DMBA-deoxyribonucleoside adducts formed by enzymatic digestion of DNA from mouse embryo cells exposed to [^{14}C]DMBA (o---o) for 24 h and of calf thymus DNA treated for 2 h in the presence of Aroclor-induced rat liver S9 fraction with (a) 740 or (b) 74 nmol [^{3}H]DMBA (●---●) per mg S9 fraction protein. The arrow is as defined in Figure 2. Labels A-F are as defined in Figure 5.

dosage in these very different biological systems, the levels of binding to DNA covered in the study in Figure 7 are lower and higher than those over which wide qualitative variations were observed in the subcellular systems (Figures 3 and 5).

DMBA-DNA Binding Catalyzed by Aroclor-Induced Microsomes from Rat, Mouse, and Hamster Liver

Figures 8 and 9 illustrate the DMBA-DNA adducts formed in the presence of microsomes from rat, mouse, and hamster liver using a high and a low substrate concentration, respectively. At the high substrate concentration (353 nmol DMBA per mg microsomal protein), binding to DNA is similar in the three systems, i.e., 11, 17, and 15 μmol DMBA per mol DNA phosphorus for rat, hamster, and mouse preparations, respectively, and in all cases binding to DNA occurs largely through the K-region epoxide of DMBA (Figure 8). The situation is somewhat more complex at the lower substrate concentrations (15, 20, and 8 nmol DMBA per mg microsomal protein for the rat, hamster, and mouse systems, respectively, in Figure 9). In each case, some products are observed that elute in coincidence with carbon-14-labeled diol-epoxide adducts from mouse embryo cells. These are accompanied by a range of other products in each case, and these appear to be present in different proportions when binding is catalyzed by the microsomal preparations from different species (Figure 9).

DMBA-DNA Binding in Intact Cellular Systems from Various Sources

Figure 10 displays Sephadex LH-20 column analyses of DMBA-DNA adducts formed in five different intact cellular systems. Four species -- human, mouse, rat and hamster -- are represented therein, and the source of tissue ranges through embryonic cells, liver, skin, and human foreskin cells. Despite quantitative differences, it seems fairly clear that qualitatively the same types of adducts are generated in these five different systems, i.e., all elute from Sephadex LH-20 columns in the same fashion as the diol-epoxide products from mouse embryo cells. Thus, while there are major differences in reactive metabolites formed and, therefore, in DMBA-DNA adducts generated when subcellular fractions are compared to whole cell systems, no such qualitative variations within a wide range of cellular systems are apparent.

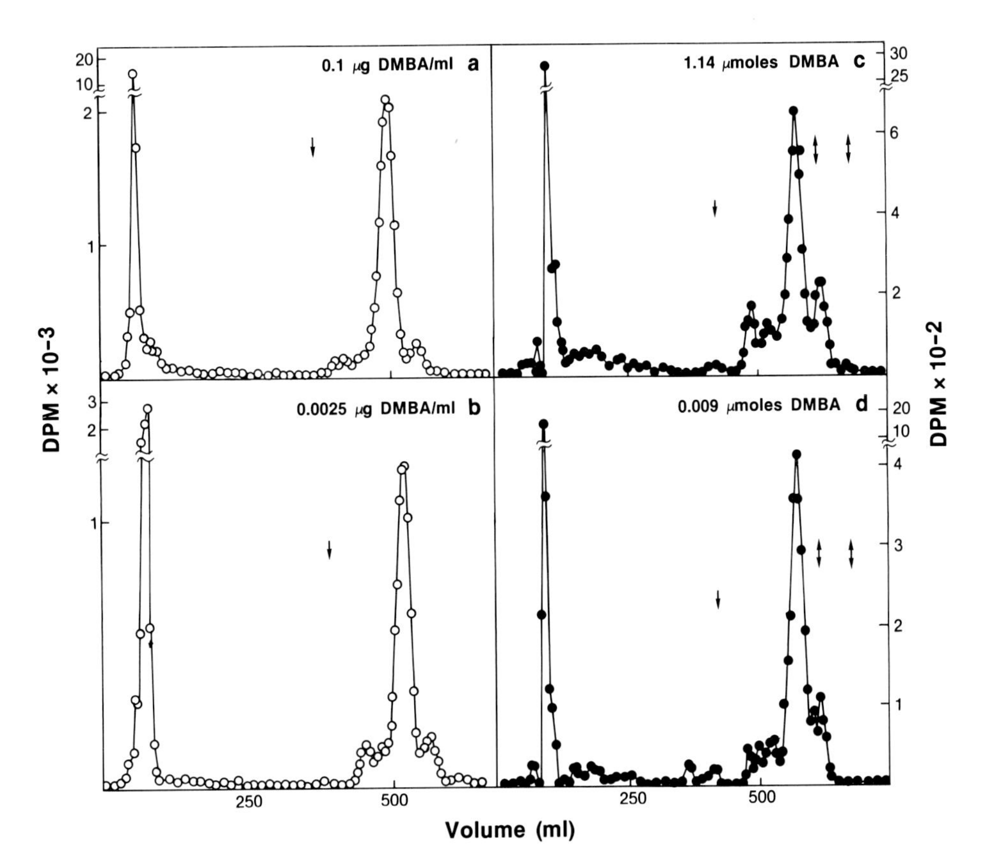

Figure 7. Comparison of Sephadex LH-20 column chromatography of DMBA-deoxyribonucleoside adducts formed by enzymatic digestion of DNA from mouse embryo cells (o---o) exposed to (a) 0.1 and (b) 0.0025 μg [^{3}H]DMBA/ml of medium for 24 h and of DNA from mouse skin (●---●) treated with (c) 1.14 and (d) 0.009 μmol [^{3}H]DMBA per mouse for 24 h. The arrows are as defined in Figure 3.

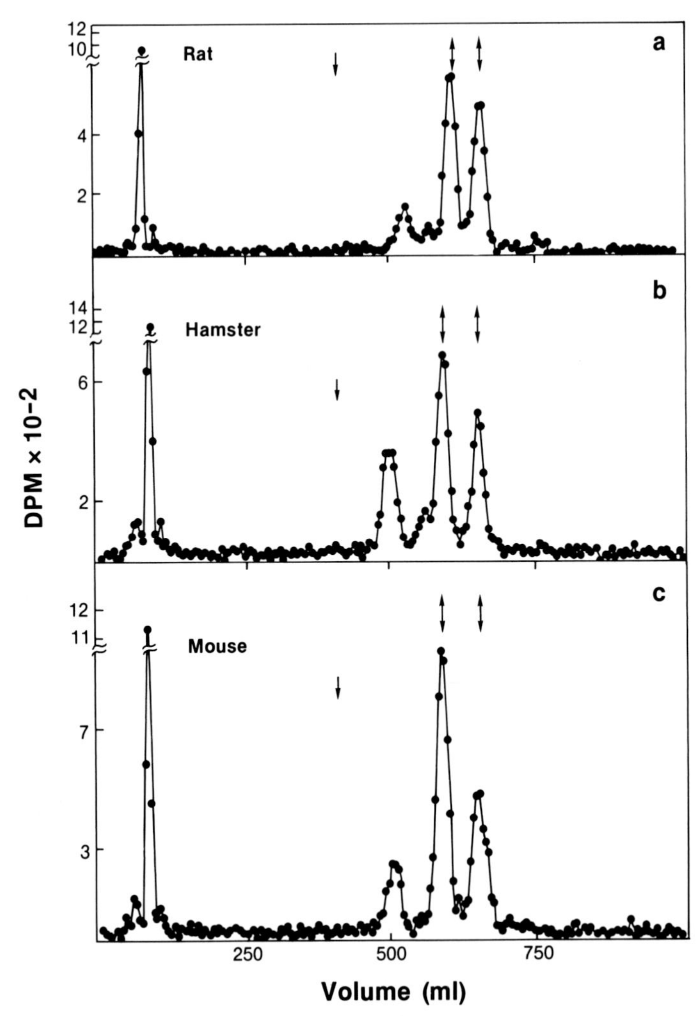

Figure 8. Comparison of Sephadex LH-20 column chromatography of DMBA-deoxyribonucleoside adducts formed by activation of DMBA at high concentration by Aroclor-induced liver microsomes from different species. Liver microsomes were prepared (11) from male Sprague-Dawley rats, Syrian golden hamsters, and NIH Swiss mice weighing approximately 150, 125, and 25 g, respectively. The [^{3}H]DMBA-deoxyribonucleoside adducts were formed by incubation of (a) rat, (b) hamster, and (c) mouse microsomes with calf thymus DNA and 353 nmol [^{3}H]DMBA per mg of microsomal protein followed by recovery, purification, and enzymatic digestion of the DNA. The arrows are as defined in Figure 3.

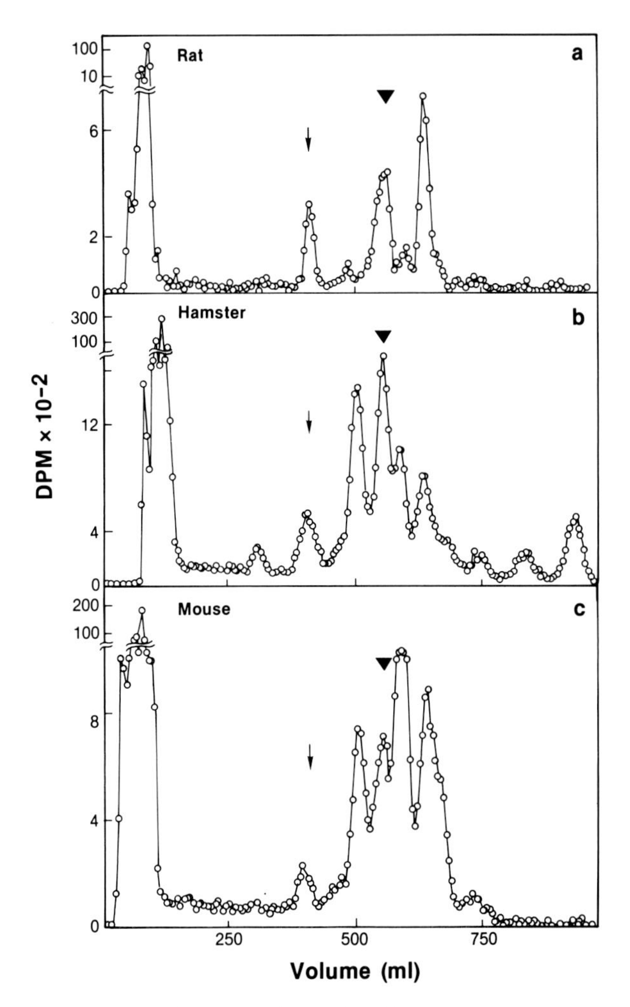

Figure 9. Comparison of Sephadex LH-20 column chromatography of DMBA-deoxyribonucleoside adducts formed by activation of DMBA at low concentration by Aroclor-induced liver microsomes from different species. Preparation of liver microsomes is described in Figure 8. The [^{3}H]DMBA-deoxyribonucleoside adducts were formed by incubation of (a) rat, (b) hamster, and (c) mouse microsomes with calf thymus DNA and (a) 15, (b) 20, and (c) 8 nmol [^{3}H]DMBA per mg of microsomal protein followed by recovery, purification, and enzymatic digestion of the DNA. The triangle denotes the position of elution in each experiment of added [^{14}C]DMBA-deoxyribonucleoside adducts formed by enzymatic digestion of DNA from mouse embryo cells exposed to [^{14}C]DMBA for 24 h. The arrow is as defined in Figure 2.

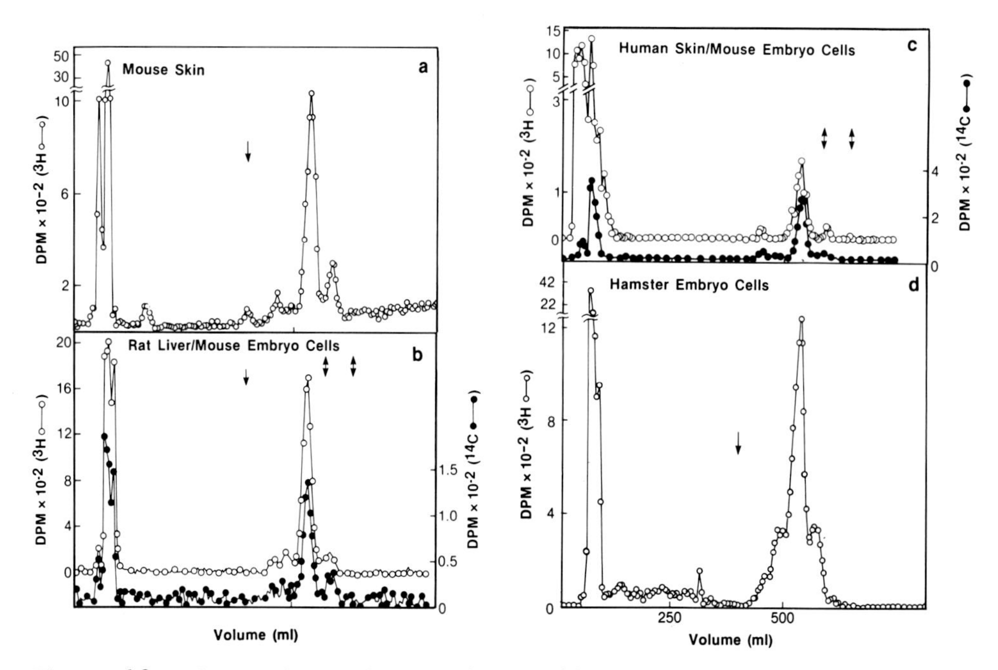

Figure 10. Comparison of Sephadex LH-20 column chromatography of DMBA-deoxyribonucleoside adducts formed by activation of DMBA in intact cells from various organs and species. DMBA-deoxyribonucleoside adducts were formed by enzymatic digestion of DNA from (a) Swiss NIH mouse skin treated with [^{3}H]DMBA for 24 h (11); (b) Sprague-Dawley rat liver cells (o---o) treated with [^{3}H]DMBA for 24 h (21) and Swiss NIH mouse embryo cells (●---●) treated with [^{14}C]DMBA for 24 h; (c) human foreskin cells (o---o) treated with [^{3}H]DMBA for 24 h (21) and Swiss NIH mouse embryo cells (●---●) treated with [^{14}C]DMBA; and (d) Syrian hamster embryo cells treated with [^{3}H]DMBA for 24 h (9). The arrows are as defined in Figure 3.

CONCLUSIONS

Our detailed investigations of the binding of DMBA to DNA in various systems indicate that the pathway(s) for metabolism of DMBA to DNA-binding metabolites: 1) are different in microsomal, S9, and whole cell systems; 2) are influenced substantially by substrate concentration in microsomal and S9 systems, following the K-region epoxide pathway predominantly at high substrate concentrations but following other pathways that lead to many different adducts -- some of which are diol-epoxide adducts -- at low substrate concentrations; 3) are not qualitatively influenced by substrate concentration in mouse embryo cells or mouse skin; and 4) follow primarily the bay region diol-epoxide pathway in the intact cellular systems examined so far, irrespective of the species or organ from which the cellular system is derived.

ACKNOWLEDGMENTS

This work was supported by contract No. N01-CO-75380 with the National Cancer Institute, National Institutes of Health, Bethesda, Maryland 20205.

REFERENCES

1. Miller, E.C., and J.A. Miller. 1976. The metabolism of chemical carcinogens to reactive electrophiles and their possible mechanisms of action in carcinogenesis. In: Chemical Carcinogens. ACS Monograph 173. C.E. Searle, ed. American Chemical Society: Washington, DC. pp. 737-762.

2. Pullman, A., and B. Pullman. 1955. Electronic structure and carcinogenic activity of aromatic molecules. In: Advances in Cancer Research, Volume 3. J.P. Greenstein, and A. Haddow, eds. Academic Press: London. pp. 117-169.

3. Sims, P., and P.L. Grover. 1974. Epoxides in polycyclic aromatic hydrocarbon metabolism and carcinogenesis. In: Advances in Cancer Research, Volume 20. G. Klein, S. Weinhouse, and A. Haddow, eds. Academic Press: London. pp. 165-274.

4. Dipple, A. 1976. Polynuclear aromatic carcinogens. In: Chemical Carcinogens. ACS Monograph 173. C.E. Searle, Ed. American Chemical Society: Washington, DC. pp. 245-314.

5. Baird, W.M., A. Dipple, P.L. Grover, P. Sims, and P. Brookes. 1973. Studies on the formation of hydrocarbon-deoxyribonucleoside products by the binding of derivatives of 7-methylbenz[a]anthracene to DNA in aqueous solution and in mouse embryo cells in culture. Cancer Res. 33:2386-2392.

6. Borgen, A., H. Darvey, N. Castagnoli, T.T. Crocker, R.E. Rasmussen, and I.Y. Wang. 1973. Metabolic conversion of benzo[a]pyrene by Syrian hamster liver microsomes and binding of metabolites to deoxyribonucleic acid. J. Med. Chem. 16:502-506.

7. Sims, P., P.L. Grover, A. Swaisland, P. Pal, and A. Hewer. 1974. Metabolic activation of benzo[a]pyrene proceeds by a diol-epoxide. Nature 252:326-328.

8. Levin, W., A.W. Wood, P.G. Wislocki, R.L. Chang, J. Kapitulnik, H.D. Mah, Y. Yagi, D.M. Jerina, and A.H. Conney. 1978. Mutagenicity and carcinogenicity of benzo[a]pyrene and benzo[a]pyrene derivatives. In: Polycyclic Hydrocarbons and Cancer: Environment, Chemistry, and Metabolism, Volume 1. H.V. Gelboin, and P.O.P. Ts'o, eds. Academic Press: New York. pp. 189-202.

9. Baird, W.M., and A. Dipple. 1977. Photosensitivity of DNA-bound 7,12-dimethylbenz[a]anthracene. Int. J. Cancer 20:427-431.

10. Moschel, R.C., W.M. Baird, and A. Dipple. 1977. Metabolic activation of the carcinogen 7,12-dimethylbenz[a]anthracene for DNA binding. Biochem. Biophys. Res. Comm. 76:1092-1098.

11. Bigger, C.A.H., J.E. Tomaszewski, and A. Dipple. 1978. Differences between products of binding of 7,12-dimethylbenz[a]anthracene to DNA in mouse skin and in a rat liver microsomal system. Biochem. Biophys. Res. Comm. 80:229-235.

12. Dipple, A., and J.A. Nebzydoski. 1978. Evidence for the involvement of a diol-epoxide in the binding of 7,12-dimethylbenz[a]anthracene to DNA in cells in culture. Chem.-Biol. Interact. 20:17-26.

13. Moschel, R.C., W.R. Hudgins, and A. Dipple. 1979. Fluorescence of hydrocarbon-deoxyribonucleoside adducts. Chem.-Biol. Interact. 27:69-79.

14. Dipple, A., J.E. Tomaszewski, R.C. Moschel, C.A.H. Bigger, J.A. Nebzydoski, and M. Egan. 1979. Comparison of metabolism-mediated binding to DNA of 7-hydroxymethyl-12-methylbenz[a]anthracene and 7,12-dimethylbenz[a]anthracene. Cancer Res. 39:1154-1158.

15. Baird, W.M., and P. Brookes. 1973. Isolation of the hydrocarbon-deoxyribonucleoside products from the DNA of mouse embryo cells treated in culture with 7-methylbenz[a]anthracene-^{3}H. Cancer Res. 33:2378-2385.

16. Meehan, T., K. Straub, and M. Calvin. 1977. Benzo[a]pyrene diol-epoxide covalently binds to deoxyguanosine and deoxyadenosine in DNA. Nature 269:725-727.

17. King, H.W.S., M.H. Thompson, and P. Brookes. 1975. The benzo[a]pyrene deoxyribonucleoside products isolated from DNA after metabolism of benzo[a]pyrene by rat liver microsomes in the presence of DNA. Cancer Res. 34:1263-1269.

18. Bigger, C.A.H., J.E. Tomaszewski, and A. Dipple. 1980. Variation in route of microsomal activation of 7,12-dimethylbenz[a]anthracene with substrate concentration. Carcinogenesis 1:15-20.

19. Ames, B.N., J.McCann, and E. Yamasaki. 1975. Methods for detecting carcinogens and mutagens with the *Salmonella*/mammalian-microsome mutagenicity test. Mutat. Res. 31:347-364.

20. Bigger, C.A.H., J.E. Tomaszewski, A.W. Andrews, and A. Dipple. 1980. Evaluation of metabolic activation of 7,12-dimethylbenz[a]anthracene *in vitro* by Aroclor 1254-induced rat liver S9 fraction. Cancer Res. 40:655-661.

21. Bigger, C.A.H., J.E. Tomaszewski, A. Dipple, and R.S. Lake. 1980. Limitations of metabolic activation systems used with *in vitro* tests for carcinogens. Science 209:503-505.

DISCUSSION

Q.: Dr. Bigger, you looked at the Aroclor-induced S9; have you ever tried phenobarbital or uninduced S9, and if so, can you get enough binding with those to study the adducts?

A.: Yes, I'm currently looking at phenobarbital-induced and uninduced microsomes. With these systems, I don't see the qualitative shifts in adduct formation with DMBA concentration that I saw with the Aroclor induced system. Binding to DNA occurs almost completely through the K-region epoxide of DMBA at high or low concentrations of DMBA.

Q.: Could you perhaps comment on why the microsomal systems do not simulate the *in vivo* situations. Is it that competing pathways which may be suppressed *in vivo* are active *in vitro*, or are you losing enzymes in the microsome isolation procedure, such as nuclear membrane enzymes?

A.: Well, I think there are a number of possible reasons, and you just mentioned some of them. Basically, one is disrupting the organization that exists in the cell and this could be altering critical spatial relationship of different enzymes in the pathway. You could be altering the absolute levels of enzymes and diluting or discarding co-factors. Probably all of these things are happening. And the result could easily be a distortion of the balance between activation and detoxification pathways which exists in the cell.

Nuclear enzyme activation appears to be qualitatively similar to microsomal, so it seems unlikely that loss of these enzymes could account for the difference. However, there may be a role played by nuclear activation. If so, the fact that in the cell the activation occurs in close proximity to the DNA may be important, because, in the cell, certain metabolites may be prevented from reacting with DNA by selective trapping or transport out of the cell. In contrast, in a test-tube mixture of DNA and microsomes presumably all reactive metabolites would have access to the DNA.

CELL SPECIFICITY IN DNA DAMAGE AND REPAIR

James A. Swenberg[1], Mary A. Bedell[1], Kathryn C. Billings[1], and James G. Lewis[2]

[1]Department of Pathology, Chemical Industry Institute of Toxicology, Research Triangle Park, North Carolina 22709 and [2]Department of Pathology, Duke University Medical Center, Durham, North Carolina 27710

INTRODUCTION

Many animal models for organ-specific neoplasia have been developed and used to investigate the pathogenesis of cancer. Studies dealing with morphologic aspects of this disease process have frequently concentrated on target cells. In contrast, most biochemical studies have employed whole organ homogenates even though tumors only develop from specific subpopulations of the target organ. For example, hepatocytes are the target cell for nitrosodiethylamine (DEN), 2-acetylaminofluorene, and dinitrotoluene, while sinusoidal lining cells represent the primary targets for vinyl chloride and 1,2-dimethylhydrazine (SDMH). Although hepatocytes comprise more than 90% of the liver's mass, they account for only 60 to 70% of its cells. The nonparenchymal cells (NPC) account for the remaining 30 to 40% of the cells and 10 to 20% of the DNA. Thus, localization of carcinogen metabolism or DNA damage and repair within susceptible and nonsusceptible cell populations requires separation of cell types.

We recently reported differential capacities for the repair of O^6-methylguanine (O^6-MG) in DNA of rat hepatocytes and NPC following oral administration of carbon 14-labeled [^{14}C]SDMH (1). Hepatocytes and NPC were collected by centrifugal elutriation, a technique that separates different cell populations on the basis of cell volume and density (2,3). Using this method, subpopulations of hepatocytes and NPC each of 95% or greater purity were separated from a mixed-cell suspension derived from collagenase perfusion of whole livers. Bile duct cells and connective tissue remained in the undigested portion of the liver. DNA was isolated from the target (NPC) and nontarget (hepatocyte) cell populations using hydroxyapatite chromatography. The DNA was dialyzed and concentrated by ultrafiltration and hydrolyzed in 0.1 N HCl at 80°C for 30 min. The purines were then separated using Sephasorb HP (Pharmacia, Piscataway, NJ) chromatography. The results are shown in Table 1.

Hepatocytes had slightly higher initial levels (at 2 h) of alkylation at both the O^6 and N-7 position of guanine. Comparable amounts of 7-methylguanine (7-MG) were lost from hepatocytes and NPC during the first 24 h after dosing with [^{14}C]SDMH. In contrast, 90% of the O^6-MG was removed from hepatocyte DNA, while only 46% was removed from NPC. This difference resulted in O^6:N-7 ratios of 0.011 for hepatocytes and 0.067 for NPC. When a second dose of [^{14}C]SDMH was administered 24 h after initial exposure and the rats were killed at 48 h, little O^6-MG was detected in hepatocytes. In contrast to hepatocytes at 48 h, a cumulative increase in O^6-MG was observed in NPC. Differential accumulation of 7-MG was also noted in the two cell populations, with less 7-MG occurring in NPC than in hepatocytes. The resulting differences in the O^6:N-7 ratios were even greater with NPC having a 28-fold higher ratio. The loss of 7-MG from NPC DNA may represent loss due to cell death or dilution of the alkylation product with newly synthesized DNA. Further support for selective cytotoxicity and cell replication is provided by the marked increase in metabolic incorporation of [^{14}C] from SDMH into normal purines (Table 1), an indication of DNA synthesis. Thus, the target cell for carcinogenesis had similar initial levels of DNA alkylation, deficient repair of the promutagenic lesion of O^6-MG, and increased cell replication due to cytotoxicity. This progression should lead to greater "fixation" of mutations due to mispairing in the target cell rather than the nontarget cell.

To more critically evaluate the influence of promutagenic DNA damage and cell replication in carcinogenesis, we examined the extent of alkylation and DNA replication during chronic administration of SDMH and DEN. Male F-344 rats were given SDMH continuously in the drinking water at 3 mg/kg/day, a regimen that induces malignant hemangioendotheliomas of the liver (4,5) or drinking water containing 40 ppm DEN, a regimen that induces hepatocellular carcinomas (6). These protocols allowed us to critically compare the responses of target and nontarget cells in the target organ, under exposure conditions that yield cell-specific carcinogenesis.

METHODS AND RESULTS

Cell Replication Studies

Rats were exposed to the carcinogen via their drinking water for 0, 1.5, 4, 8, or 16 days. On the day of sacrifice, a 300-mg

Table 1. Alkylation of Hepatocyte and NPC DNA Following Oral Exposure of Rats to (^{14}C)SDMH[a].

Cell Type	No. of Doses	Time of Posttreatment (h)	Alkylation of DNA/10^6 Guanine			Metabolic Incorporation of [^{14}C] from [^{14}C]SDMH	
			O^6-MG	7-MG	O^6:7-MG	Guanine (DPM/μM)	Adenine (DPM/μM)
Hepatocyte	1	2	89.0 ± 7.5[b]	1032 ± 70	.086	N.D.[c]	N.D.
NPC	1	2	65.4 ± 8.4	783 ± 78	.083	N.D.	N.D.
Hepatocyte	1	24	8.9 ± 2.5	753 ± 80	.011	7.6 ± 7.7	18.3 ± 10.4
NPC	1	24	34.6 ± 0.7	525 ± 60	.067	79.4 ± 46.8	78.7 ± 15.3
Hepatocyte	2[d]	48	4.6 ± 3.6	1362 ± 54	.003	8.1 ± 8.1	21.5 ± 13.6
NPC	2	48	56.3 ± 4.3	689 ± 90	.085	375.6 ± 35.9	369.3 ± 53.8

[a]Reference 1.
[b]Mean ± standard error of three rats.
[c]N.D. = not detectable.
[d]Second dose administered 24 h after first.

pellet of bromodeoxyuridine (BrdU) was implanted subcutaneously. Five hourly injections of [^{3}H]thymidine (0.5 μCi/g) were administered intraperitoneally beginning 1 h later. One hour after the fifth injection of [^{3}H]thymidine, animals were anesthetized with phenobarbital, their livers perfused with collagenase solution, the hepatocytes and NPC separated, and DNA isolated as previously described (1). The DNA was then subjected to cesium chloride density gradient ultracentrifugation to separate BrdU-labeled DNA, representing scheduled DNA synthesis, from normal density DNA and any repair synthesis. Examples of gradient profiles are shown in Figure 1, and a summary of such data for SDMH and DEN is presented in Figure 2. A marked increase in NPC replication resulted from chronic administration of SDMH. A much lesser response was exhibited by the nontarget cell, the hepatocyte. Increased labeling of normal density DNA with [^{3}H]thymidine was demonstrated only in hepatocytes and is thought to represent unscheduled DNA repair synthesis. The extent of cell replication increased moderately in both the hepatocyte and the NPC following similar administration of DEN.

Chronic Alkylation Studies

Additional rats were similarly exposed to SDMH for chronic DNA alkylation studies. Since the cost of using radioisotopes for such studies would be prohibitive, we modifed the cation exchange high-pressure liquid chromatography method of Herron and Shank (7) and analyzed the levels of guanine, adenine, and 7-MG with ultraviolet absorbance (254 nm) and O^{6}-MG using fluorescence spectrophotometry. Hepatocytes consistently had higher levels of 7-MG than did NPC (see Figure 3). A decrease in 7-MG levels was evident after 4 days of SDMH administration. This decrease was followed by increased levels of 7-MG at 8 days and a slow decline thereafter. Subsequent experiments using a somewhat lower dose of SDMH (30 ppm) confirmed these data; however, the decrease occurred at 6 days and was less pronounced (8). The exact mechanisms involved in these changes are unknown. The lower levels of 7-MG may be due to a wave of cell necrosis, followed by compensatory cell replication. It may also be due to decreased water consumption, which would result in a lower exposure. The secondary increase occurred after readjusting the concentration of SDMH in the drinking water to achieve the targeted dose of 3 mg/kg/day. From this increase and the subsequent study, a slow decrease in 7-MG seems to occur between 8 and 28 days. The failure to achieve a true steady state may reflect partial induction of DNA repair enzymes for the removal of 7-MG (9,10,11).

In contrast to 7-MG, O^{6}-MG levels were always greater in the target cell for SDMH carcinogenesis, the NPC (see Figure 4). Hepatocyte levels of O^{6}-MG were greatest after 1.5 days of exposure

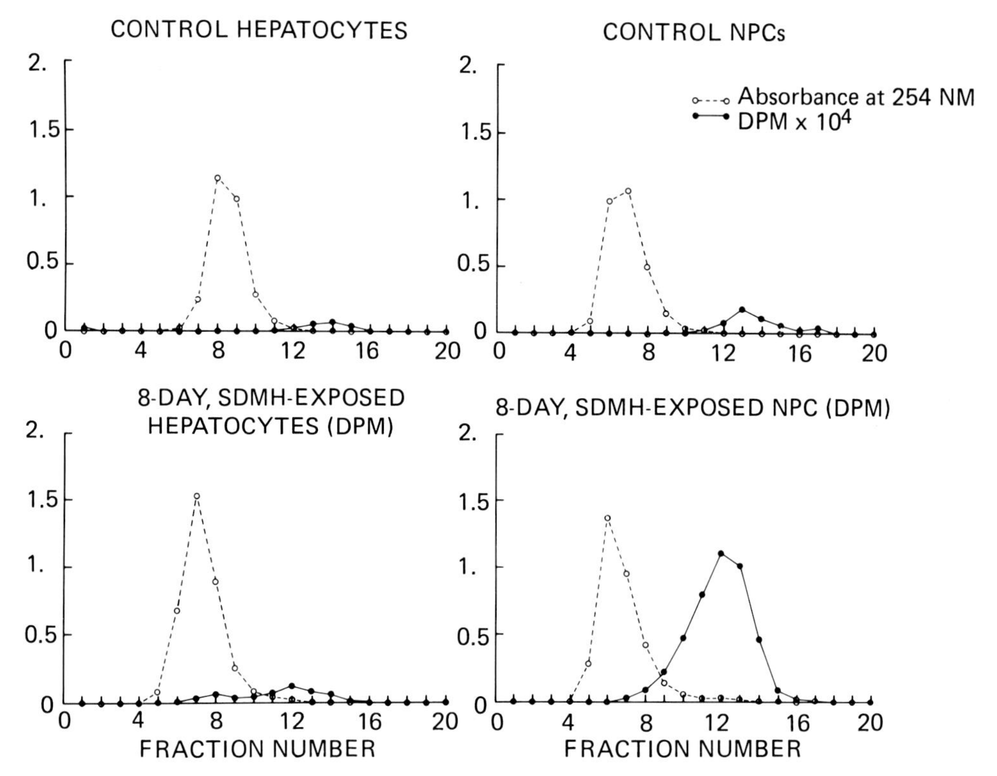

Figure 1. UV absorbance and radioactivity profiles of DNA from control and 8-day SDMH-exposed hepatocytes and NPC subjected to cesium chloride density gradient ultracentrifugation.

and decreased thereafter. In fact, O^6-MG was not detectable in hepatocytes at 4, 16, or 28 days. The values shown in Figures 4 through 6 assume the normalized limits of detection (5 pmol/injection) per milligram DNA on these days. We have subsequently increased the limit of detection at least 10-fold and can now demonstrate low levels of O^6-MG (~1 pmol/mg DNA) in hepatocytes through 28 days (8). A decrease in O^6-MG similar to that of 7-MG was evident at 4 days of exposure. The greatest amount of alkylation at the O^6 position of guanine was evident in NPC after 8 days of SDMH administration. Levels of O^6-MG in NPC decreased between 8 and 28 days. This decrease may be the result of O^6-demethylase induction (12-16).

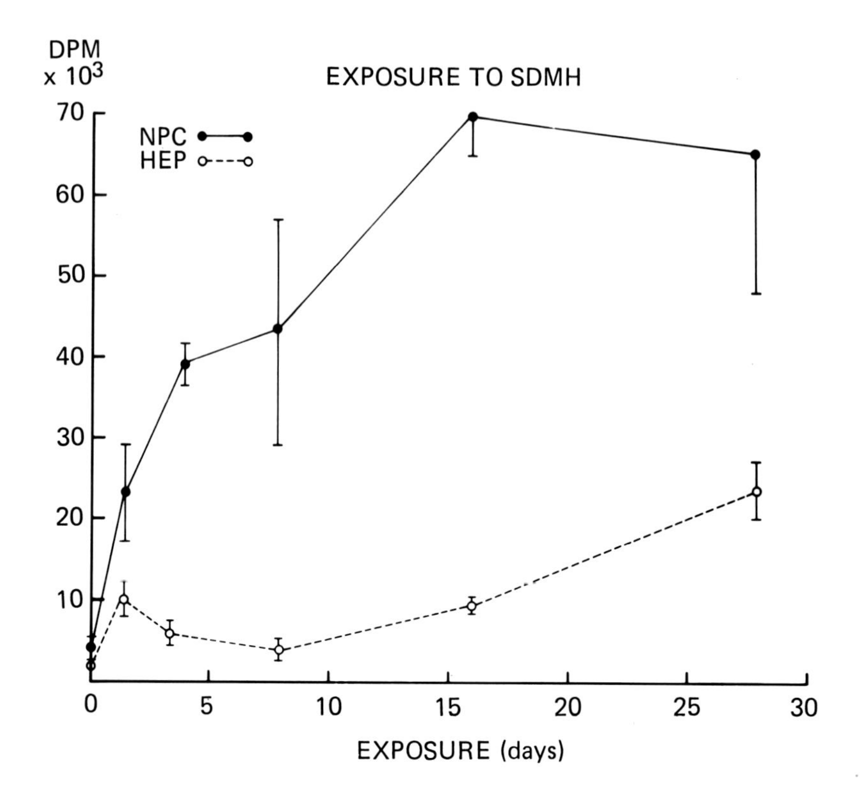

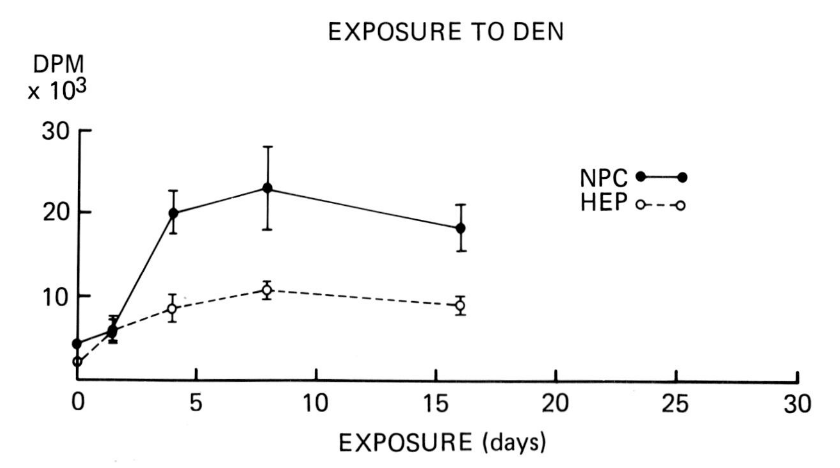

Figure 2. Differential effects of SDMH and DEN exposure on cell replication. Each point represents the mean ± S.E.M. for three rats.

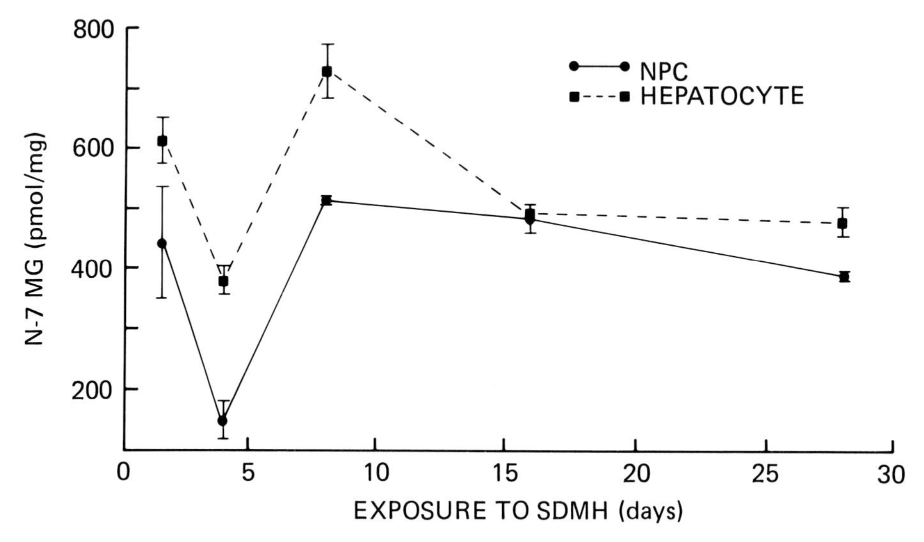

Figure 3. Levels of 7-MG in hepatocyte and NPC DNA following exposure to 3 mg/kg/day SDMH for up to 28 days.

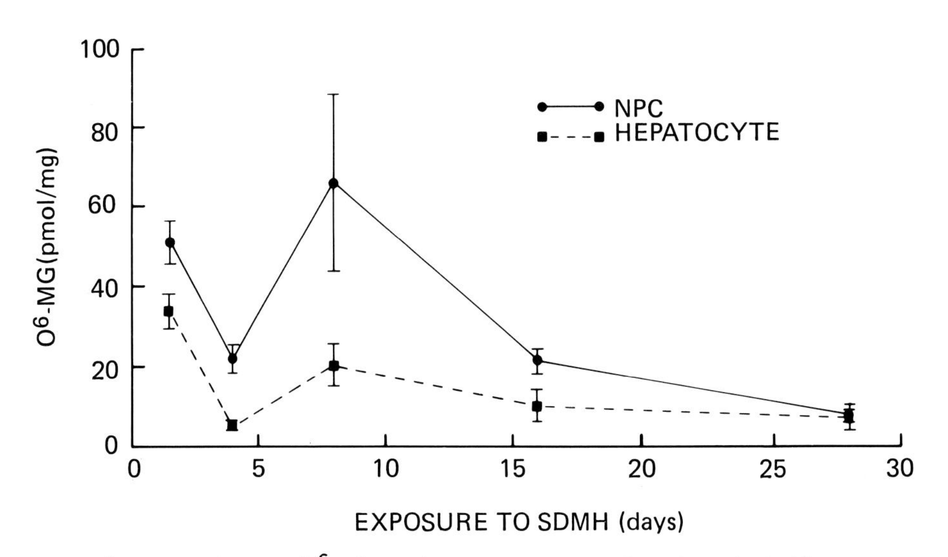

Figure 4. Levels of O^6-MG in hepatocytes and NPC DNA following exposure to 3 mg/kg/day SDMH for up to 28 days. Data for hepatocytes at days 4, 16, and 28 are presented as the maximum possible using the detection limit of 5 pmol/injection and normalizing the data per milligram.

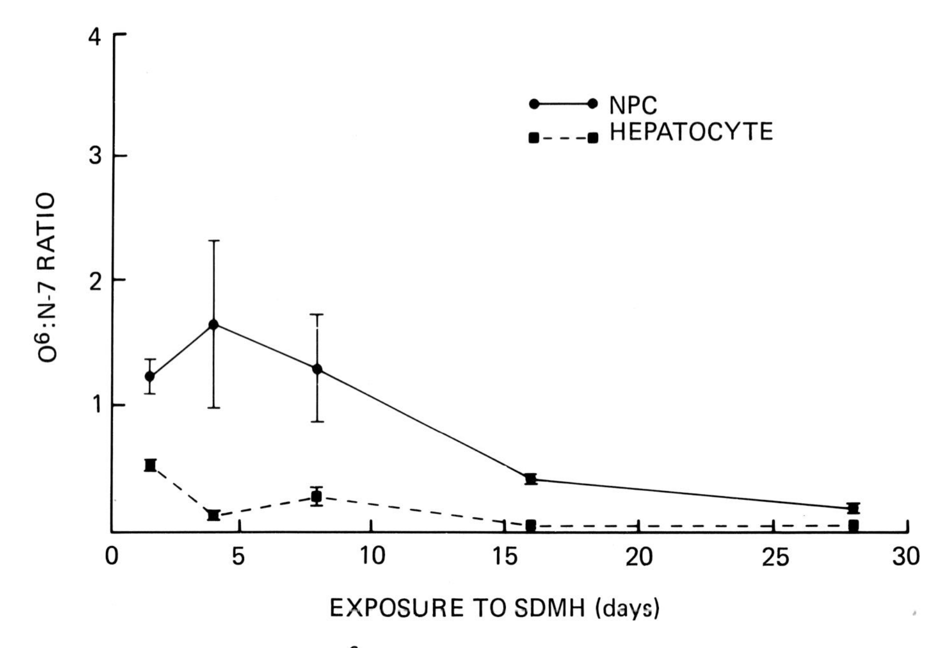

Figure 5. Ratios of O ^{6}:N-7 for hepatocyte and NPC DNA following continuous SDMH exposure for up to 28 days.

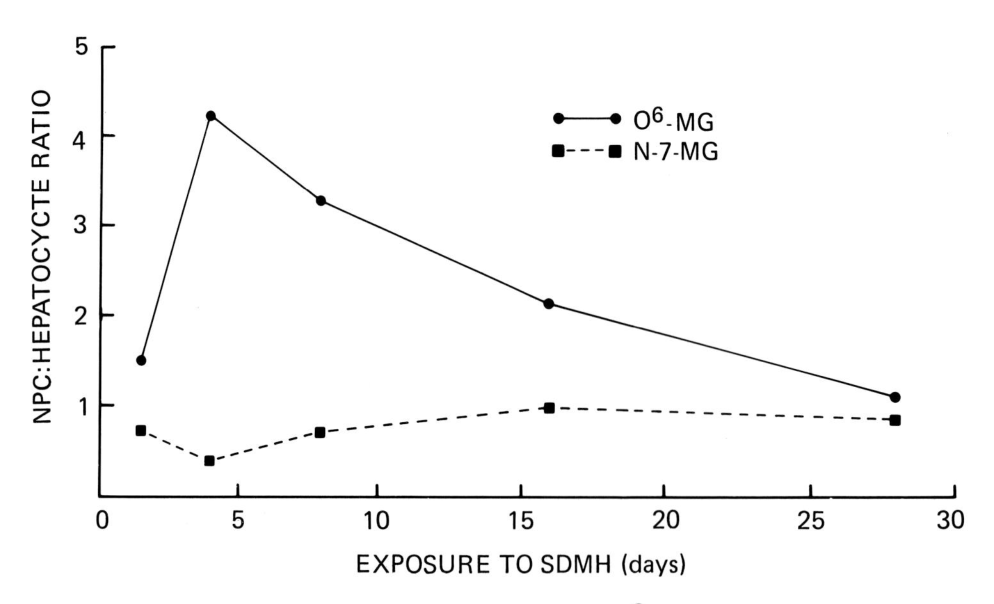

Figure 6. Ratios of NPC:hepatocyte for O ^{6}-MG and 7-MG in DNA following continuous SDMH exposure.

Distinct differences in formation and removal of DNA alkylation products exist between the target (NPC) and nontarget (hepatocyte) cell. Figure 5 compares the O^6-MG:7-MG ratios for hepatocytes and NPC. Clearly, hepatocytes are much more efficient at removing O^6-MG than are NPC. The decreasing O^6-MG:7-MG ratio in both cell types supports induction of repair systems for O^6-MG removal. Figure 6 illustrates the NPC:hepatocyte ratios for O^6-MG and 7-MG. Whereas the ratio is approximately 1 for 7-MG, it is several-fold greater for O^6-MG.

CONCLUSIONS

Our working hypothesis states that cell replication in the presence of promutagenic DNA damage results in a mutational, initiating event and initiation followed by promotion leads to carcinogenesis. Assuming that O^6-MG is the major promutagenic adduct and using the cell replication and alkylation data obtained during chronic SDMH administration, we can now examine our basic hypothesis for target and nontarget cell populations.

Figure 7 illustrates this relationship for hepatocytes and NPC following SDMH administration. The "initiation index" is expressed for each cell population as the normalized replication index (DPM in heavy DNA per milligram total DNA times picomoles O^6-MG per milligram DNA). Clearly, the potential for initiation is markedly greater in the target cell than in the nontarget cell. Furthermore, the data suggest that even though carcinogenicity requires chronic exposure for months to years, the vast majority of initiation may be confined to the first weeks of administration. If subsequent carcinogen exposure is necessary for tumor formation, the additional exposure may exert its primary effect through promotion. In view of recent advances in our understanding of hepatic promotion (17,18), it should now be possible to evaluate the promoting abilities of simple alkylating agents.

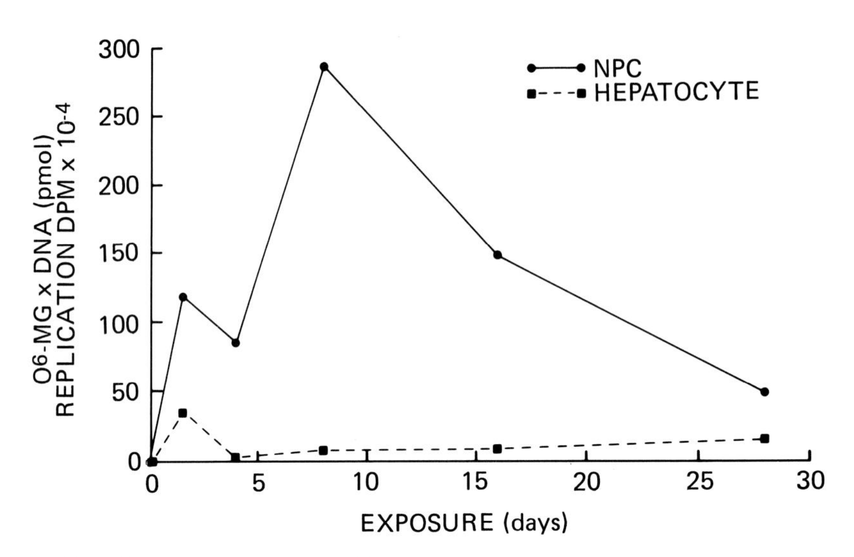

Figure 7. "Initiation index" for NPC and hepatocytes during a 28-day exposure to 3 mg/kg/day SDMH in drinking water.

REFERENCES

1. Lewis, J.G., and J.A. Swenberg. 1980. Differential repair of O^6-methylguanine in DNA of rat hepatocytes and nonparenchymal cells. Nature 288:185-187.

2. Sanderson, R.J., and K.E. Bird. 1977. Cell separations by counterflow centrifugation. In: Methods in Cell Biology, Volume 15. D.M. Prescott, ed. Academic Press: New York. pp. 1-14.

3. Wisse, E., and D.L. Knook. 1979. The investigation of sinusoidal cells: A new approach to the study of liver function. In: Progress in Liver Disease, Volume VI. H. Popper and F. Schaffner, eds. Grune and Stratton: New York. pp. 153-171.

4. Druckrey, H. 1972. Organospecific carcinogenesis in the digestive tract. In: Topics in Chemical Carcinogenesis. W. Nakahara, S. Takayama, T. Sugimura, and S. Odashima, eds. University Park Press: Tokyo. pp. 73-101.

5. Druckrey, H. 1970. Production of colon carcinomas by 1,2-dialkylhydrazines and azoalkanes. In: Carcinoma of the Colon and Antecedent Epithelium. W.J. Burdette, ed. Charles C. Thomas: Springfield. pp. 267-279.

6. Weisburger, J.H., R.M. Madison, J.M. Ward, C. Viguera, and E.K. Weisburger. 1975. Modification of diethylnitrosamine liver carcinogenesis with phenobarbital but not with immunosuppression. J. Natl. Cancer Inst. 54:1185-1188.

7. Herron, D.C., and R.C. Shank. 1979. Quantitative high pressure liquid chromatographic analysis of methylated purines in DNA of rats treated with chemical carcinogens. Anal. Biochem. 100:58-63.

8. Lewis, J.G., M.A. Bedell, K.C. Billings, and J.A. Swenberg. 1981. Differences in DNA alkylation, repair and replication in hepatocytes and nonparenchymal cells (NPC) following chronic administration of 1,2-dimethylhydrazine (SDMH). Proc. Am. Assoc. for Cancer Res. 22:75.

9. Laval, J., J. Pierre, and F. Laval. 1981. Release of 7-methylguanine residues from alkylated DNA by extracts of _Micrococcus luteus_ and _Escherichia coli_. Proc. Natl. Acad. Sci. 58:852-855.

10. Singer, B., and T.P. Brent. 1981. Human lymphoblasts contain DNA glycosylase activity excising N-3 and N-7 methyl and ethyl purines but not O^6-alkylguanines or 1-alkyladenines. Proc. Natl. Acad. Sci. 78:856-860.

11. Margison, G.P., and A.E. Pegg. 1981. Enzymatic release of 7-methylguanine from methylated DNA by rodent liver extracts. Proc. Natl. Acad. Sci. 78:861-865.

12. Pegg, A.E. 1978. Enzymatic removal of O^6-methylguanine from DNA by mammalian cell extracts. Biochem. Biophys. Res. Comm. 84:166-173.

13. Pegg, A.E., and G. Hui. 1978. Formation and subsequent removal of O^6-methylguanine from deoxyribonucleic acid in rat liver and kidney after small doses of dimethylnitrosamine. Biochem. J. 173:739-748.

14. Pegg, A.E. 1980. Formation and subsequent repair of alkylation lesions in tissues of rodents treated with nitrosamines. Arch. Toxicol. Suppl. 3:55-68.

15. Montesano, R., H. Brisel, G. Planche-Martel, G.P. Margison, and A.E. Pegg. 1980. The effect of chronic treatment of rats with dimethylnitrosamine on the removal of O^6-methylguanine from DNA. Cancer Res. 40:452-458.

16. Medcalf, A.S.C., and P.D. Lawley. 1981. Time course of O^6-methylguanine removal from DNA of N-methyl-N-nitrosourea-treated human fibroblasts. Nature 289:796-798.

17. Farber, E. 1980. The sequential analysis of liver cancer induction. Biochim. Biophys. Acta 605:149-166.

18. Pitot, H.C., and A.E. Sirica. 1980. The stages of initiation and promotion in hepatocarcinogenesis. Biochim. Biophys. Acta 605:191-215.

DISCUSSION

Q.: Can I argue with your speculation? I think it's very interesting; however, you have to be very careful to make enough measurements. If you're only making measurements of O^6-methylguanine every 12 h or every 24 h, you may underestimate the amounts of potential insult.

What you really ought to do is integrate the area under the curve.

A.: We're looking at the total amount of O^6 that's present in animals that are continuously exposed, duplicating the exposure that induces the tumors.

We're taking these animals in the morning, and rat notoriously have greater activity in drinking and feeding during the evening, so we're really looking at some of the highest levels of alkylation that are present.

Q.: I'm really not sure that you know that because I think if you look just a few minutes after the animal had drunk, then you would find some.

A.: What I think is happening is that we're maintaining an induced state of demethylase activity, so that O^6-methylguanine is removed almost as fast as it's formed. It is true that the more data points one has, the better the estimate will be.

Q.: On your promotion theory, I'm wondering if the DMH repetitive treatment couldn't itself be the promoting agent. I'd like to ask a general question: Has anyone ever shown that nitrosamines do or don't have promoting activity in any of the systems?

A.: I clearly agree with you that the DMH may be a promoting agent. The question is, which effect of DMH? Is it the 7-methylguanine? Is it toxicity due to protein alkylation? We really don't know yet, but I think that we need to investigate the questions. Nitrosamines can probably act as promoting agents, initiating agents, or complete carcinogens. I can't cite any specific investigations of their promoting potential, however.

DNA ADDUCT FORMATION AND REMOVAL IN N-ACETOXY-2-ACETYLAMINOFLUORENE-EXPOSED CULTURED CELLS AND IN ORGANS FROM RATS FED 2-ACETYLAMINOFLUORENE

Miriam C. Poirier[1], Stuart H. Yuspa[1], B'Ann True[2], and Brian A. Laishes[2]

[1]Laboratory of Experimental Pathology, National Cancer Institute, Bethesda, Maryland 20205, and [2]McArdle Laboratory for Cancer Research, University of Wisconsin Medical School, Madison, Wisconsin 53709

INTRODUCTION

The development of carcinogen DNA-adduct antibodies has made possible a new approach to investigate carcinogen-DNA interactions (1). To quantitate adducts of a particular carcinogen, highly-avid rabbit antibodies have been employed to allow detection by radioimmunoassay (RIA) of one adduct in 10^5 DNA bases (1). The studies described here employed the antiserum anti-guanosin-(8-yl)-acetylaminofluorene (anti-G-8-AAF) elicited against the nucleoside-adduct coupled covalently to bovine serum albumin and injected into rabbits (2). The antiserum is specific for the acetylated and deacetylated C-8 adducts of 2-acetylamino-fluorene (2-AAF) with DNA (dG-8-AAF and dG-8-AF) (see Figure 1). It does not cross-react with the minor adduct, 3-deoxyguanison-(N^2-yl)-acetylaminofluorene (dG-N^2-AAF) (see Figure 1), the carcinogen alone, or DNA (2,3). Since the C-8 adducts comprise the major proportion (80 to 90%) of adducts formed upon interaction of 2-AAF, or its activated derivative N-acetoxy-2-acetylaminofluorene (N-Ac-AAF) with DNA *in vivo* (3,4,5), the anti-G-8-AAF was considered appropriate for initial studies. The antibody has been utilized to distinguish between the acetylated and deacetylated C-8 adducts of 2-AAF in DNA, and to quantitate the proportions of each in DNA extracted from either cultured cells exposed to N-Ac-AAF or from livers and kidneys of male rats fed 2-AAF.

N-(Deoxyguanosin-8-yl)-2-Acetylaminofluorene
(dG-8-AAF)

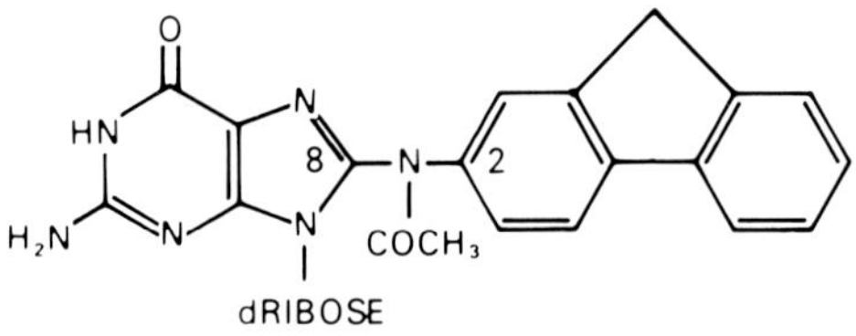

N-(Deoxyguanosin-8-yl)-2-Aminofluorene
(dG-8-AF)

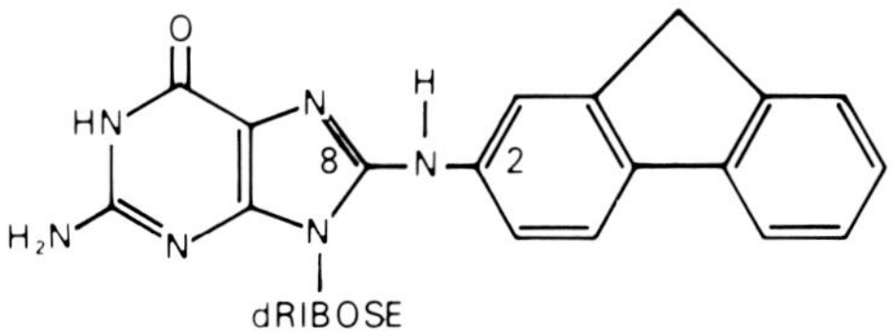

3-(Deoxyguanosin-N^2-yl)-2-Acetylaminofluorene
(dG-N^2-AAF)

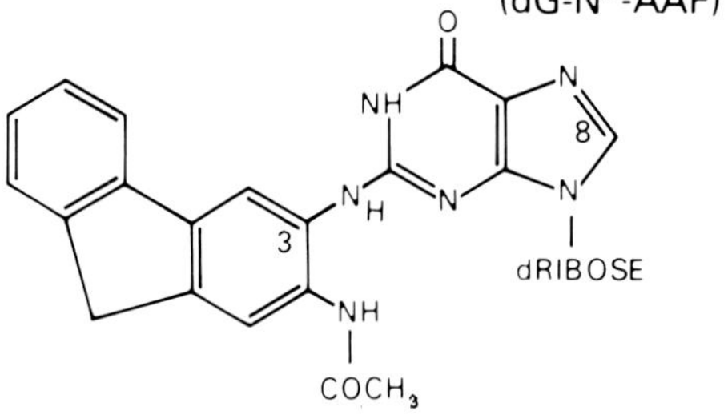

1-[6-(2,5-Diamino-4-Oxypyrimidinyl-N^6-Deoxyriboside)]-3-(2-Fluorenyl)Urea
(Diamino-Py-FU)

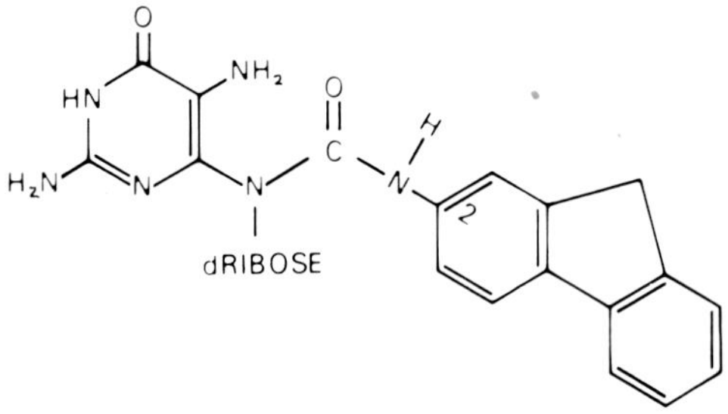

Figure 1. Structures of the adducts formed *in vivo* and *in vitro* upon interaction of 2-AAF or N-Ac-AAF with DNA.

MATERIALS AND METHODS

Cell Cultures

Details concerning primary culture preparation, cultured cell maintenance, and exposure techniques for various pharmacologic agents (including the carcinogen N-Ac-AAF) have been published (6). The preparation of DNA from cultured cells has been described in detail (7) and is basically similar to that outlined below for rat tissues.

Animals and Diets

Young adult male Wistar-Furth rats, weighing 130 to 150 g, were obtained from Microbiological Associates, Bethesda, MD. Groups of 3 to 4 rats were housed in hanging wire or plastic cages. All animals were maintained on a 12-h light cycle (7:00 AM to 7:00 PM), permitted free access to tap water, and fed the standard control diet *ad libitum* until they reached a mean body weight of 185 to 188 g (inclusive) with a standard deviation of no more than ±8 g.

All animals on a control diet received the purified, semi-synthetic basal diet Bio-Mix No. 101 (Bio-Serv, Inc., Frenchtown, NJ). The composition of the diet has been described (8).

2-AAF (m.p. 192 to 196°C, Aldrich Chemical Co., Milwaukee, WI) was added to the control diet (Bio-Mix No. 101) at a concentration of 0.02% (w/w).

Preparation of DNA from Rat Tissues

Tissues were homogenized in 0.32 M sucrose containing 0.001 M potassium phosphate (pH 7.5), 0.0015 M calcium chloride and 1% Triton X-100 with a Polytron homogenizer. Homogenized samples were prepared for cesium chloride isopycnic centrifugation and centrifuged as previously described (7). After fractionation of the gradients, absorbance for each tube was read at λ260 and the DNA-containing fractions were pooled and dialyzed against deionized water. The amount of DNA was determined by absorbance at λ260 and a portion was taken for enzymatic hydrolysis and RIA. Adducts frozen in the unhydrolyzed condition were stable for several months.

Radioimmunoassay

Procedures for synthesizing all adducts for both immunization and RIAs, immunization procedure details, and characterizing antibody specificity have been described previously (2,7). DNA samples for RIA were denatured and hydrolyzed by S_1 nuclease. (See reference 3 for discussion of DNA hydrolysis and performance of the RIAs.)

Two types of RIA have been employed in experiments described in this report. First, equal amounts of the same DNA were assayed simultaneously with [^{3}H]G-8-AAF and [^{3}H]G-8-AF, and the binding levels were determined by comparison with appropriate standard curves. The difference in percent inhibition observed in the two assays is defined as percent inhibition with [^{3}H]G-8-AF minus percent inhibition with [^{3}H]G-8-AAF. It indicates the degree of deacetylation (6): the larger the difference in percent inhibition is, the larger the proportion of deacetylated adduct in the mixture is. Second, increasing amounts of modified DNA competing against [^{3}H]G-8-AAF as tracer was assessed. When standard unlabeled dG-8-AF competes against [^{3}H]G-8-AAF at an antibody dilution of 1:24000, a saturation of the inhibition profile occurs around 40% inhibition (see Figure 2) (3). Standard mixtures of acetylated and deacetylated adducts have been shown to saturate at higher percentage inhibition levels, the magnitude of increase being proportional to the percentage of dG-8-AAF in the mixture (6). A precise quantitation of the proportion of acetylated and deacetylated C-8 adducts is obtained using a linear regression equation with a particular DNA competition profile assayed simultaneously with appropriate standards (6,9).

RESULTS

Sensitivity and Specificity of the G-8-AAF Antiserum

Four months after initial immunization of rabbits with G-8-AAF, all three rabbits produced antibodies of similar characteristics with affinity constants in the range of 10^9 l/mol. The antibodies did not cross-react with deoxyguanosine, DNA, 2-AAF, 2-aminofluorene (2-AF), N-Ac-AAF, dG-N^2-AAF or the ring-opened deacetylated adduct 1[6-(2,5 diamino-4-oxypyrimidinyl-N^6-deoxyriboside)]-3(2-fluorenyl)urea (diamino-Py-Fu) (Figure 1) (10). With a [^{3}H]G-8-AAF tracer competing against dG-8-AAF as inhibitor, 50% inhibition was observed at 06. pmol under non-equilibrium conditions (see Figure 2). A similar, but slightly less sensitive curve is obtained at the same antibody concentration with a [^{3}H]G-8-AF tracer competing against dG-8-AF (data not shown), indicating that antiserum has near equivalent

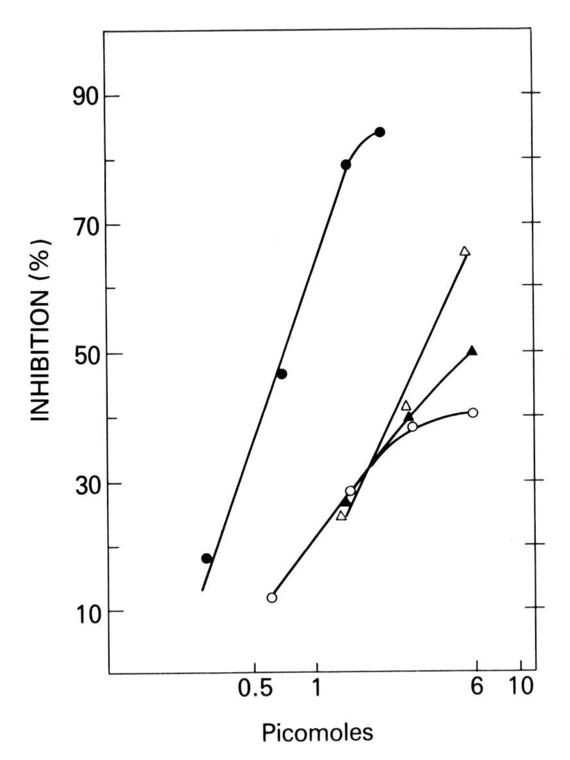

Figure 2. RIA standard curves (non-equilibrium conditions, final serum dilution 1:2400) in competition assay with [^{3}H]G-8-AAF and a series of mixtures of nonradioactive dG-8-AAF and/or dG-8-AF. The curves are as follows: ● --- ●, dG-8-AAF; O --- O, dG-8-AF; Δ --- Δ, 8.7% dG-8-AAF, 91.3% dG-8-AF; ▲ --- ▲, 5% dG-8-AAF, 95% dG-8-AF.

affinity for the acetylated and deacetylated C-8 adducts (3). The sensitivity limit of the assay is defined by the maximum amount of DNA that can be added to each tube without giving substantial nonspecific inhibition. Using an equivalent amount of control DNA added to the standard curve tubes, it is possible to accurately assay tubes with as much as 40 μg of DNA, bringing the lower sensitivity limits in the range of 10 fmol/μg DNA.

A most interesting feature of antibody specificity is that only a portion of the antibody population is truly specific for both acetylated and deacetylated adducts. In cross-competition assays with the acetylated adduct as tracer and the deacetylated adduct as inhibitor, a saturation of the inhibition curve occurs at about 40% inhibition (see Figure 2), and has proven to be a useful property of the antiserum. If small amounts of dG-8-AAF are added with substantially larger amounts of dG-8-AF as inhibitor (keeping the total adduct concentration constant), the curve with [^{3}H]G-8-AAF as tracer will saturate at proportionally higher percentage inhibition levels. When profiles of an unknown DNA sample are compared to profiles of the standard mixtures using [^{3}H]G-8-AAF as tracer, the proportion of acetylated adduct (between 0 and 10% of the total) can be calculated within ±0.7% from a linear regression equation (9). For mixtures in which the acetylated C-8 adduct is greater than 10%, a less precise estimation of each C-8 adduct proportion in the mixture can be obtained by assaying the same amount of DNA in RIAs with both [^{3}H]G-8-AAF and [^{3}H]G-8-AF tracers (6). Appropriate standard mixtures run simultaneously will indicate within ±3% the percent acetylated C-8 adduct in the mixture (see Materials and Methods).

Determination of Acetylated and Deacetylated C-8 Adducts Acetylaminofluorene in Cultured Cells

Previous studies suggested that deacetylation of 2-AAF may be a determinant in its ultimate mutagenic or carcinogenic effect (4,14). Using RIA procedures, the natural binding pattern in a number of cell types was explored in detail to determine if adduct formation could be altered pharmacologically. Mouse (BALB/c) epidermal cells were exposed to increasing concentrations (10^{-6}, 10^{-5} and 10^{-4} M) of N-Ac-AAF (3,7,11). The levels of bound DNA adducts, after a 1-h exposure (2 to 30 μmol AAF/mol DNA-P), reflected the dose and resembled those observed in cells by other investigators using radioactively-labeled N-Ac-AAF (12,13). DNA profiles assayed by RIA with [^{3}H]G-8-AAF as tracer revealed that C-8 adducts on the DNA of mouse epidermal cells exposed to 10^{-5} M N-Ac-AAF were primarily deacetylated (see Figure 3) and the linear regression equation yielded a value of 3.3 ± 0.3% dG-8-AAF for several experiments (6). To confirm this finding, primary mouse epidermal cells were exposed to 10^{-5} M [^{3}H]N-Ac-AAF, the DNA were isolated and hydrolyzed, and the individual adducts were chromatographed by high pressure liquid chromatography (HPLC) and compared with standard markers. Of the total radioactivity eluted with markers of the acetylated and deacetylated C-8 adducts, 3.5% co-chromatographed with dG-8-AAF and 96.5% eluted with dG-8-AF, thus substantiating the RIA results (M.C. Poirier and F.A. Beland, unpublished observations).

Having determined that most C-8 adducts formed in N-Ac-AAF-exposed primary mouse epidermal cells were deacetylated, interest developed in investigating DNA binding in other epithelial cells and fibroblasts of mouse, human, and rat origin. The results

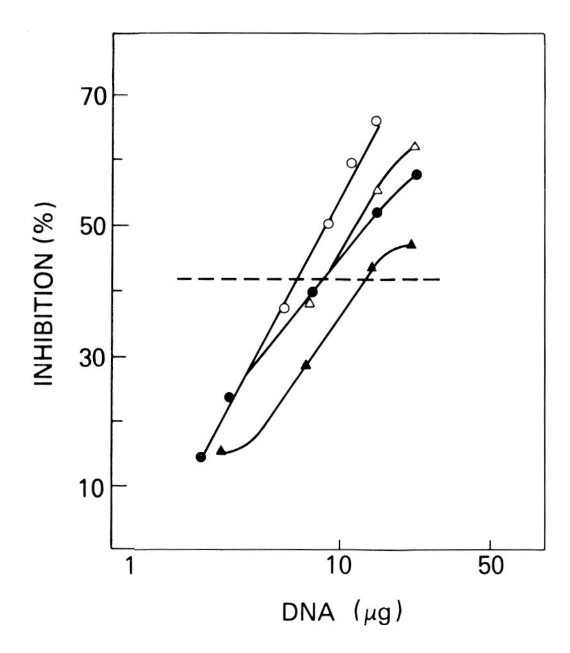

Figure 3. RIA of increasing concentrations of DNA assayed under the same conditions as shown in Figure 2 with [^{3}H]G-8-AAF tracer. Cells were exposed to 10^{-5} M N-Ac-AAF; DNAs were prepared on cesium chloride gradients, dialyzed, and assayed by RIA. The curves are as follows: 0 --- 0, primary rat hepatocyte; ▲ --- ▲, BALB/c epidermal cells; ● --- ●, normal human fibroblasts (YDF); and Δ --- Δ, SENCAR epidermal cells.

of these studies appear in Table 1 and Figure 3. All cells investigated, except primary rat hepatocytes, formed ≥90% of the C-8 adducts as dG-8-AF. This outcome did not appear to be a function of the species or the cell culture medium, but an intrinsic property of the cells themselves (6). Further studies with primary BALB/c epidermal cells showed that the percentage of acetylated C-8 adducts and total binding levels increased approximately threefold when N-Ac-AAF exposure occurred in the absence of serum, indicating that a small proportion of the deacetylation could be attributed to the presence of 10% serum during carcinogen treatment. In addition, pretreatment of primary mouse and rat epidermal cells with 10^{-8} to 10^{-5} M paraoxon, a microsomal deacetylase inhibitor (14,15), blocked most of the binding and formation of the deacetylated C-8 adduct. Adduct levels were 0.5 to 7% (1 to 15 fmol/μg DNA) of those observed in the controls (100 to 200 fmol/μg DNA), and the adducts formed were acetylated (6). These studies suggest that in mouse, rat, and human cells of dermal or epidermal origin microsomal deacetylation of N-Ac-AAF is critical for its binding to DNA.

Table 1. Acetylated and Deacetylated C-8 Adducts Formed in N-Ac-AAF-Exposed Cells

Cells	dG-8-AAF (%)	dG-8-AF (%)
Mouse		
BALB/c epidermal	3.3 ± 0.3[a]	96.7
SENCAR epidermal	8.0 ± 0.3	92.0
BALB/c fibroblast	5.0	95.0
SENCAR fibroblast	5.0	95.0
Human		
YDF dermal fibroblast	4.5	95.5
Rat		
Epidermal	9.0 ± 0.3	91.0
Fibroblast	5.4 ± 0.3	94.5
Hepatocyte	80.0	20.0

[a]Linear regression analysis applies to all entries with mean ± confidence limits expressed as % dG-8-AAF.

In contrast, primary rat hepatocytes exposed to either 10^{-5}M N-Ac-AAF for 1 h or 10^{-5}M 2-AAF for 5 h formed primarily acetylated C-8 adducts. No inhibition occurred in the [^{3}H]G-8-AF RIA with up to 20 μg DNA (6). Calculations based on the amount of DNA in the RIA and simultaneously-run standard curves indicated that at least 80% of the C-8 adducts formed were acetylated. In addition, the slope of the hepatocyte DNA profile differed from DNA profiles of the other cells (see Figure 3). Since paraoxon does not inhibit binding in primary hepatocytes (16), activation appears to proceed by a metabolic pathway yielding primarily an acetylated C-8 adduct, such as the sulfotransferase enzyme known to be present in rat liver (17).

These data indicated considerable similarity in extent and pattern of 2-AAF binding in analogous cells of three species, although rat liver may be an exception. Further studies compared adduct removal by DNA repair since this is an important determination of survival, mutagenesis, and transformation. Human fibroblasts assayed after N-Ac-AAF exposure in several laboratores are remarkably efficient in removing radiolabeled 2-AAF adducts from DNA (12,13,128,19). When C-8 adduct repair was monitored in normal human fibroblasts (YDF3) by RIA, the results were comparable to those obtained in other laboratories (50% remaining at 24 h); similar studies with differentiating primary mouse epidermal cells indicated that approximately 60% of C-8 adducts remained at the end of a 24-h repair period (3). Thus, the mouse cells formed approximately the same proportion of C-8 adducts as the human cells and were able to remove them with comparable efficiency. These results suggest a quantitatve similarity between the two species, but do not prove similar mechanisms are used to affect the carcinogen removal in different species.

Formation amd Removal of dG-8-AAF and dG-8-AF in Liver and Kidney DNA of Male Rats Fed 0.02% 2-AAF

Male Wistar-Furth rats were fed 0.02% 2-AAF continuously for up to 60 days and the C-8 adduct levels in liver and kidney DNA was monitored by RIA. After only one day on the 0.02% 2-AAF-containing diet, an average of 80 fmol C-8 adduct/μg DNA was observed in the livers of three rats, and the binding to kidney DNA was below the limits of detectability by RIA (see Table 2). After three days of feeding, 135 fmol of adduct/μg DNA were found in liver, while kidney DNA contained approximately 10% of the liver values. With continuous AAF feeding, C-8 adducts bound to liver DNA increased for 30 days and reached a plateau at about 240 fmol/μg DNA (Table 2). Subsequently (at 60 days and 16 weeks), the amount of C-8 adduct in liver DNA did not increase above the 30-day value. Binding of 2-AAF to kidney DNA never exceeded about 10 to 15% of the values observed in liver. The lower overall adduct formation in kidney may be related to the insensitivity of this organ to the carcinogenic effects of 0.02% 2-AAF.

Differences in the proportions of acetylated and deacetylated C-8 adducts were investigated at various times during continuous 2-AAF administration. Liver DNA adduct profiles at days 3, 5, 7, and 15 had similar slopes (see Figure 4) and gave a difference in percentage inhibition values (see Materials and Methods) comparable to those for a mixture of 20% dG-8-AAF, 80% dG-8-AF. Profiles for DNA at days 30 and 60 showed a high degree of deacetylation, with the difference in percentage of inhibition values similar to a mixture of 3% dG-8-AAF, 97% dG-8-AF. A dramatic difference in the proportion of deacetylated adducts between 15 and 31 days of feeding appeared, evident from the slope of the DNA profiles (see Figure 4), and the proportion of deacetylated C-8 adducts appeared to increase with time of continuous feeding.

Table 2. 2-AAF C-8 Adducts in Liver and Kidney DNA from Male Rats Fed 0.02% 2-AAF[a]

Exposure (days)	Liver/DNA (fmol/μg)	Kidney/DNA (fmol/μg)
1	80 ± 3.6[b]	ND[c]
3	135 ± 1.4	14.9 ± 1.2
5	132 ± 8.4	--
7	148 ± 11.9	--
15	156 ± 17.9	22.8 ± 0.1
31	236 ± 13.6	29.4 ± 4.3
60	238 ± 15.7	31.3 ± 3.2

[a]There was one control animal at each time point and all were negative for C-8 adducts in both liver and kidney DNA.
[b]Mean ± S.E. of 3 animals.
[c]ND = Non-detectable.

To investigate the efficiency of C-8 adduct removal in rat liver and kidney, male Wistar-Furth rats were fed 0.02% 2-AAF for 7 or 28 days followed by control diet for 1, 7 and 28 days. Three animals were sacrificed at each of these time points and liver and kidney DNA was assayed for C-8 adducts by RIA (see Table 3). Following 7 or 28 days of feeding (with no removal period), C-8 adduct binding levels were 100 fmol/μg DNA and DNA profiles (not shown) were similar to those observed at 7 (20% acetylated) and 30 (3% acetylated) days in the continuous feeding experiment. In animals fed 2-AAF for 7 days, the C-8 adduct level in liver and kidney decreased consistently with time on carcinogen-free diet so that by 28 days, 64% of these adducts were removed from liver and kidney. In animals fed 2-AAF for 28 days, the C-8 adduct levels in liver and kidney remained relatively constant with time on the control diet. These results were substantiated in a second experiment of similar design in which, after 26 days on the control diet, the C-8 adduct level was 65% of that observed at the end of 28 days of 0.02% 2-AAF feeding (data not shown). Thus, the persistence of high levels of C-8 adduct, or apparent loss in the ability to remove C-8 adducts is associated with the feeding of 0.02% 2-AAF for 28 days.

DISCUSSION

The antiserum against G-8-AAF used in these studies is a sensitive and specific probe for the presence of acetylated and

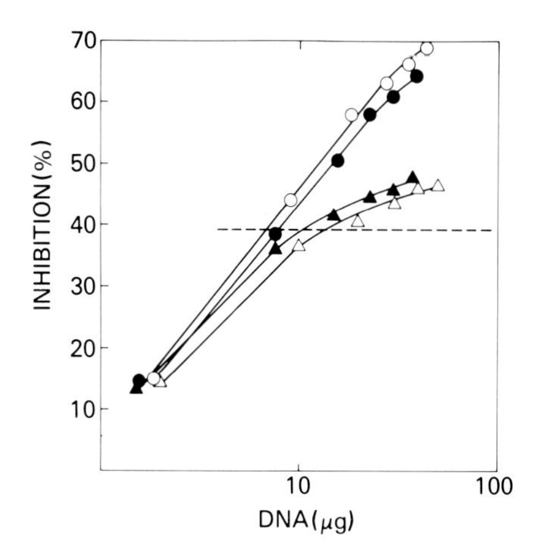

Figure 4. RIA profiles of increasing concentrations of DNA extracted from livers of rats fed 0.02% 2-AAF for 7 (O --- O), 15 (● --- ●), 31 (▲ --- ▲), and 60 (Δ --- Δ) days. The tracer was [^{3}H]G-8-AAF and (----) indicates the dG-8-AF saturation in the same assay. Compared with the appropriate standards, the 7- and 15-day samples are approximately 20% dG-8-AAF, 80% dG-8-AF. The 31- and 60-day samples are 3% dG-8-AAF, 97% dG-8-AF.

deacetylated 2-AAF C-8 adducts on DNA; it has been used to detect 1 carcinogen molecule in 3 x 10^5 nucleotides by RIA. The antiserum does not cross-react with the carcinogen alone, nucleosides, or 2-AAF-DNA adducts having markedly different structures (dG-N^2-AAF and diamino-Py-FU). It has been employed to measure both total C-8 adducts and the relative proportions of acetylated and deacetylated C-8 adducts and the relative proportions of acetylated and deacetylated C-8 adducts in the DNA of cultured cells exposed to N-Ac-AAF and the livers and kidneys of rats fed 2-AAF. The results are comparable to those obtained when radioactively-labeled N-Ac-AAF and 2-AAF were used to expose cultured cells or animals (3,4,5,12,13,16 and C. Irving, personal communication, University of Tennessee, Memphis, TN).

Table 3. Removal of C-8 Adducts in Liver and Kidney DNA of Male Rats Fed 0.02% 2-AAF[a]

Exposure (days)	Removal (days)	Liver/DNA (fmol/μg)	Kidney/DNA (fmol/μg)
7	0	99.9 ± 8.6[b]	21.0 ± 0.98
7	1	70.0 ± 4.2	16.6 ± 1.75
7	7	64.2 ± 7.2	16.6 ± 0.13
7	28	35.7 ± 2.0	8.9 ± 3.57
28	0	95.8 ± 0.8	29.3 - 1.71
28	1	115.7 ± 3.3	29.8 ± 4.81
28	7	75.0 ± 4.7	27.5 ± 5.91
28	28	118.3 ± 25.1	23.2 ± 2.12

[a]There was one control animal at each time point and all were negative for C-8 adducts in liver and kidney DNA.
[b]Mean ± S.E. of 3 animals.

RIA allowed us to compare the formation of C-8 adducts in DNA from epidermal cells and dermal fibroblasts of mouse, human, and rat origin exposed to N-Ac-AAF. The fact that $\geq$90% of C-8 adducts found in these DNAs were deacetylated, coupled with the marked inhibition of DNA binding by paraoxon, a microsomal deacetylase inhibitor, provide compelling evidence for activation through a deacetylase enzyme. Supporting evidence is provided by experiments indicating that the sulfotransferase and arylhydroxamic acid transferase enzymes (17,20) are absent in skin. In contrast, rat liver appears to metabolize 2-AAF through these other mechanisms as well. Paraoxon does not diminish the binding of 2-AAF to DNA in primary rat hepatocytes (16), indicating that microsomal deacetylation is not an obligate pathway. However, the presence of a high proportion of acetylated C-8 adduct (60 to 80%) in DNA from primary hepatocytes (5,6,16) suggests that sulfotransferase is a major activating enzyme in these cells. This enzyme appears to play an important role *in vivo* where acetylated dG-8-AAF comprises about 20% of the total C-8 adduct of liver (4,5). The liver *in vivo* also contains substantial amounts of arylhydroxamic acid transferase (20), which could account for the high proportion (80%) of deacetylated C-8 adducts observed in rats upon continuous feeding of 2-AAF. Thus, cell- or tissue-specific differences in metabolic capabilities within the same organism are responsible for the type of adduct formed. Of ultimate interest is the biological significance of specific adducts, particularly regarding carcinogenesis.

Our studies represent the first experiments monitoring specific DNA adducts during prolonged continuous 2-AAF feeding. The quantitative pattern of total C-8 adduct formation agrees with unpublished data (C. Irving, personal communication, University of Tennessee, Memphis, TN), obtained by continuously feeding radioactive 2-AAF for 8 weeks. Irving's studies, as well as our own, show evidence for increasing adduct formation at early times, followed by a plateau beyond which binding did not increase. This constant adduct level at later times suggests that an equilibrium is reached between new DNA damage and repair. However, we found that after 28 days of 0.02% 2-AAF feeding, the ability to remove C-8 adducts appears to be impaired during an additional 28 days on a carcinogen-free diet. This outcome could indicate diminished repair capacity caused by carcinogen damage. Since rats were already mature (180 g) when 2-AAF administration was begun, the mitotic index during the feeding and post-feeding period is expected to be less than 0.01% (21). After 28 days of 2-AAF-containing diet, we found an average of 5 γ-glutamyl transpeptidase positive foci per liver when sectioning each lobe once, and the small cell population was less than 5%, indicating no large populations of highly-altered cells in these livers. Mature hepatocytes would not be expected to become refractory to 2-AAF metabolism until 6 to 8 weeks of 2-AAF feeding, the time at which the first nodules appear (22). Possibly repair mechanisms are relatively intact after prolonged feeding, but carcinogen binding to DNA continues withdrawal of 2-AAF from the diet by metabolic recycling. The impact of such a mechanism on the host would be dramatic and extremely important for determining true dose-response data in carcinogenesis studies. Using immunological methods offers a unique opportunity to pursue such studies *in vivo*.

ACKNOWLEDGMENTS

Dr. I.B. Weinstein, Dr. D. Grunberger, and Dr. S. Blobstein synthesized the original G-8-AAF antigen for these studies, and we are grateful to them for many thoughtful discussions.
Dr. G.M. Williams provided the primary rat hepatocytes,
Dr. R. Connor derived the linear regression equation, and
Dr. E. Kriek gave us samples of dG-N^2-AAF and diamino-Py-FU to test the antibody cross-reactivity. The technical assistance of Marc Dubin, Brigitte Former, Curt Thill, and Elroy Patterson is gratefully acknowledged.

REFERENCES

1. Poirier, M.C. 1981. Antibodies to carcinogen-DNA adducts. J. Natl. Cancer Inst. 67:515-519.

2. Poirier, M.C., S.H. Yuspa, I.B. Weinstein, and S. Blobstein. 1977. Detection of carcinogen-DNA adducts by radioimmunoassay. Nature 270:186-188.

3. Poirier, M.C., M.A. Dubin, and S.H. Yuspa. 1979. Formation and removal of specific acetylaminofluorene-DNA adducts in mouse and human cells measured by radioimmunoassay. Cancer Res. 39:1377-1381.

4. Kriek, E. 1972. Persistent binding of a new reaction product of the carcinogen N-hydroxy-N-2-acetylaminofluorene with guanine in rat liver DNA _in vivo_. Cancer Res. 32:2042-2048.

5. Beland, F.A., K.L. Dooley, and D.A. Casciano. 1979. Rapid isolation of carcinogen-bound DNA and RNA by hydroxyapatite chromatography. J. Chromatog. 174:177-186.

6. Poirier, M.C., G.M. Williams, and S.H. Yuspa. 1980. Effect of culture conditions, cell type, and species of origin on the distribution of acetylated and deacetylated deoxyguanosine C-8 adducts of N-acetoxy-2-acetylaminofluorene. Molec. Pharmacol. 18:234-240.

7. Poirier, M.C. 1981. Measurement of the formation and removal of DNA adducts of N-acetoxy-2-acetylaminofluorene. In: DNA Repair: A Laboratory Manual of Research Procedures, Volume 1A. E.C. Friedberg and P.C. Hanawalt, eds. Marcel Dekker, Inc.: New York. pp. 143-153.

8. Laishes, B.A., and P.B. Rolfe. 1980. Quantitative assessment of liver colony formation and hepatocellular carcinoma incidence in rats receiving intravenous injections of isogeneic liver cells isolated during hepatocarcinogenesis. Cancer Res. 40:4133-4143.

9. Poirier, M.C., and R.J. Connor. (in press). A radioimmunoassay for 2-acetylaminofluorene-DNA adducts. In: Immunochemical Techniques, Volume 2. H. Van Vunakis and J. Langone, eds. Academic Press: New York.

10. Kriek, E., and J.G. Westra. 1980. Structural identification of the pyrimidine derivatives formed from N-(deoxyguanosin-8-yl)-2-acetylaminofluorene in aqueous solution at alkaline pH. Carcinogenesis 1:459-467.

11. Yuspa, S.H., and C.C. Harris. 1974. Altered differentiation of mouse epidermal cells treated with retinyl acetate _in vitro_. Exp. Cell Res. 86:95-105.

12. Amacher, D.E., J.A. Elliott, and M.W. Lieberman. 1977. Differences in removal of acetylaminofluorene and pyrimidine dimers from the DNA of cultured mammalian cells. Proc. Natl. Acad. Sci. USA 74:1553-1557.

13. Amacher, D.E., and M.W. Lieberman. 1977. Removal of acetylaminofluorene from the DNA of control and repair-deficient human fibroblasts. Biochem. Biophys. Res. Comm. 74:285-290.

14. Sakai, S., C.E. Reinhold, P.J. Wirth, and S.S. Thorgiersson. 1978. Mechanism of in vitro mutagenic activation and covalent binding of N-hydroxy-2-acetylaminofluorene in isolated liver cell nuclei from rat and mouse. Cancer Res. 38-2058-2067.

15. Schut, H.A., P.J. Wirth, and S.S. Thorgiersson. 1978. Mutagenic activation of N-hydroxy-2-acetylaminofluorene in the salmonella test system: The role of deacetylation by liver and kidney fractions from mouse and rat. Molec. Pharmacol. 14:682-692.

16. Howard, P.C., F.A. Beland, and D.A. Casciano. 1981. Quantitation of N-hydroxy-2-acetylaminofluorene-mediated DNA adduct formation and the subsequent repair in primary rat hepatocyte cultures. J. Supra Struct. Cell. Biochem. Suppl. 5, Abstract 534, p. 197.

17. DeBaun, J.R., E.C. Miller, and J.A. Miller. 1970. N-hydroxy-2-acetylaminofluorene sulfotransferase: Its probable role in carcinogenesis and in protein (methion-S-yl) binding in rat liver. Cancer Res. 30:577-595.

18. Cerutti, P.A. 1978. Repairable damage in DNA. In: DNA repair mechanisms: ICN-UCLA Symposia on Molecular and Cellular Biology, IX. P.C. Hanawalt, E.C. Friedberg, and C.F. Fox, eds. Academic Press: New York. pp. 1-14.

19. Levinson, J.W., B. Konze-Thomas, V.M. Maher, and J.J. McCormick. 1979. Evidence for a common rate-limiting step in the repair process of ultraviolet light and N-acetoxyacetylaminofluorene-induced damage in the DNA of human fibroblasts. Proc. Am. Assoc. Cancer Res. 20:105.

20. King, C.M., and C.W. Olive. 1975. Comparative effects of strain, species, and sex on the acyltransferase- and sulfotransferase-catalyzed activations of N-hydroxy-N-2-fluorenylacetamide. Cancer Res. 35:906-912.

21. Albert, R.E., F.J. Burns, L. Bilger, D. Gardner, and W. Troll. 1972. Cell loss and proliferation induced by N-2-fluorenylacetamide in the rat liver in relation to hepatoma induction. Cancer Res. 32:2172-2177.

22. Stout, D.L., and F.F. Becker. 1978. Alteration of the ability of liver microsomes to activate N-2-fluorenyl-acetamide to a mutagen of *Salmonella typhimurium* during hepatocarcinogenesis. Cancer Res. 38:2274-2278.

DISCUSSION

Q.: I recently heard in a seminar that the acetylated and deacetylated adducts have very different positions in the DNA. One is the minor groove and one is the major groove. Would you comment on that in relationship to your studies?

A.: Approximately six or seven years ago Kriek first observed in rat liver that there was repair of the acetylated and that deacetylated C-8 adducts, and that these adducts distort the DNA helix. He felt that the N^2 adduct which lies in the minor groove did not perturb the DNA helix and was therefore not subject to repair.

Since that time the studies of Grunberger, Kriek and others have shown that the deacetylated C-8 adduct does not perturb the helix very much. By S1 nuclease digestion these workers have shown that the helical distortion extends only to two or three base pairs on either side of the adduct. Kriek, Beland and others have shown that this adduct is easily repaired *in vivo* and so the relationship between DNA-hilical distortion and repair capability remains unclear.

Q.: What do you think of the possibility that the continued feeding simply serves as an inhibitor of the repair processes?

A.: You know, I think that's a possibility. I'm really not willing to speculate about the mechanism of this until I do some more experiments and I think there are several possibilities.

If you look at the literature there are extensive data on the fate of the liver during 2-AAF feeding. I think that we need to look at this in detail.

Q.: How old were the animals that you were working with?

A.: Our animals were about eight months old; they weighed about 180 g; at this point the mitotic index is about 0.01 percent. The question is, does the carcinogen induce mitosis and we have to look at it further before we make any claims.

TRANS-SPECIES AND TRANS-TISSUE EXTRAPOLATION OF CARCINOGENICITY ASSAYS

David B. Clayson

Eppley Institute for Research in Cancer and Allied Diseases, University of Nebraska Medical Center, Omaha, Nebraska 68105

From earliest times, mankind has endowed animals with specific human attributes. Language reflects many of these attributes in phrases such as "wise as an owl," "cunning as a fox," or "assinine." Soothsayers have used the detailed morphological examination of outbred animals to predict man's fate in the future. It is relevant to our present society that none of these attributions were scientific absolutes; they could be manipulated to suit the current political exigencies. Our current mysticism dictates that we regard all agents that induce cancer in animals as having the same effect in man. Although some evidence for this theory exists, and it represents a cautious view, it is again by no means a scientific absolute.

Today, it is prudent and politically expedient to believe that an agent that induces tumors in any species of animal will be a potent and therefore regulatable carcinogen in man. My purpose in this paper is to ask how we, as a society, might take apart the assumptions underlying this prudent concept and replace it with something scientifically better defined.

Gross Differences Between Humans and Laboratory Animals

Table 1 lists some of the more apparent differences between man and laboratory animals. Because the values in this table will be used in potency calculations, they are given as single numbers and not ranges. The factors shown here tell us little about likely relative potencies of an agent in different species. For example, longevity might lead us to suspect that man may be more sensitive to carcinogens, because in a long-living animal tumors have much longer to develop. However, the proportion of men and animals that develop tumors in old age is not too dissimilar. So, we have to look to differences in DNA repair systems and the efficacy of immune processes to counteract the effects of species variations in longevity and tumor development. The effect of man's size relative to rodents indicates that in man many more cells are at risk. Again, restorative processes must be invoked to explain similar spontaneous tumor incidences. The menstrual cycle in women and non-human primates might be predicted to affect hormone-responsive tumor development in a qualitatively or quantitatively different manner from the estrous cycle in rodents. However, no evidence for this difference exists, probably because so little work has been done on non-human primates. If the menstrual cycle can indeed be compared to pseudo-pregnancy in mice, then perhaps some more definite statements might be made.

Table 1. Differences Between Humans and Laboratory Animals

Factor	Man	Mouse	Rat
Life span[a]	70	2.5	3.0
Gestation[b]	270	21	21
Weight[c]	70,000	25-40	100-500
Estrous cycle	No	Yes	Yes
Menstrual cycle	Yes	No	No
Quadriped	No	Yes	Yes
Biped	Yes	No	No
Mammal	Yes	Yes	Yes
Gall bladder	Yes	Yes	No
Vitamin C-dependent	Yes	No	No

[a]Years.
[b]Days.
[c]Grams.

Even when we consider the detail of the mechanisms of chemical induction of cancer and compare metabolic activation of procarcinogens, electrophile interaction with critical targets, DNA repair or replication to lock in chemically-induced lesions, as well as the development of tumor progenitor cells to frank clinical cancer, we fail to observe many significant qualitative differences between species. The guinea pig, for example, is resistant to 2-acetylaminofluorene (2-AAF) carcinogenesis: when 2-AAF is applied *in vivo*, the guinea pig fails to convert a significant proportion of this procarcinogen to its proximate form, N-hydroxy-2-AAF. Even though this series of observations is one key to the development of the current electrophilic activation theory of chemical carcinogens, the evidence is by no means conclusive. Although a total of 60 guinea pigs was used to test the lack of carcinogenicity of 2-AAF (2), the maximum survivals of 2.5 to 3.0 years may be somewhat less than desirable for a negative experiment in this species. Takeishi et al. (3) showed that perhaps the guinea pig can N-hydroxylate 2-AAF after all, and that the guinea pig differs from other species in its pronounced ability to detoxify the active metabolite *in vivo*. Even this one well-documented example of a species difference in metabolism corresponding to a species difference in carcinogenesis must be regarded with some suspicion. I do not believe that such differences are, at this stage, likely to help in attaining meaningful criteria for trans-species extrapolation of carcinogenicity tests.

Potency

The observation that there are few gross physiological conditions that help us explain, let alone predict, qualitative interspecies differences in carcinogenesis means that we must make our judgments on a quantitative basis. In other words, our task is to explain differences in potency of carcinogens in species A compared to species B. First, we must define potency in a measurable and meaningful way. The potency or strength of a carcinogen is reflected in five different sets of observations: probability that a tumor is formed, dose rate of carcinogen used, mean time to tumor, multiplicity of tumor in a tissue, and quality of pathologic diagnosis. The first three observations are key points and the latter two relatively marginal to our discussion. Therefore, to define the potency or strength of a carcinogen, we will use only probability of tumor formation, dose rate, and time to tumor. The use of only these three observations is logical, because multiplicity becomes less important at low doses and is an extension of the concept of probability of a tumor. I do not choose to question the adequacy of pathologic diagnosis.

As a start, examine the premise:

$$\text{Potency of a carcinogen} = 7 - \log_{10} D_{E50}$$

where, using a standard experimental protocol, potency is the negative of the logarithm of the dose D_{E50} (in μmol/week/kg) required to induce a 50% incidence of tumors in a life span experiment. The constant, 7, ensures that all values are positive.

This definition has several advantages. First, no need exists to extrapolate the dose requirement to one tumor in a population of 10^6 or some other equally meaningless figure. In many cases, the figure for 50% tumor induction will be an interpolation of the data, rather than an extrapolation, and can be approached using some rough-and-ready approximations. Second, because we demand a full lifetime experiment, toxic doses that markedly shorten longevity will often be discarded using this definition. I have used log dose simply to compress the range of values and to avoid any undue emphasis on small differences. It will be seen to have other advantages later. I would have liked to use the mean plasma concentration rather than dose rate for systemic tumor induction, because it might allow a range of protocols to be compared meaningfully. However, for standard carcinogens, plasma concentrations are seldom available. Therefore, the experimental protocol used to assess potency must be stated. Typical potencies of experimental carcinogens fed to rats or mice are shown in Table 2. These potencies are very approximate but serve to indicate their wide range.

Table 2. The Potency of a Range of Carcinogens to Rat or Mouse Liver Following Continuous Feeding

Chemical	Species	Potency
Aflatoxin	Rat	9.18
Michler's ketone	Rat	4.62
Nitrosodimethylamine	Rat	4.00
Carbon tetrachloride	Rat	3.87
2-Aminoanthraquinone	Rat	4.44
Trichlorethylene	Mouse	2.12
Saccharin	Rat[a]	1.92

[a]Bladder.

Now let us compare the potencies of 4-aminobiphenyl in the dog, rat, and mouse (Table 3). Where tests have been performed only at one level, we can make a linear plot to zero, or the control incidence of tumors, and extrapolate or interpolate the data. I think these values, although only as accurate as my rough calculations and the carcinogenicity assays that generated them, go some way to provide meaningful data for interspecies comparison. The model suggested can be modified for use with any series of standard assays, and where more accurate data exists, can be refined. A similar approach to potency was adopted by Meselson and Russell (4).

Table 3. Potency of 4-Aminobiphenyl Following Administration to Different Species

Species	Route of Administration	Tissue	Potency
Dog	Oral	Bladder	6.22
Mouse	Gavage	Liver	4.52
Rat	Subcutaneous	Intestine	4.37

Multistage Model of Carcinogenesis

Defining carcinogenic potency is only a very small part of the problem of interspecies extrapolation of carcinogenesis results. A chemical carcinogen possesses many properties relevant to carcinogenesis, each of which may vary independently and possibly even in opposite directions. Thus, the physical properties of a carcinogen may affect its distribution in the body and its plasma concentration and protein binding, i.e., its availability. Physical properties may also affect its affinity for activating and deactivating metabolizing enzymes. The stability of the ultimate electrophile or its transport form may influence its ability to reach the critical receptors and its interaction. I visualize sites on DNA as the most likely critical receptors. The configuration and placement of the carcinogen adduct on the DNA may affect the ability of DNA repair enzymes to act, while the original carcinogen or any of its metabolic products may be toxic to repair or other enzymes. Toxicity to the immune system, hormonal systems, or proliferative systems may influence the ultimate tumor yield. Clearly, we cannot at this stage summate each and every one of these biochemical or physiologic-biologic properties to achieve an exact explanation of potency differences between species. The amount of work required would be horrendous for even a single chemical, and the weighting to be given to different factors would be the subject of seemingly endless and probably fruitless argument. We would be as well employed debating the number of angels that might dance on the eye of a needle as to attempt to line up our limited mechanistic knowledge in such a comprehensive way.

Simplification is clearly needed. The best established explanation is the two-phase mechanism of carcinogenesis for mouse skin put forward by Berenblum and Shubik (5-7). It is now being tested experimentally in other tissues, such as liver by Peraino (8-10), bladder by Cohen (11), pancreas by Pour et al. (12), and so on. The interaction or initiation phase is a composite of all factors up to and including the DNA repair stage. The development or promotion phase includes all these factors that may influence tumor development.

Evaluation of Initiation Potency

For mouse skin and a few other model systems, we have whole-animal data on the initiating ability of a few chemical carcinogens. However, in my opinion, whole-animal experiments are not the most appropriate model for gaining a general insight into the initiating potency of chemical carcinogens that can be applied to trans-species extrapolations. I take this view because 1) we have adequate models for only a few tissues in a very few species, 2) strong and correct ethical objections to experimentation in man, the species of primary concern, exist, and 3) the cost of whole-animal experiments is often prohibitive.

The present range of short-term prescreening tests for carcinogens in general is, I believe, designed to reflect the initiating ability of a carcinogen. For quantitative results, the Ames *Salmonella* test is, in my view, less than suitable, because the rough treatment involved in the preparation of the S9 metabolizing fraction may damage or dissociate activating from deactivating enzymes, and because cell-free systems lack the membranes that may help to maintain enzyme co-factors at their proper levels. Many examples of qualitatively correct, but quantitatively inexact, results exist from attempts to correlate results of these tests with the results of carcinogenesis assays. In addition, microbial mutation tests, such as the Ames test (13-15), appear insensitive to specific carcinogens such as hydrazines, estrogens, possibly metals, and even nitrosamines.

In my opinion, the mammalian cell-mediated mammalian cell mutagenesis system as developed by Langenbach and Huberman (16,17) may provide much more reliable answers. The suggestion is a relatively safe one, because this approach has not been used or tested to the same extent as the Ames or other microbial mutation systems. The test consists of co-cultivating primary explants of cells from the chosen tissue as a metabolic activating system with Chinese hamster V79 lung cells that are mutable to resistance to the lethal effects of drugs such as azaguanine, thioguanine, or ouabain. The use of primary explants of mammalian cells has several advantages over the S9 fraction. No disturbance of metabolizing enzymes or intracellular membranes occurs; therefore, much greater similarity to *in vivo* metabolism should exist. Primary explants appear to retain the metabolizing characteristics of the tissue of origin to a greater extent than either the S9 fraction or continuously cultured cells. Cell suspensions of any tissue may be utilized; preparation of S9 fraction from some of these tissues may be difficult. Langenbach and Malick, of the Eppley Institute, have successfully exploited liver, kidney, bladder epithelial, and lung tissue and have shown that each metabolically activates major groups of carcinogens. Human cells from specific tissues urgently need to be used.

Further work is required to illustrate fully the precision of this technique; however, in a preliminary series of studies, Langenbach (18) has found that when S9 fraction from liver is used to activate metabolically a series of four pancreatic carcinogens, the results are almost inversely related to the *in vivo* pancreatic carcinogenic potency, and with the liver cell-mediated assay, a good correlation is obtained. Such evidence is encouraging, but as yet, by no means conclusive (Figure 1).

If this method or some other technique is used to obtain quantitative values for the initiating potency of a series of carcinogens, we might be able to establish a potency equation:

$$\text{Potency for initiation} = X - \log ad_m + R$$

where d_m is the dose required to initiate a standard number of mutations or other events in the chosen system, X and a are constants designed to line up the scale of potency with *in vivo* studies, and R is a factor that reflects the ability of the particular tissue and species to repair its DNA from the effects of the carcinogen before they are locked in by replication. The latter factor is introduced because the V79 cell system does not reflect either tissue or species-specific activity of DNA repair systems or the rate of replication occurring in a specific tissue *in vivo*.

PROMOTION

Such a wide variety of biological processes are presently believed to affect tumor development. Proposals on how the potency of an agent for tumor development may be quantitated are exceedingly difficult to formulate. If we wish to include man in our trans-species extrapolation net, *in vitro* methods are needed. Presently available whole-animal models are limited to one species and tissue. For example, phorbol esters appear to exert their

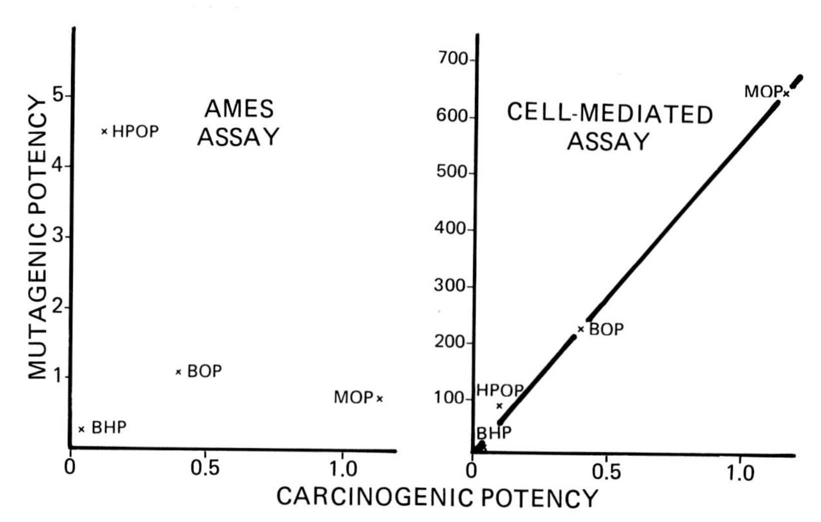

Figure 1. Relationship of carcinogenicity with mutagenicity in the Ames Salmonella and cell-mediated assays. Carcinogenic potency is expressed as the reciprocal of the lowest weekly dose that produced a tumor incidence of at least 60 to 70%. BHP stands for N-nitrosobis(2-hydroxy propyl)amine, HPOP for N-nitroso-2-hydroxypropyl-2-propylamine, BOP for N-nitrosobis(2-oxopropyl)amine, and MOP for N-nitroso-methyl-2-oxopropylamine. (Reproduced with permission from reference 18.)

major effects only in mouse skin (19), and phenobarbital mainly affects rat and mouse liver (8-10,20). Some attempts have been made to reproduce initiation-promotion in vitro, but to the best of my knowledge, no really general approaches have been devised. The reason is simply that we have not yet decided what we are looking for -- we have little idea of the mechanisms involved. Therefore, we cannot begin to judge whether any in vitro test is adequate.

At the risk of being accused of vastly oversimplifying a very complex problem, I suggest that two major considerations underlying the tumor development phase of carcinogenesis exist. The first consideration is the effect of the overall proliferative stimulus the agent gives to the tissue and the second is the selective stress that the agent applies between untransformed and tumor progenitor cells.

Examples of the importance of the general proliferative stimulus would be expected in tissues such as liver and bladder, which normally have a very low rate of proliferation. Peraino et al. (8-10) have demonstrated that phenobarbital stimulates rat liver cell proliferation; this result may explain its promoting action on 2-AAF-initiated rats. Over the years, my colleagues and I have shown that bladder carcinogens fed continuously in the diet lead to hyperplasia, increased DNA synthesis, and enhanced cell proliferation (21). Similarly, physical irritation by stone or urothelial infections also leads to these effects (22).

Although not yet rigorously proven, such stimulation is regeneration in response to chemically-induced cell loss or necrosis. I assume that the induction of cell proliferation will be related in some way to the dose of the agent. I suspect that for cells from tissues that have a built-in tendency to retain their mass or integrity within the whole animal, such as the liver or bladder, a good approximation to cell proliferation induction may be obtained from the level of cell killing induced by the agent.

Among the factors believed to influence tumor development, cell proliferation, induced for example by hormones and other humoral effects, may have an influence on the proliferative aspects of tumor development. Hormonal, other humoral, and possibly immunologic influences will play key roles in the selection process if the normal and transformed cells differ in either their receptor molecules or the efficiency with which they act.

Comparison of the toxicity of an agent to normal cells and those incubated in the presence of the agent itself may help quantify the selection pressure induced by the agent. For example, cells from cultures maintained in the presence of carbon tetrachloride were reported to be no longer as responsive to the necrotizing effects of this agent as untreated cells. Similarly, James Miller and Elizabeth Miller (23) determined that rat liver neoplasia induced by 4-dimethylaminoazobenzene has lost the ability to activate this carcinogen and is therefore "protected" against it. I suspect that both the proliferative and selection processes in any given tissue are likely to be dose-related. We may postulate:

$$\text{Potency for development} = Y - \log bd_p - \log cd_s$$

where Y, b, and c are constants, d_p is the dose required to produce a defined proliferative stimulus, and d_s is the dose required to produce a given degree of selection. Unfortunately, we will need defined methods to determine d_p and d_s.

Putting all our speculations together, we arrive at the following:

$$\text{Potency of a carcinogen} = 7 - \log_{10} D_{E50}$$

$$= \text{Potency of initiation + potency for development}$$

$$= Z - \log ad_m + R - \log nd_p - \log cd_s$$

$$\text{Potency of a carcinogen} = f(Rdm \cdot d_p \cdot d_s)$$

where D_{E50} and dm, but not yet d_p and d_s, can be measured by presently devisable techniques using either whole animals or cell culture.

This model assumes that initiation and promotion are independently dose related. In the initiation phase, dose determines the level of DNA change responsible for initiation in the tissue; in the development phase, dose determines the magnitude of the proliferative or selection processes. This model has some rather striking consequences that affect risk assessment. If we consider a "pure" initiator in which tumor development is due only to natural body processes, we obtain a more linear dose-response model clearly demonstrated by single-dose irradiation experiments. Likewise, if we consider a "pure" tumor developer, we would also expect to obtain a more nearly linear relationship between dose and tumor response than we would if we consider a complete carcinogen possessing both initiating and promoting capabilities. The ED_{01} experiment, sometimes known as the mega-mouse experiment, performed at the National Center for Toxicological Research, suggests this view may be correct (24).

The ED_{01} Experiment

The ED_{01} experiment examined the effect of low doses of 2-AAF on the incidence of liver and bladder tumors in BALB/c mice. In all, about 22,000 animals were used, and at "low" doses marked differences in the response of these two tissues seemed to occur. The bladder showed an apparent threshold, but the liver did not (Figure 2). Various statistical manipulations led to claims that this difference is more apparent than real, and that if the mice had lived for 6 to 10 years, this difference would have disappeared (24). This assumption is ridiculous, since mice do not live that long.

The first thing about these results that strikes me forcibly is that an appreciable incidence of liver neoplasia in untreated BALB/c mice occurred, but an exceedingly low spontaneous incidence

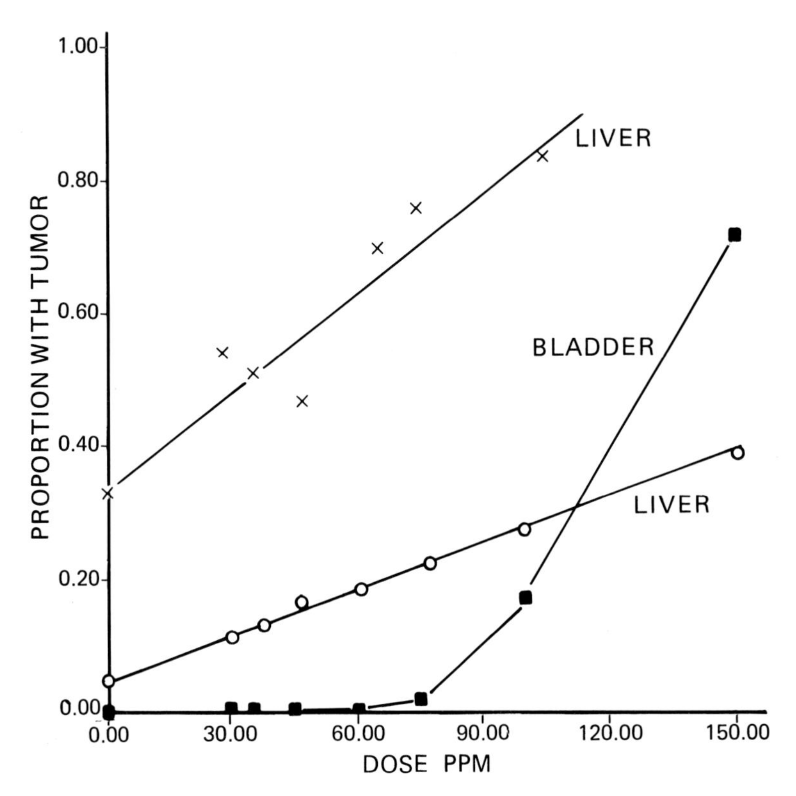

Figure 2. Effect of various doses of 2-acetylaminofluorene on tumor response in male BALB/c mice. O-O shows liver carcinoma response after 24 months and X-X after 33 months. ■-■ shows total bladder carcinoma response.

of bladder tumors occurred (between 0 and 0.1%). In other words, liver tumor incidence might be increased, especially at low dose levels, just by enhancement.

The key question is, what happens if we repeat this experiment in a strain of mice that without treatment has an exceptionally low liver tumor incidence? I predict that the dose-tumor incidence curve may come to resemble the one seen in the bladder in the ED_{01} experiment. At the higher dose levels, the liver tumor rate appears to be exceeding its apparent linearity. This result suggests that at these higher dosages, possibly both the initiating and promoting effects of 2-AAF come into play in the liver as in the bladder. Pursuing this kind of argument further may lead to some rather striking conclusions.

I have discussed trans-species extrapolation in terms of practicalities. What can we measure that is relevant at this time? What else do we need to know? I believe that my approach is more likely to provide a meaningful insight into the problems posed by such extrapolations than a detailed listing of differences between species that may or may not be relevant to carcinogenesis. The problem is a matter of obtaining quantitative parameters on which to base firm judgments; a mere listing of divergent properties between species will get us nowhere. The detailed mechanistic interpretation of why A is a much weaker carcinogen than B can be attempted more easily when we know whether the difference is in the tumor initiation or tumor development stage. Regulatory decisions to protect public health will probably be easier with broadly based but quantitated information than with detailed mechanistic studies that neither the public, the regulators, nor many scientists really understand.

ACKNOWLEDGMENTS

This paper was first presented to the Toxicology Forum at its 1980 Winter Meeting in Arlington, VA (February 28, 1980 through March 3, 1980).

REFERENCES

1. Miller, J.A. 1970. Chemical carcinogenesis - an overview. G.H.A. Clowes Memorial Lecture. Cancer Res. 30:559-576.

2. Miller, E.C., J.A. Miller, and M. Enomoto. 1964. The comparative carcinogenicities of 2-acetylaminofluorene and its N-hydroxy metabolite in mice, hamsters, and guinea pigs. Cancer Res. 24:2018-2031.

3. Takeishi, K., S.O. Kaneda, and T. Seno. 1979. Mutagenic activation of 2-acetylaminofluorene by guinea-pig liver homogenates: Essential involvement of cytochrome P-450 mixed-function oxidases. Mutat. Res. 62:425-437.

4. Meselson, M., and K. Russell. 1977. Comparisons of carcinogenic and mutagenic potency. In: Origins of Human Cancer. Proceedings of the Cold Spring Harbor Conference. H. Hiatt, J.D. Watson, and J.A. Winsten, eds. pp. 1473-1481.

5. Berenblum, I., and P. Shubik. 1947. The role of croton oil applications, associated with a single painting of a carcinogen, in tumor induction of the mouse's skin. Brit. J. Cancer 1:379-383.

6. Berenblum, I., and P. Shubik. 1947. A new, quantitative approach to the study of the stages of chemical carcinogenesis in the mouse's skin. Brit. J. Cancer 1:384-386.

7. Berenblum, I., and P. Shubik. 1949. The persistence of latent tumour cells induced in the mouse's skin by a single application of 9,10-dimethyl-1,2-benzanthracene. Brit. J. Cancer 3:384-386.

8. Peraino, C., R.J.M. Fry, and E. Staffeldt. 1971. Reduction and enhancement by phenobarbital of hepatocarcinogenesis induced in the rat by 2-acetylaminofluorene. Cancer Res. 31:1506-1512.

9. Peraino, C., R.J.M. Fry, E. Staffeldt, and J.P. Christopher. 1975. Comparative enhancing effects of phenobarbital, amobarbital, hydantoin, and dichlorodiphenyltrichloromethane on 2-acetylaminofluorene-induced hepatic tumorigenesis in the rat. Cancer Res. 35:2884-2890.

10. Peraino, C., R.J.M. Fry, E. Staffeldt, and W.E. Kisieleski. 1973. Effects of varying the exposure to phenobarbital on its enhancement of 2-acetylaminofluorene-induced hepatic tumorigenesis in the rat. Cancer Res. 33:2701-2705.

11. Cohen, S.M., M. Arai, J.B. Jacobs, and G.H. Friedell. 1979. Promoting effect of saccharin and DL-tryptophan in urinary bladder carcinogenesis. Cancer Res. 39:1207-1217.

12. Pour, P., R.G. Runge, D. Birt, R. Gingell, T. Lawson, D. Nagel, L. Wallcave, and S. Salmasi. 1980. Current knowledge of pancreatic carcinogenesis in the hamster and its relevance to the human disease. Cancer Res. 40:3585-3590.

13. Ames, B.N., W.E. Durston, E. Yamasaki, and F.D. Lee. 1973. Carcinogens are mutagens - a simple test system combining liver homogenates for activation and bacteria for detection. Proc. Natl. Acad. Sci. USA 70:2281-2285.

14. Ames, B.N., F.D. Lee, and W.E. Durston. 1973. An improved bacterial test system for the detection and classification of mutagens and carcinogens. Proc. Natl. Acad. Sci. 70:782-786.

15. Ames, B.N. 1977. Environmental chemicals causing cancer and genetic birth defects: Developing a strategy for minimizing human exposure. CA Policy Seminar. pp. 1-37.

16. Langenbach, R., H.J. Freed, and E. Huberman. 1978. Liver cell-mediated mutagenesis of mammalian cells by liver carcinogens. Proc. Natl. Acad. Sci. USA 75:2864-2867.

17. Langenbach, R., H.J. Freed, D. Raveh, and E. Huberman. 1978. Cell specificity in metabolic activation of aflatoxin B_1 and benzo[a]pyrene to mutagens for mammalian cells. Nature 276:277-279.

18. Langenbach, R., R. Gingell, C. Kuszynski, B. Walker, D. Nagel, and P. Pour. 1980. Mutagenic activities of oxidized derivatives of N-nitrosodipropylamine in the liver cell-mediated and *Salmonella typhimurium* assays. Cancer Res. 40:3463-3467.

19. Berenblum, I., and V. Lonal. 1970. The leukemogenic action of phorbol. Cancer Res. 30:2744-2478.

20. Rossi, L., M. Ravera, G. Repetti, and L. Santi. 1976. Long-term administration of DDT or phenobarbital-Na in Wistar rats. Int. J. Cancer 19:19-185.

21. Clayson, D.B., and E.H. Cooper. 1970. Cancer of the urinary tract. Adv. Cancer Res. 13:271-381.

22. Clayson, D.B. 1979. Bladder cancer in rats and mice: Possibility of artifacts. In: Aspects of Cancer Research, 1971-1978. Natl. Cancer Inst. Monographs 52:519-524.

23. Miller, J.A., and E.C. Miller. 1953. The carcinogenic aminoazo dyes. Adv. Cancer Res. 1:339-396.

24. Staffa, J.A., and M.A. Mehlman, eds. 1979. Innovations in cancer risk assessment (ED_{01} study). Pathotox Publishers: Park Forest South, IL. pp. 1-246.

DISCUSSION

Q.: I'm interested in finding out how you cope with one of the difficult problems in trying to correlate experimental data with some general assessments, that is, the kind of tumor response that one can get with a given carcinogen and dose.

You suggested in your numerical approach an index of potency. As you know, I'm pretty skeptical about the applicability of such numerical indices. One of the reasons is that, for example, you may have a substance like aflatoxin which, as we know, is extremely active in rats in certain circumstances, but almost inactive in certain strains of mice. Many other such examples of these differences have been reported at this meeting.

I find it difficult to come out with a numerical response, for example, a 50% increase of lung adenomas in mice, which you could get in some strains with great ease with very low doses, as opposed to 50% of increase of carcinoma of the pancreas in another type of animal, to which one would intuitively give more weight.

A.: Well, as to your first question, we get very wide species variation; that is, in any meaningful form of index (and I'm not going to pretend that I've got the right one yet), these will show up as values at different heights.

We probably don't want to know that aflatoxin is a pretty poor carcinogen in the mouse; rather, we want some way of predicting what it does in man to compare with our epidemiological data.

As far as different tumor types are concerned, we are on much more difficult ground. But I wonder. I am coming more and more to the conclusion, as I'm sure many of you are, that there is a difference between genotoxic and non-genotoxic carcinogen.

When you're working in a system like the lung, mouse lung, which you mentioned, you're often working against an appreciable background of tumors, and just as that AAF which I showed might just be enhancing a spontaneous tumor yield, I think you've got to look very carefully at some of these carcinogens to convince yourself that maybe their major purpose is not just the development of tumors -- I'll avoid the word "promotion" since I think that's a specialized word -- rather than the full induction and initiation of tumors.

I think the sort of approach I've been describing to you -- working out the inducing power and the tumor-developing power -- will, in fact, illuminate that point far better than our present approach of just looking down a microscope, counting the tumors, and saying how wonderful we are.

CARCINOGENIC RISK ASSESSMENT—THE CONSEQUENCES OF BELIEVING MODELS

Edmund A. C. Crouch

Energy and Environmental Policy Center, Jefferson Physics Laboratory, Harvard University, Cambridge, Massachusetts 02138

INTRODUCTION

To estimate risks to humans from carcinogens requires extrapolation from animal or other data. Any such extrapolation must be made in the context of a model or models, but no current consensus exists as to which models are correct. There is no shortage of suggested models for this task, each motivated by theoretical arguments, but the differences among them can lead to enormously different predictions. Furthermore, they often lack any practical demonstration of validity.

If we limit ourselves to the problem of extrapolating to humans the results of carcinogenicity tests in animals, at least three major hurdles must be overcome. First, which model should be used to represent the dose-response curves in the animal studies? Given such a model, the animal results allow estimation of the parameters of the model and hence extrapolation to different doses. Second, how should a dose-response curve estimated for one species be extrapolated to another species, strain, or sex? There is no prior reason to believe (although probably most people would believe) that the dose-response curves in two different species should be of the same form. Even with this assumption, many arguments arise over the correct relationship of the parameters of the dose-response curves in the two species. Third, rarely emphasized but essential for practical risk assessment, what are the magnitudes of the uncertainties introduced in making such extrapolations? Too often no allowance at all is made for such uncertainties. Likewise, statistical confidence limits (based on numbers of animals used in tests) are frequently used as uncertainty estimates, while such a major uncertainty-introducing step as extrapolation between species is treated as exact.

One way to approach the problems outlined above is to choose a set of plausible assumptions or models and observe the consequences when they are applied to available data. Evidently, if we get inconsistent results our assumptions are wrong somewhere, but if we get consistent, aesthetically pleasing results, we might even begin to believe in the assumptions. This paper summarizes one approach that appears capable of giving a consistent and useful method of estimating carcinogenic risks in humans by extrapolation from animal tests.

METHODOLOGY

Initial Assumptions

As a start, the following is a list of assumptions from which we can begin, together with a short justification for each.

(a) A suitable measure of response for our dose-response model is lifetime probability (p) of cancer. This is a function of dose measure d, so p = p(d). This measure is chosen since it is comparatively easy to measure, comparatively unambiguous and of interest when applied to humans.

(b) A suitable measure of dose is the lifetime total consumption of carcinogen expressed in body weights of the consuming animal. Again, this measure is easily obtained, and the normalization to body weight is suggested by any theory that gives cancer induction rates proportional to average carcinogen concentrations in tissue. As a practical matter, the measure actually used in the comparisons discussed below is an average dose rate:

$$d = \frac{1}{T}\int_0^{T'} \frac{m(t)}{w(t)}\,dt$$

where d = dose measure (mg kg^{-1} day^{-1})
T = nominal lifetime (days)
T′ = actual lifetime (days)
m(t) = actual dose rate of carcinogen at age t (mg day^{-1})
w(t) = weight of animal at age t (kg)

(c) The relation between p and d is linear at low dosages, and satisfies

$$p(d) = 1 - (1 - \alpha) \exp [- \beta d/(1 - \alpha)]$$

with $0 \leqslant \alpha \leqslant 1$ and $\beta \geqslant 0$ for all doses. Note that $p \simeq \alpha + \beta d$ at low dosages, so that β measures the slope of the dose-response curve at low dosages. The dose-response curve is assumed linear at low dosages, being the simplest _a priori_ guess. Furthermore, for human risk assessment one will probably always be required to use a confidence bound of some form. It has been shown for a wide variety of models that such confidence bounds are always linear at low enough dosages (1). The high-dose form was chosen as the simplest single formula yielding the required behavior over $0 \leqslant d \leqslant \infty$ ($p \to 1$ as $d \to \infty$; $p \to \alpha + \beta d$ as $d \to 0$). The parameter α is the natural background lifetime cancer probability, while the parameter β (measured in mg^{-1} kg day) is defined to be the potency of the carcinogen.

(d) In any animal experiment performed in which each animal receives a dose of measure d, the number of animals getting cancer is binomially distributed with an expected fraction p(d). This is an often unstated assumption widely used in analyzing the results of such experiments. If the probability p is the same for each animal, and the animals behave independently, then it is a correct assumption, but neither of these is necessarily true. In practice, we usually cannot be sure that each animal received the same dose d, only that the average dose was d.

These assumptions represent a plausible set that may be used to analyze experiments, even though individual experiments cannot by themselves prove or disprove any one of them. They are a set of initial biases that all the experiments together may strengthen or possibly disprove.

Consequences

Given these assumptions, we can extract estimates for the parameters α and β from carcinogenicity tests in animals (2). These parameters may be expected to vary between chemicals, between species, between sexes and possibly, if we are unlucky in our choice of assumptions, will show no consistency or pattern. A suitable method of analysis (others could no doubt be used) is a maximum likelihood technique described below.

If for experiment i ($i = 1,2,.....N$) at dose d_i, r_i out of n_i animals are found to have cancer of a particular type or at a particular site, then the parameters α and β for this cancer are those that maximize

$$\pounds = \prod_{i=1}^{N} \binom{n_i}{r_i} p_i^{r_i} (1 - p_i)^{n_i - r_i}$$

where $p_i = 1 - (1 - \alpha) \exp [- \beta d_i/(1 - \alpha)]$

This problem is straightforward and may be solved rapidly on a pocket calculator.

The main interest is in the parameter β for various carcinogens in different species (the actual values used in [2] are the maximum values of β found for various combinations of types of cancer and/or sites of occurrence). Does it give a measure of the strength of a carcinogen (as suggested by the name 'potency') that is repeatable in the same species and consistent between species? Unfortunately, few good tests of carcinogens are repeated in the same species, but we can test for consistency between sexes. Figure 1 shows the correlation between the potencies estimated for various chemicals in male and female B6C3F1 mice. Evidently, very good correlation exists over a wide range of potencies (note the logarithmic scale). Similar correlations were found between males and females for the other species that we tested (see below). Thus far we have been analyzing the National Cancer Institute (NCI) series of Carcinogenesis Bioassays, since they provide a series with relatively consistent experimental design. Figures 2 and 3 show similar plots of the potencies of the same chemicals measured in different species. Each point represents a single chemical tested in the two species; the values of potency plotted are the geometric means of those found in male and female. (Logarithmic plots appear most natural here, hence the use of a geometric mean.) The dotted lines on the various plots are of unit slope -- that on Figure 1 being the line of equal potencies, while those on Figures 2 and 3 are least-squares unit slope fits with the identified outliers omitted. (Note: With larger numbers of chemicals included in the analysis, and computations of significance and confidence limits taken into account, probably only piperonyl sulfoxide may be considered an outlier.)

There is no reason (apart from one's own biases) to expect that the potencies as measured above should be equal, or even well correlated, between two species. Even if one admits the possibility of correlations, such a simple relation as proportionality (corresponding to the dotted lines) might be

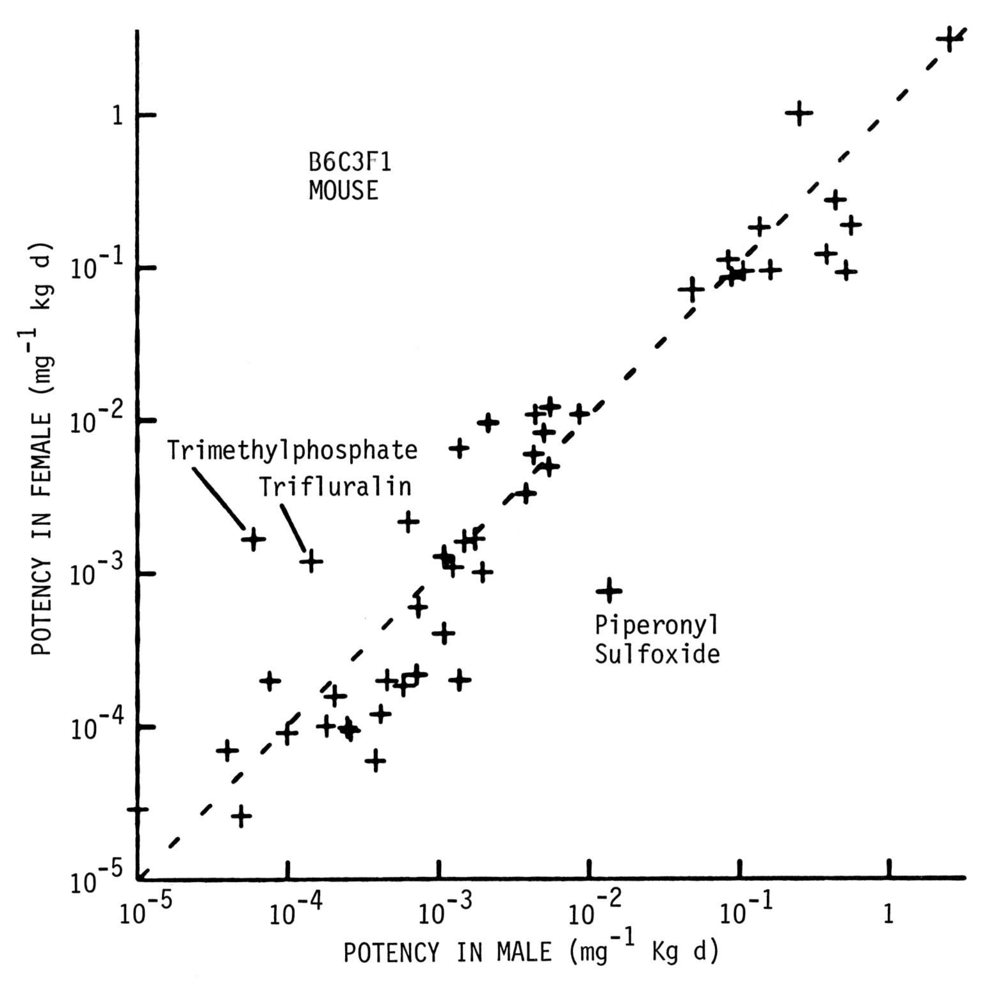

Figure 1. Carcinogenic potencies of various chemicals in male and female B6C3F1 mice. The dashed line, with unit slope, indicates the line of equal potencies. The best least squares linear fit of these points indicates that the potency in females is approximately 0.8 the potency of males.

surprising. Fits to plots such as Figures 1, 2, and 3, unconstrained with respect to slope, turn out to have slopes that do not differ significantly from unity; therefore, proportionality seems to be the simplest hypothesis. The observation of these good correlations suggests that the approach taken so far may be fruitful, and that it may be advantageous to investigate why some outliers appear that do not follow the pattern (e.g., drastic

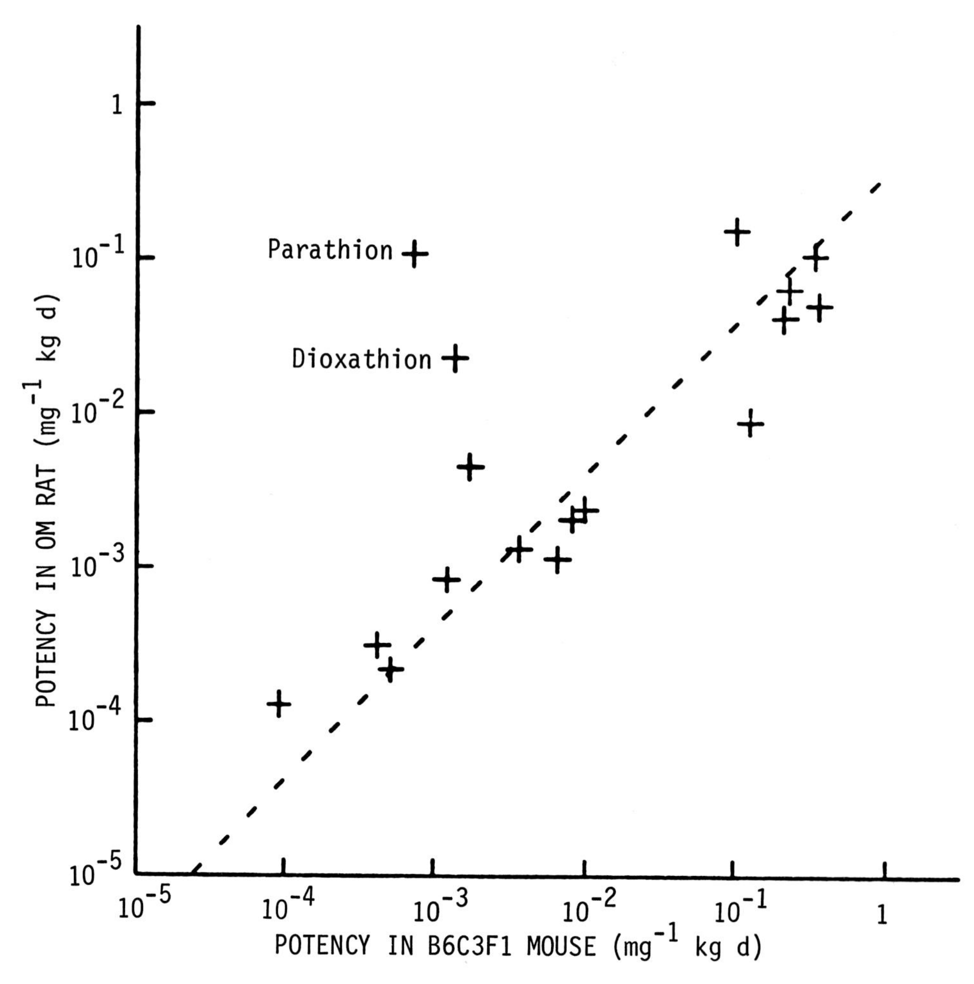

Figure 2. Carcinogenic potencies of various chemicals in OM rats and B6C3F1 mice. The dashed line represents the best least squares linear fit of these points with the two identifies outliers omitted. The intercept of this line with the axes indicates the potency in OM rats is approximately 0.4 the potency in B6C3F1 mice.

metabolic differences for these particular species administered these chemicals).

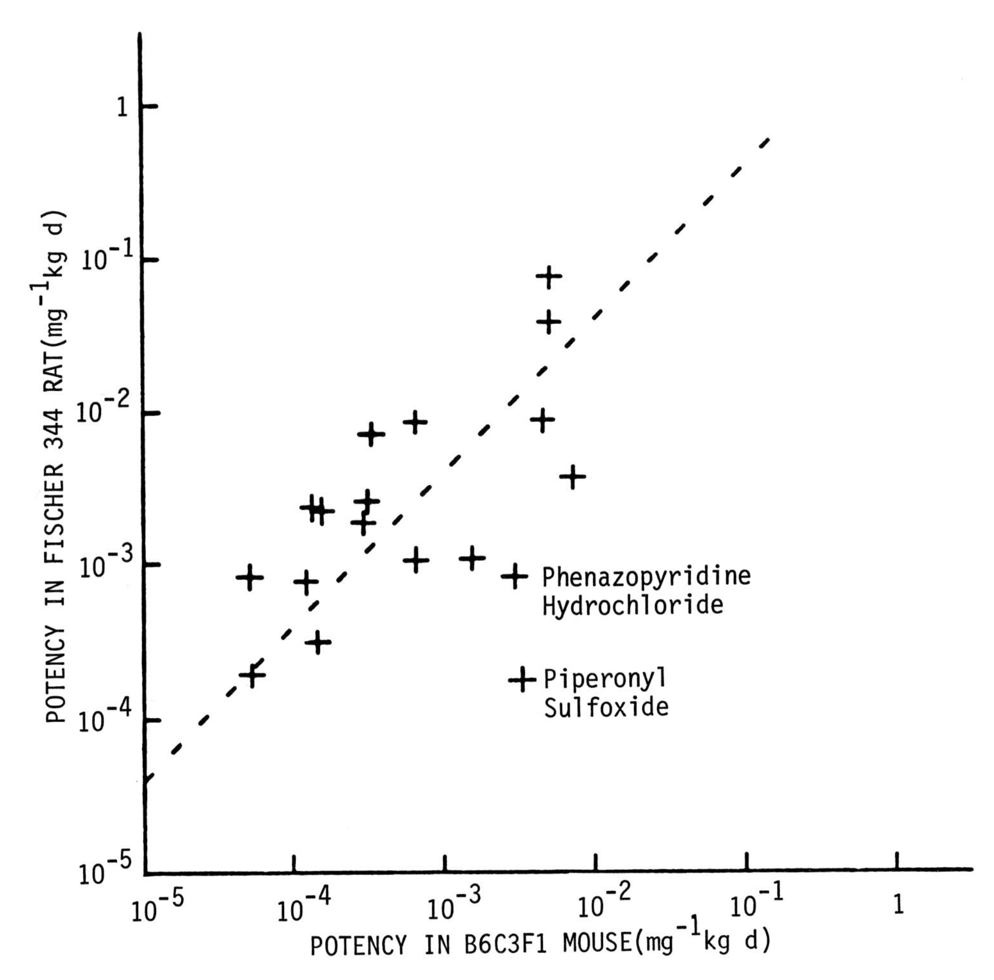

Figure 3. Carcinogenic potencies of various chemicals in Fischer 344 rats and B6C3F1 mice. The dashed line represents the best least squares linear fit of these points with the two identified outliers omitted. The intercept of this line with the axes indicates the potency in Fischer 344 rats is approximately four times the potency in B6C3F1 mice.

Further Assumption

Continuing in the spirit of this approach, let us now introduce a further assumption.

(e) If β_1 represents the potency of a carcinogen in one species (or strain or species/strain/sex combination) and β_2 is similarly defined for the same carcinogen in another species, then

$$\ln \beta_1 = \ln k_{12} + \ln \beta_2 + e_{12}$$

where k_{12} is an interspecies factor to be obtained by experiment, e.g., from plots like Figures 1 and 2, and e_{12} is a random error term, normally distributed with zero mean and standard deviation σ_e to be estimated experimentally. (k_{12} is chosen to give e_{12} zero mean, and the normality assumption on e is for simplicity).

Applying this assumption to the data set used for Figures 1 and 2 gives the estimates for k and σ_e shown in Table 1, although these values are sensitive to the treatment accorded the outliers on the graphs.

Table 1. Values of k and σ_e Obtained from Comparisons of Potencies in Different Sexes or Species for Various Sets of Chemicals[a]

Species 1	Species 2	k	σ_e	No.[b]
Female OM rat	Male OM rat	1.1	0.7	18
Female Fischer 344 rat	Male Fischer 344 rat	0.5	1.0	21
Female B6C3F1 mouse	Male B6C3F1 mouse	0.8	0.9	40
OM rat[c]	B6C3F1 mouse[c]	0.4	1.0	15
Fischer 344 rat[c]	B6C3F1 mouse[c]	4.5	1.2	16

[a]With a larger data set and a more satisfactory selection criterion for inclusion in the comparisons (a significance ≤ 0.05 for every potency calculated), the figures in this table become:

k	σ_e	No.[b]
1.3	0.9	17
0.6	0.8	38
1	0.7	58
0.6	1.7	10
2.7	1.6	18

[b]Number of chemicals for which comparisons were available for this correlation.

[c]Geometric mean of potency evaluated in male and female.

These estimates of σ_e include at least three components. First, the statistical uncertainty is introduced into the estimation of the values of β by the finite size of the animal experiments. While this part could be treated more completely, simple examples suggest that it is small compared with the other components. Second, other uncertainties arise from uncontrolled experimental variability, e.g., in food and water supply, crowding, temperature control, or lighting. That such variations exist may be seen from Table 2, which gives data on incidences of one particular cancer (hepatocellular carcinoma) in the untreated control groups of male B6C3F1 mice used in about 180 of the NCI Carcinogenesis Bioassays. Third, deviations from the assumptions we have made so far should be included. These are discussed further below.

Table 2. Incidence of Hepatocellular Carcinoma in Untreated Control Groups of Male B6C3F1 Mice in Various Laboratories and from Two Suppliers

Laboratory	Supplier 1	Supplier 2
A	13/272 = 0.048	5/39 = 0.12
B	42/508 = 0.083	12/60 = 0.20
C	23/222 = 0.104	---
D	45/356 = 0.126	42/145 = 0.29
E	25/170 = 0.147	52/216 = 0.24
F	80/396 = 0.202	38/104 = 0.37
G	33/98 = 0.337	---
H	---	100/407 = 0.246

Extension to Humans

The treatment of humans according to the scheme outlined so far presents a problem no different in principle from any other species. However, in order to estimate potencies of carcinogens in humans from the potencies in test animals, it is necessary to know the value of k for animal-human correlations. The little data we have suggest that for mouse-human or rat-human correlations, $k \simeq 1$ (see [2] and [3]). In human risk assessment, it is often required that a conservative risk measure be adopted, e.g., by using a confidence limit. This confidence limit may be established by estimating σ_e for the human-animal correlation and using it to obtain a probability distribution for human potency from the animal test data. Since insufficient human-animal comparison data exist to estimate σ_e directly, we suggest that the value $\sigma_e \simeq 1.25 \simeq \ln 3.5$ be used, corresponding to the largest value observed in Table 1. The details are described elsewhere (3).

To summarize, the use of assumptions (a) through (e) appears to be supportable from the data thus far analyzed, and appears to give a method for estimating one measure of human risk, together with uncertainties on that measure, from animal carcinogenicity tests.

DISCUSSION

We have outlined a set of assumptions and some of the consequences of those assumptions when they are combined with suitable data. Here we discuss in more detail some of those assumptions, and in some cases suggest alternatives and ways of attempting to confirm or deny them.

Most of the analysis so far has been performed on carcinogenesis tests involving feeding of the carcinogen (either in the diet or by gavage) to the test animals. It is moot whether the same approach may be taken for inhalation, injection, and dermal testing methods. The few experiments analyzed in which injection was the application method seem to follow a similar pattern, but too few have been analyzed to be sure. The relation to tests of the same carcinogens applied in food or by gavage also needs to be explored. Where one can compare results from different testing methods, it is encouraging that one usually finds results that may be interpreted as quantitative agreement in the values of the potency (suitably defined in different situations). However, until a wide range of carcinogens can be evaluated, this finding must be considered highly subjective.

While lifetime probability of cancer is one measure of risk, it is not the only one. Some other measures, such as age-specific rates, may be more useful. However, no other way has been found of relating such rates to the total lifetime probability. While theories such as that of Armitage and Doll (4) may be used to obtain such a relationship, they would still probably require estimates of age-specific incidence rates in the test animals, and hence tests on much larger numbers of animals. With animal testing as currently practiced, the use of the simplest supportable models -- those with the fewest parameters to estimate -- seems essential.

The dose measure used is not claimed to be optimum in any sense. With this measure, an extra (empirical) factor k must be introduced to relate lifetime cancer probabilities for the mouse and rat species studies. In other words, if animals of the two species are dosed at the same rate (using this measure), their lifetime cancer probabilities differ by a factor k (assuming low doses). However, it is straightforward to show from the data of Table 1 that a similar factor must be introduced, if the other commonly touted dose measure (mass consumed/body surface area) is used. Such a factor will in general be needed for any dose measure. The optimum measure to search for will be one that minimizes the standard deviation σ_e. The value of k then may be estimated from a large set of comparisons, or from a few high-precision experiments on standard carcinogens.

The introduction of the empirical factor k (together with a random component) overcomes another of the arbitrary assumptions usually made in choosing between dose measures. It takes into account possible differences due to lifetime differences, thus bypassing the argument over whether one should equate lifetimes of different species or years in real time.

The dose measure used here preferentially weights doses at low ages, since $m(t)/w(t)$ is largest then. Some weighting factor other than $1/w(t)$ may give a dose measure closer to the optimum defined above; indeed, age-dependence models of carcinogenesis could be tested in this way, since for any such model the expected effect of doses at given ages can be computed, allowing the definition of an age-related weighting factor. It may also turn out that one should use actual rather than nominal lifetime as the divisor in the given dose measure, another possible modification to the weighting factor.

Some find objectionable the dose-response curve used. However, the correlations observed may not necessarily depend on the low-dose behavior of this curve. They are actually correlations between convenient parameters of data taken at comparatively high doses. There is no reason why a similar attempt may not be made using some other model, although, at least in the data set used thus far, the values $\beta d/(1 - \alpha)$, which must be small to obtain the linear approximation in the model chosen, vary over a wide range, corresponding to effective linearity up to strong non-linearity. When it comes to extrapolation to humans for risk assessment, however, current practice requires the assumption of a linear low-dose hypothesis. Even with such a constraint, the choice of a "wrong" model for the dose-response curve may have a large effect on the evaluated uncertainty σ_e (if, indeed, any correlations are seen at all, to allow its evaluation with other models). It is plausible, for example, that at low doses one should write $p \simeq \alpha (1 + \beta d)$ rather than the assumed $p \simeq \alpha + \beta d$. Table 2 shows that α can easily vary by a factor of five, which could account for at least some of the uncertainty σ_e. Using the technique outlined, we can test various such assumptions on the specific form of the dose-response curve in the same way as for variations of the age weighting applied in defining the dose measure: look for the smallest attainable values of σ_e.

Animal experiments are usually analyzed by assuming binomially distributed results at a fixed dose. Several circumstances could upset this assumption. If the animals interact (e.g., intergroup interaction in the groups of typically five animals per cage used in current tests), an analysis by group may be more appropriate. If different individuals dosed at the same rate actually have different probabilities of cancer (e.g., there is a probability distribution for cancer induction at each dose), the resulting distribution of results may have larger higher moments than a binomial distribution. In the latter case, the mean estimates of potency would hardly be affected by the techniques of this paper, since the extra variance will appear in the random error term e, not as a bias on the factor k. However, the uncertainty in extrapolating to a different species (in particular, humans) could be underestimated substantially, as an extra component would be added to the variance due to this individual variability. Such a possibility must certainly be taken into account in extrapolation to humans, since animal testing is performed on highly inbred strains, whereas humans are, as a whole, highly diverse. The presence or absence of such effects might be found by running animal tests on outbred strains of test animals (where any such individual variability should be undiminished if it exists at all), or perhaps by using test groups of animals made up of several inbred strains.

CONCLUSIONS

We have outlined a procedure for extrapolating the results of carcinogenesis bioassays between species that glosses over organ and species specificity in chemical carcinogenicity -- perhaps contrary to the spirit of the meeting -- in order to have a generally applicable result. Although different chemicals may affect different organs specifically, the target organs may be different in different species. The procedure described may give a way of looking for consistent patterns in such specificity. It is possible to define the potency in particular organs, and then look for patterns like "liver in mouse implies thyroid in rats" among a large number of chemicals. Species specificity for particular carcinogens will show up as the outliers on plots such as Figures 2 and 3. This procedure may have some application here, in addition to its use for extrapolation.

ACKNOWLEDGMENTS

It is a pleasure to acknowledge continuing collaboration with Professor Richard Wilson. This work is currently supported by the Department of Energy under contract no. DE-AC02-81EV10598.

REFERENCES

1. Guess, H., K. Crump, and R. Peto. 1977. Uncertainty estimates for low-dose-rate extrapolations of animal carcinogenicity data. Cancer Res. 37:3475-3483.

2. Crouch, E., and R. Wilson. 1979. Interspecies comparison of carcinogenic potency. J. Toxicol. Environ. Hlth. 5:1095-1118.

3. Crouch, E., and R. Wilson. 1981. The regulation of carcinogens. Risk Analysis 1:47-57.

4. Armitage, P., and R. Doll. 1954. The age distribution and a multi-stage theory of carcinogenesis. Brit. J. Cancer VIII:1-12.

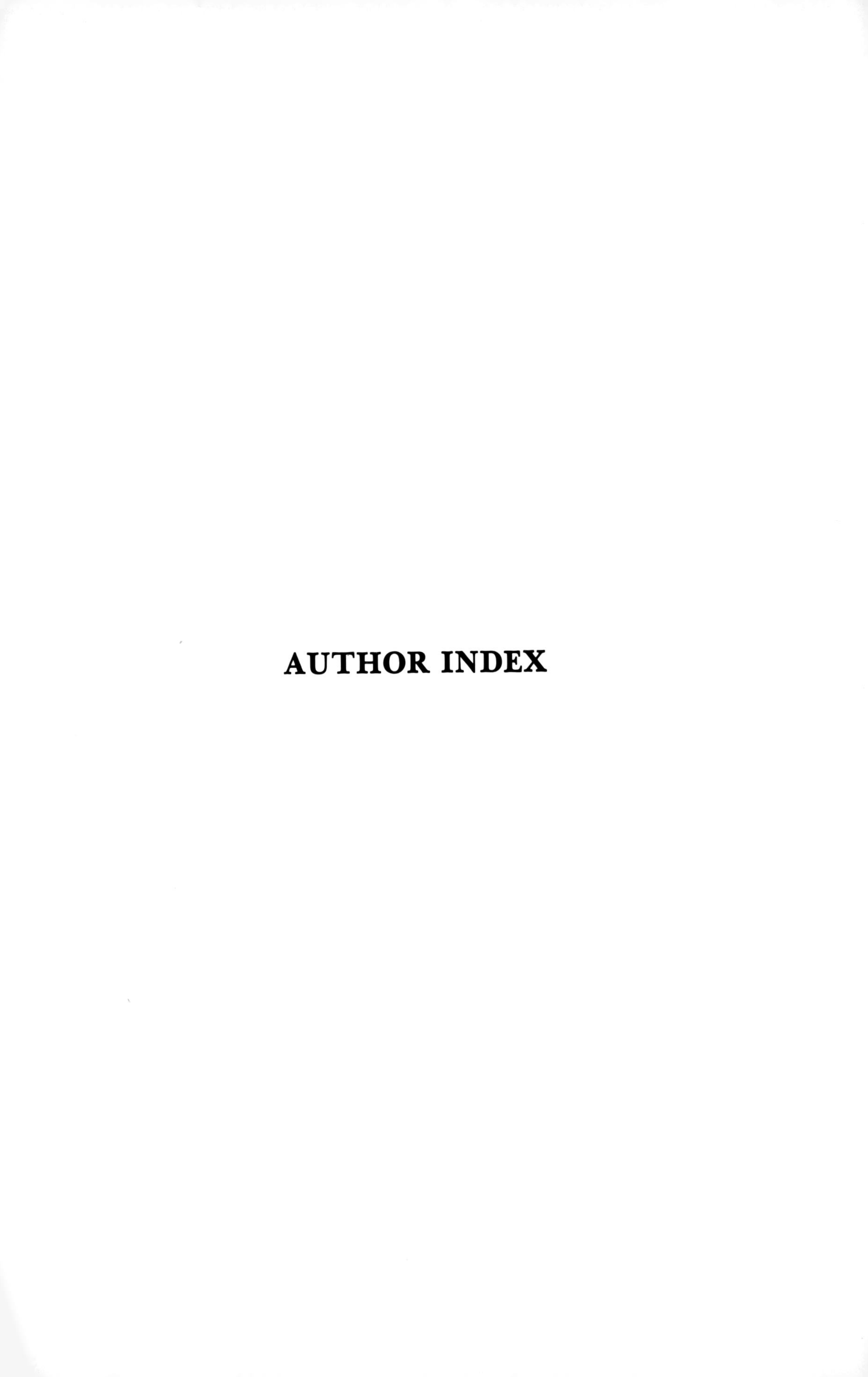

AUTHOR INDEX

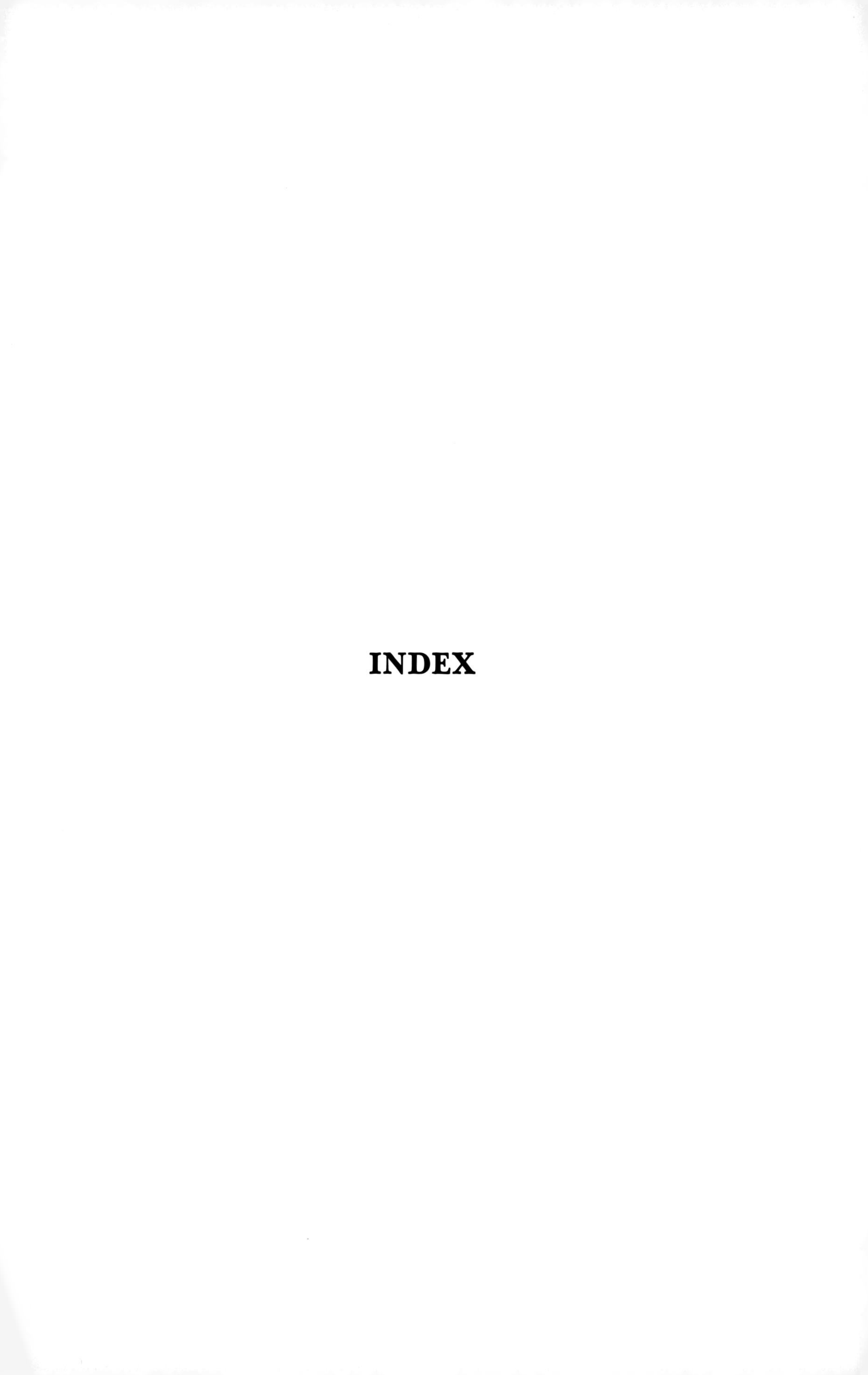

INDEX

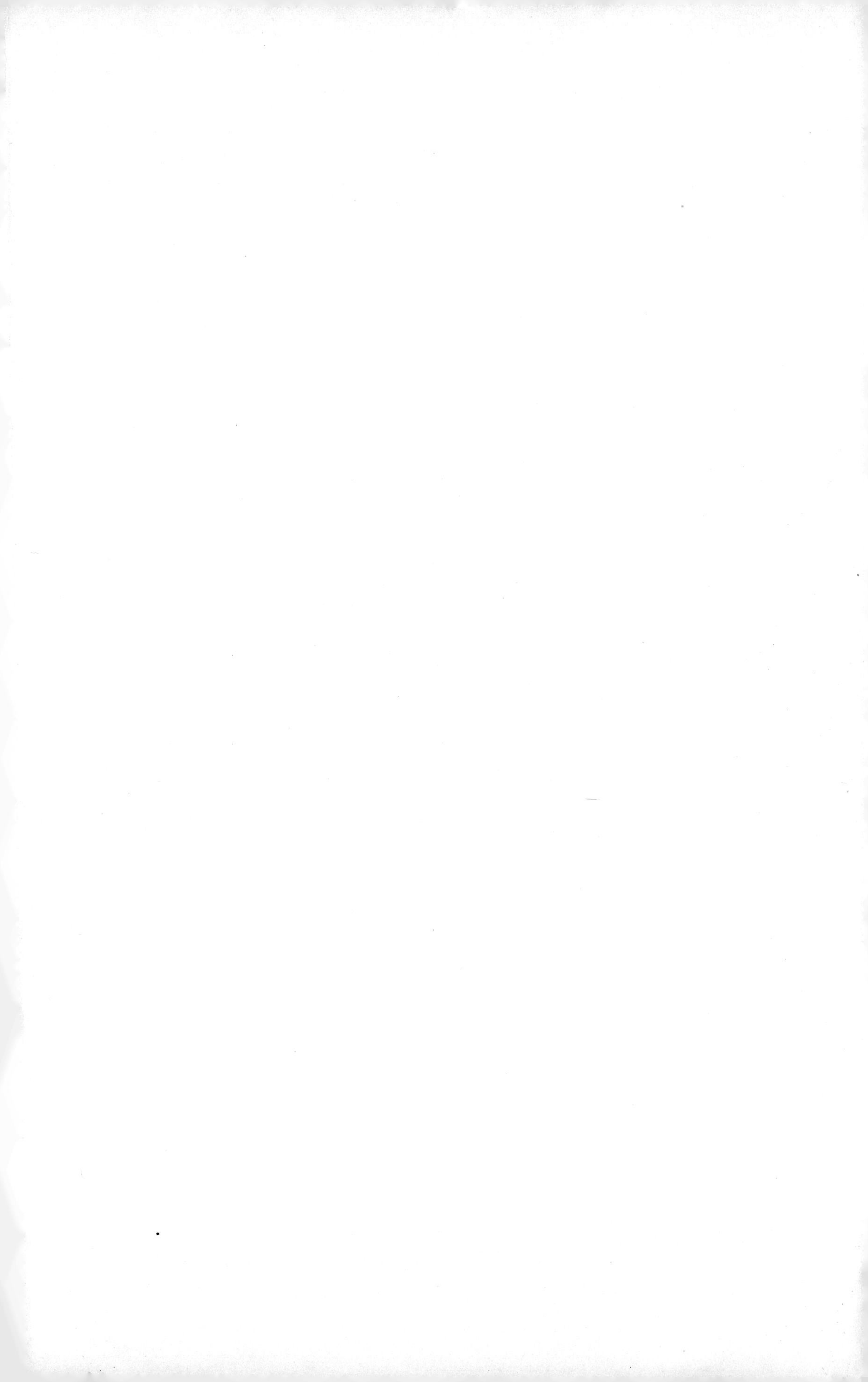